Perioperative Two-Dimensional Transesophageal Echocardiography

Annette Vegas

Perioperative Two-Dimensional Transesophageal Echocardiography

A Practical Handbook

Second Edition

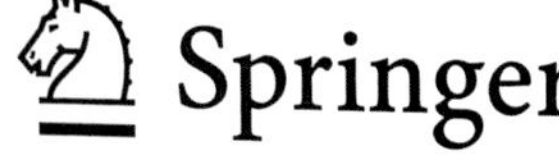

Annette Vegas
Professor of Anesthesiology
Former Director of Perioperative TEE
Department of Anesthesia
Toronto General Hospital
University of Toronto
Toronto, Ontario, Canada

ISBN 978-3-319-60178-6 ISBN 978-3-319-60902-7 (eBook)
https://doi.org/10.1007/978-3-319-60902-7

Library of Congress Control Number: 2017959343

Printed on acid-free paper

This Springer imprint is published by Springer Nature
The registered company is Springer International Publishing AG
The registered company address is: Gewerbestrasse 11, 6330 Cham, Switzerland

To my parents, Patrick and Lena, and my brother Derek for their love and support throughout my life

To colleagues who have helped me better understand echocardiography

To Dr. Andre Denault of the Montreal Heart Institute who has inspired me to be a better clinician, echocardiographer, and educator

To current and former fellows, residents, and students who have challenged me to become a better educator

Preface

The role of transesophageal echocardiography (TEE) continues to expand as a valuable diagnostic tool used during cardiac surgery and in the intensive care unit. Clinicians from different specialties, including anesthesiology, cardiology, and critical care, train in TEE to provide this added skill to their practice in these venues. Learning to become a proficient echocardiographer can be daunting, particularly within the time pressures of the operating room. The skills and expertise of the echocardiographer must constantly evolve to provide timely accurate information which may impact patient management and outcome.

The first edition of the handbook was initially created to fulfill the need for an illustrative synopsis of common cardiac pathology encountered in cardiac surgery patients. It was designed to provide a compact portable reference for using TEE to recognize cardiac pathology in the perioperative period. The ongoing challenge for the echocardiographer is to integrate new technology, techniques, and updated echocardiography guidelines into everyday practice. The second edition of this handbook meets this need by providing updated reference material readily at hand to confirm echocardiographic findings. This edition has been completely rewritten to better explain new concepts and provide examples for the current use of TEE in clinical practice. The second edition has expanded to over 325 pages, with 4 new chapters and over 200 additional figures, but retains its compactness and portability. It will appeal to anesthesiologists, cardiac surgeons, and cardiologists with a range of experience from novice to expert echocardiographers.

This handbook is a compilation of echocardiography information and TEE images from perioperative TEE studies performed at Toronto General Hospital (TGH), Toronto, ON, Canada. As with all written texts, it does not do justice to the cardiac activity seen in live or recorded TEE. The reader is referred to other sources for video recordings of TEE. The TEE website, http://pie.med.utoronto.ca/TEE/ developed by the Perioperative Interactive Education (PIE) group at Toronto General Hospital, is a rich online free resource for TEE educational material.

Learning and practicing echocardiography is a career-long process. In the words of Galileo Galilei, "You cannot teach a man anything; you can only help him find it within himself." I hope this handbook will help you along your journey.

Toronto, ON, Canada

Annette Vegas, MD, FRCPC, FASE

Acknowledgments

To members of the current TGH Perioperative Echocardiography Group (PEG), all talented anesthesiologists and proficient echocardiographers.

To the Perioperative Interactive Education (PIE) group at Toronto General Hospital, under the direction of Gordon Tait, and current and former members, in particular Willa Bradshaw, Michael Corrin, and Jodi Crossingham. I have had the good fortune of working with these imaginative and talented people who have enabled me to indulge my passion for developing free educational tools with a global impact. Their outstanding work is on display throughout this book.

To my colleagues from the Division of Cardiac Surgery, consummate professionals who attract a varied practice that keeps TGH cardiac anesthesiologists challenged to provide exemplary patient care.

To members of the TGH cardiology echocardiography lab, under the direction of Dr. Anna Woo and former directors Dr. Sam Siu and Dr. Harry Rakowski who generously share their knowledge.

To Dr. Gian-Marco Busato, a former summer student, medical student, and now an ENT surgeon, for the extraordinary artistic talent he used to draw the illustrations for this handbook.

Finally to Ms. Willa Bradshaw, B.Sc., M.Sc.B.M.C., medical illustrator, who precisely assembled all the detailed figures and added many of her own fine illustrations to this book.

Abbreviations

These are the common abbreviations used throughout the book. Other abbreviations are defined in the context in which they are used.

A	Anterior
AC	Anterior commissure
ACHD	Adult congenital heart disease
AI	Aortic insufficiency
AL	Anterolateral
AMVL	Anterior mitral valve leaflet
Ao	Aorta
ARVD	Arrythmogenic right ventricular dysplasia
AS	Aortic stenosis or antero-septal
ASD	Atrial septal defect
ASE	American Society of Echocardiography
At	Acceleration time
AV	Aortic valve
AVA	Aortic valve area
A-V	Atrioventricular
BAV	Bicuspid aortic valve
BPM	Beats per minute
BSA	Body surface area
C	Chamber
CAD	Coronary artery disease
CO	Cardiac output
CPB	Cardiopulmonary bypass
CS	Coronary sinus
CSA	Cross-sectional area
CT	Computer tomography
CVP	Central venous pressure
Cx	Circumflex artery
CW	Continuous wave
D	Dimension or diameter
DBP	Diastolic blood pressure
DS	Deceleration slope
DT	Deceleration time
DVI	Dimensionless valve index
ED	End diastole
EDA	End diastolic area

EDD	End diastolic diameter
EDP	End diastolic pressure
EDV	End diastolic volume
EF	Ejection fraction
EI	Eccentricity index
EROA	Effective regurgitant orifice area
ES	End systole
ESA	End systolic area
ESD	End systolic diameter
ESV	End systolic volume
ET	Ejection time
FAC	Fractional area change
FR	Frame rate
FS	Fractional shortening
GE	Gastroesophageal
GLPSS	Global longitudinal peak systolic strain
HBP	High blood pressure
HF	Heart failure
HOCM	Hypertrophic obstructive cardiomyopathy
HR	Heart rate
HV	Hepatic vein
HVF	Hepatic vein flow
I	Inferior
IABP	Intra-aortic balloon pump
IAS	Inter-atrial septum
ICT	Isovolumic contraction time
IE	Infective endocarditis
IL	Infero-lateral
IPPV	Intermittent positive pressure ventilation
IS	Infero-septal
IVC	Inferior vena cava
IVRT	Isovolumic relaxation time
IVS	Interventricular septum
JA	Jet area
JH	Jet height
L	Left or lateral or length
LAA	Left atrial appendage
LA	Left atrium
LAD	Left anterior descending
LAP	Left atrial pressure
LAX	Long axis
LCA	Left coronary artery
LCC	Left coronary cusp
LCCA	Left common carotid artery
LLPV	Left lower pulmonary vein
LMCA	Left main coronary artery
LSVC	Left superior vena cava
LUPV	Left upper pulmonary vein
LV	Left ventricle
LVAD	Left ventricular assist device
LVH	Left ventricular hypertrophy
LVM	Left ventricular wall mass
LVID	Left ventricle internal diameter
LVOT	Left ventricular outflow tract
MAC	Mitral annular calcification
MAPSE	Mitral annular plane systolic excursion
MC	Mitral commissural

ME	Mid-esophageal
MI	Myocardial infarction
MPI	Myocardial performance index
MR	Mitral regurgitation
MRI	Magnetic resonance imaging
MS	Mitral stenosis
MV	Mitral valve
MVA	Mitral valve area
MVI	Mitral valve inflow
N	Non
NSR	Normal sinus rhythm
P	Pressure or posterior
PA	Pulmonary artery
PAC	Pulmonary artery catheter
PAP	Pulmonary artery pressure
PAPVD	Partial anomalous pulmonary venous drainage
PASP	Pulmonary artery systolic pressure
PDA	Patent ductus arteriosus
PFO	Patent foramen ovale
PHT	Pressure half-time
PI	Pulmonic insufficiency
PISA	Proximal isovelocity surface area
PM	Papillary muscles or posteromedial
PMVL	Posterior mitral valve leaflet
Pr	Prosthetic
PS	Pulmonic stenosis
PSS	Peak systolic strain
PV	Pulmonic valve
PVF	Pulmonary vein flow
PVR	Pulmonary vascular resistance
PW	Pulsed wave
Qp	Pulmonary blood flow
Qs	Systemic blood flow
R	Right
RA	Right atrium
RAA	Right atrial appendage
RAP	Right atrial pressure
RCA	Right coronary artery
RCC	Right coronary cusp
RLPV	Right lower pulmonary vein
RPA	Right pulmonary artery
RUPV	Right upper pulmonary vein
RV	Right ventricle
RVH	Right ventricular hypertrophy
RegF	Regurgitant fraction
RegV	Regurgitant volume
RVH	Right ventricular hypertrophy
RVOT	Right ventricular outflow tract
RVSP	Right ventricular systolic pressure
RWMA	Regional wall motion abnormality
SAM	Systolic anterior motion
S	Systole
SAM	Systolic anterior motion
SAX	Short axis
SC	Saline contrast
SCA	Society of Cardiovascular Anesthesiology
SLE	Systemic lupus erythematosus

SOVA	Sinus of Valsalva aneurysm
SR	Strain rate
STE	Speckle tracking echocardiography
STJ	Sinotubular junction
SV	Stroke volume
SVi	Stroke volume index
SVC	Superior vena cava
SVR	Systemic vascular resistance
TAH	Total artificial heart
TAPSE	Tricuspid annular plane systolic excursion
TDI	Tissue Doppler imaging
TEE	Transesophageal echocardiography
TG	Transgastric
TGC	Time gain compensation
TOF	Tetralogy of Fallot
TGA	Transposition of the great arteries
TR	Tricuspid regurgitation
TS	Tricuspid stenosis
TTE	Transthoracic echocardiography
TV	Tricuspid valve
TVI	Tricuspid valve inflow
UE	Upper esophageal
VAD	Ventricular assist device
VSD	Ventricular septal defect
VTI	Velocity time integral
W	Width

Contents

1
TEE Views

A. Vegas, *Perioperative Two-Dimensional Transesophageal Echocardiography*, https://doi.org/10.1007/978-3-319-60902-7_1

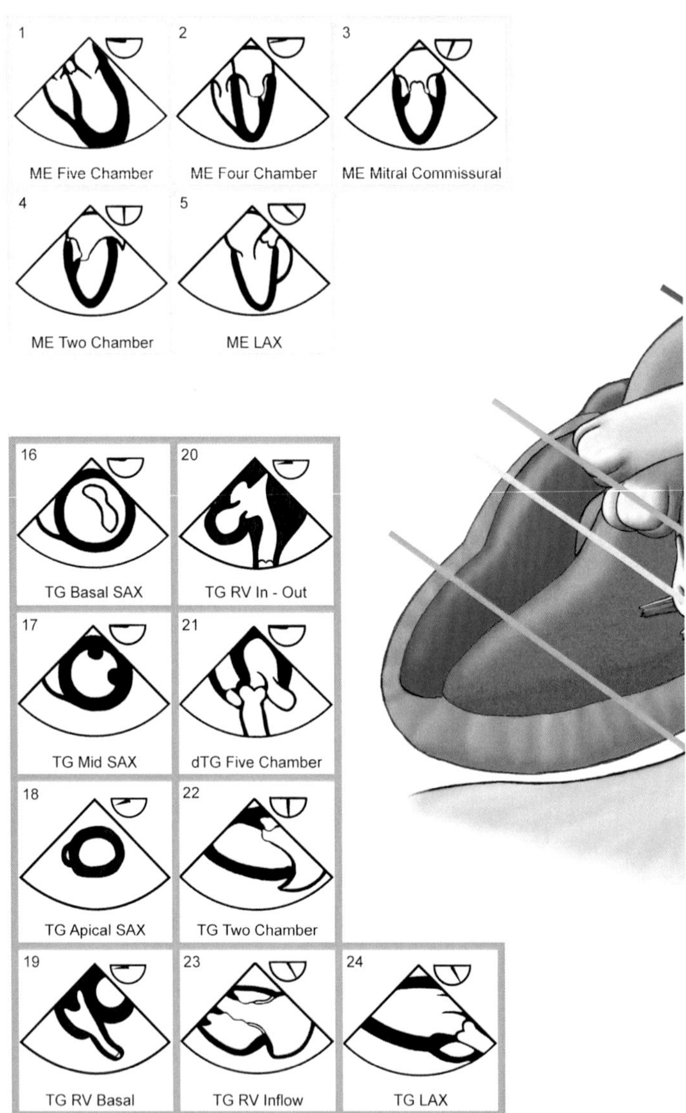

Standard Views

- The original standard 20 TEE views that comprise a comprehensive TEE exam as described by the SCA/ASE (1999) have been augmented by 8 additional views.
- Conveniently, all views can be grouped together by the probe level in the esophagus and the structures being interrogated as diagrammed here:
  - **Yellow**: mid-esophageal (ME) views that examine the LV and MV
  - **Green**: ME views that examine the AV, TV, bicaval, and pulmonary veins
  - **Blue**: ME and upper-esophageal (UE) views for different regions of the aorta
  - **Orange**: transgastric (TG) views that examine the LV, RV, and AV with good spectral and tissue Doppler alignment

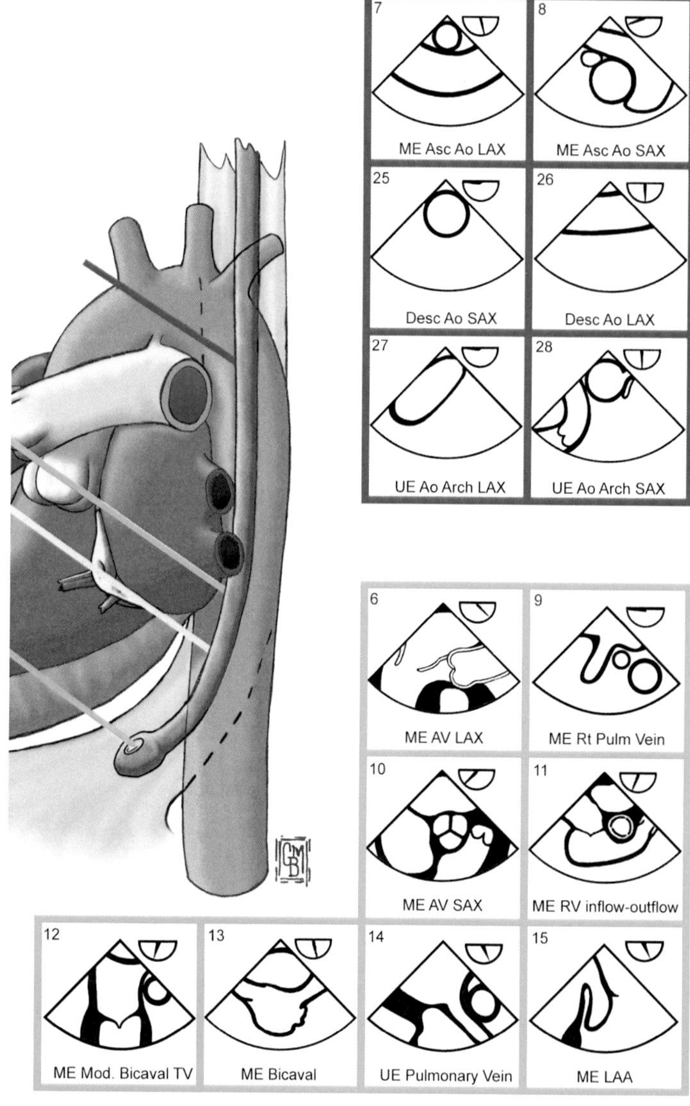

Sources

- Hahn R, Abraham T, Adams MS, et al. Guidelines for Performing a Comprehensive Transesophageal Echocardiographic Examination: Recommendations from the ASE and the SCA. J Am Soc Echocardiogr 2013;26:921–64.
- Shanewise JS, Cheung AT, Aronson S, et al. ASE/SCA Guidelines for performing a comprehensive intraoperative multiplane transesophageal echocardiography examination. Anesth Analg 1999;89:870–84.
- Flachskampf FA, Decoodt P, Fraser AG, et al. Guideline from the Working Group: Recommendations for Performing Transesophageal Echocardiography. Eur J Echocardiograph 2001;2:8–21.

TEE Probe Manipulation

Probe movements (entire probe moves)

1. Advance or withdraw
2. Turn right or left

Knob movements (only probe tip moves)

3. Flex right or left
4. Anteflex or retroflex

Transducer movements (probe stays still)

5. Rotate angle forward (0–180°)
6. Rotate angle back (180–0°)

Transducer Planes

- Transverse (0°)
- Longitudinal (90°)
- Multiplane (0–180°)

Image Display

- Pie-shaped sector
- Display right (R), left (L)
- Near field (closest to probe)
- Far field (farthest from probe)

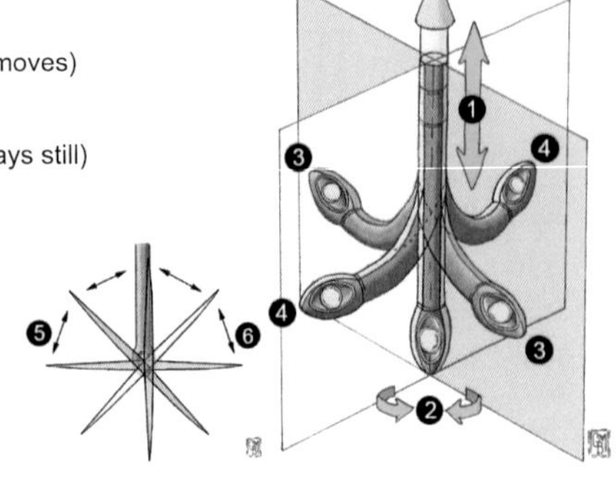

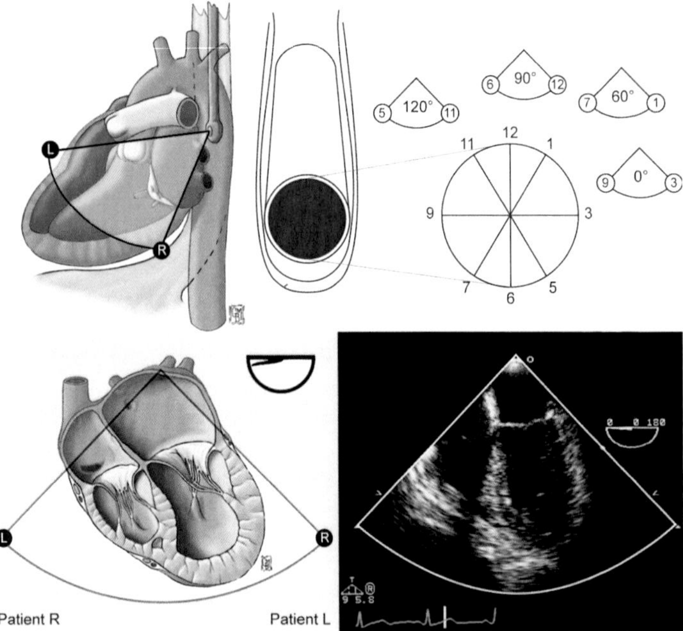

- Standard terminology describes TEE probe manipulation, the imaging plane, and the image display. The 2D TEE probe displays a pie-shaped sector with the top of the display designated as the sector apex or the near field that is closest to the probe. The far field contains structures (often the most anterior ones) that are furthest from the probe. Machine settings can invert the image, positioning the sector apex at the bottom or switch right and left (like imaging at 180°).
- As the TEE probe is held still, the transducer angle can be rotated through 180°. Correlation of the image plane and 3D aspect of the heart is complex. It is convenient to draw an analogy between the sector plane and a clock face to understand the structures that may be displayed. At 0°, the display right corresponds to the patient's left side and the display left to the patient's right side. At 90°, superior structures appear on the display right and inferior structures to the display left.

There are several approaches to performing a TEE study:

- View-based approach is the most frequently used and relies on obtaining most of the standard TEE views in an organized way.
- Structure-based approach provides a detailed examination of a structure of interest using different TEE planes. This focused TEE study is useful if time is limited.
- Sequential-segmental approach looks at the arrangement of the atria, ventricles, and great vessels in congenital heart patients (see p. 223).
- This graphic map from the VIRTUAL TEE website, developed by the Perioperative Interactive Education (PIE) group at the University of Toronto, shows a structured and logical description of the relationships between ASE/SCA 20 standard views and serves as a tool for navigating to the desired views.

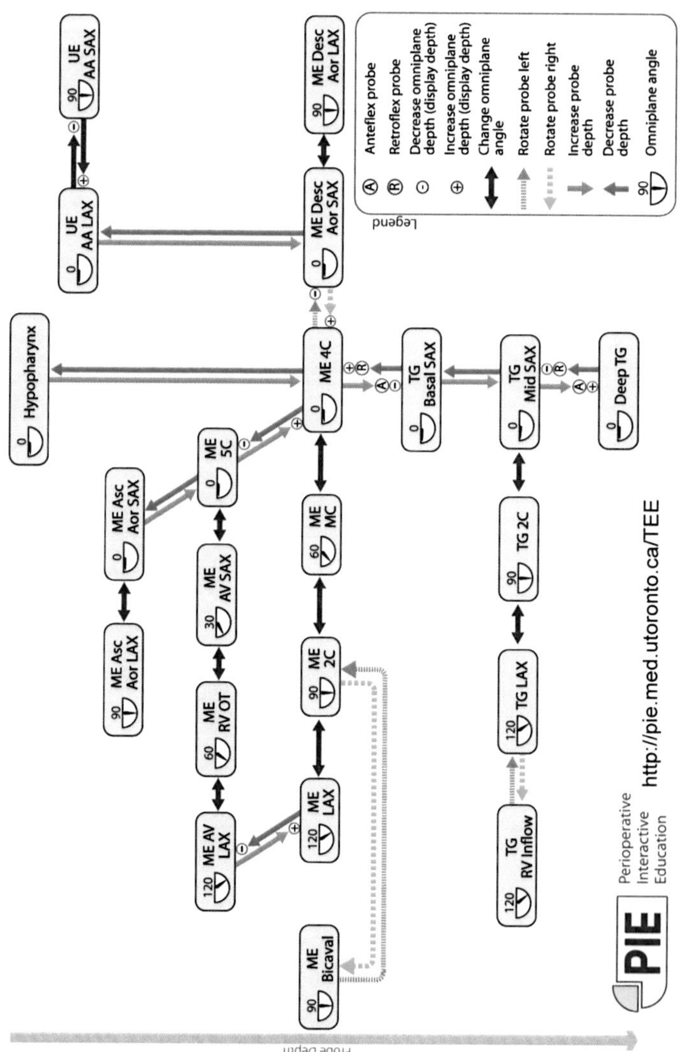

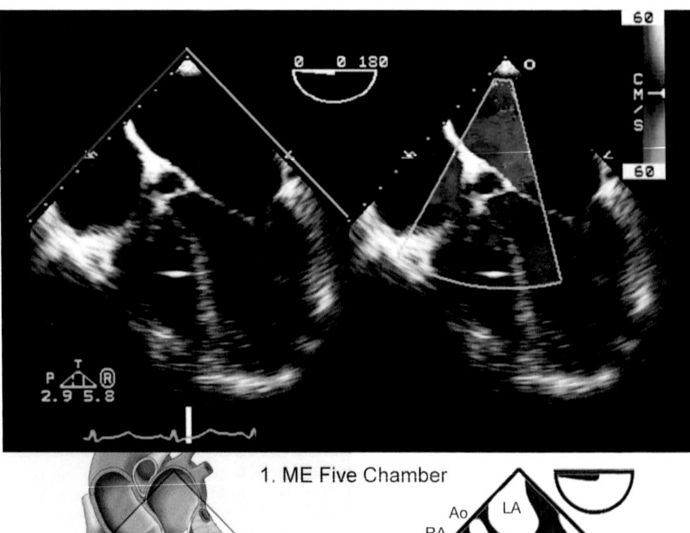

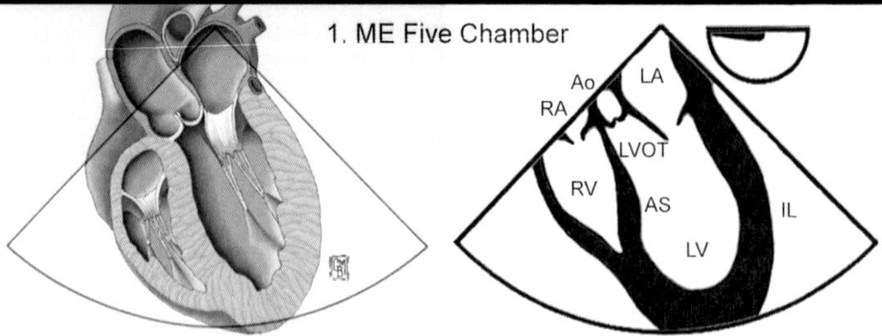

The ME 5 Chamber (5C) view is obtained by withdrawing the probe from the ME 4C view (0°) until the aortic valve (AV) and aortic root are brought into view. Similar structures as in the ME 4C view are seen; the 5th chamber is the left ventricular outflow tract (LVOT) and the AV in the center of the screen. Color Doppler box is positioned over the LVOT and AV with Nyquist 50–70 cm/s to assess flow. Turbulent systolic flow is LVOT pathology; turbulent diastolic flow is aortic insufficiency.

http://pie.med.utoronto.ca/TEE

Imaged Structures

Left Atrium (LA)
Left Ventricle (LV)
  Antero-Septal (AS), Infero-Lateral (IL)
Right Atrium (RA)
Right Ventricle (RV)
Mitral Valve (MV):
  A2/P2 or A1/P1
  Doppler: color, PW spectral
Tricuspid Valve (TV):
  Anterior + septal leaflets
Left Ventricular Outflow Tract (LVOT)
Aortic Valve (AV):
  Non/right coronary cusps
  Color Doppler
Interventricular Septum (IVS): Color
Inter-Atrial Septum (IAS): Color

Diagnostic Issues

Same as 4 Chamber view
HOCM
  Septal measurements (end-diastole)
Ventricular Septal Defect (VSD)
  Perimembranous
  Muscular
LVOT turbulent flow
  Aortic insufficiency (diastole)
  Septal hypertrophy (systole)

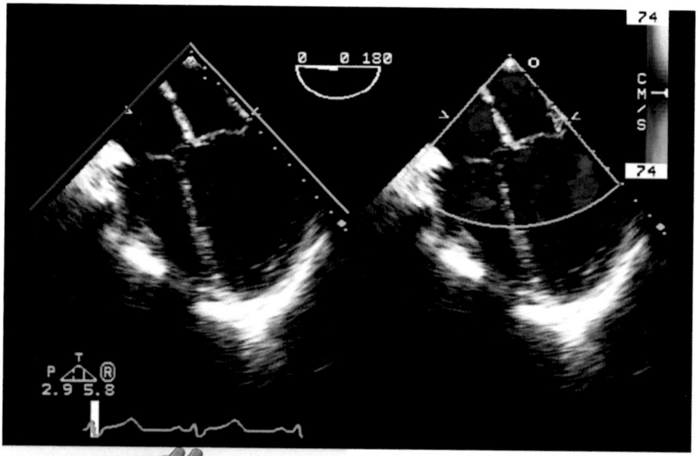

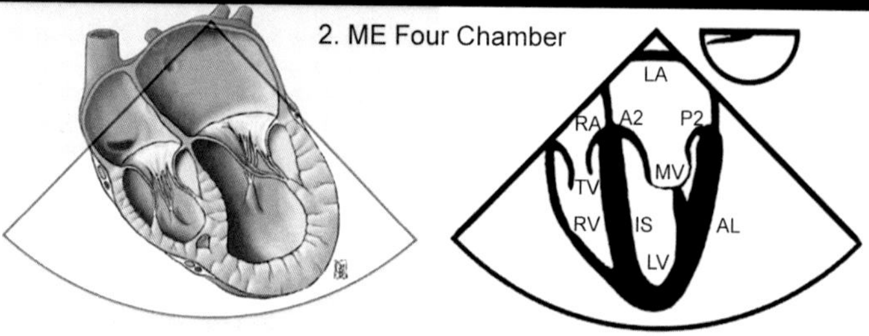

2. ME Four Chamber

The ME 4 Chamber (4C) view (0–20°) is obtained by positioning the probe in the mid-esophagus behind the LA. The imaging plane is directed through the LA, center of the MV and LV apex. Adjustments are made to the (a) transducer angle to maximize the TV diameter, (b) image depth to include the LV apex, and (c) probe tip retroflexion to avoid foreshortening the LV apex. This snapshot of the heart includes all 4 chambers (LA, RA, LV, RV), 2 valves (MV, TV), and the septae (IAS, IVS). Color Doppler box over the TV and MV with Nyquist 60–70 cm/s shows laminar antegrade (blue) diastolic flow. Turbulent (red mosaic) retrograde systolic flow is valvular regurgitation (shown as trace MR above).

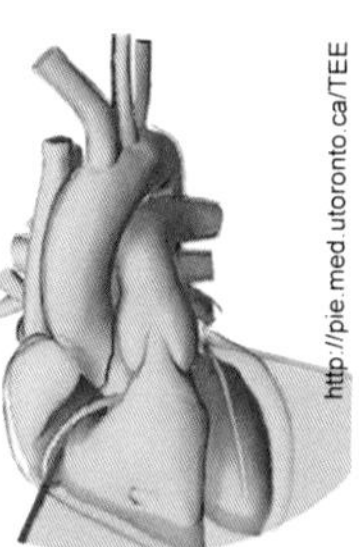

http://pie.med.utoronto.ca/TEE

Imaged Structures	Diagnostic Issues

Left Atrium (LA)
Left Ventricle (LV):
  Infero-Septal (IS), Antero-Lateral (AL)
  Antero-Lateral (AL) papillary muscle
Mitral Valve (MV): A2/P2 segments
  Doppler: Color, PW spectral
Tricuspid Valve (TV):
  Anterior/posterior + septal leaflets
  Color Doppler
Right Atrium (RA)
Right Ventricle (RV)
Inter-Atrial Septum (IAS): Color
Interventricular Septum (IVS): Color
	Chamber enlargement and function
	LV systolic function
	MV pathology
	TV pathology
	  Maximize annulus (28 mm ± 5)
	Atrial Septal Defect (ASD)
	  Primum ASD
	Ventricular Septal Defect (VSD)
	  Muscular VSD
	  Inlet VSD
	Pericardial effusion

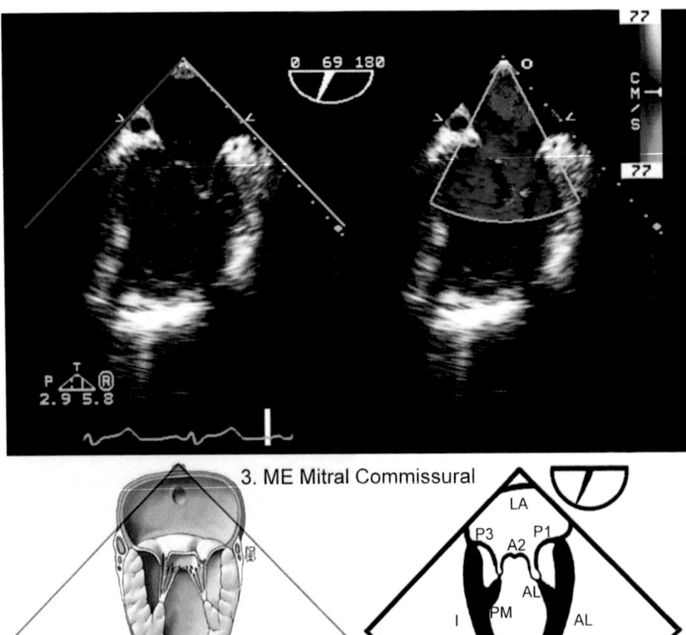

In the ME Mitral Commissural (ME MC) view, the probe transducer is now imaging at 50–70° through the LA, center of the MV and LV apex. An accurate view is less dependent on the transducer angle, but instead relies on identifying the correct anatomy. Careful probe manipulation is required to image (a) 3 MV segments, (b) 2 coaptation points, (c) both papillary muscles, and (d) LV apex without foreshortening. The P3 scallop (left), P1 scallop (right), and A2 segment in the middle form the intermittently seen "trap door" of the MV. Color Doppler box over the MV with Nyquist 60–70 cm/s shows laminar antegrade (blue) diastolic flow. Turbulent (red mosaic) retrograde systolic flow is mitral regurgitation (MR); multiple MR jets and commissural MR jets may be identified. The high Nyquist of 77 cm/s shown above will underestimate the severity of MR. Spectral Doppler at the point of leaflet tip coaptation can assess transvalvular mitral flow.

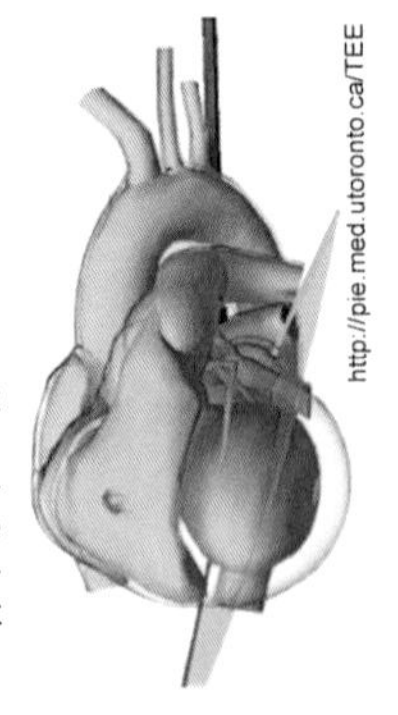

Imaged Structures	Diagnostic Issues
Left Ventricle (LV):	LA: mass, thrombus
Inferior (I) + Antero-Lateral (AL) walls	LV systolic function
Papillary muscles:	LV pathology
Posteromedial (PM), Antero-Lateral (AL)	MV pathology
Mitral Valve (MV):	Coronary sinus flow
P3/A2/P1 segments	Pericardial effusion
Doppler: Color, PW spectral commissural	
Left Atrium (LA)	
Coronary Sinus	
Circumflex Artery	

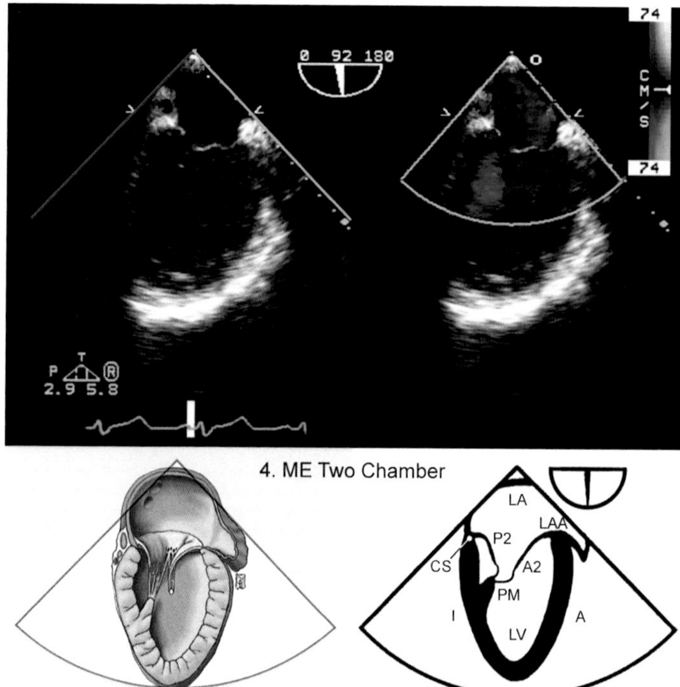

The ME 2 Chamber (ME 2C) view is obtained by increasing the transducer angle to 80–100° from the ME 4C (0°) or ME Mitral Commissural (50–70°) views. The RA and RV are eliminated from the display. This view is orthogonal to the ME 4C view. The image is displayed with the cephalad part (anterior wall) to the right and the caudad part (inferior wall) to the left. The probe tip might need to be retroflexed to avoid foreshortening the LV. The left atrial appendage (LAA) is often seen. The MV has the longer anterior leaflet (A3-A1) on the display right and shorter posterior leaflet (P3 or P2) on the left with a single coaptation point. Color Doppler box over the MV with Nyquist 50–70 cm/s (slightly high as seen above) shows laminar antegrade (blue) diastolic flow. The coronary sinus (CS) is seen in short-axis above the posterior MV annulus with laminar flow (blue).

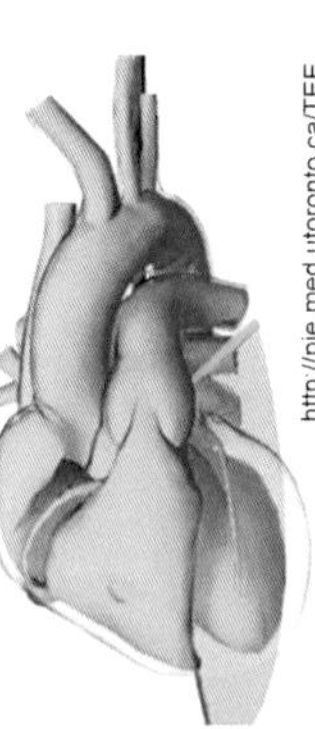

http://pie.med.utoronto.ca/TEE

Imaged Structures	Diagnostic Issues
Left Ventricle (LV):	LAA
Inferior (I) + Anterior (A) walls + LV apex	Mass, thrombus
Posteromedial (PM) papillary muscle	LAA velocity
Mitral Valve (MV):	LA pathology, size
P2/A2 A1 segments	LV systolic function
Doppler: Color, PW Spectral	LV apex pathology
Left Atrium (LA):	MV pathology
Left Atrial Appendage (LAA)	Coronary sinus flow
Doppler: Color, PW Spectral	
Coronary Sinus (CS)	

5. ME Long-Axis

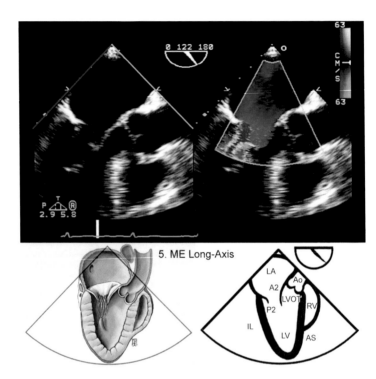

The ME Long-Axis (ME LAX) view is obtained by increasing the transducer angle to 120–140° from the ME 4C (0°) or ME MC (45–70°) or ME 2C (90°) views. The more cephalad structures including the LVOT, AV, and proximal ascending aorta are lined up on the display right. The depth is adjusted to include the entire LV (it is too shallow above). The A2 and P2 MV segments with a single coaptation point are reliably seen in this view. Color Doppler box over the MV, LVOT, and AV with Nyquist 50–70 cm/s shows laminar antegrade (blue) diastolic flow through the MV and systolic flow (red) through the LVOT and AV. Flow acceleration is shown here during diastole through this open MV. Spectral Doppler at the point of coaptation of the MV leaflet tips assesses transmitral flow, but is poorly aligned for flow in the LVOT and AV.

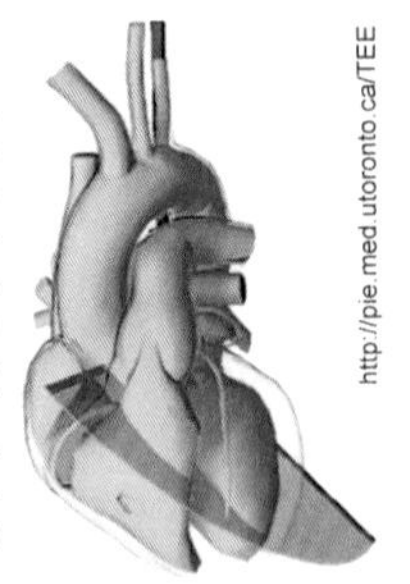

http://pie.med.utoronto.ca/TEE

Imaged Structures	Diagnostic Issues

Left Atrium (LA)
Mitral Valve (MV): P2/A2 segments
  Doppler: Color, PW spectral
Left Ventricle (LV):
  Infero-Lateral (IL) + Antero-Septal (AS)
Interventricular Septum (IVS)
  Color Doppler
Left Ventricular Outflow Tract (LVOT)
Right Ventricular Outflow Tract (RVOT)
Aortic Valve (AV):
  Color Doppler
Aortic Root and Ascending Aorta (Ao)
	MV pathology
	LV systolic function
	Ventricular Septal Defect (VSD)
	  Perimembranous VSD
	LVOT pathology
	AV pathology
	Aortic root pathology
	LA pathology

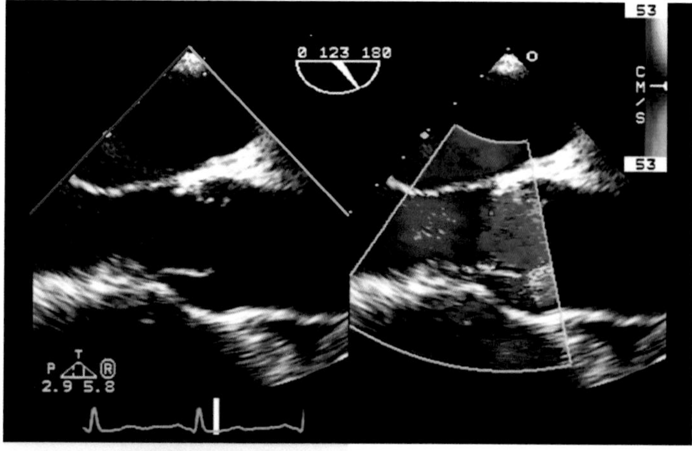

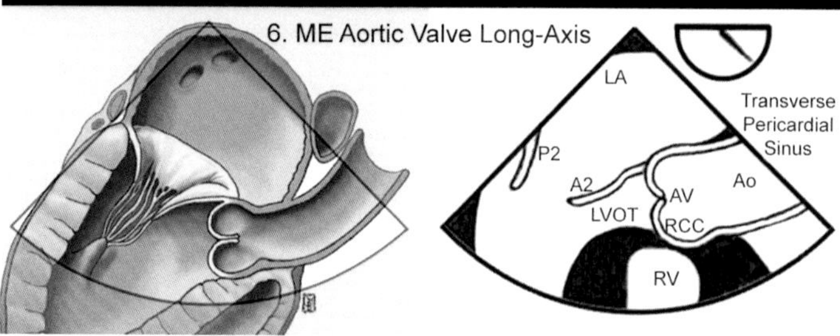

The ME Aortic Valve Long-Axis (ME AV LAX) view is obtained at 120–140° by decreasing the depth from the ME LAX view (120°). The LVOT, AV, and proximal ascending aorta are lined up on the display right and some of the MV and LV are eliminated from the display. Withdrawing the probe shows more of the AV and aortic root; advancing the probe better images the posterior MV annulus and MV morphology. The AV is seen in long-axis with the anterior positioned cusp always the right coronary cusp, the other is either the non- or left coronary cusp. Color Doppler box over the AV with Nyquist 50–70 cm/s shows unidirectional laminar antegrade systolic flow, which, in relation to the probe, appears red through the LVOT and blue through the AV and ascending aorta.

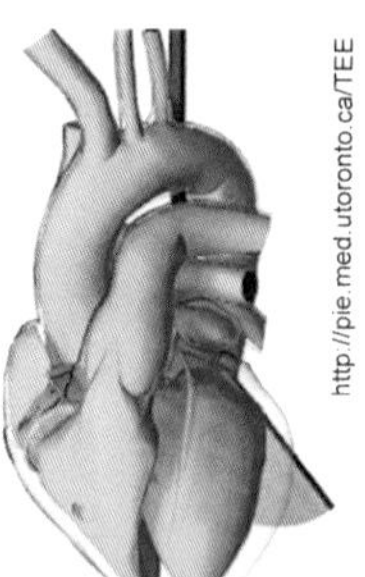

http://pie.med.utoronto.ca/TEE

Imaged Structures	Diagnostic Issues
Left Atrium (LA)	AV pathology
Left Ventricular Outflow Tract (LVOT)	Ventricular Septal Defect (VSD)
Right Ventricular Outflow Tract (RVOT)	Perimembranous VSD
Aortic Valve (AV):	LVOT pathology
Right Cusp (RCC), left or non-cusps	MV pathology
Color Doppler	Aortic root pathology
Mitral Valve (MV): P2/A2 segments	LA pathology
Doppler: Color, PW spectral	
Interventricular Septum (IVS): Color	
Aortic Root + Ascending Aorta (Ao)	
Measurements	
Right coronary artery	
Transverse Pericardial Sinus	

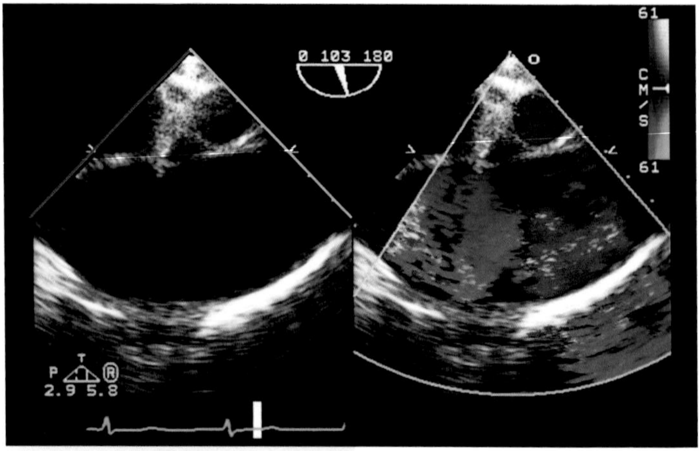

7. ME Asc Aortic LAX

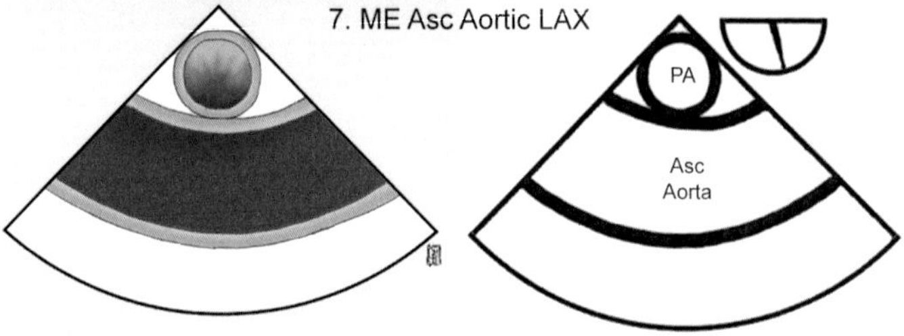

PA

Asc Aorta

The ME Ascending Aortic Long-Axis (LAX) view is visualized from the ME AV LAX (120°) by withdrawing the probe and decreasing the transducer angle slightly (100–110°). An adequate view may be difficult to obtain due to poor tissue contact. The walls of the ascending aorta should appear parallel and the right pulmonary artery (RPA) is seen in short-axis in the center of the display. Color Doppler box over the aorta and RPA with Nyquist 50–70 cm/s shows laminar antegrade systolic flow. Though flow is continuous and unidirectional during systole, in relation to the probe, it appears red through the proximal and blue through the distal ascending aorta. In late systole and early diastole, flow is in the opposite direction to facilitate closure of the AV. Black color indicates the probe is perpendicular to flow. Turbulent systolic flow suggests aortic stenosis. Continuous flow during systole and diastole in the aorta indicates aortic insufficiency.

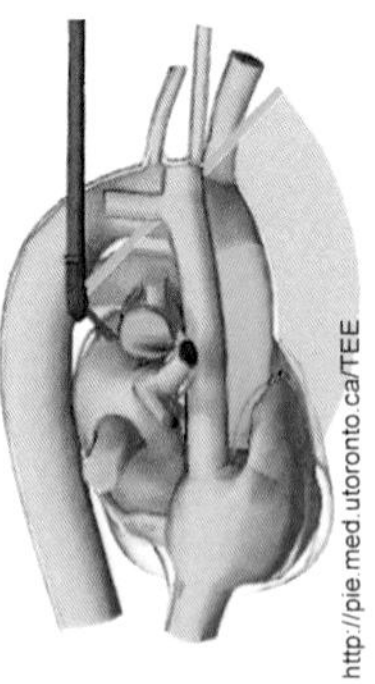

Imaged Structures	Diagnostic Issues
Ascending (Asc) Aorta	Aorta pathology:
Color Doppler	Atherosclerosis
Right Pulmonary Artery (RPA)	Dissection
Transverse pericardial sinus	Aneurysm
	Aortic Insufficiency flow
	Aortic Stenosis flow
	Pulmonary artery catheter in RPA
	Pulmonary embolism
	Pericardial effusion

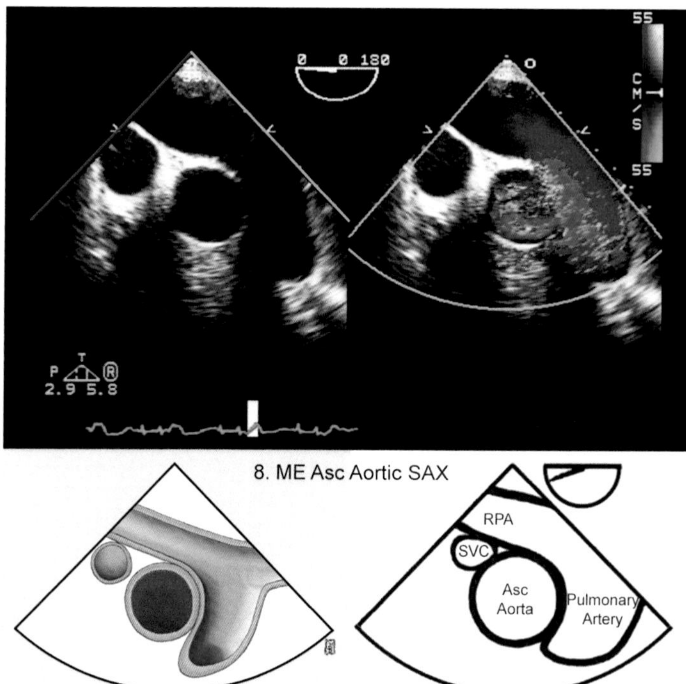

8. ME Asc Aortic SAX

The ME Ascending Aortic Short-Axis (SAX) view (0–10°) is obtained by withdrawing the probe from the ME Aortic Valve SAX view (30°) and rotating the transducer angle back to 0°. This view can also be obtained from the ME Ascending Aortic LAX (110°) view by decreasing the transducer angle to 0–10° to image the superior vena cava (SVC) in SAX, Ascending Aorta in SAX, and right and main pulmonary arteries in LAX. Color Doppler box is positioned over the pulmonary artery (PA) and aorta with Nyquist 50–70 cm/s to show laminar antegrade systolic flow. The color Doppler box can be separately positioned over the SVC with a lower Nyquist of 30 cm/s to show flow. Shown above is systolic flow acceleration in the main PA and turbulent flow in the ascending aorta.

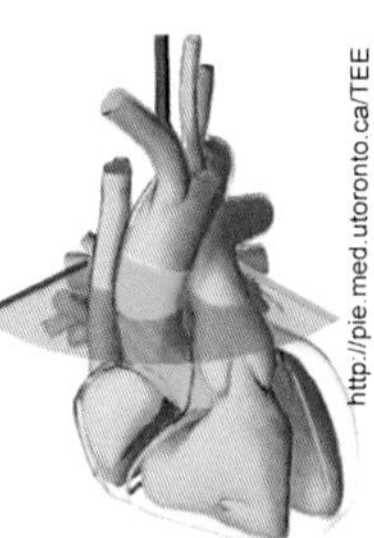

Imaged Structures	Diagnostic Issues
Ascending (Asc) aorta	Aorta pathology:
Color Doppler	Atherosclerosis
Main Pulmonary Artery (PA)	Dissection
Measure size	Aneurysm
Doppler: Color, PW spectral	Aortic Insufficiency flow
Right Pulmonary Artery (RPA)	Aortic Stenosis flow
Superior Vena Cava (SVC)	Pulmonary embolism
	Pulmonary artery catheter position
	SVC catheter
	PA cardiac output

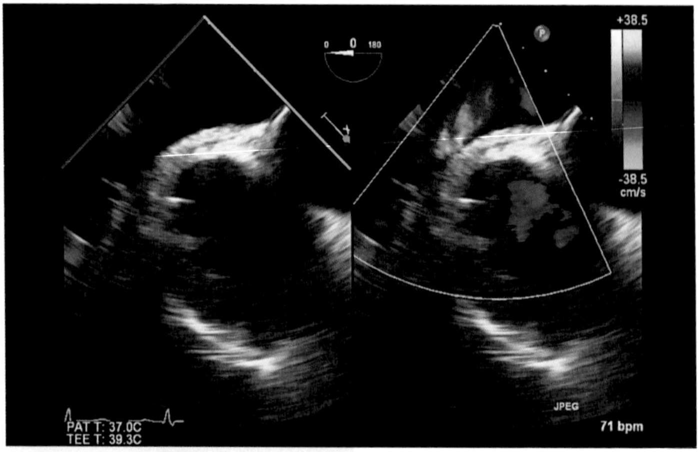

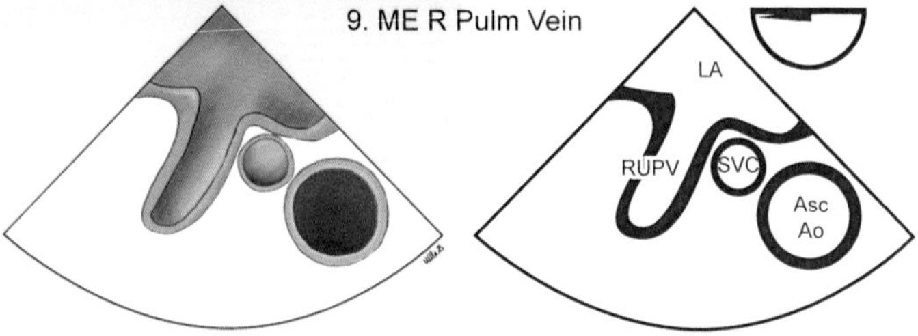

9. ME R Pulm Vein

The ME right pulmonary vein view is obtained by rotating the probe right (clockwise) from the ME Ascending Aorta SAX view (0–10°). The right upper pulmonary vein (RUPV) is easily identified by color Doppler (Nyquist 40 cm/s) as it enters the LA adjacent to the superior vena cava (SVC). The right lower pulmonary vein (RLPV) enters the LA at a right angle above the RUPV, often making it difficult to identify with color Doppler as blood flow is perpendicular to the probe. Increasing the transducer angle to 30° improves visualization of both right pulmonary veins (see p. 53) with color Doppler. The RUPV is well-aligned for spectral Doppler interrogation, the RLPV is not. Note also, both the SVC and ascending aorta are seen in short-axis.

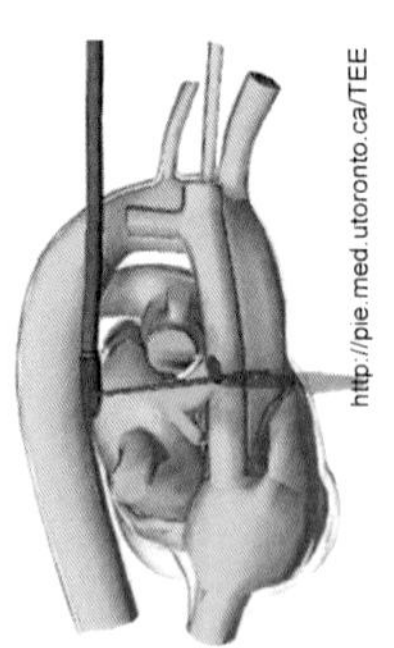

Imaged Structures	Diagnostic Issues
Right Upper Pulmonary Vein (RUPV) Doppler: Color, PW Spectral Right Lower Pulmonary Vein (RLPV) Superior Vena Cava (SVC) Doppler: Color Ascending Aorta (Asc Ao) Left Atrium (LA)	Pulmonary vein flow Anomalous pulmonary venous drainage SVC catheter

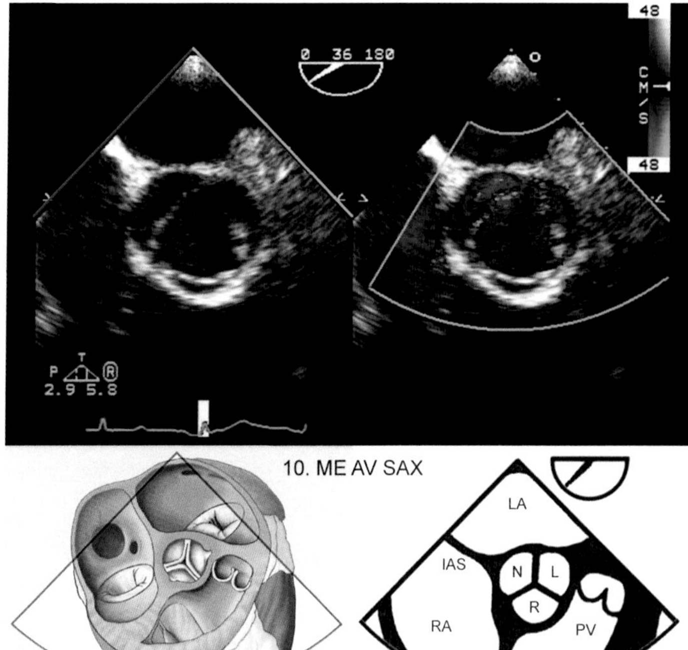

From the ME 4C view, the probe is withdrawn until the AV is centrally positioned in the display. To obtain the ME AV SAX view, increase the transducer angle to 30–45° with slight anteflexion to align the imaging plane parallel to the AV annulus. All three AV cusps should appear symmetric. Withdraw the probe to image the orifices of the left main and right coronary arteries arising from the aorta. Color Doppler box over the AV with Nyquist 50–70 cm/s shows laminar (red) systolic flow through the AV. Continuous flow during systole and diastole suggests aortic insufficiency. The PV and RVOT are seen and may be sufficiently aligned to obtain spectral Doppler information. Color Doppler box over the IAS with lower Nyquist (30 cm/s) may identify a defect.

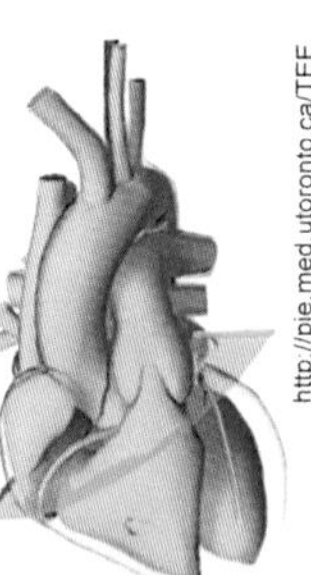

http://pie.med.utoronto.ca/TEE

Imaged Structures	Diagnostic Issues
Aortic Valve (AV):	AV morphology
3 cusps: Non (N), Right (R), Left (L)	AV pathology
Commissures, coaptation points	AV area planimetry
Color Doppler	Aortic insufficiency location
Coronary arteries (withdraw probe):	IAS pathology:
Left Coronary Artery (LCA)	Secundum ASD
Right Coronary Artery (RCA)	Patent Foramen Ovale (PFO)
Inter-Atrial Septum (IAS):	LA size (anterior-posterior diameter)
Color Doppler (low velocity)	
Left Atrium (LA): measure size	
Right Atrium (RA)	
Right Ventricular Outflow Tract (RVOT)	
Pulmonic Valve (PV)	

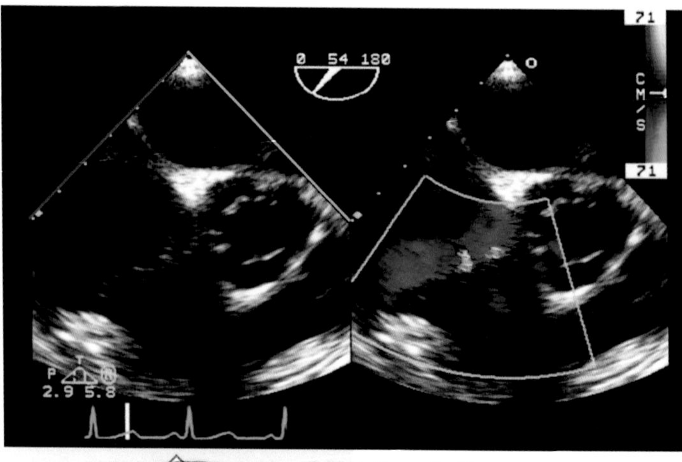

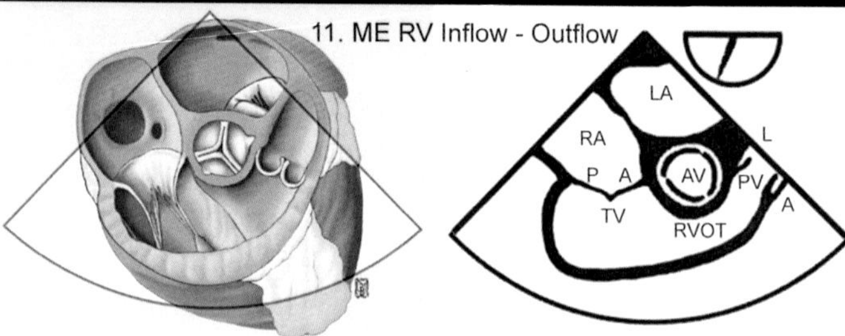

Aptly named, this view images the RV inflow from the tricuspid valve (TV) on the display right and RV outflow tract (RVOT) through to the pulmonic valve (PV) on the display left in a single view. This view is obtained from the ME AV SAX view (30°) by increasing the transducer angle to 50–75°. An off-axis image of the aortic valve (AV) is displayed centrally. Color Doppler box is positioned separately over the TV and PV with Nyquist 50–70 cm/s to show laminar antegrade (blue) diastolic flow through the TV and systolic flow (red) through the PV. Pulsed-wave (PW) spectral Doppler sample volume at the TV and PV assesses flow through these valves.

http://pie.med.utoronto.ca/TEE

Imaged Structures

Tricuspid Valve (TV):
  Posterior + anterior/septal leaflets
  Doppler: Color, PW/CW spectral
Pulmonic Valve (PV):
  Measure annulus 2.0 ± 0.3 cm
  Anterior + left cusps
  Color Doppler
Right Ventricular Outflow Tract (RVOT):
  1 cm proximal to PV: 1.7 ± 0.2 cm
Pulmonary Artery (PA):
  Main PA 1 cm distal to PV: 1.8 ± 0.3 cm
Inter-Atrial Septum (IAS)
Right Atrium (RA)
Left Atrium (LA)
Transverse pericardial sinus

Diagnostic Issues

Pulmonic valve pathology
Pulmonary artery pathology
RVOT pathology
TV pathology
TV Doppler
  PW: antegrade flow
  CW: retrograde flow (TR)
Atrial Septal Defect (ASD secundum)
Ventricular Septal Defect (VSD)

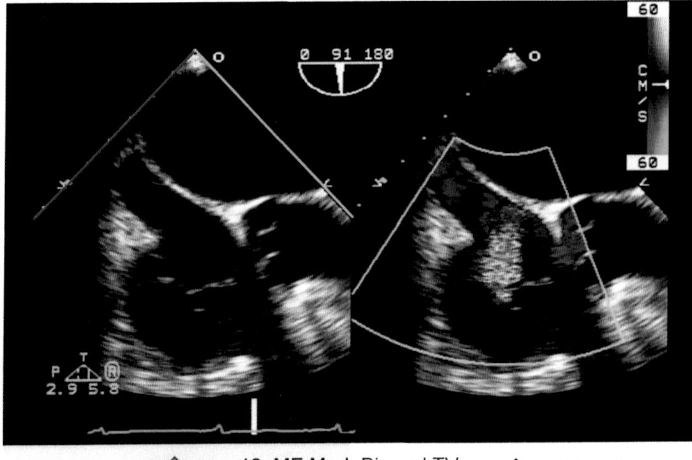

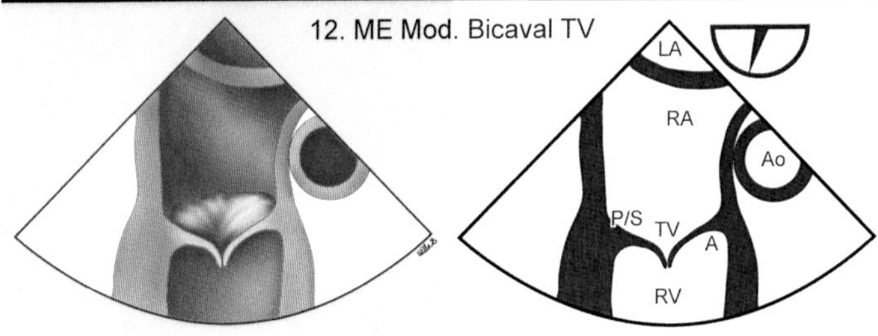

12. ME Mod. Bicaval TV

The ME Modified Bicaval Tricuspid Valve (TV) view (50–70°) is obtained from the ME RV inflow-outflow view (50–70°) with the TV in the display center by turning the probe to the right (clockwise). The imaging plane is directed through the LA to image the right heart including the RA, TV, RV, and inter-atrial septum (IAS). Two TV leaflets are seen, the anterior leaflet is on the display right and the septal or posterior leaflet (advance probe) on the display left. Color Doppler (Nyquist 50–70 cm/s) over the TV may demonstrate tricuspid regurgitation (TR). CW spectral Doppler alignment may be adequate to obtain a complete spectral trace of the TR jet. The peak TR velocity can estimate the right ventricular systolic pressure (RVSP).

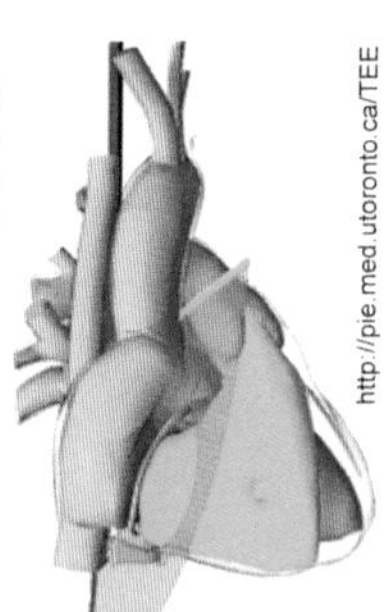

http://pie.med.utoronto.ca/TEE

Imaged Structures	Diagnostic Issues
Left Atrium (LA)	Tricuspid Regurgitation (TR)
Right Atrium (RA)	RVSP
Tricuspid Valve (TV):	Atrial Septal Defect (ASD)
Posterior/septal + anterior	Venous catheters
Doppler: Color (TR), PW/CW spectral	Pacemaker wires
Superior Vena Cava (SVC)	Venous cannula position (SVC/IVC)
Inferior Vena Cava (IVC)	
Inter-Atrial Septum (IAS):	
Mid-portion IAS	
Color Doppler (low velocity)	
Ascending aorta	
Coronary Sinus (CS)	

13. ME Bicaval

LA
IVC
IAS
SVC
RA
RAA

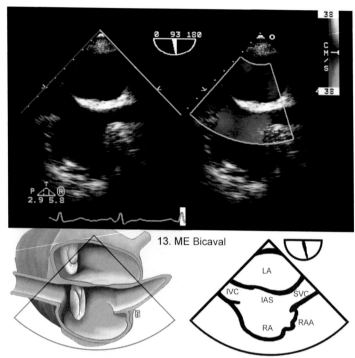

The ME Bicaval view (90°) is obtained from the ME 2 Chamber view (90°) by turning the entire probe to the patient's right (clockwise) towards the superior vena cava (SVC) and inferior vena cava (IVC). The transducer plane cuts longitudinally through the LA, RA, and both the IVC and SVC. The structures are displayed with the LA at the sector apex (closest to probe), RA in the far field, caudad IVC (left), and cephalad SVC (right). The imaging plane is perpendicular to the IAS, making the assessment of any defects in septal tissue more reliable than the ME 4 Chamber view. Color Doppler box is positioned over the IAS and proximal IVC and SVC with Nyquist 30–50 cm/s. Laminar antegrade flow is present in the cava. Any flow across the IAS is abnormal suggesting an ASD or PFO.

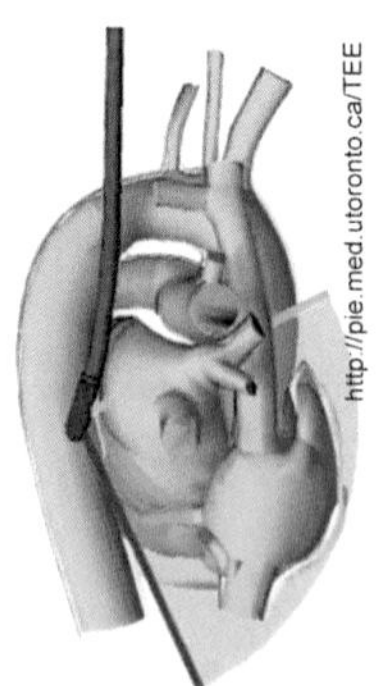

Imaged Structures	Diagnostic Issues
Left Atrium (LA)	IAS pathology
Right Atrium (RA):	Defects
Free wall, appendage (RAA)	Secundum ASD
Eustachian valve	Sinus venosus defect
Crista terminalis	Patent Foramen Ovale (PFO)
Superior Vena Cava (SVC):	Lipomatous Hypertrophy
Measure: 1.4 ± 0.2 cm	Mass
Inferior Vena Cava (IVC):	SVC/IVC flow
Measure: 1.6 ± 0.2 cm	Venous catheters, Pacemaker wires
Inter-Atrial Septum (IAS):	Venous cannula position (SVC/IVC)
Color Doppler (low velocity)	Pericardial effusion

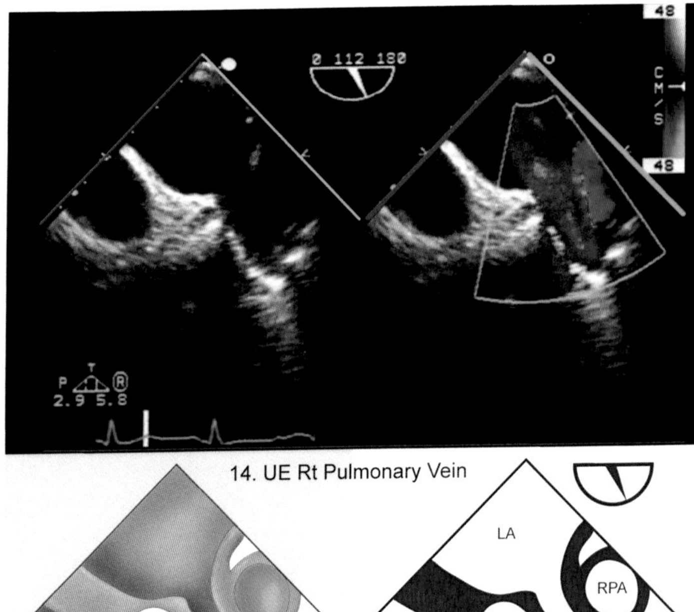

14. UE Rt Pulmonary Vein

The right upper pulmonary vein (RUPV) can be easily identified in a modified bicaval view (90–110°) by withdrawing the probe slightly and increasing the transducer angle from the ME bicaval view (90°). Color Doppler (Nyquist 40–60 cm/s) helps locate the RUPV as it drains into the left atrium (LA) between the right pulmonary artery (RPA) and right atrium (RA). There is good spectral Doppler alignment for RUPV interrogation.

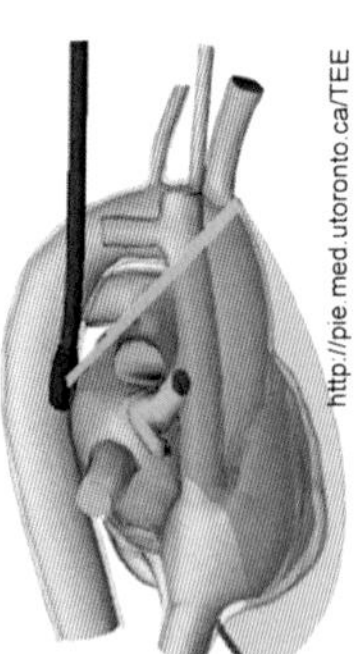

Imaged Structures	Diagnostic Issues

Right Upper Pulmonary Vein (RUPV)
  Doppler: Color, PW Spectral
Right Pulmonary Artery (RPA)
Left Atrium (LA)
Right Atrium (RA)
	Pulmonary Vein
	  Doppler flow
	  Stenosis
	Sinus Venosus defect
	Anomalous Pulmonary Venous Drainage

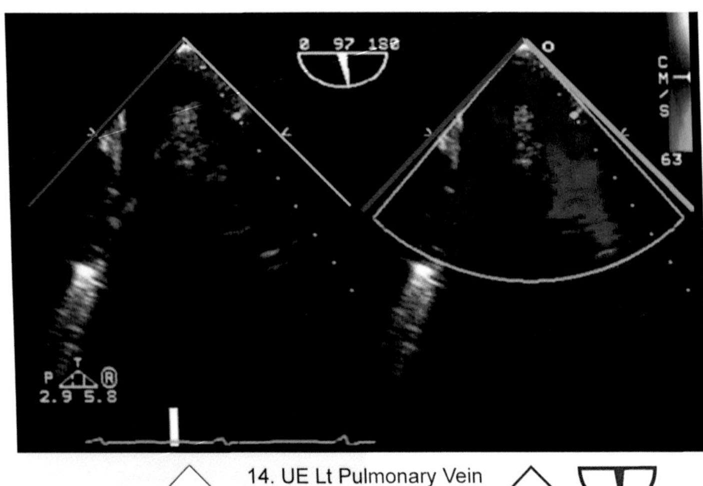

14. UE Lt Pulmonary Vein

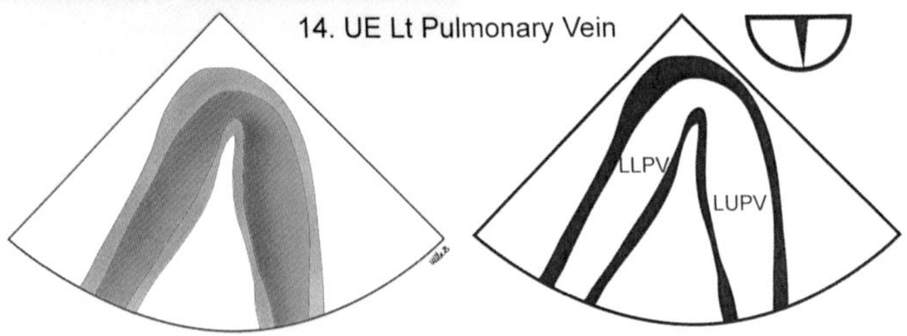

Both left pulmonary veins can be imaged in the same UE left pulmonary veins view (90–110°). In this view, the veins appear as an inverted "v" as they enter the left atrium (LA). The left upper/superior pulmonary vein appears on the display right and the left lower/inferior pulmonary vein is on the display left. The addition of color Doppler (Nyquist 50–70 cm/s) and changing the transducer angle by 10° increments can aid in identifying both veins. Both left pulmonary veins are well-aligned for spectral Doppler interrogation. The main pulmonary artery may be seen in short-axis in the display.

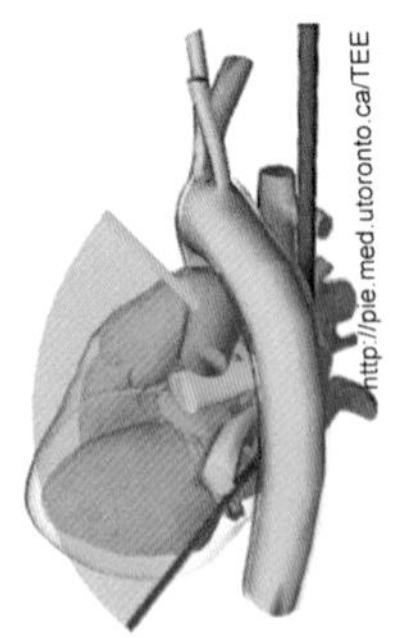

Imaged Structures	Diagnostic Issues

Left Atrium (LA)
Left Upper Pulmonary Vein
  Doppler: Color, PW spectral
Left Lower Pulmonary Vein
  Doppler: Color, PW Spectral
	Pulmonary vein flow
	Anomalous Pulmonary Venous Drainage

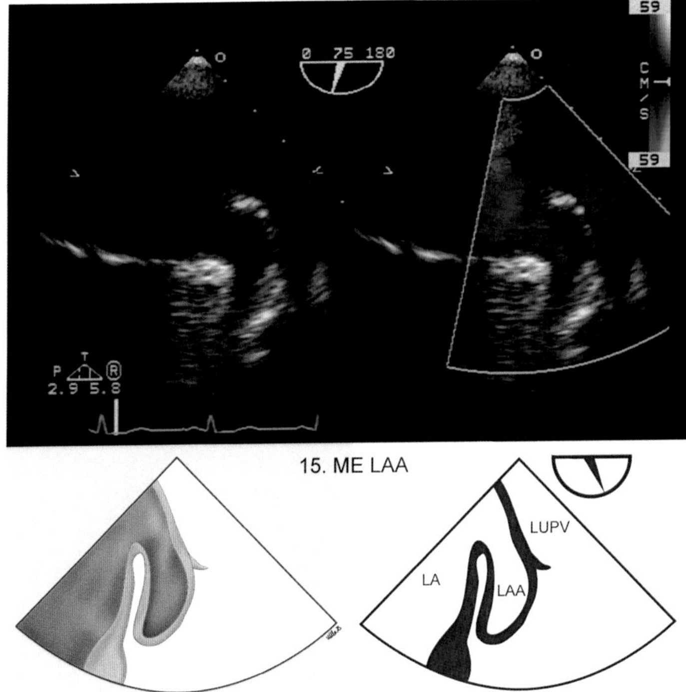

15. ME LAA

The ME left atrial appendage (LAA) view (80–110°) is obtained by identifying the mitral valve (MV) in the ME 2C view (90°), reducing the sector depth and turning the probe to the left (counter-clockwise) to better image the LAA. The LAA is seen from 30 to 110° in multiple ME views as shown above. Withdrawing the probe slightly images the left upper pulmonary vein (LUPV), which is more posterior to the LAA and closer to the probe. Color Doppler (Nyquist 50-70 cm/s) shows laminar flow in both systole (blue flow, see above) as the LAA fills and diastole (red flow) as the LAA empties. Pulsed-wave spectral Doppler is well-aligned to assess LAA velocities (see p. 50). The presence of spontaneous echo contrast and low velocity (<20 cm/s) makes the diagnosis of LAA thrombus more likely.

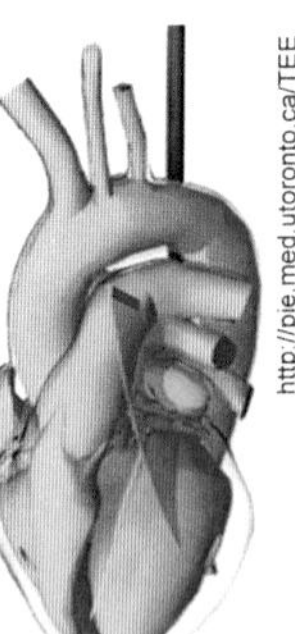

Imaged Structures	Diagnostic Issues

Left Atrial Appendage (LAA):
  Size:
    Diameter 1.6 ± 0.5 cm
    Length 2.9 ± 0.5 cm
  Doppler: Color, PW spectral
Left Upper Pulmonary Vein (LUPV)
  Doppler: Color, PW spectral
Mitral Valve (MV)
	LAA thrombus
	LUPV flow
	LAA flow

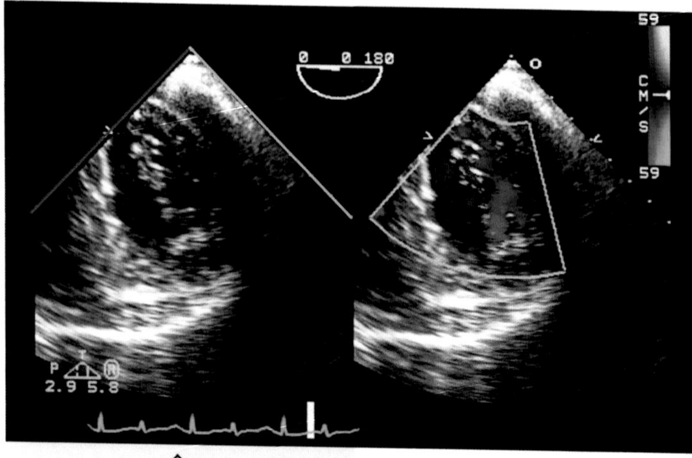

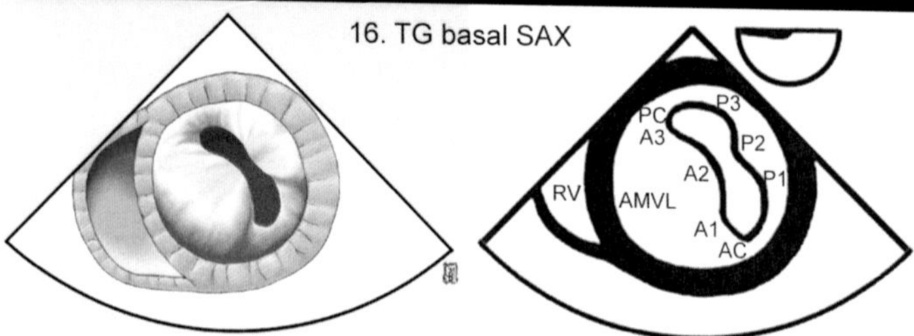

16. TG basal SAX

The transgastric basal Short-Axis (TG basal SAX) view (0°) is obtained as the probe is advanced into the stomach or by withdrawing the probe from the TG mid-SAX view (0°). This permits a view of the MV from the stomach that is parallel to the annulus with the posterior leaflet on the display right and the anterior leaflet to the left. The posterior commissure, A3, and P3 are closest to the probe. Color Doppler box is positioned over the MV with Nyquist 50–70 cm/s to show laminar (blue) diastolic flow through the MV. Continuous flow during systole and diastole suggests mitral regurgitation (MR) with accurate identification of the location. Each of the 6 basal LV segments can be analyzed for systolic function.

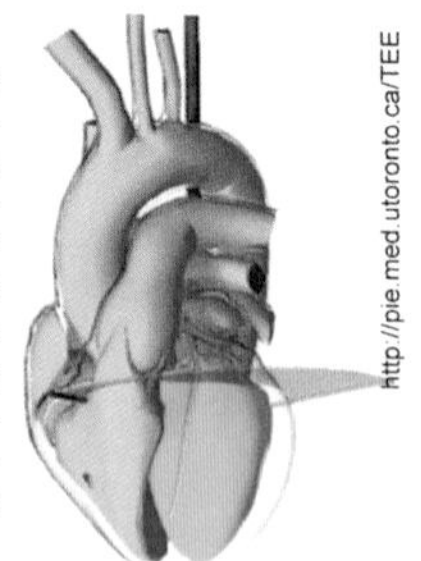

Imaged Structures	Diagnostic Issues
Left Ventricle (LV): 6 basal segments Inferior (I) ↔ Anterior (A) Infero-Lateral (IL) ↔ Antero-Septal (AS) Antero-Lateral (AL) ↔ Infero-Septal (IS) Mitral Valve (MV): leaflets, 6 segments Posterior (PMVL): P1, P2, P3 Anterior (AMVL): A1, A2, A3 Commissures: Anterior/lateral (AC) Posterior/medial (PC) Color Doppler Right Ventricle (RV) Interventricular Septum (IVS)	MV: Pathology Site of MR LV: basal segment function Ventricular Septal Defect (VSD) Pericardial effusion

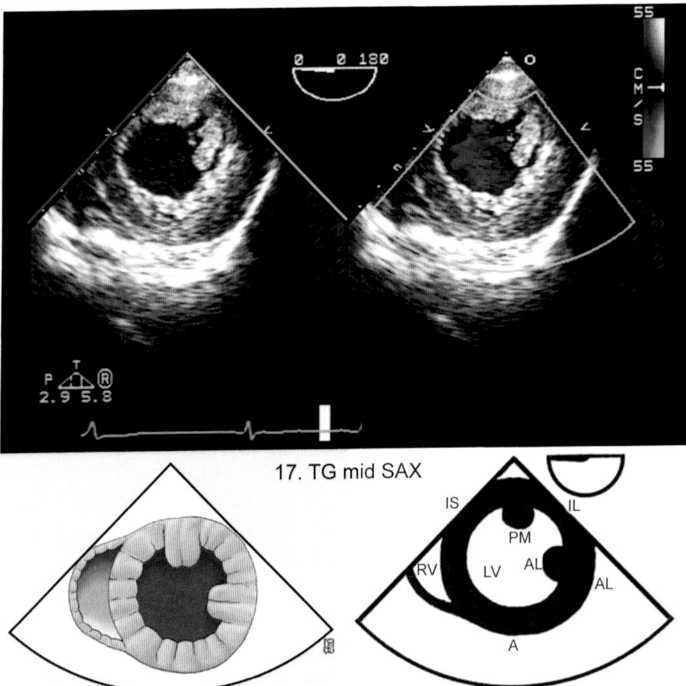

The transgastric (TG) views are obtained by advancing the TEE probe in a neutral position into the stomach and applying varying degrees of anteflexion to the probe tip. In the TG mid-SAX view (0°), the left ventricle (LV) is imaged in short-axis (SAX) with all 6 LV segments viewed at once. The probe tip is manipulated (a) by gentle anteflexion to increase contact with gastric mucosa, (b) left flexion to center the LV cavity, and (c) slightly increasing the transducer angle to obtain a symmetrical circular LV with both papillary muscles present. Though not frequently used in this view, color Doppler with Nyquist 50–70 cm/s can be used to show flow across the interventricular septum (IVS), suggesting a ventricular septal defect (VSD).

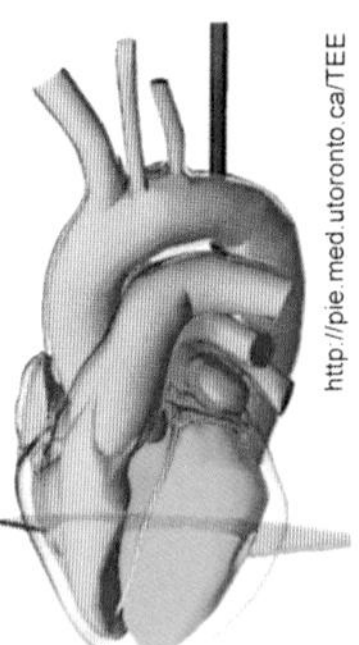

Imaged Structures	Diagnostic Issues
Left Ventricle (LV): 6 opposing mid segments Inferior (I) ↔ Anterior (A) Infero-Lateral (IL) ↔ Antero-Septal (AS) Antero-Lateral (AL) ↔ Infero-Septal (IS) Papillary muscles: Antero-Lateral (AL) Posteromedial (PM) Right Ventricle (RV) Interventricular Septum (IVS)	LV cavity size LV wall thickness LV systolic function Global, regional IVS motion Ventricular Septal Defect (VSD) Pericardial effusion

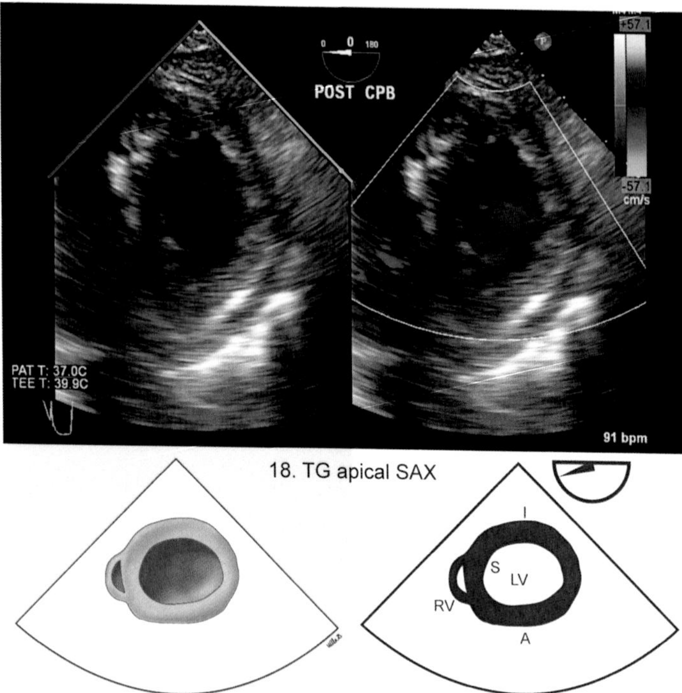

The transgastric apical Short-Axis (TG Apical SAX) view (0–20°) is obtained by advancing the probe with gentle anteflexion along the gastric mucosa from the TG mid-SAX view (0–20°). A short-axis view of the left ventricle (LV) is seen with a small cavity and without papillary muscles. Turning the probe to the right shows a short-axis view of the right ventricular apex.

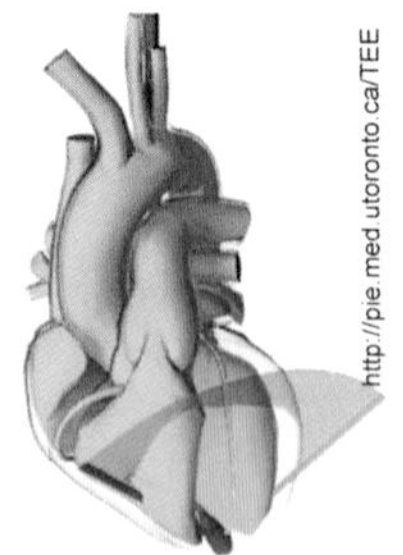

http://pie.med.utoronto.ca/TEE

Imaged Structures	Diagnostic Issues
Left Ventricle (LV): 4 apical LV segments: Anterior ↔ Inferior Septal ↔ Lateral Right Ventricle (RV) Interventricular Septum (IVS)	LV: Apical segment function Apical aneurysm Ventricular Septal Defect (VSD) Pericardial effusion

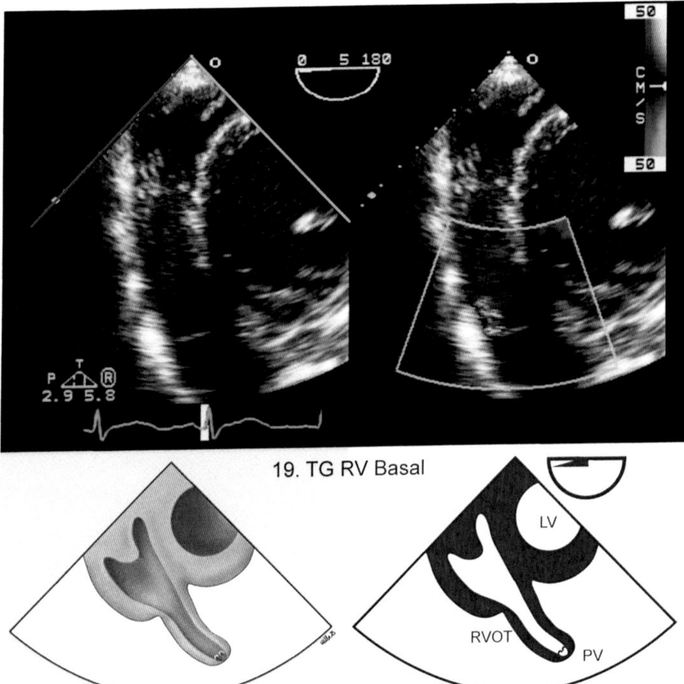

19. TG RV Basal

The transgastric right ventricular basal (TG RV basal) view (0–20°) is obtained by turning the probe right (clockwise) from the TG basal SAX view (0–20°). The imaging plane is adjusted to see the tricuspid valve (TV) in short-axis and the right ventricular outflow tract (RVOT) in long-axis. Increasing the transducer angle to between 0 and 30° shows the pulmonic valve (PV) in long-axis in the lower display right, similar to the UE arch SAX view. This view allows good alignment for spectral Doppler assessment of the PV and RVOT. Color Doppler box (Nyquist 50 cm/s) can be positioned over the PV to show pulmonic insufficiency and turbulence in the RVOT.

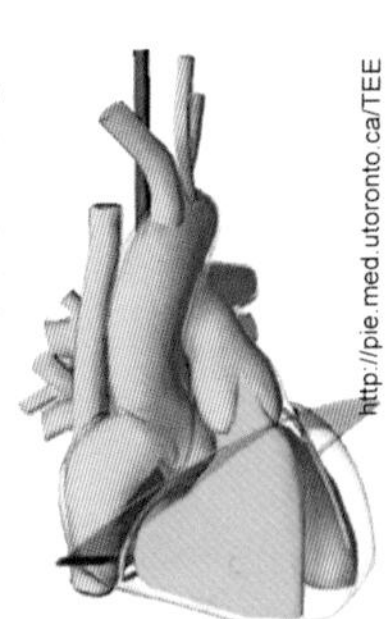

Imaged Structures	Diagnostic Issues
Left Ventricle (LV): Basal segments Right Ventricle (RV): Basal segments Right Ventricular Outflow Tract (RVOT) Tricuspid Valve (TV): SAX Anterior, posterior, septal leaflets Pulmonic Valve (PV) Interventricular Septum (IVS)	TV pathology PV pathology RVOT Ventricular Septal Defect (VSD)

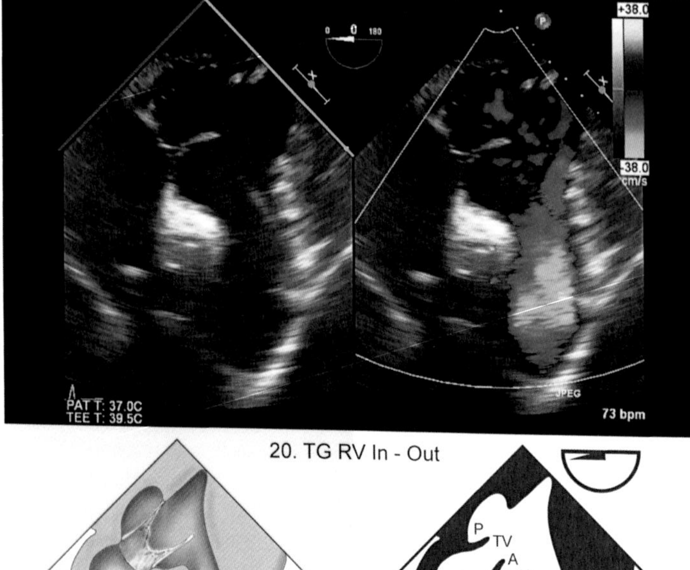

The transgastric right ventricular inflow-outflow (TG RV In-Out) view (0–20°) is obtained from the TG RV basal view by right flexing the probe tip. This is a challenging view to obtain in a normal heart and similar information can be obtained from other TG views. The imaging plane is adjusted to image the pulmonic valve (PV), right atrium (RA), right ventricle (RV), right ventricular outflow tract (RVOT), and tricuspid valve (TV). In this view, typically the anterior and posterior leaflets of the TV are imaged, as well as the left and right cusps of the PV. Advancing the probe may be necessary to align RVOT flow for optimal spectral Doppler interrogation. Color Doppler box with Nyquist of 50 cm/s can be positioned over the TV and PV to assess flow.

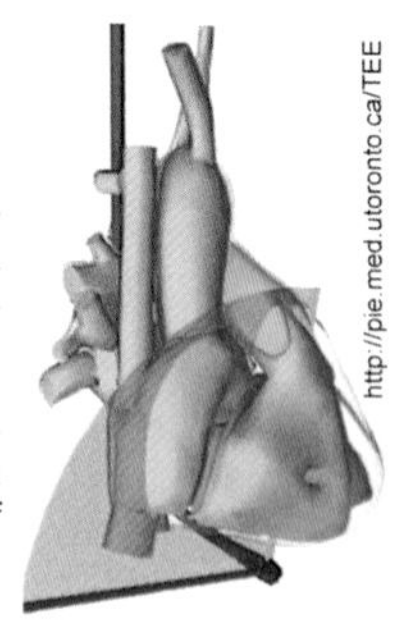

Imaged Structures	Diagnostic Issues

Right Atrium (RA)
Right Ventricle (RV)
Right Ventricular Outflow Tract (RVOT)
  Doppler: Color, PW Spectral
Pulmonary Valve (PV)
  Right, left cusps
  Doppler: Color, CW spectral
Tricuspid Valve (TV)
  Anterior, posterior leaflets
  Color Doppler
	TV pathology
	PV pathology
	PV spectral Doppler
	RVOT color Doppler
	RVOT pathology

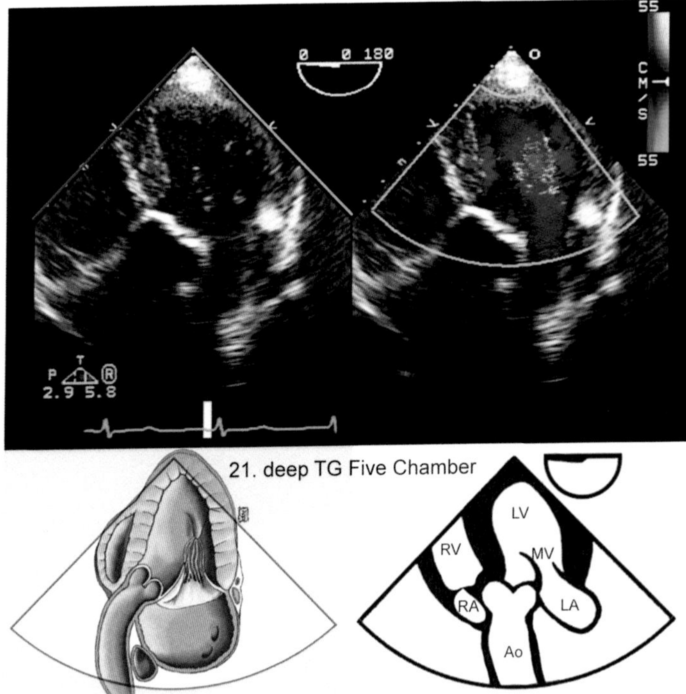

The deep transgastric five-chamber (Deep TG 5C) view (0°) is obtained by advancing the probe with anteflexion in the stomach from the TG mid- or apical SAX views. Leftward probe tip flexion may be necessary to place the LVOT and aortic valve (AV) in the display center with the LV apex at the sector apex. A common mistake in obtaining this view is to extremely anteflex the probe tip from the TG basal SAX view, which places the LV apex at 2 o'clock on the display and not at the sector apex. Spectral Doppler alignment is good to measure flow velocity across the AV and in the LVOT. Color Doppler box positioned over the AV and MV with Nyquist 50–70 cm/s shows laminar antegrade systolic flow (blue) through the AV and diastolic flow (red, as seen above) through the MV. Retrograde flow through either valve suggests regurgitation and appears as the opposite color to antegrade flow.

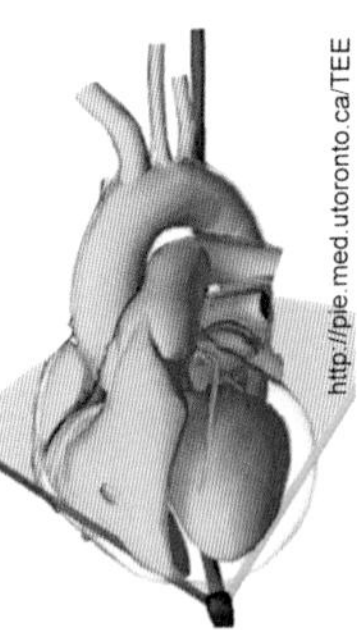

Imaged Structures	Diagnostic Issues
Left Ventricle (LV):	AV pathology:
Apex, Antero-Septal, Infero-Lateral	Stenosis, Insufficiency
Left Ventricular Outflow Tract (LVOT):	AV spectral Doppler
Doppler: Color, PW Spectral	Prosthetic AV function
Aortic Valve (AV):	LVOT:
Doppler: CW Spectral	Pathology
Ascending Aorta	Spectral Doppler
Mitral Valve (MV)	Ventricular Septal Defect (VSD)
Interventricular Septum (IVS)	MV pathology
Left Atrium (LA)	

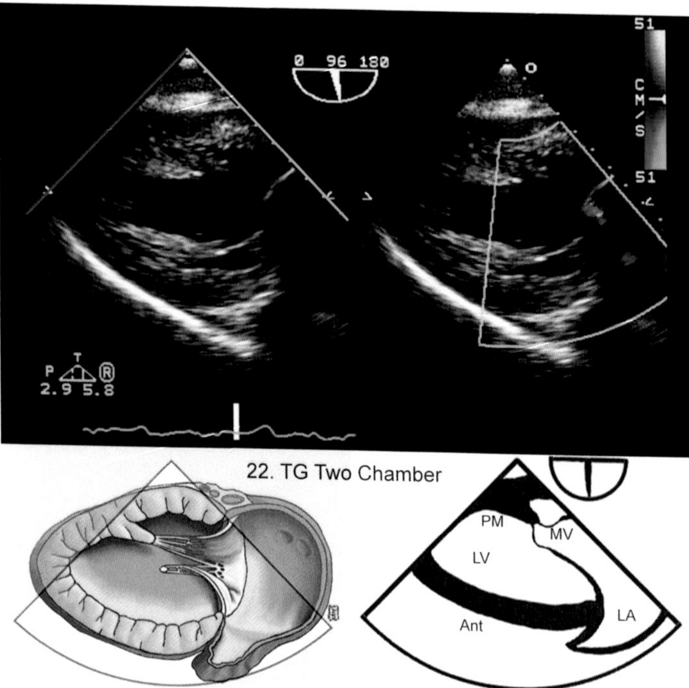

The transgastric two-chamber (TG 2C) view is obtained from the TG mid-SAX view (0°) by increasing the transducer angle to 90–110°. This images the left ventricle (LV) in long-axis and the subvalvular structures of the mitral valve (MV). This view is similar to the ME 2 Chamber view now turned 90° with the probe closest to the inferior wall of the LV, which appears at the sector apex of the display. Color Doppler box is positioned over the MV with Nyquist 50–70 cm/s. Laminar diastolic flow occurs through the MV. Retrograde systolic flow suggests mitral regurgitation (MR).

http://pie.med.utoronto.ca/TEE

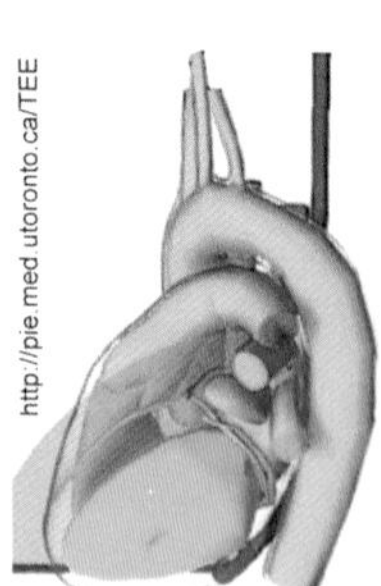

Imaged Structures	Diagnostic Issues
Left Ventricle (LV): Apex Anterior (Ant) + Inferior (I) walls (basal + mid-segments) Posteromedial papillary muscle (PM) Left atrium (LA): Left Atrial Appendage (LAA) Mitral Valve (MV): Anterior and posterior leaflets Subvalvular apparatus (chordae) Color Doppler	LV systolic function MV subvalvular apparatus MV pathology Pericardial effusion

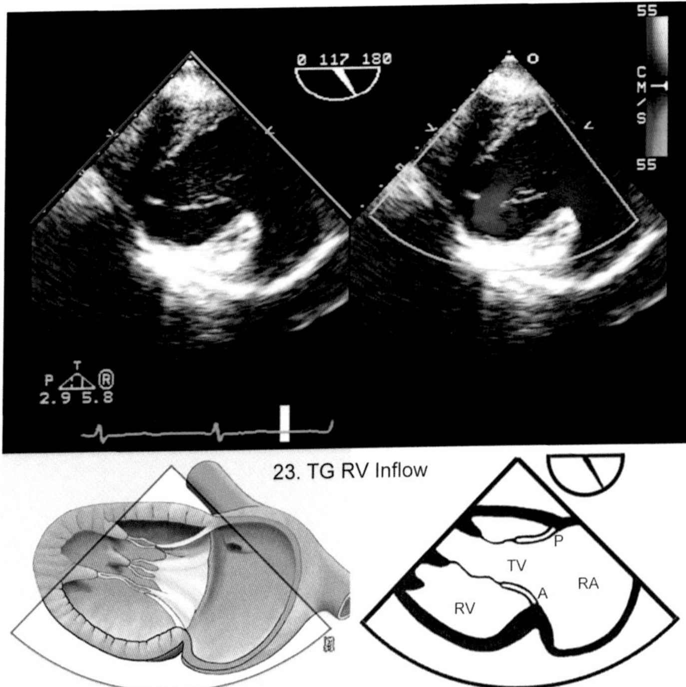

23. TG RV Inflow

The transgastric right ventricular inflow (TG RV Inflow) view (90–120°) is obtained from the TG basal SAX view (0°), by turning the probe to the right to center the tricuspid valve (TV) and increasing the transducer angle to 110–130°. This view shows the RV in long-axis, with the RV apex on the display left, the inferior RV wall in the near field, and the anterior RV free wall in the far field. Color Doppler box is positioned over the TV with Nyquist 50–70 cm/s to show laminar antegrade diastolic flow. Continuous unidirectional diastolic flow, in relation to the probe as shown above, appears red from the right atrium (RA) through the TV and blue when filling the RV. Retrograde systolic TV flow appears blue or turbulent and suggests tricuspid regurgitation (TR).

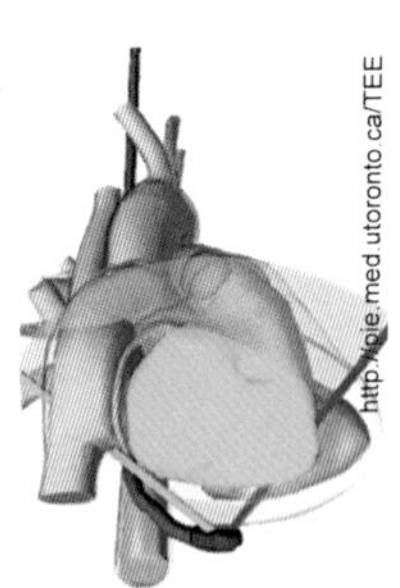

Imaged Structures	Diagnostic Issues
Tricuspid Valve (TV): Posterior (P) + Anterior (A) leaflets Subvalvular apparatus Tricuspid Annular Plane Systolic Excursion (TAPSE) Color Doppler Right Ventricle (RV): Inferior + Anterior walls Tissue Doppler inferior wall Right Atrium (RA)	TV pathology RV systolic function RA mass Tissue Doppler Imaging (TDI) RV Inferior wall Pericardial effusion

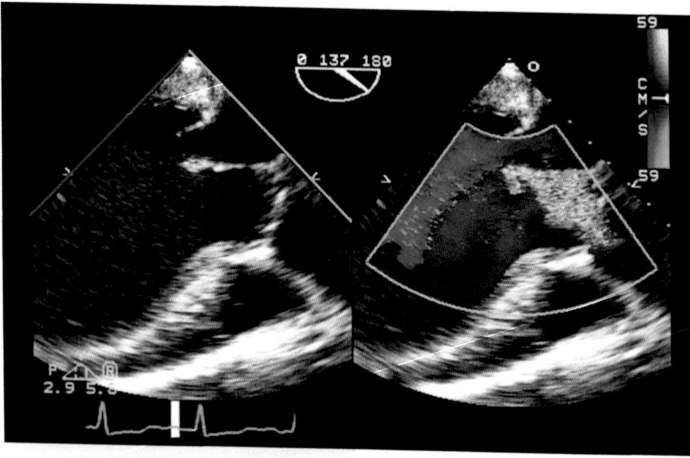

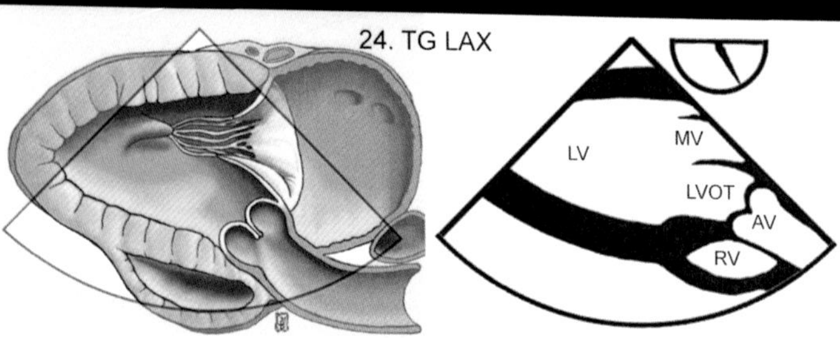

The transgastric Long-Axis (TG LAX) view is developed from the TG 2 Chamber view (90°) by increasing the transducer angle to 120–140°. The left ventricular outflow tract (LVOT) and aortic valve (AV) appear on the display right in the far field. This view is similar to the ME AV LAX view, but permits adequate spectral Doppler alignment. Color Doppler box is positioned over the MV, LVOT, and AV with Nyquist 50–70 cm/s to show laminar antegrade systolic flow through the LVOT (red) and AV (blue). Turbulent diastolic flow through the AV suggests aortic insufficiency (AI) as shown above. Systolic flow through the interventricular septum (IVS) is a ventricular septal defect (VSD).

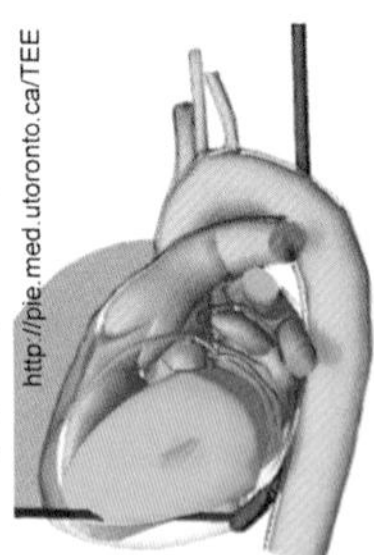

Imaged Structures	Diagnostic Issues
Left Ventricle (LV): Antero-Septal + Infero-Lateral walls (basal + mid-segments) Left Ventricular Outflow Tract (LVOT): PW Doppler Interventricular Septum (IVS) Mitral Valve (MV): Anterior + posterior leaflets Subvalvular apparatus Doppler: Color Aortic Valve (AV): Doppler: Color, CW Spectral Cusps	MV: Leaflets, subvalvular Mitral Regurgitation (MR) LV systolic function AV Doppler gradient LVOT Doppler gradient Ventricular Septal Defect (VSD) Prosthetic AV function Pericardial effusion

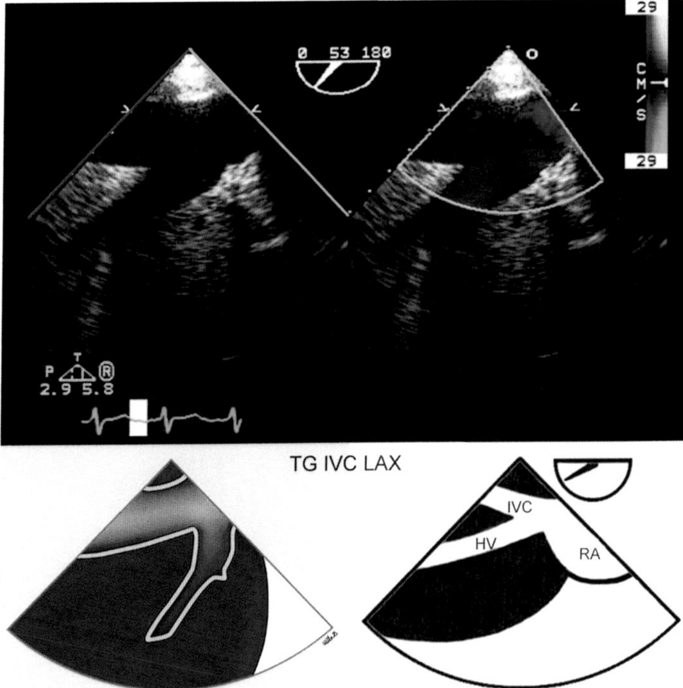

The transgastric inferior vena cava Long-Axis (TG IVC LAX) view is obtained by finding the TG mid-SAX view (0°). Turn the probe right to find the liver; withdraw to find the IVC as it enters the right atrium (RA). Adjust the probe and transducer angle (30–50°) to identify the hepatic vein (HV) as it enters the IVC. Color Doppler box is positioned over the hepatic vein and IVC with a low Nyquist 30 cm/s to show laminar antegrade flow. In relation to the probe, flow appears red through the proximal IVC and hepatic vein and blue into the right atrium (RA). Pulsed-wave spectral Doppler analysis can also be performed on the hepatic vein (see p. 51).

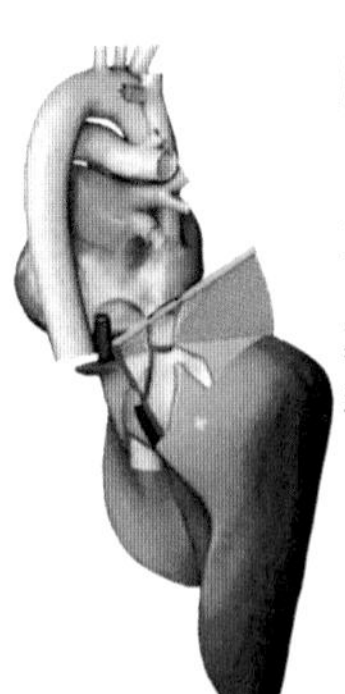

http://pie.med.utoronto.ca/TEE

Imaged Structures	Diagnostic Issues
Inferior Vena Cava (IVC): Size 1.6 ± 0.2 cm Color Doppler (low velocity) Hepatic Vein (HV): Size 0.8 ± 0.3 cm Color Doppler (low velocity) PW Doppler Liver Right Atrium (RA)	Tricuspid Regurgitation IVC: Mass (tumor, thrombus) IVC cannula position IVC respiratory variation in size Liver pathology

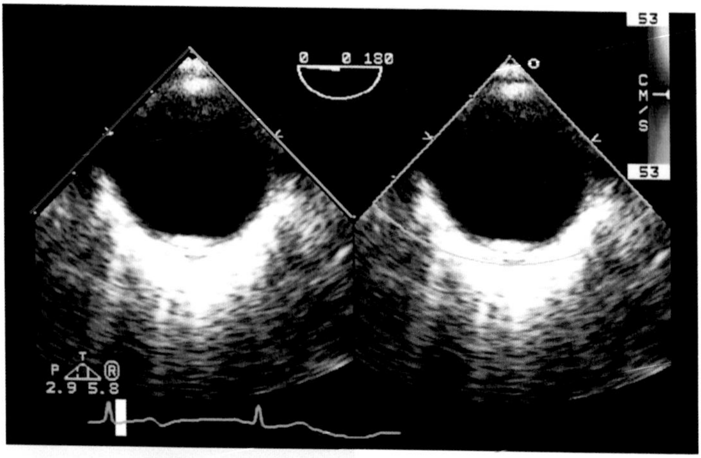

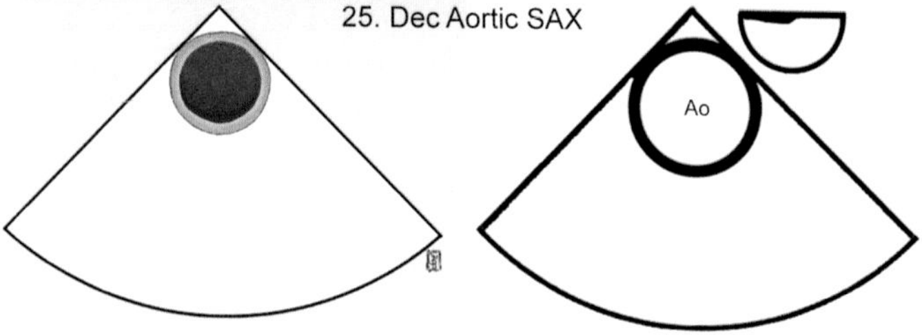

25. Dec Aortic SAX

Ao

The descending thoracic aorta is visualized in SAX (0°) by turning the probe to the left from the ME 4 Chamber view (0°). The image sector is reduced to better examine the aortic walls. The near field image of the circular aorta represents the right anterior wall of the aorta. Advance and withdraw the probe to image more of the descending aorta. Color Doppler box is positioned over the aorta with Nyquist 50–70 cm/s to show intermittent laminar antegrade systolic flow (red) as shown above. Continuous flow during systole and diastole in the aorta suggests aortic insufficiency (AI).

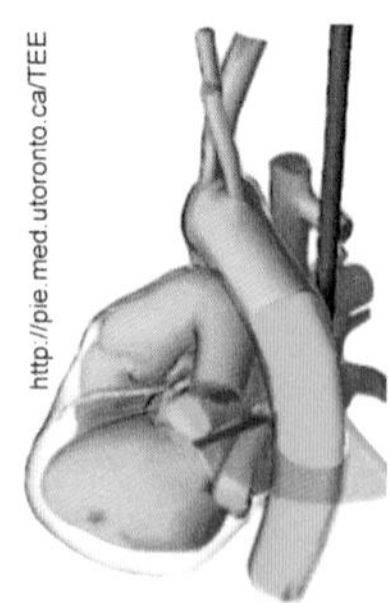

http://pie.med.utoronto.ca/TEE

Imaged Structures	Diagnostic Issues
Descending Aorta (Ao): Size Doppler: Color, PW Spectral Left pleural space	Aorta pathology: Atherosclerosis Dissection Aneurysm Left pleural effusion AI severity PW Doppler IABP position

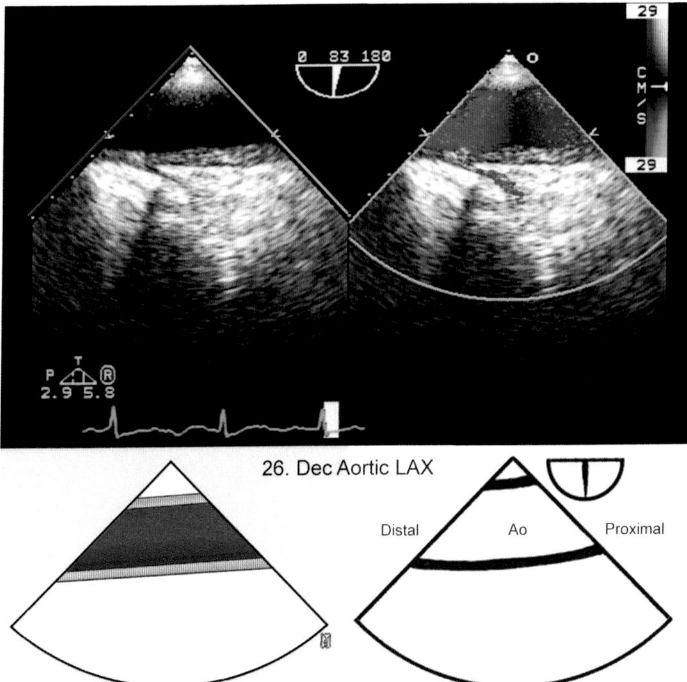

26. Dec Aortic LAX

From the descending thoracic aortic SAX view (0°), the transducer angle is increased to 90°, to obtain the descending aortic LAX view. The distal aorta is to the display left and the proximal aorta to the display right. The walls of the aorta should appear in parallel. Color Doppler box is positioned over the aorta with Nyquist 50–70 cm/s to show laminar antegrade systolic flow. Though flow is continuous and unidirectional, in relation to the probe, it appears red through the proximal and blue through the distal descending aorta. Black color indicates the probe is perpendicular to flow. A lower Nyquist limit as shown above can help identify intercostal branches at different aortic levels.

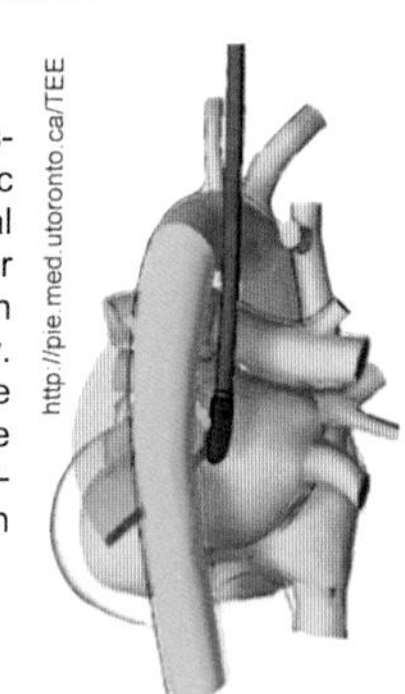

http://pie.med.utoronto.ca/TEE

Imaged Structures	Diagnostic Issues
Descending Aorta (Ao): Size Doppler: Color, PW Spectral Intercostal arteries Left pleural space	Aorta pathology: Atherosclerosis Dissection Aneurysm AI severity PW Doppler IABP position Left pleural effusion

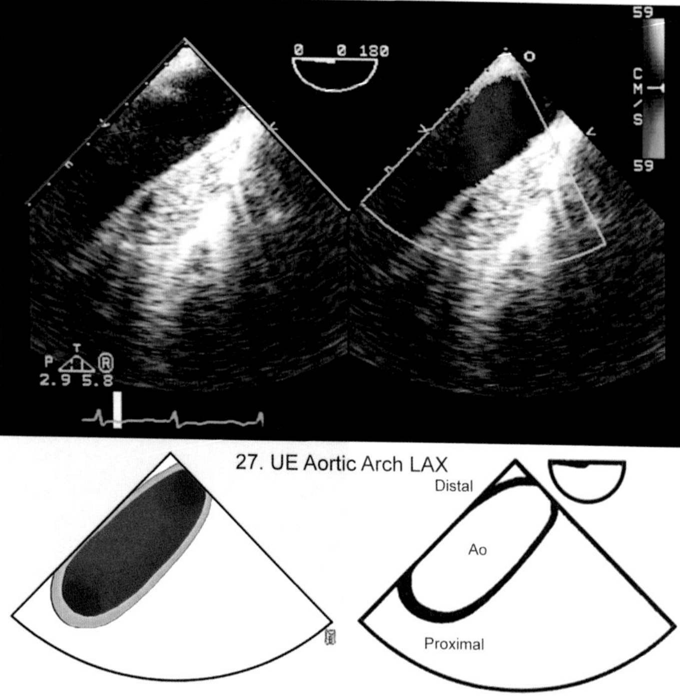

From the thoracic Descending Aortic SAX view (0°), the probe is withdrawn cephalad with a slight right (clockwise) turn. The circular shape of the thoracic descending aorta changes to an oblong shape of the transverse Aortic Arch LAX view (0°). The proximal aortic arch is to the display left and the distal arch to the right. Further withdrawal may image the great vessels of the head and neck. Color Doppler box is positioned over the aorta with Nyquist 50–70 cm/s to show laminar antegrade systolic flow. Though flow is continuous and unidirectional during systole, in relation to the probe, it appears red through the proximal and blue through the distal aortic arch (compare with Descending Aortic LAX view). Black color indicates the probe is perpendicular to flow. Continuous flow during systole and diastole in the aortic arch suggests aortic insufficiency (AI). Pulsed-wave spectral Doppler of the distal arch can help assess AI severity.

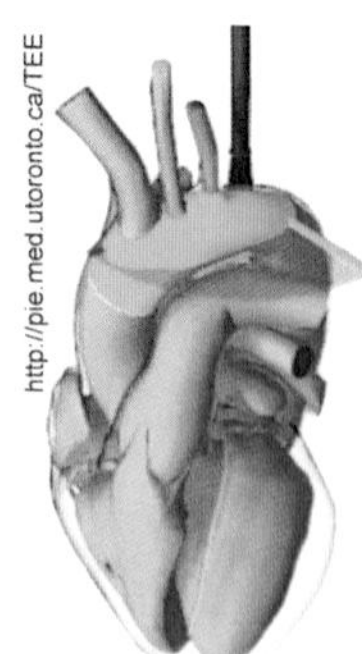

Imaged Structures	Diagnostic Issues
Distal Ascending Aorta Aortic Arch (Ao arch) Size Doppler: Color, PW Spectral Innominate vein	Aorta pathology: Atherosclerosis Dissection Aneurysm Right Aortic Arch AI severity PW Doppler

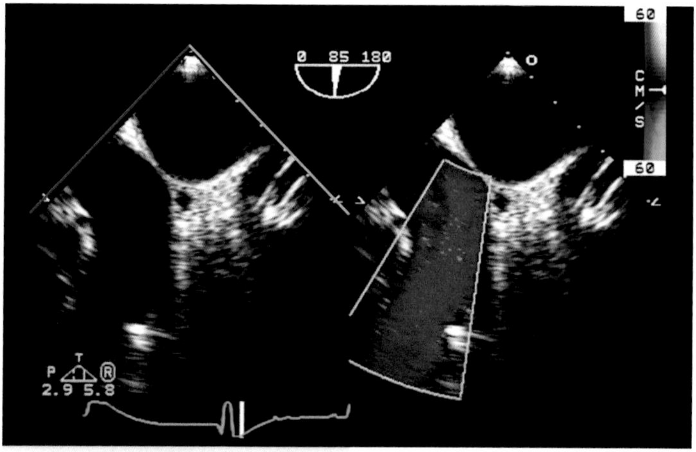

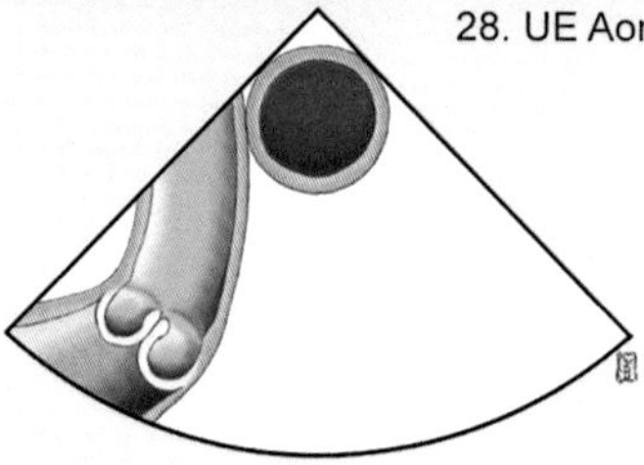

28. UE Aortic Arch SAX

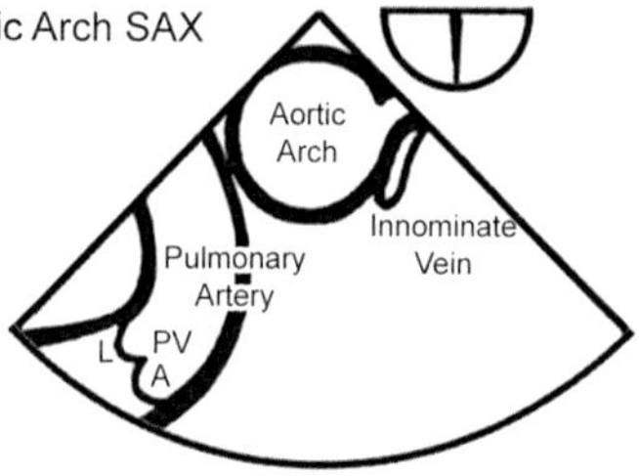

From the upper-esophageal Aortic Arch LAX view (0°), increasing the transducer angle to 70–90° obtains the UE Aortic Arch SAX view. This shows the proximal origin of the left subclavian artery and innominate vein in the upper right display. The pulmonic valve (PV) and main pulmonary artery (PA) in long-axis are seen in the lower left display. Color Doppler box is positioned over the right ventricular outflow tract (RVOT), PV, and PA with Nyquist 50–70 cm/s to show laminar antegrade systolic flow. Retrograde diastolic flow suggests pulmonic insufficiency. The color Doppler box can be separately positioned over the aortic arch with Nyquist of 70–90 cm/s and a lower Nyquist of 30 cm/s over the innominate vein to demonstrate flow.

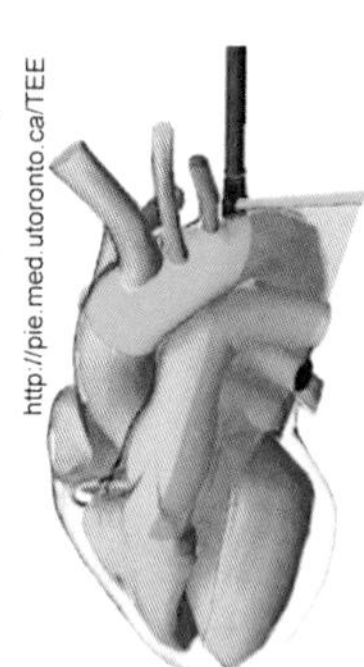

Imaged Structures	Diagnostic Issues
Aortic Arch	Aorta pathology:
Pulmonary Artery (PA):	Atherosclerosis
Size	Dissection
Doppler: Color, PW Spectral	Pulmonic Valve:
Pulmonic Valve (PV):	Pathology
Left (L) and Anterior (A) cusps	Pulmonic stenosis gradient
PV annulus measure	Pulmonic insufficiency
Doppler: Color, PW Spectral	PV/PA cardiac output
Innominate vein	Patent Ductus Arteriosus (PDA)
Catheter	Pulmonary artery catheter position

These additional views are reproduced courtesy of A. Vegas, and available at http://pie.med.utoronto.ca/TEE/TEE_content/TEE_alternativeViews.html

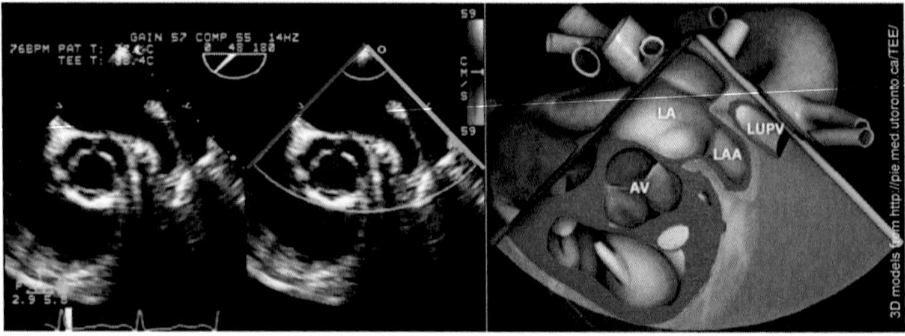

Mid-esophageal Left Atrial Appendage

Another view of the left atrial appendage (LAA) is obtained by reducing the image depth from the ME RVOT view and adjusting the transducer angle between 60 and 80°. The LAA is seen above the AV with the left upper pulmonary vein (LUPV) above as it is more posterior and closest to the probe. Color Doppler box positioned over the LAA and LUPV with Nyquist 50–70 cm/s shows laminar flow, here during systole. This view is similar to the ME LAA view (80–110°) as described on p. 21.

Imaged Structures	Diagnostic Issues
Left Atrial Appendage (LAA): Size: diameter 1.6 ± 0.5 cm length 2.9 ± 0.5 cm Color Doppler PW Doppler Left Upper Pulmonary Vein (LUPV) Color Doppler PW Doppler Aortic Valve (AV)	LAA thrombus LUPV flow LAA flow Aortic aneurysm Aortic Insufficiency

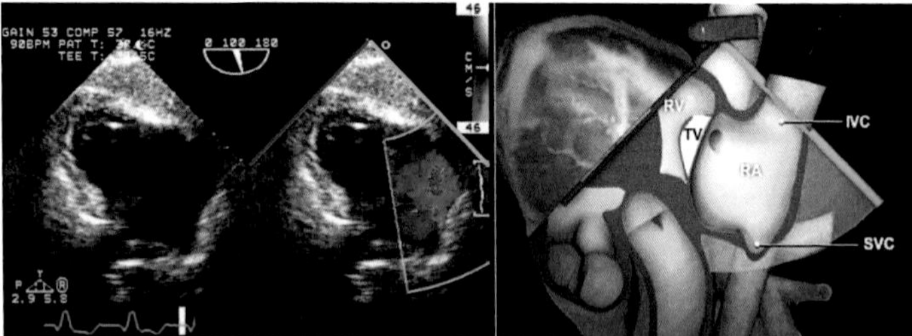

Transgastric Superior and Inferior Vena Cava

This transgastric view of both cava is obtained from the TG RV Inflow view (90–120°) by adjusting the transducer angle and/or rotating the probe slightly. In this view, the inferior vena cava (IVC) appears at the display top and the superior vena cava (SVC) and aorta at the bottom. Color Doppler box (Nyquist 50 cm/s) positioned over both cava shows laminar flow into the right atrium (RA) from the IVC (blue) and SVC (red). This view gives alignment for spectral Doppler of both vena cava.

Imaged Structures	Diagnostic Issues
Right Atrium (RA) Right Ventricle (RV) Tricuspid Valve (TV) Inferior Vena Cava (IVC) Superior Vena Cava (SVC)	TV pathology IVC PW Doppler SVC PW Doppler

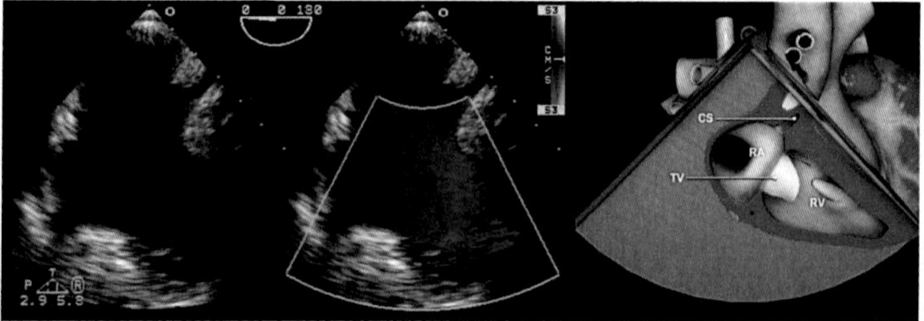

Coronary Sinus

The coronary sinus long-axis view (0°) is obtained at the gastroesophageal junction by advancing the probe from the ME 4 Chamber view (0°) or withdrawing the probe from the TG basal SAX view (0°). The coronary sinus (CS) is seen in long-axis entering the right atrium (RA) above the tricuspid valve (TV). The valve of Thebesius may be present at the orifice of the CS making insertion of catheters difficult.

Imaged Structures	Diagnostic Issues
Right Atrium (RA)	Coronary sinus:
Right Ventricle (RV)	Dilated (>2 cm), persistent left SVC
Tricuspid Valve (TV):	PW Spectral Doppler:
Septal (S) + Posterior (P) leaflets	Retrograde flow in TR
Color Doppler	Cardioplegia catheter
Coronary sinus (CS):	Pacer
Size: diameter 0.7 ± 0.2 cm	TV pathology
Color Doppler	
PW Spectral Doppler	
Valve of Thebesius	

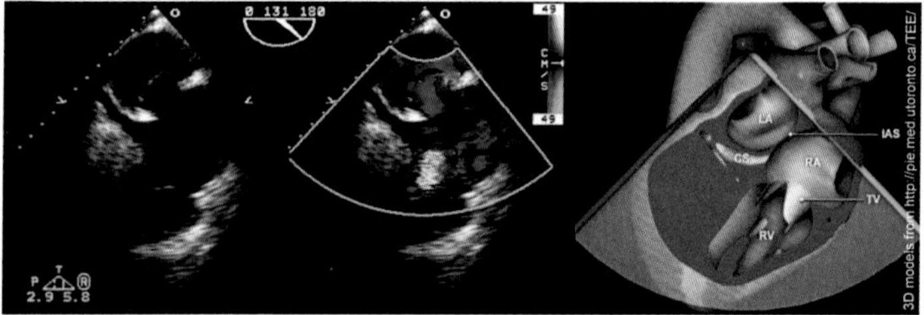

Mid-esophageal Tricuspid Valve

This modified mid-esophageal view of the tricuspid valve (TV) is obtained from the ME bicaval view (90°) by increasing the transducer angle to 120–150°. This view allows imaging of the anterior and posterior leaflets of the TV and often gives optimal alignment for spectral Doppler of the TV. The coronary sinus (CS) is seen in the upper left of the display as it wraps around the left atrium (LA), which differentiates it from the inferior vena cava.

Imaged Structures	Diagnostic Issues
Right Atrium (RA):	TV pathology
Appendage (RAA)	CW Doppler tricuspid regurgitation
Right Ventricle (RV)	CS color flow
Tricuspid Valve (TV):	SVC color flow
Anterior + posterior leaflets	Inter-Atrial septum flow
Color/CW or PW Doppler	
Coronary Sinus (CS)	
Superior Vena Cava (SVC)	
Left Atrium (LA)	
Inter-Atrial Septum (IAS)	

http://pie.med.utoronto.ca/TEE/TEE_content/TEE_standardViews_intro.html

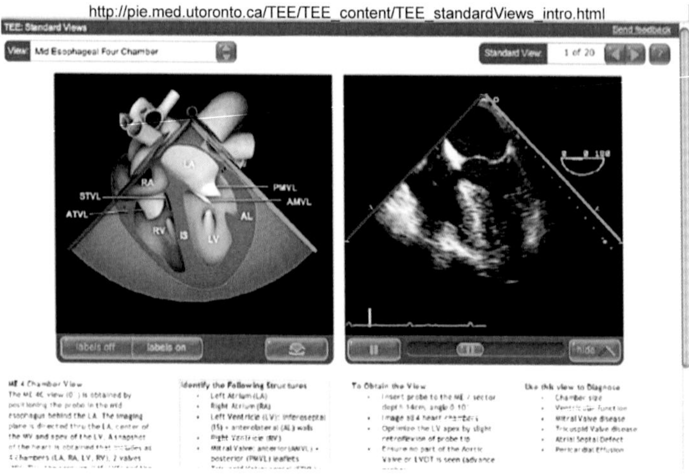

The Perioperative Interactive Education (PIE) Group at the University of Toronto has developed a series of free interactive online modules to help the novice echocardiographer learn TEE. In the Standard Views module, the user can view video clips of each of the original 20 standard TEE views alongside a 360° rotatable static 3D heart model showing the position of the TEE probe and the ultrasound plane. Rotation of the heart from the anatomic to the TEE orientation helps trainees make the mental rotation when viewing TEE images.

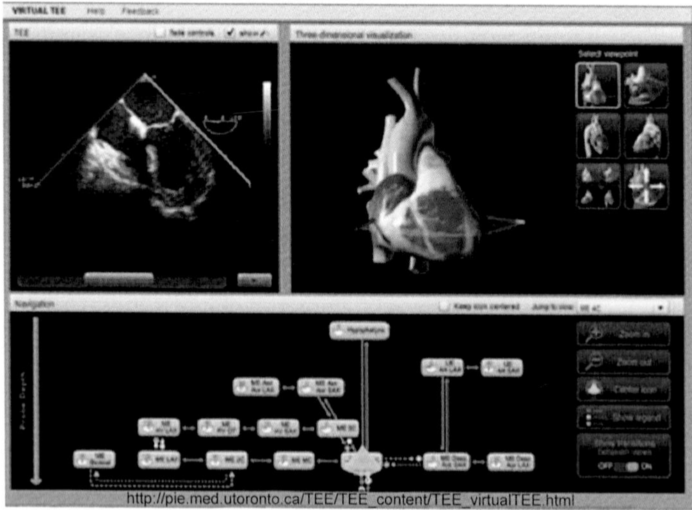

http://pie.med.utoronto.ca/TEE/TEE_content/TEE_virtualTEE.html

Visual Interactive Resource for Teaching, Understanding And Learning Transesophageal Echocardiography (VIRTUAL TEE) is an online teaching aid designed by the Perioperative Interactive Education (PIE) group at the University of Toronto. This web module describes a structured and logical relationship between the ASE/SCA original 20 standard views. There are video clips of each of the 20 standard TEE views, as well as clips of the transitional movements between them. A static 3D heart model demonstrates the ultrasound probe and plane position, which is animated and moves with the movement in the video clips. The 3D heart can be viewed from one of four views (anterior, superior, left, right) at all times.

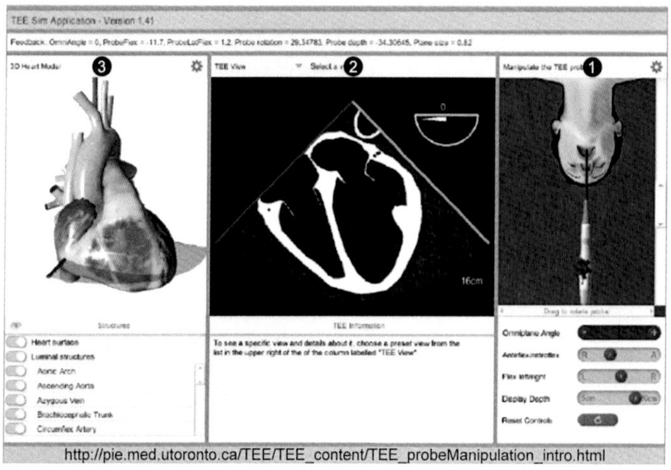

http://pie.med.utoronto.ca/TEE/TEE_content/TEE_probeManipulation_intro.html

The online TEE simulation module designed by Michel Corrin of the PIE group at the University of Toronto is a low fidelity TEE simulator that aims to imitate TEE probe manipulation required to produce real-time TEE imaging of a static heart.

➊ In the "manipulate the TEE probe" pane, the user can adjust the TEE probe position by advancing, withdrawing, or turning the probe right or left and changing the transducer angle through 0-180°. Using sliders, the probe tip can be anteflexed, retroflexed, or flexed to the right or left.

➋ The ultrasound pane shows the results of any changes in probe manipulation as a real-time computer-generated TEE image in the "TEE view." Structures displayed in the TEE image can be identified by moving the mouse pointer over the structure. Each of the 20 recommended TEE views can be selected and displayed from the "Select a view" option within this pane.

➌ The "3D Heart Model" pane has a freely rotatable static 3D heart model with TEE sector plane that correlates TEE probe manipulation with the exterior heart surface. Removing the exterior surface can show casts (luminal structures) of various cardiac structures. By highlighting a 3D heart model structure, the TEE imaging plane can then be manipulated to appear in the TEE view.

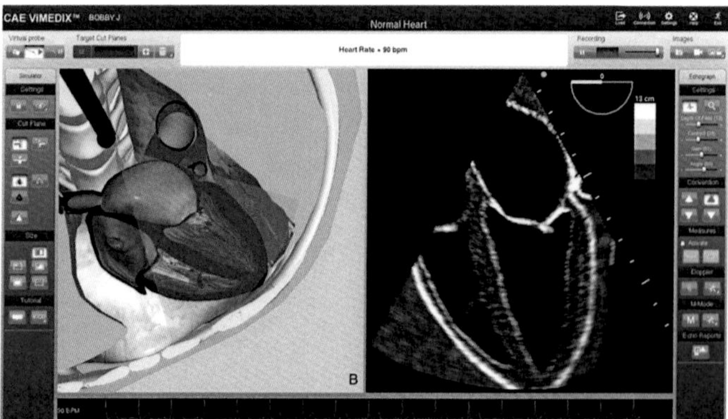

High fidelity ultrasound simulators such as the Vimedix™ (CAE Healthcare, Quebec, Canada) and HeartWorks (Inventive Medical, London, UK) are commercially available. These simulators consist of a mannequin and replica ultrasound probe connected to a computer and high-resolution monitor that displays a dynamic 3D-augmented reality and computer-generated TEE image.

2 Doppler and Hemodynamics

A. Vegas, *Perioperative Two-Dimensional Transesophageal Echocardiography*, https://doi.org/10.1007/978-3-319-60902-7_2

Color Maps

- Color Doppler is a form of pulsed Doppler that displays returning echoes as color superimposed on a 2D image. Frequency shift (or Doppler shift) between successive transmitted and returned sample points is processed using "autocorrelation".
- Color is assigned based on the direction of flow and mean velocity in the sampled area, so unlike spectral Doppler, alignment with flow is not required.
- By convention, the color displayed depends on blood flow direction relative to the transducer: **B**lue is flow **A**way, and **R**ed is flow **T**owards (**BART**). The zero velocity baseline in the center is black as there is no frequency shift (no flow).
- Color Doppler is displayed using different color maps. The enhanced velocity color map shows higher velocity flows as brighter colors. The variance color map uses additional colors (yellow and green) to indicate turbulent flow, thus displaying a mosaic of colors. Variance expresses the degree to which velocities within a given sample volume differ from the mean velocity within that sample.

Shown here is normal color Doppler flow in the ME AV LAX view with different color maps (A) enhanced velocity and (B) variance. Yellow (in A) or red (in B) indicates flow towards the probe in the LVOT, black is no flow in relation to the probe, and blue (in A, B) is flow away from the probe through the AV and aortic root.

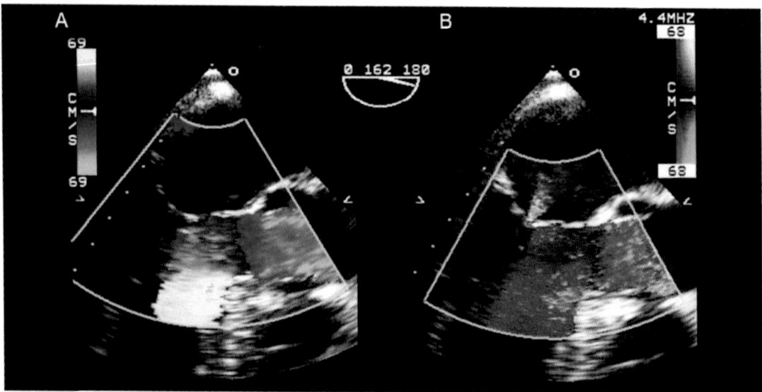

Color Scale (Nyquist Limit)

- To accurately display the flow velocity, an appropriate velocity scale (Nyquist limit) must be selected: high (aorta), moderate (valves), or low (venous structures).
- An inappropriately high Nyquist limit may miss flow through a structure, while a low Nyquist limit may overestimate or suggest turbulent flow.
- The velocity scale can be crudely adjusted (increased or decreased) by using the "color scale" knob on the ultrasound machine. The display depth that the structure of interest appears also influences the velocity scale. Positioning the color box in the near field increases the scale, while in the far field the scale is lower.
- Flow velocity exceeding the Nyquist limit appears aliased (see next page).

In this ME AV LAX view of aortic insufficiency (AI), the (A) low Nyquist limit of 30 cm/s overestimates the AI severity compared with (B) a Nyquist limit of 71 cm/s.

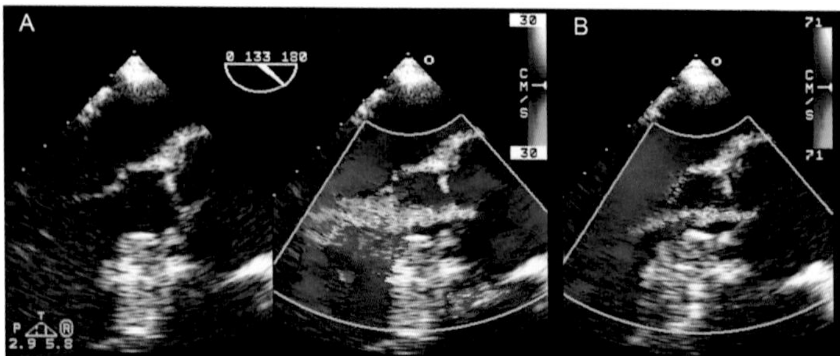

Parameters That Can Be Adjusted in Color Doppler Mode Include

- Choice of color map: velocity or variance
- Color scale: changes range of color flow velocities, crudely adjust Nyquist limits
- Baseline: shift up/down to change range of color flow velocities in one direction
- Size and depth of color box: influences Nyquist limit
- Color gain: adjusts system sensitivity to received color flow signals (preset 50%)

Turbulent Flow

Laminar flow exists when blood flows at the same velocity. Turbulent flow is characterized by flow at many different speeds and directions which results in greater difference (or variance) around the mean velocity. The difference in mean velocities can be displayed using a variance color map.

Aliasing/Flow Acceleration

Aliasing in color Doppler occurs when flow exceeds the Nyquist limit and appears side by side as an opposite color, suggesting a change in direction of flow. In reality, flow is still in the same direction. Unlike spectral Doppler, aliasing in color Doppler is a useful way to assess pathology. The presence of flow acceleration within any valve indicates valve pathology, as shown here for (A) mitral stenosis and (B) mitral regurgitation.

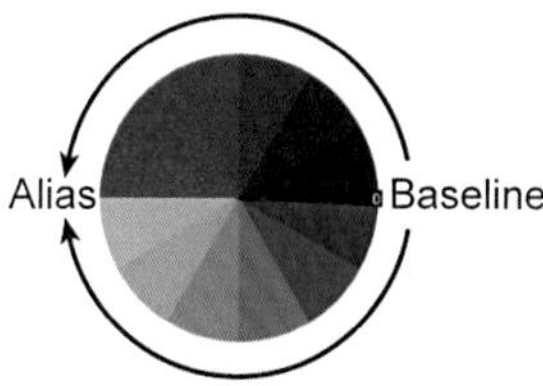

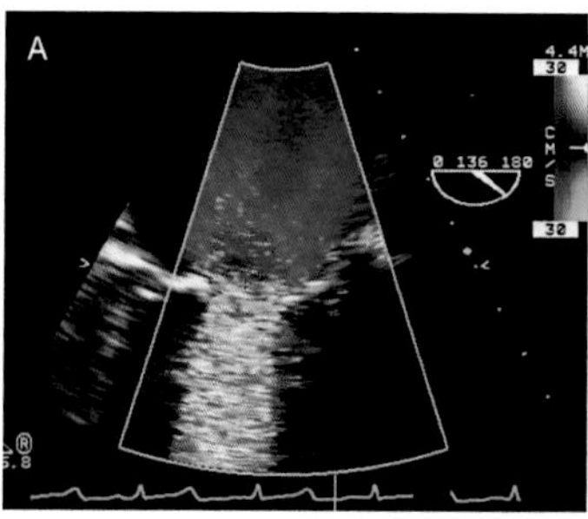

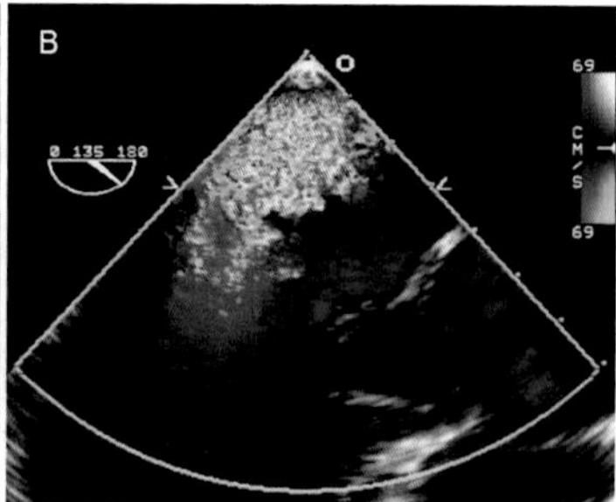

Color Doppler Artifacts

- Shadowing: an absence of color
- Ghosting: brief flashes of color
- Noise: excessive gain (below)
- Absence color: low color gain (below)
- Aliasing: flow acceleration (above)
- Electrical interference: cautery

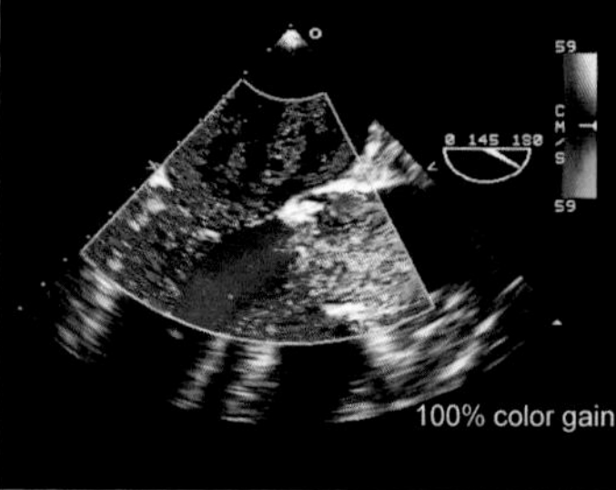

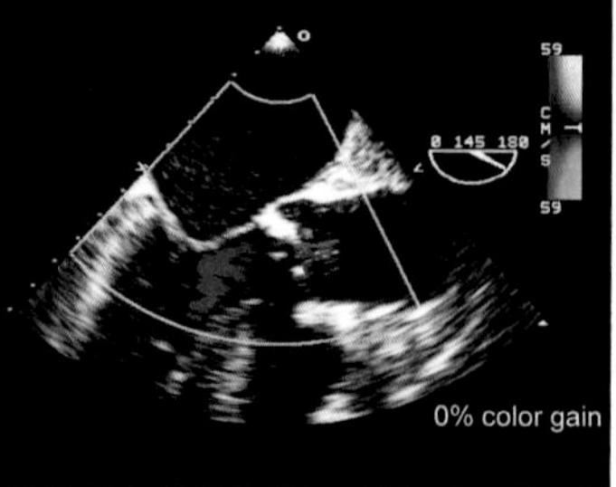

Color Doppler Assessment Examines

- Anatomic structure (underlying 2D image, or use color suppress)
- Blood flow direction (toward or away from transducer based on color map)
- Mean velocity (frequency shift, set Nyquist limit)
- Timing with ECG (systole or diastole, better assess using color m-mode)
- Laminar or turbulent flow

Doppler Effect: The frequency of sound emitted from a moving object is shifted in proportion to the velocity of the moving object.
Doppler Shift (Fd): The difference in frequencies of source (Ft) and receiver (Fr)

$$Fd = (Fr - Ft)$$

which is (+) when moving towards and (−) when moving away. Typical ultrasound Doppler shifts of −10 to +20 KHz are audible.
Doppler Equation: relationship of Doppler shift (Fd) and blood flow velocity (V)

$$V = c(Fd)/2Ft \ \cos\theta$$

where c = speed of sound in tissue, Ft = transducer frequency, cos θ = angle between the ultrasound beam and the path of the moving object
Bernoulli Equation: relates blood flow velocity to pressure gradient, full equation $P_1 - P_2 = 4(V_1 - V_2)^2$, which if small V_2, is simplified to $P_1 - P_2 = 4\ V_1^2$

Spectral Doppler

- Returning echoes from moving objects are complex signals with many varied Doppler-shifted frequencies. Analysis by Fast Fourier Transformation (FFT) is used to identify individual frequencies for display as a grey pixel at any time point.
- By convention, FFT shows the frequency shift/Doppler velocity (y-axis) against time (x-axis) in a spectral display. Doppler traces vary depending on the transducer position in relation to blood flow. Flow towards the transducer (+ frequency shift) is above the baseline and flow away from the transducer (– frequency shift) is below the baseline. The zero velocity baseline is in the center.
- The amplitude (y-axis) is directly proportional to the measured RBC velocity (Doppler shift). Multiple frequencies exist at any time point, each frequency signal is displayed as a pixel. The magnitude (z-axis) of the Doppler signal is determined by the number of RBCs traveling at each of those velocities and is displayed using various shades of grey. The greyer (or denser) the display the more RBCs.

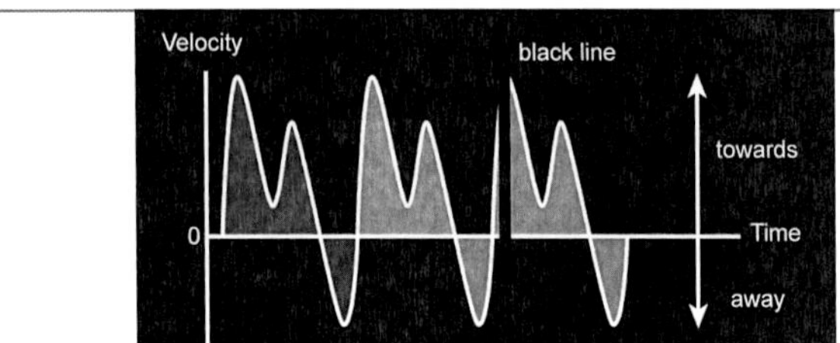

At each time point, the spectral display shows:

- Blood flow direction (toward or away from the transducer)
- Velocity (frequency shift)
- Signal magnitude (grayness)
- Timing with ECG (systole or diastole)

Black line represents an absence of Doppler information as the 2D image is updated.

Controls can be adjusted to alter the spectral trace in the spectral Doppler mode:

- **Scale**: adjusts the range of velocities displayed. It is set so the highest and lowest velocities are not cut-off and the spectral trace fills the display.
- **Baseline**: adjusts the zero baseline velocity up or down within the spectral display. It is helpful to position the baseline in one of the extreme positions (top or bottom) in order to display as much of the abnormal velocity as possible.
- **Doppler Gain**: alters the overall strength of returning signals. Increasing the gain will better display weak signals. Use the lowest gain setting that allows the recording of adequate signals.
- **Grey scale**: alters the various ranges of grey displayed
- **Wall filter**: sets the threshold below which low frequency signals are removed from the display (preset at 500 Hz). Setting a high wall filter eliminates more of the lower velocities, providing a cleaner baseline.
- **Sweep speed**: changes the ECG rate (25, 50, 100, 150 mm/s), which affects the number of individual cycles that are displayed. A slow speed displays more cycles and is useful to assess respiratory variation.

Pulsed Wave Doppler (PWD)	Continuous Wave Doppler (CWD)
• Uses one crystal in the transducer to intermittently send + receive signals • Allows sampling of blood velocity at a specific depth (range resolution) • Limit on the maximum velocity seen (aliasing) due to the Nyquist limit (PRF = 2 × transmitted frequency). Velocities >2 m/s will appear aliased. • The spectral trace often appears as a thin line with a clear curve. This suggests that the velocities sampled in this particular region are similar.	• Uses two crystals in the transducer to continuously send + receive signals • Sampling occurs along the entire Doppler beam (range ambiguity). The main disadvantage of CW Doppler is its lack of depth discrimination. • Unlimited maximum velocity displayed (no Nyquist limit), accurately measures high velocities without aliasing. • The spectral trace will often appear filled in as different velocities are sampled along the entire sample line.

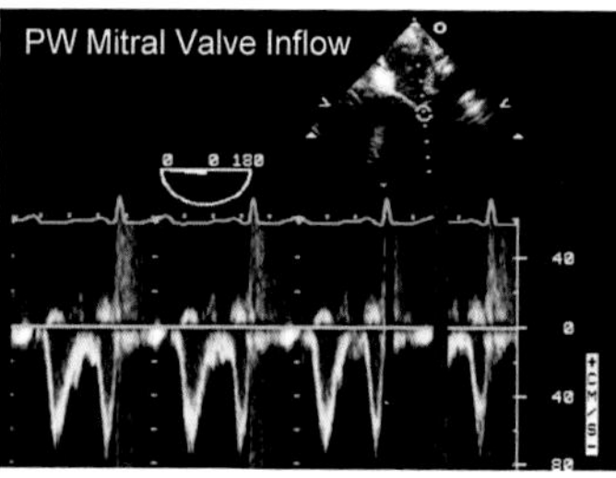

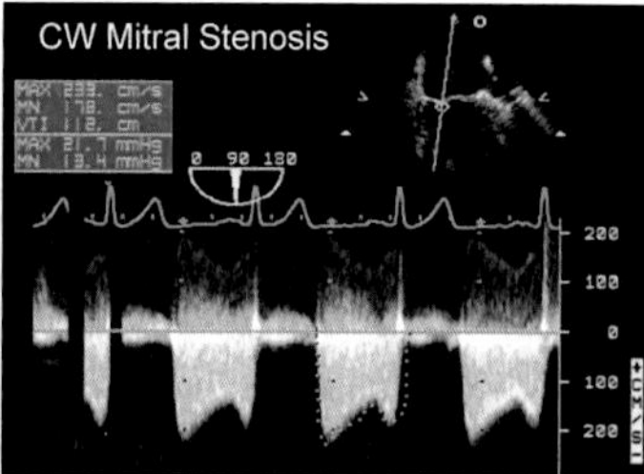

Velocity Measurements

- Accurate velocity measurement requires optimal Doppler alignment of the sample volume parallel to blood flow.
- Different velocities can be measured directly from the Doppler trace:
  - Mean is the average velocity obtained by tracing the outer edge. This is the peak velocity at a given time divided by the number of peak velocities sampled.
  - Modal is most common velocity, frequency with the darkest spectral trace (PW).
  - Peak is the highest velocity at a given time.

Aliasing

- Aliasing in spectral Doppler occurs when the velocity exceeds the rate at which the PW Doppler can properly record it. The PW Doppler spectral trace is cut-off and appears on the opposite side of the baseline.

(A) MV inflow PW with an aliased mitral regurgitation signal that is better displayed by (B) using CW, shifting the baseline down, or adjusting the scale.

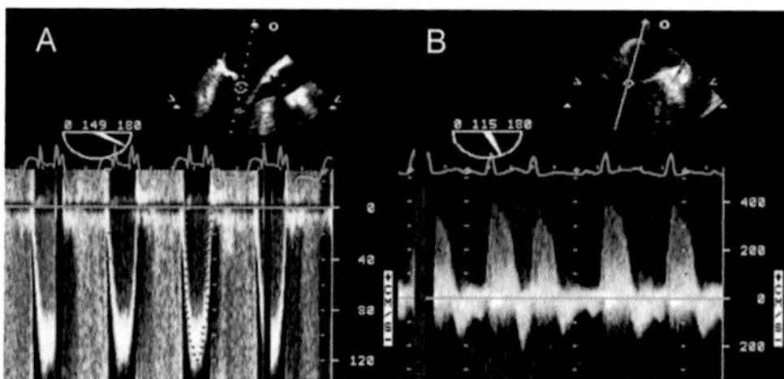

Doppler Indications (Spectral and Color)

Use to diagnose and quantify normal and pathological blood flow involving:

- Valves: aortic, mitral, pulmonic, and tricuspid
- Great Vessels: SVC, IVC, aorta, PA, hepatic veins, pulmonary veins
- Defects (ASD, VSD), abnormal connections (fistula, conduits)
- Aortic dissection

- The appearance of spectral Doppler profiles will vary with abnormal flow and technical considerations. Ideally, the transducer should be positioned as parallel to flow as possible with the sample volume or cursor through the middle of flow.
- Baseline, scale, and gain should be adjusted to ensure the entire spectral trace fills the space and a well-defined outline is seen.

Flow through a narrowed orifice shows:
A. Laminar flow with similar velocities before the stenosis.
B. Stenosis flow has high peak velocity that often requires CW Doppler to record.
C. Turbulent flow occurs in the post-stenotic area with eddies of different flows.

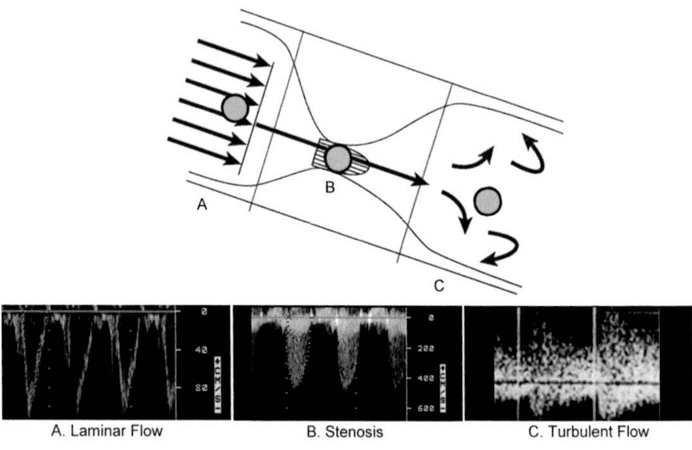

A. Laminar Flow B. Stenosis C. Turbulent Flow

Spectral Doppler Artifacts

Crosstalk Artifact
This appears as a symmetric-shaped signal on both sides of the baseline, but with different spectral intensities. It results from high Doppler gain and is reduced by lowering power output of the US machine or reducing spectral gain.

Mirroring Artifact
This is a symmetric signal of the same intensity on both sides of the baseline. It results from sampling flow at a near perpendicular Doppler angle. Shown here is a PW spectral Doppler trace from a sample volume positioned perpendicular to flow in the descending aorta LAX view.

Spectral Broadening
Implies the presence of a wide range of velocities and appears as a filled-in spectral display. While most commonly associated with CW Doppler, it may also occur in PW Doppler. In PWD, this is related to irregular flow as in this example of PW MV inflow or pulmonary vein flow if the Doppler sample volume is positioned too close to the vessel wall.

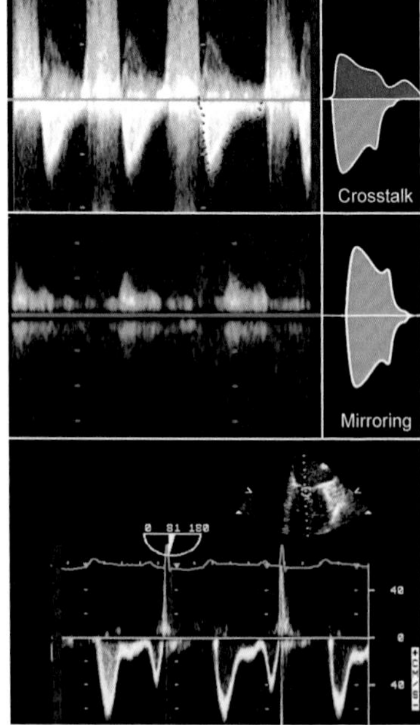

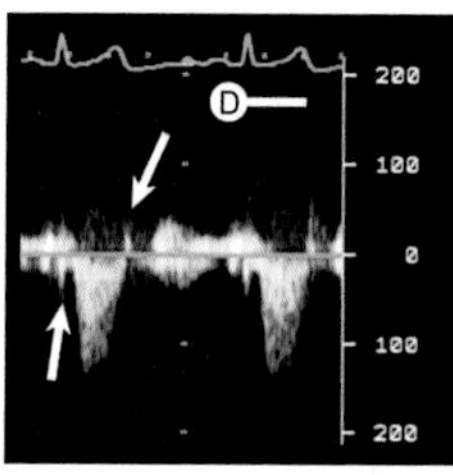

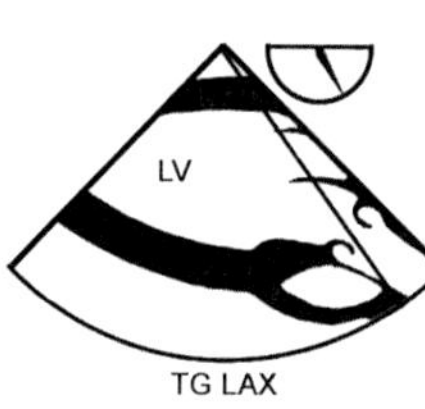

Aortic Valve

Antegrade
Systolic flow (Ao → LV)
CW Doppler
Flow below baseline
Doppler velocity 1–1.3 m/s
Identify opening and closing valve clicks (arrows)
Rapid rate of acceleration
Diagnostic issues:
- Aortic stenosis
- Aortic insufficiency

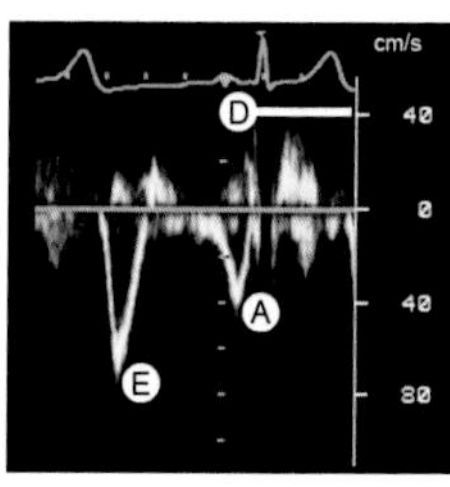

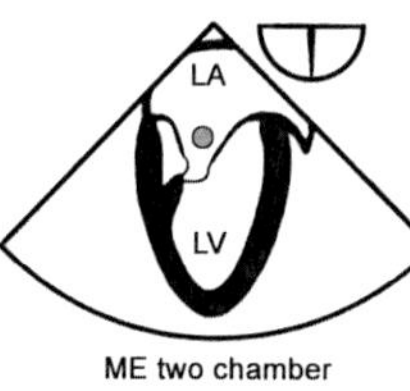

Mitral Valve

Antegrade
Diastolic flow (LA → LV)
PW Doppler
Leaflet tips or annulus
Flow below baseline
Doppler velocity (<1 m/s)
- Emax 0.6–0.8 m/s
- Amax 0.2–0.4 m/s

Diagnostic issues:
- Diastology
- Mitral stenosis
- Pericardial tamponade

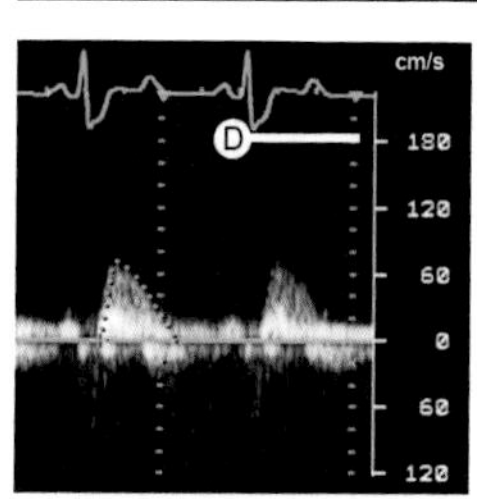

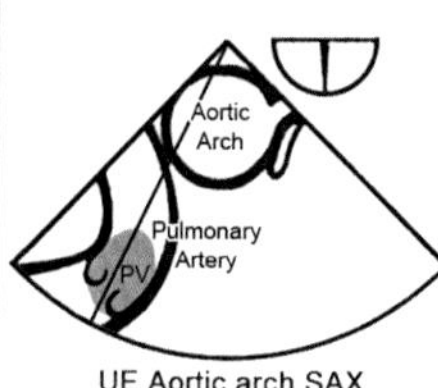

Pulmonic Valve

Antegrade
Systolic flow (RV → PA)
CW Doppler
Flow above baseline
Doppler velocity 0.8–1 m/s
Slower acceleration rate (≥130 ms) compare to AV
Diagnostic issues:
- Pulmonic stenosis

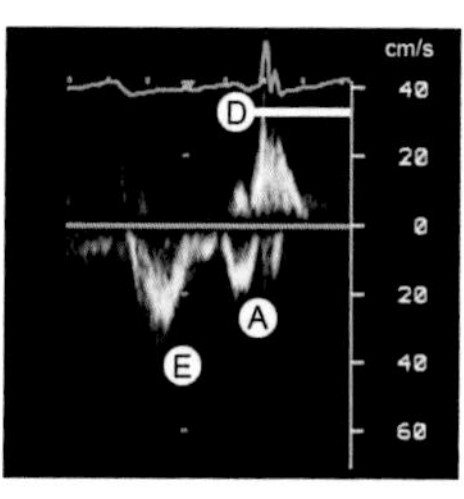

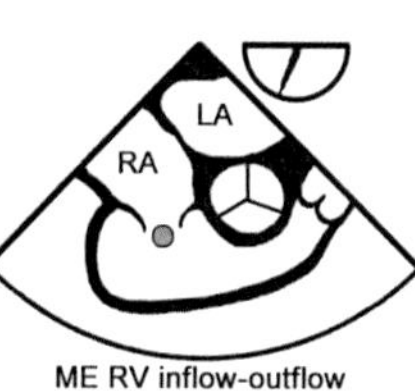

Tricuspid Valve

Antegrade
Diastolic flow (RA → RV)
PW Doppler
Flow below baseline
Doppler velocity (<0.7 m/s)
- Emax 0.4 ± 0.098 m/s
- Amax 0.2 ± 0.075 m/s
- Respiratory variation so average several cycles

Diagnostic issues:
- Tricuspid stenosis
- Pericardial tamponade

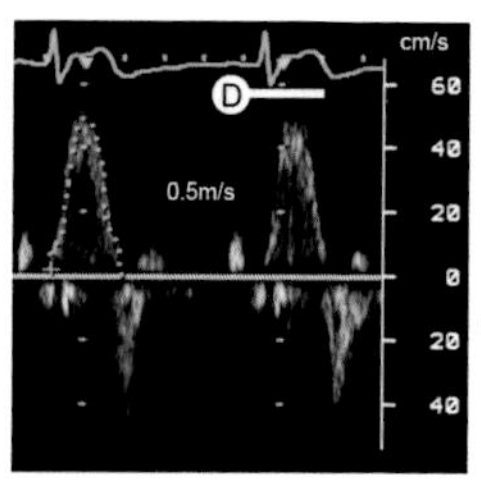

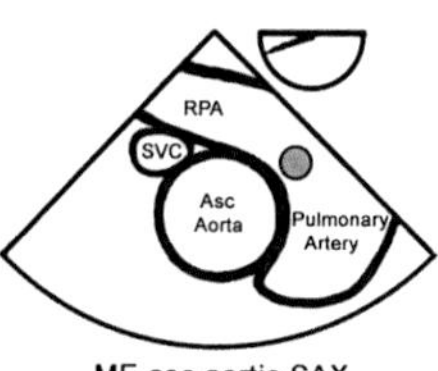

Pulmonary Artery

Doppler alignment
- UE arch SAX or
- ME Asc aortic arch

PW Doppler
Doppler above baseline
Systolic flow
Doppler velocity 50 cm/s
VTI for cardiac output
Acceleration time (AT)

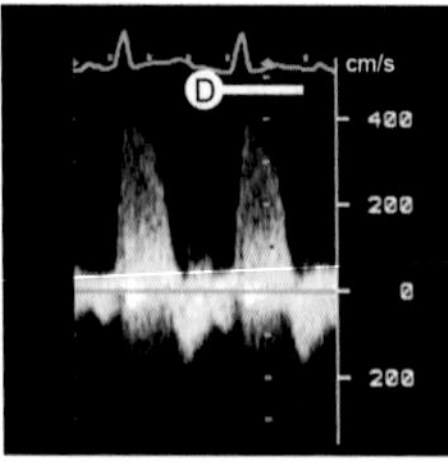

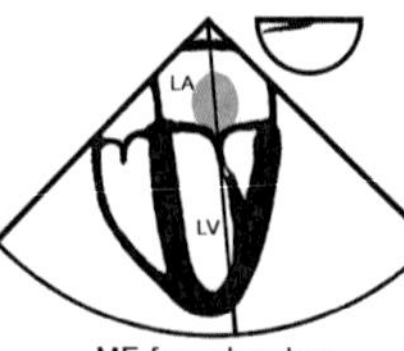

ME four chamber

Mitral Regurgitation

Retrograde (mosaic)
Systolic flow (LV → LA)
CW Doppler
Flow above baseline
Doppler velocity 4–6 m/s
Signal intensity ∝ MR

Estimate
LAP = $Aortic_{SBP} - 4(MR_{peak})^2$

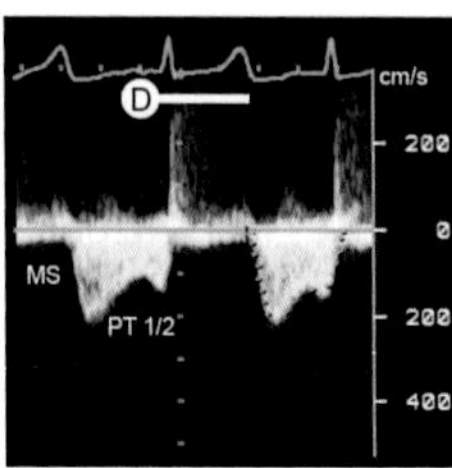

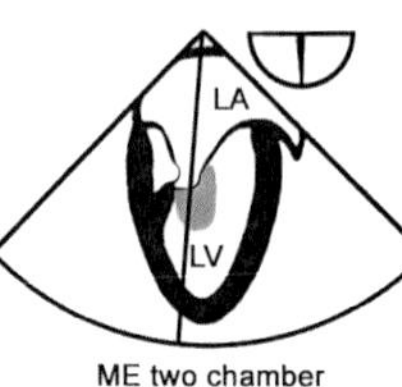

ME two chamber

Mitral Stenosis

Antegrade (mosaic)
Diastolic flow (LA → LV)
PW/CW Doppler
Flow below baseline
Doppler velocity > 3 m/s
High mean
pressure > 12 mm Hg
PT1/2 MV area

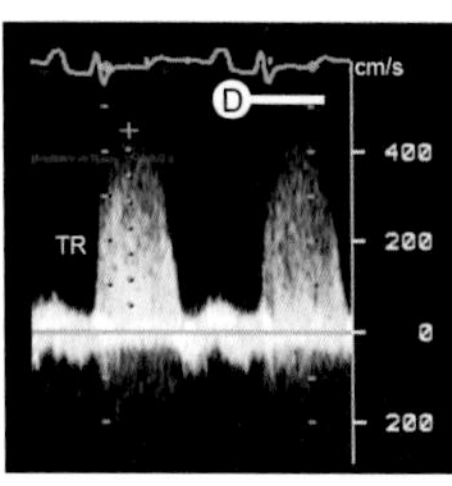

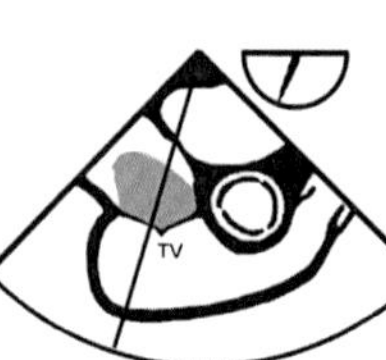

ME RV inflow-outflow

Tricuspid Regurgitation

Retrograde (mosaic)
Systolic flow (RV → RA)
CW Doppler
Flow above baseline
Doppler velocity > 2.5 m/s
Signal intensity ∝ TR
Estimate RVSP
(PASP) = $4(TR_{peak})^2$ + RAP

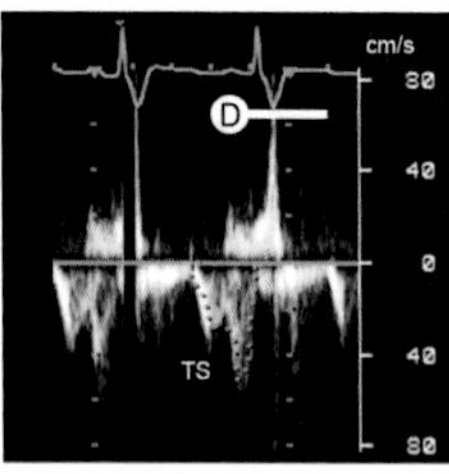

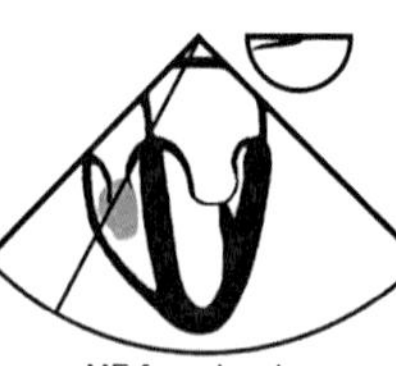

ME four chamber

Tricuspid Stenosis

Antegrade (mosaic)
Diastolic flow (RA → RV)
PW/CW Doppler
Flow below baseline
Doppler velocity > 1.5 m/s
Mean pressure gradient
>6 mmHg
PT1/2 TV area

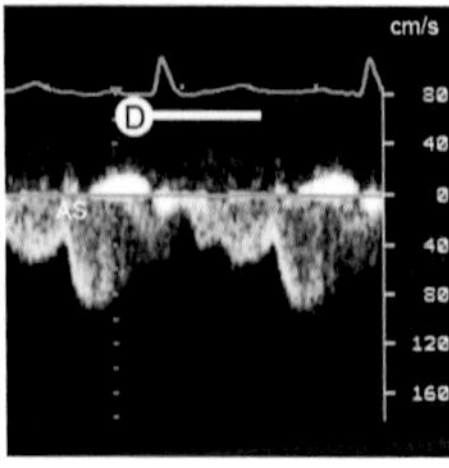

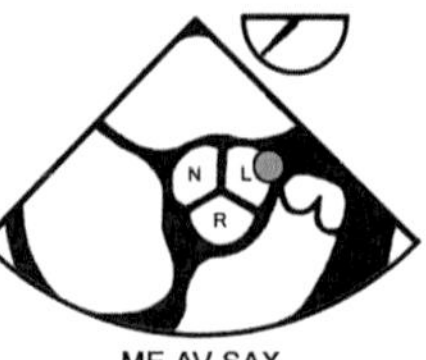

ME AV SAX

Coronary Artery

Doppler alignment try:
RCA (AV LAX)
LCA (AV SAX)
PW Doppler
Doppler below baseline
Systolic (S) + diastolic (D)
LMCA (D) 71 ± 19 cm/s
LMCA (S) 36 ± 11 cm/s
RCA (D) 39 ± 12 cm/s
RCA (S) 25 ± 8 cm/s

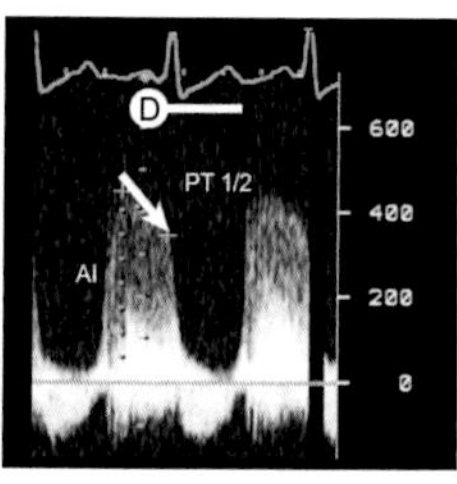

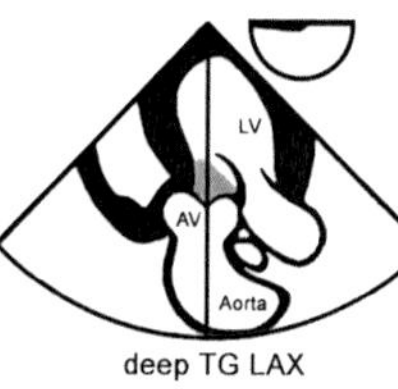

deep TG LAX

Aortic Insufficiency

Retrograde (mosaic)
Diastolic flow (Ao → LV)
CW Doppler
Flow above baseline
Doppler velocity 3–5 m/s
Signal intensity ∝ AI
Deceleration slope
PT1/2
Estimate
$LVEDP = Aortic_{dbp} - 4(AI_{end})^2$

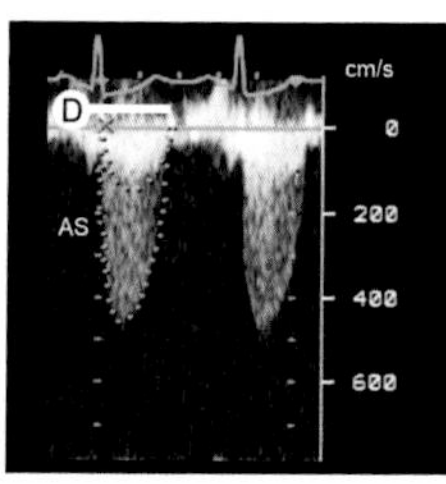

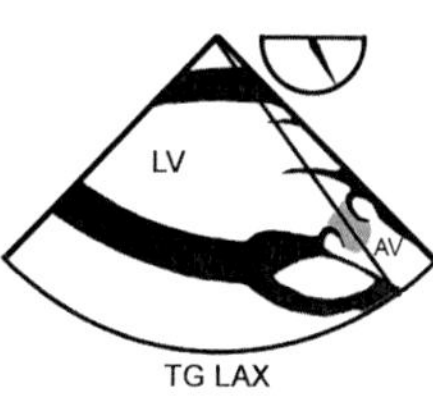

TG LAX

Aortic Stenosis

Antegrade (mosaic)
Systolic flow (LV → Ao)
CW Doppler
Flow below baseline
Doppler velocity > 2 m/s
Peak/mean P gradients
VTI for AV area using continuity equation

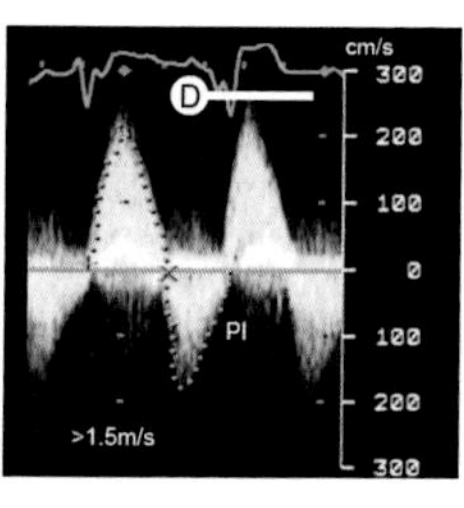

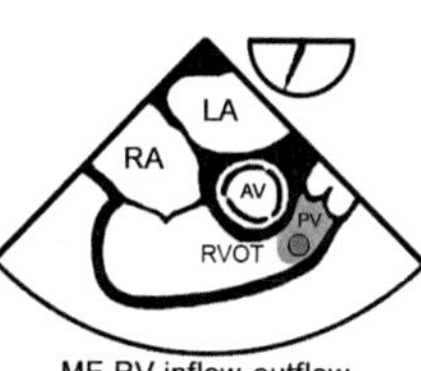

ME RV inflow-outflow

Pulmonic Insufficiency

Retrograde (blue)
Diastolic flow (PA → RV)
PW or CW Doppler
Flow below baseline
Doppler velocity > 1.5 m/s
Signal intensity ∝ PI
Estimate
$PADP = 4(PI_{end})^2 + RAP$

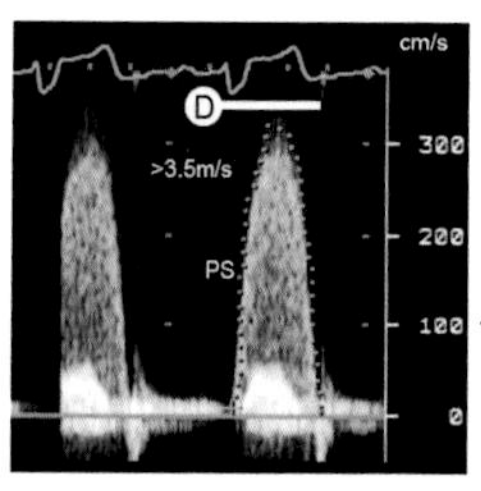

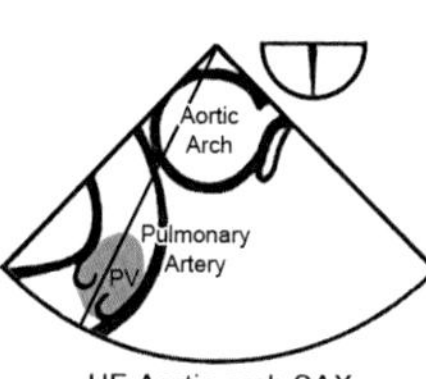

UE Aortic arch SAX

Pulmonic Stenosis

Antegrade (red/mosaic)
Systolic flow (RV → PA)
PW/CW Doppler
Flow above baseline
Doppler velocity > 3.5 m/s
Peak P grad >80 mm Hg
VTI for PV area using continuity equation

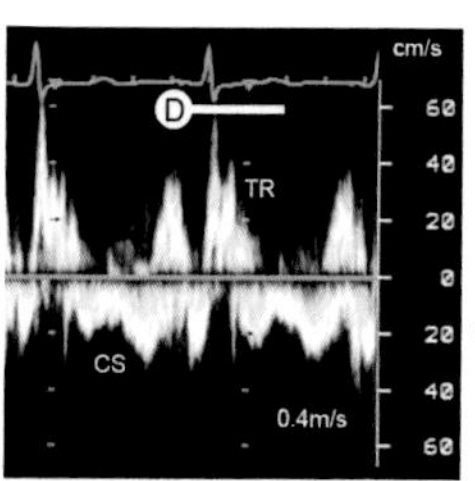

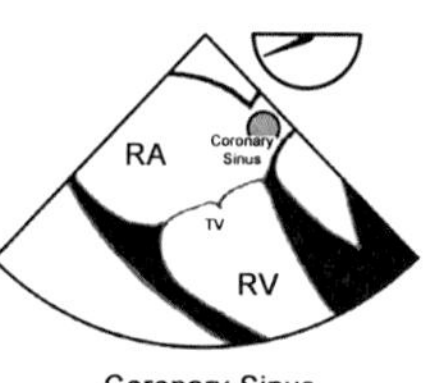

Coronary Sinus

Coronary Sinus

CS view at GE junction before stomach
Flow from CS to RA
Laminar flow
PW Doppler
Doppler below baseline
Systolic + diastolic flow
Low velocity < 50 cm/s
Flow reversal in TR

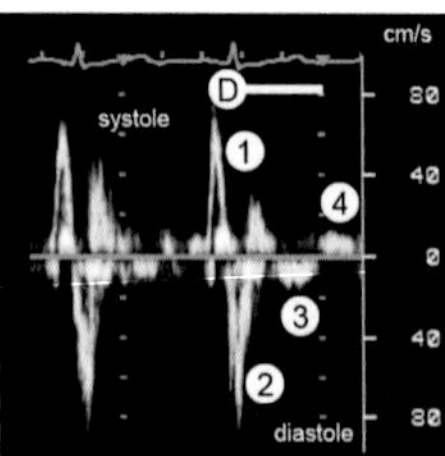

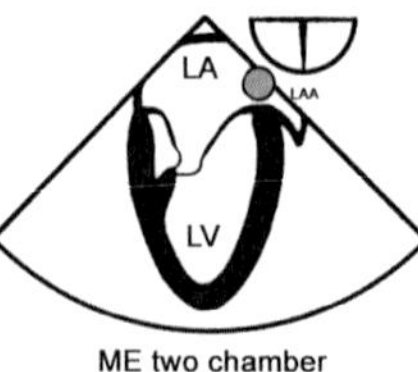

ME two chamber

Left Atrial Appendage

Use ME 2C view
PW Doppler LAA
Flow pattern depends on rhythm, in NSR: 4 waves
1. LAA contraction
   Atrial systole
   60 ± 8 cm/s
2. LAA filling, early
   Atrial diastole
   52 ± 13 cm/s
3. Passive LAA filling, late
4. LAA emptying early
   velocity 20 ± 11 cm/s

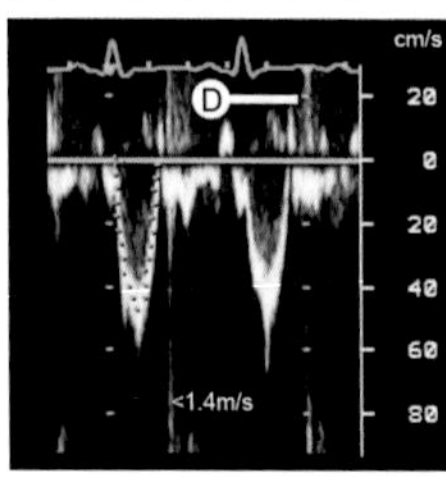

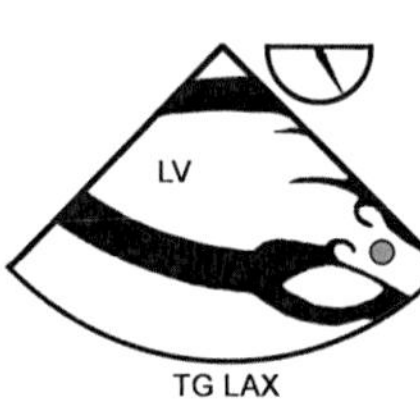

TG LAX

Ascending Aorta

Use TG LAX view
Systolic flow
PW Doppler
Doppler below baseline
Max velocity of 1.4 m/s
VTI for continuity equation

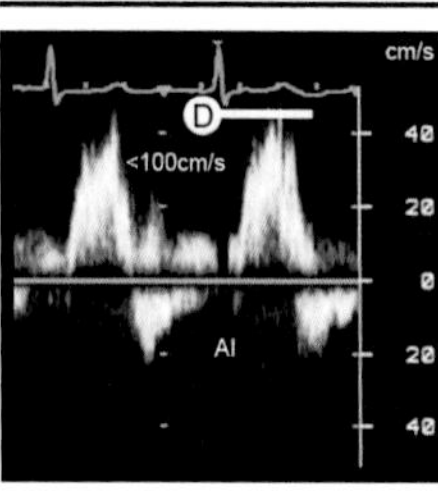

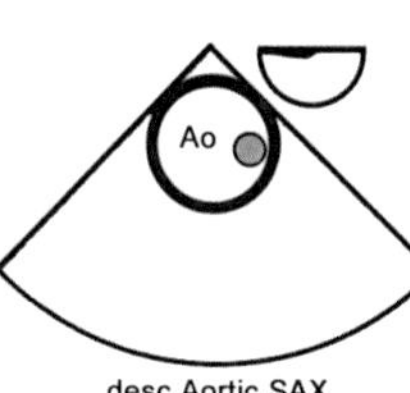

desc Aortic SAX

Descending Aorta

Use Desc Aortic SAX
Systolic flow
PW Doppler
Doppler above baseline
Velocity 100 cm/s (1 m/s)
Diastolic flow reversal
   Indicates Aortic Insufficiency (AI)
More distal in the descending aorta the flow reversal, the more severe the AI

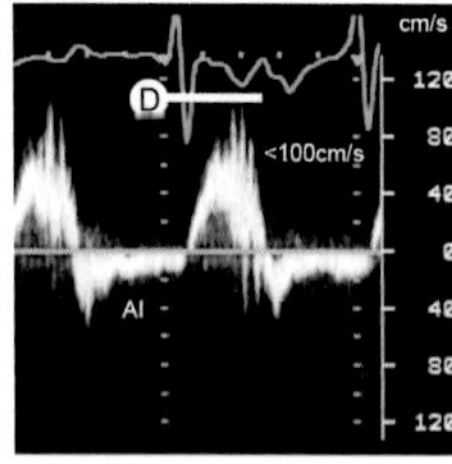

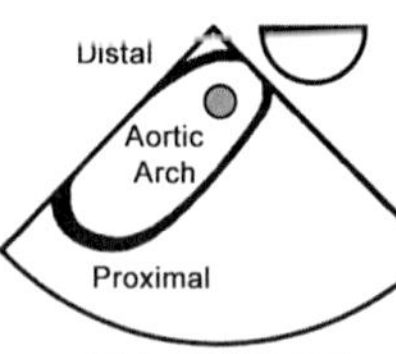

UE Aortic Arch LAX

Distal Aortic Arch

Use UE aortic arch LAX
Systolic flow
PW Doppler
Doppler above baseline
Velocity 100 cm/s (1 m/s)
Diastolic flow reversal
   Indicates Aortic Insufficiency (AI)

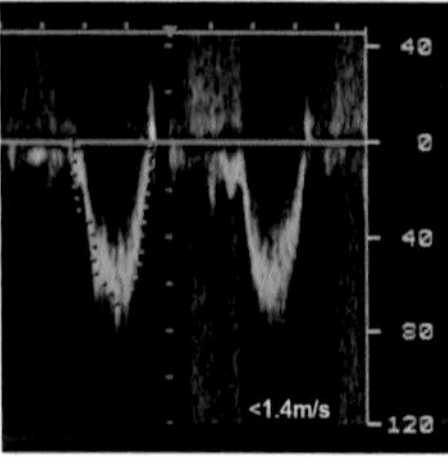

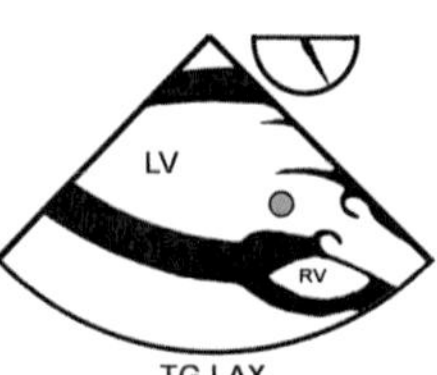

TG LAX

Left Ventricular Outflow Tract

Use TG LAX view
Systolic flow
PW Doppler in LVOT
Doppler below baseline
Max velocity of 1.4 m/s
VTI for continuity equation

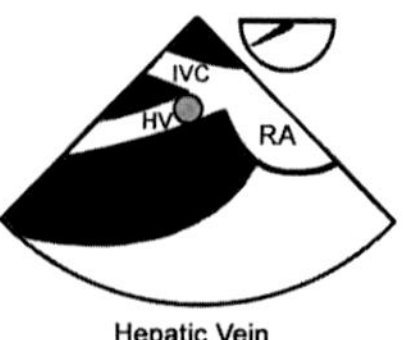

- Hepatic vein flow is obtained from the transgastric inferior vena cava view (TG IVC) at 0–30° (see p. 31). The probe tip and transducer angle are manipulated to obtain parallel alignment for PW Doppler in the hepatic vein and a clean spectral trace.
- This represents right atrial (RA) inflow as there is no valve between the IVC and hepatic vein.
- The waveform is affected by respiration, so record at end-inspiration during spontaneous ventilation.
- Waveform has four phases/waves: **A, S, V, and D** as described below.
- The "**C**" wave is retrograde flow after the "A" wave and is a normal variant as a result of the TV bulging into the RA as the RV contracts against a closed PV.
- Abnormal hepatic vein flow (HVF):
  - ↓ HVF: ↑ RAP, liver disease, ↑ intra-abdominal P
  - Reverse "S": severe TR, Blunted "S": RV dysfunction
  - ↑ "A" wave: tricuspid stenosis, complete heart block
  - Irregular pattern: arrhythmia (AF)
  - Constrictive pericarditis: retrograde wave between "D" and "A" waves

Hepatic Vein

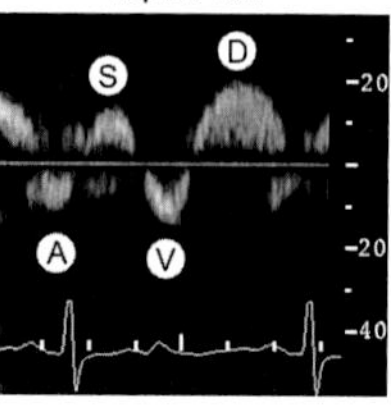

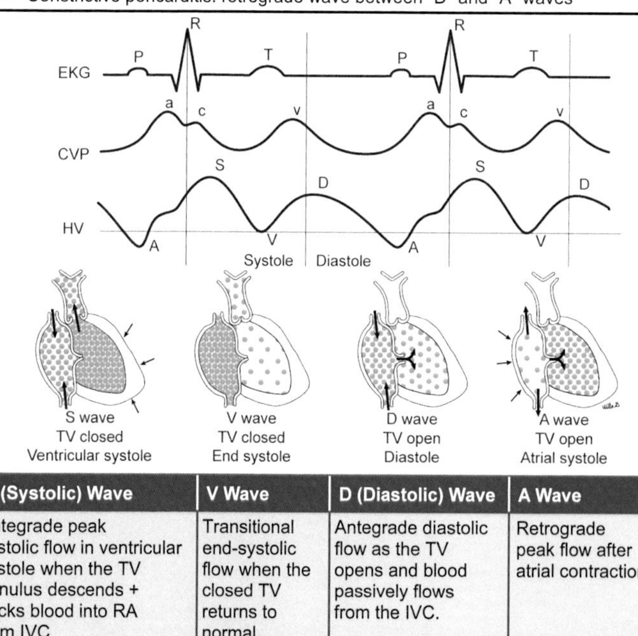

S wave
TV closed
Ventricular systole

V wave
TV closed
End systole

D wave
TV open
Diastole

A wave
TV open
Atrial systole

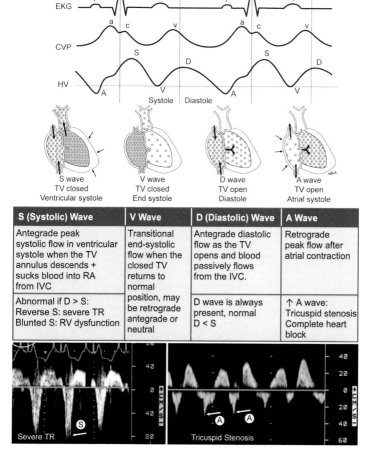

S (Systolic) Wave	V Wave	D (Diastolic) Wave	A Wave
Antegrade peak systolic flow in ventricular systole when the TV annulus descends + sucks blood into RA from IVC	Transitional end-systolic flow when the closed TV returns to normal position, may be retrograde antegrade or neutral	Antegrade diastolic flow as the TV opens and blood passively flows from the IVC.	Retrograde peak flow after atrial contraction
Abnormal if D > S: Reverse S: severe TR Blunted S: RV dysfunction		D wave is always present, normal D < S	↑ A wave: Tricuspid stenosis Complete heart block

Severe TR

Tricuspid Stenosis

- Can image all four pulmonary veins using TEE
- Doppler alignment is best for the LUPV (ME 2C) and RUPV (modified bicaval).
- PWD sample volume is positioned 1–2 cm from vein orifice, to obtain a clean trace.
- Pulmonary vein flow (PVF) represents LA filling.
- Tri-phasic or quadra-phasic pattern
- PVF is affected by:
  - LA contraction and relaxation
  - LV relaxation
  - MV pathology
  - Heart rhythm
- Diagnostic issues:
  - S reversal (MR)
  - Diastolic dysfunction (see p. 120)

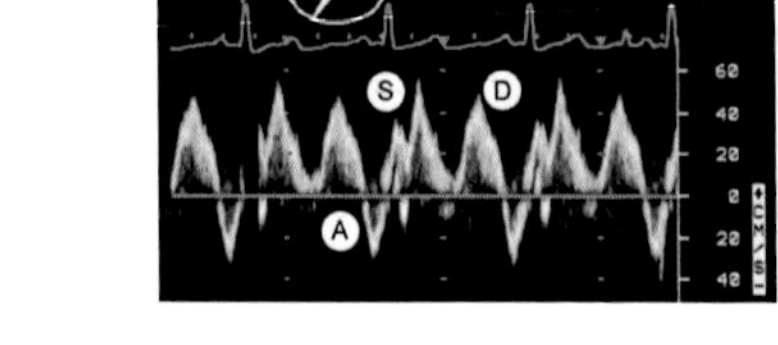

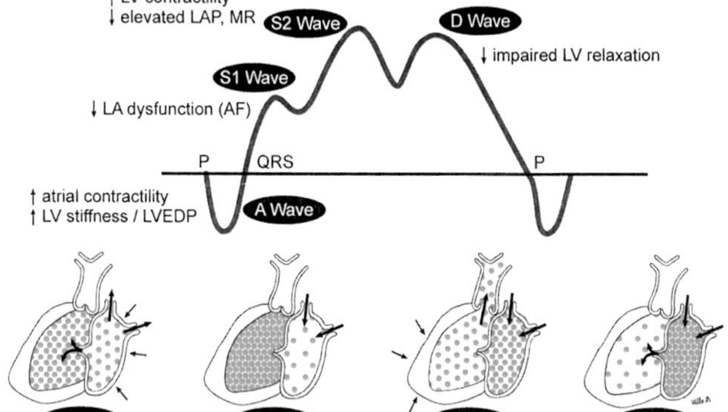

A (Atrial) Wave (14–25 cm/s)	S (Systolic) Wave (28–82 cm/s)	D (Diastolic) Wave (27–72 cm/s)
Result of atrial contraction Resistance to atrial forward flow, changes "A" velocity + duration	Biphasic S1 relates to atrial relaxation S2 mitral annulus descent	Relates to LV relaxation MV open with LV inflow Corresponds to MV E
↑ A velocity with: ↑ LVEDP (if A ≥ 35 cm/s) Mitral stenosis Complete heart block ↓ A velocity with atrial arrhythmia ↑ A wave duration compared MV A, ↑ LVEDP if Δ > 20–30 ms	↑ S1 with: LA dysfunction atrial fibrillation ↑ S2: better LV contractility ↑ LAP "blunts" S flow (S/D < 1) MR may result in S reversal	↓ D with impaired LV relaxation

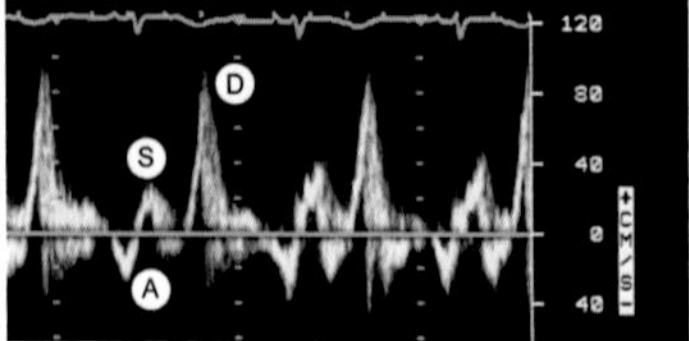

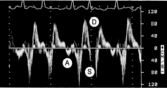

Blunted Pattern

Peak ratio of S to D < 1

- Not specific for moderate MR
- Diastolic function:
  - S < D: pseudonormal
  - S << D: restricted filling

Systolic Reversal

Peak ratio of S to D < 0

Retrograde flow in mid/late systole

- Highly specific for severe MR

LUPV (ME 60° view)
Easiest pulmonary vein to image. Find left atrial appendage (LAA) in ME 60°, withdraw probe slightly, LUPV lies above (posterolateral) to the LAA and coumadin ridge. Laminar color Doppler flow.

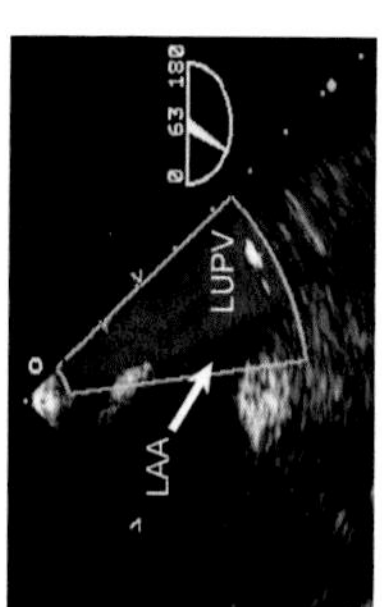

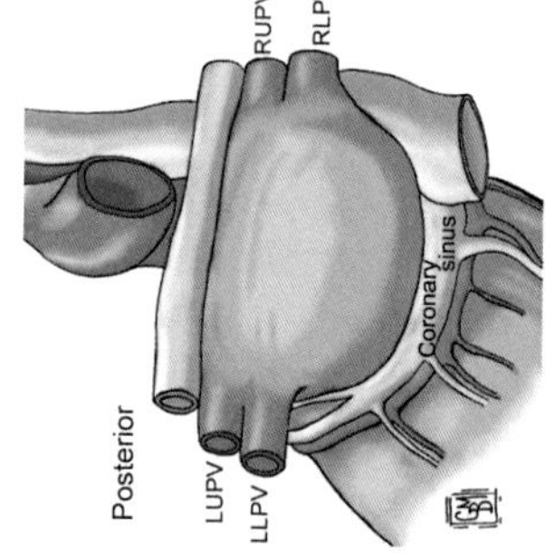
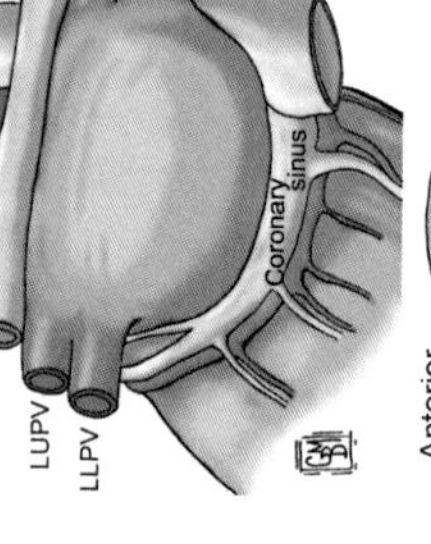

RUPV (ME 120° view)
The RUPV is easily imaged in the modified ME bicaval view at 110–120°. From the bicaval view increase the omniplane angle to 120°, the RUPV appears in the display right near the right pulmonary artery (RPA).

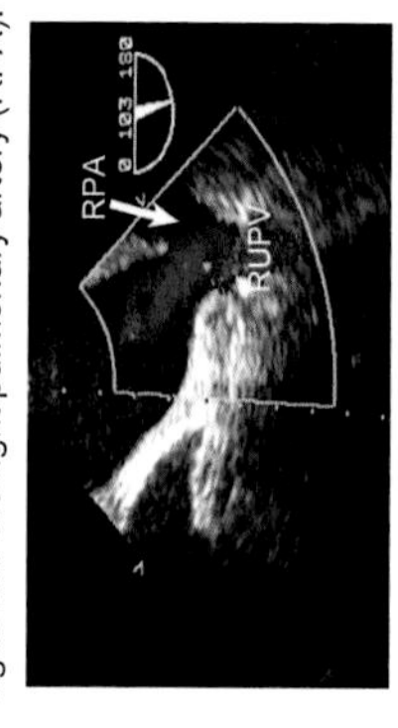

LLPV + LUPV (ME 90° view)
The LLPV is the most difficult pulmonary vein to image. One technique is to image the LUPV, keeping it in view, increase the omniplane angle to 90°. The left-sided veins appear as an inverted "V."

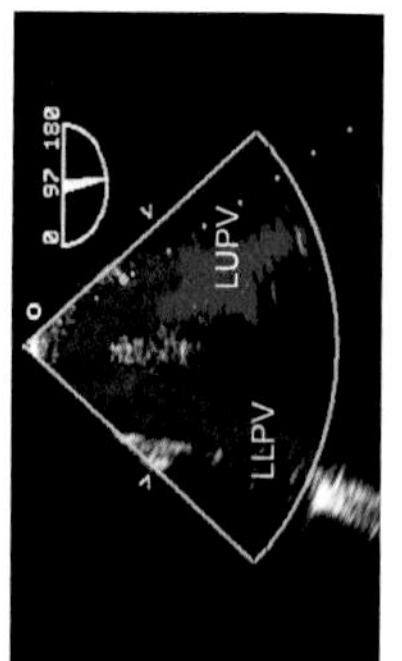

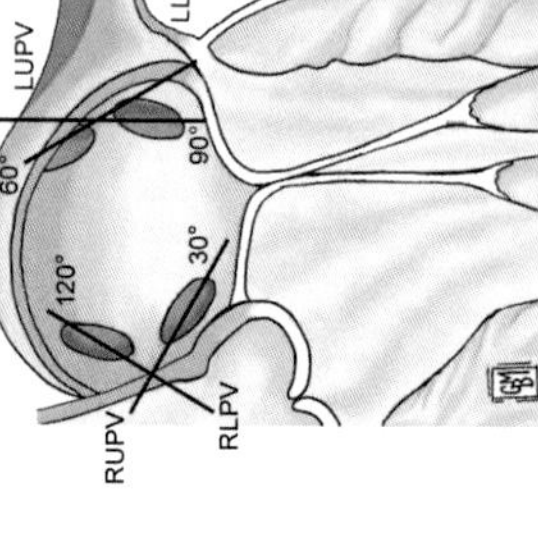

RLPV + RUPV (ME 30° view)
Turn the probe to image the right side of the LA. The RLPV is imaged from 0–30° above (posterior) and perpendicular to the LA. The RUPV is imaged at 30°, below (anterior) to the RLPV.

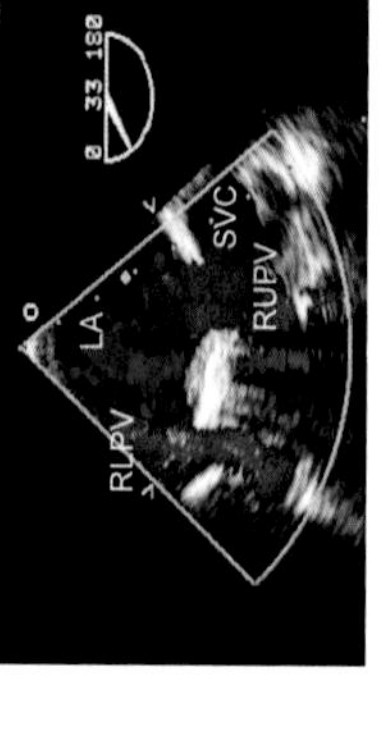

Turbulent Pulmonary Vein Flow

Pulmonary Vein Anastomosis
Turbulent antegrade color flow is seen (*arrow*) within a stenotic left upper pulmonary vein (LUPV) anastomosis during a lung transplant. Peak velocity is elevated. Note high velocity color scale and flow acceleration.

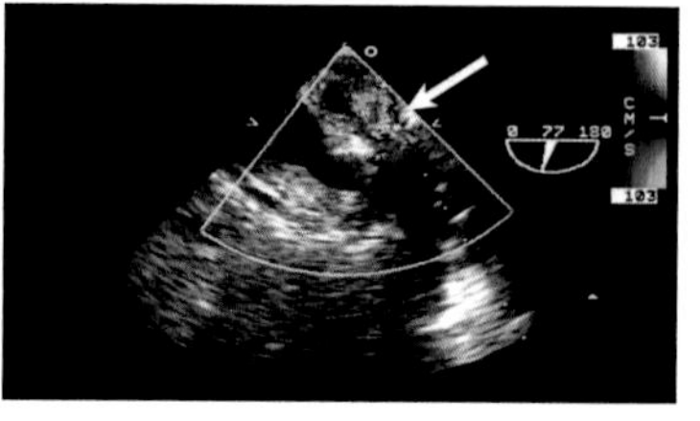

Tissue Doppler Imaging (TDI)

- TDI records and displays Doppler signals produced by the movement of tissue.
- There is analysis of structural motion or myocardial deformation for: displacement, velocity, strain, and strain rate.
- Compared with normal blood flow (60–100 cm/s), TDI has much lower velocity signals (−20 to +20 cm/s). TDI can be displayed using spectral or color Doppler.

Color TDI

- Provides real time color-coded scheme of mean tissue (myocardial) velocities with a low Nyquist scale (12 cm/s) superimposed over 2D image.
- Blue represents movement away from the probe and red towards the probe (BART like blood flow).
- Excellent spatial resolution as whole ventricle is assessed but poor temporal resolution.
- M-mode cursor on color TDI shows velocities from base (*top*) to apex (*bottom*) improving temporal resolution but without a 2D image.
- Offline processing of multiple myocardial locations can display averaged velocity, displacement, strain, strain rate in a spectral display.

Spectral TDI

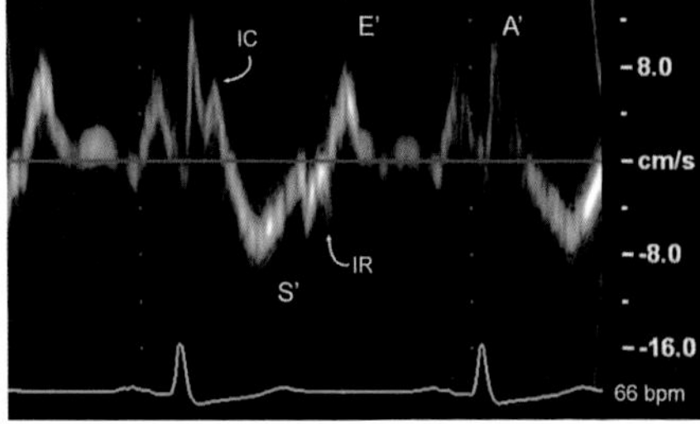

- Measure and displays peak myocardial velocity with a low velocity scale (12 cm/s), and good temporal but poor spatial resolution as only one area is sampled.
- Spectral TDI used for myocardial assessment has the subscript "m" as in Sm', Am' and Em'. Differentiates TDI of mitral valve (MV) annulus which uses Sa', Ea', Aa'.
- Timed to the ECG, the TDI spectral display of the mitral annulus comprises a systolic velocity (S′) and two opposite directed velocities, in early diastole (E′) before MV opening and after atrial contraction (A′). This trace appears opposite in direction to the PW spectral Doppler trace of MV inflow as the ventricle myocardium moves upwards during diastole. E' occurs slightly before E of MV inflow. During isovolumic contraction (IC) and isovolumic relaxation (IR), biphasic low velocity signals occur which are most likely related to local shape changes as well as cardiac rotation and torsion. No velocity is recorded during diastasis.
- Measurements providing the most information using TDI include peak velocity E', A', S' (cm/s), time intervals (ms), and the E'/A' ratio.

To Obtain Spectral TDI Traces

- TDI preset uses PW sample volume positioned over any myocardial segment with high FR (>100), but not a high wall filter, thus recording low velocity waves.
- Maximize FR, narrow sector + reduce depth over LV segment in ME 4C view
- Activate TDI preset to display myocardial Doppler color shift (Nyquist ±15 cm/s). Colorized tissue better identifies tissue boundaries for the TDI sample volume.
- Align probe for parallel interrogation of tissue motion.
- Activate cursor, position sample volume (3–5 mm).
- Activate PW Doppler to obtain a spectral display of peak tissue velocities.
- Adjust scale (20 cm/s), Doppler gain, and sweep speed 50–100 mm/s to optimize the spectral trace.

Applications of Tissue Doppler Imaging (TDI)

Left Ventricle
- Global systolic function: S' velocity estimate EF, normal S': **> 5.4 cm/s** (ME lateral)
- Regional systolic function: detect subendocardial ischemia
- Ischemic response with Dobutamine stress test diagnoses CAD
- Diastolic function: classification of diastolic pattern, E' is preload-independent
- Estimation of LV filling pressure

Valvular Disease
- Detects subclinical ventricular dysfunction
- Volume lesions (AI, MR) ↑ **E'**

Cardiomyopathy
- Differentiate restrictive cardiomyopathy (↓ **E'**) and constrictive pericarditis
- Prognosis in systolic heart failure

Right Ventricle
- Global systolic function: tricuspid annulus normal **S' > 10–11.5 cm/s**

Myocardial TDI

- Cardiac myocytes are organized in parallel sheets that have different orientations: circumferential (middle) and longitudinal (endocardial and epicardial).
- The heart contracts in systole using three movements (see p. 64):
  - longitudinal shortening of base to apex by the subendocardium (ME views)
  - radial thickening (40%) inwards of the subepicardium (TG views)
  - circumferential torsion of base clockwise + apex counterclockwise (TG views)

Transverse TDI (circumferential fibers) from the TG anterior and inferior LV segments are in opposite directions, hence the mirror image of velocities.

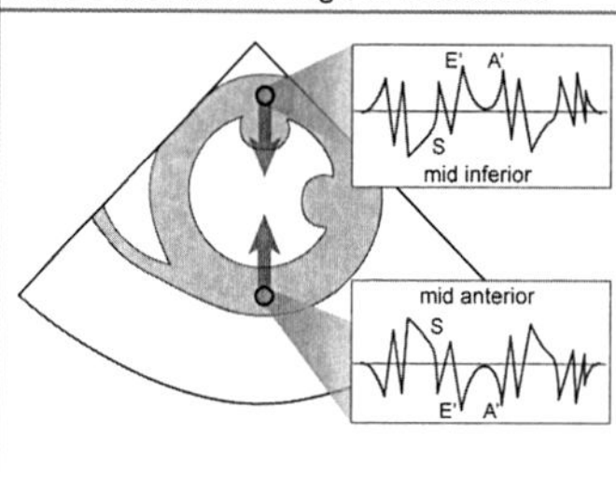

Longitudinal TDI (longitudinal fibers) is obtained from ME views of different LV walls. Lengthening occurs during diastole and shortening during systole

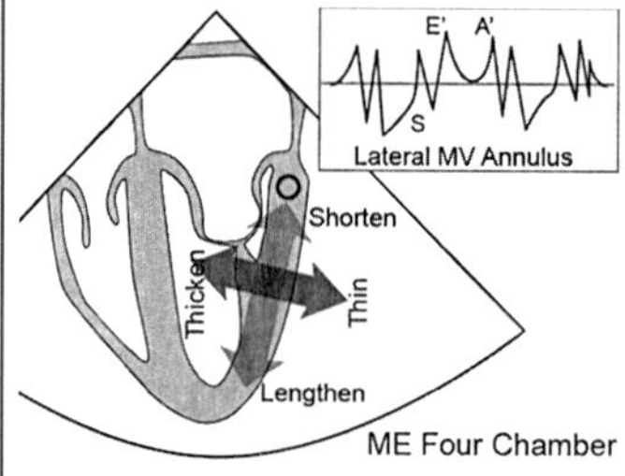

Factors Affecting TDI Velocities

- The number of contracting myocytes and myocardial α-adrenergic receptors density gives higher S' and E'. These are lowest in the septum, and decrease from basal to mid-apical segments. Right-sided annular velocities are higher than left.
- Annular velocity is invalid with valve prosthesis and annular calcification.
- A higher heart rate results in ↑ S'.
- Advancing age has more fibrous tissue so ↑ A', ↓ S' and ↓ E' velocities.
- S' and E' velocities are directly dependent on preload, A' less so.
- Acute increases in afterload → ↓ E' velocity, chronic increases → ↓ S' and ↓ E'.
- Pericardiotomy and mechanical ventilation have little effect.

Limitations of TDI Velocity
- TDI recordings not comparable between TTE and TEE (values lower with TEE).
- TDI requires a parallel Doppler alignment to tissue motion.
- Spectral TDI records both longitudinal and transverse cardiac motion and is unable to differentiate between them (low spatial resolution).
- TDI is unable to differentiate active from passive motion (tethering).

- Echocardiography does not directly measure pressures, but does measure velocity of blood flow and relates both by the Bernoulli equation.
- To measure intra-cardiac pressures, one can use Doppler velocity measurements of regurgitant jets across valves and apply the modified Bernoulli equation ($\Delta P = P_1 - P_2 = 4(V_2^2 - V_1^2)$) to determine the pressure gradient between chambers.
- Limitation of these measurements includes:
  - Requires a regurgitant jet across the valve
  - Maximal regurgitant velocity signal (obtain a complete spectral trace)
  - Accurate Doppler measurement (angle of Doppler beam <30°)
  - Absence of valvular or subvalvular obstruction

Tricuspid Regurgitation (TR) to Estimate RVSP (PASP)

A systolic pressure gradient exists between the RV (P_1) and RA (P_2), across a closed tricuspid valve. Estimate the pressure drop from the peak velocity of TR jet.

- $P_1 - P_2 = 4v^2 \rightarrow P_1 = 4v^2 + P_2 \rightarrow \text{RVSP} = 4(\text{peak TR})^2 + \text{RAP}$

The RAP is estimated from CVP or use an empiric value of 5–10 mmHg.
Important clinically as is a noninvasive estimate of PASP that reflects the severity of pulmonary hypertension (in the absence of pulmonic stenosis or RVOT obstruction).

Pulmonic Insufficiency (PI) to Estimate PA Diastolic Pressure (PADP)

In the setting of PI, the pulmonic valve is closed and a pressure gradient exists across the PA and RV. Measure the end-diastolic PI velocity. This provides the pressure gradient between the PA and RV at end-diastole and, by adding RAP, can estimate PADP.

- $\text{PADP} = 4 \times (\text{PI end-diastolic velocity})^2 + \text{RAP}$
- $\text{Mean PAP} = 4 \times (\text{PI peak velocity})^2$

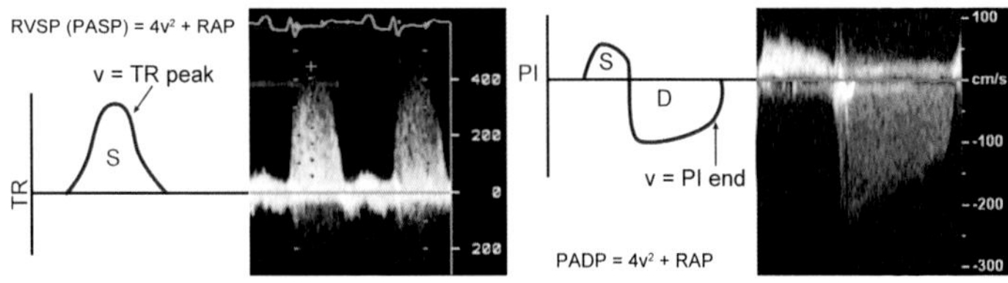

Aortic Insufficiency (AI) to Estimate LVEDP

In the setting of AI, the aortic valve is closed and a pressure gradient exists between the aorta and the LV. Measure the end-diastolic AI peak velocity. Knowing the aortic diastolic blood pressure, use the peak end-diastolic AI velocity to estimate LVEDP

- $P_1 - P_2 = 4v^2 \rightarrow \text{Aortic}_{DBP} - \text{LVEDP} = 4(\text{AI}_{end}\ V)^2$
- $\text{LVEDP} = \text{Aortic}_{DBP} - 4(\text{AI}_{end}\ V)^2$

Mitral Regurgitation (MR) to Estimate LAP

The peak velocity of the MR jet represents the gradient between the LV and the LA during systole across a closed MV. Assuming no AV pathology or LVOT obstruction, the aortic systolic blood pressure represents the LV systolic pressure and can be used to calculate the LAP.

- $P_1 - P_2 = 4v^2 \rightarrow \text{Aortic}_{SBP} - \text{LAP} = 4(\text{peak } V_{MR})^2$
- $\text{LAP} = \text{Aortic}_{SBP} - 4(\text{peak } V_{MR})^2$

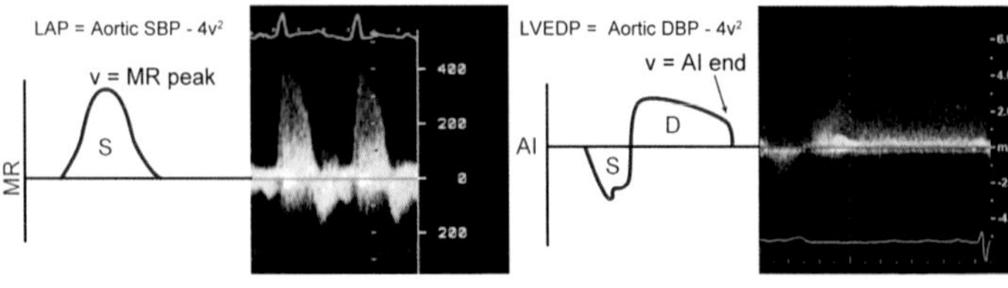

Aortic Valve Area (AVA) Continuity Equation

$$A2 = \frac{V1 \quad A1}{V2} = \frac{VTI_{LVOT} \quad 0.785\ d^2_{LVOT}}{VTI_{AV}} = AVA$$

- In theory, to calculate AVA can use the ratio of peak velocities, mean velocities, or VTI multiplied by LVOT CSA.
- Use ME AV LAX (120°) view to obtain LVOT "d" measurement in mid-systole just below the aortic valve (not at AV annulus) or can estimate LVOT area as 2.0 cm² (± 0.2 cm²). Calculate area (A):
  $A = \pi r^2 = \pi(d/2)^2 = 0.785d^2$
- Use TG LAX (120°) view, place CW sample cursor through LVOT/AV/ root and trace to obtain the VTI.
- Use TG LAX (120°) view, to place PW sample at the LVOT level (below AV), trace the spectral envelope to obtain the VTI. Start the PW sample volume in the AV outflow and move back towards the LVOT to obtain a smooth well-defined velocity trace with minimal spectral broadening.

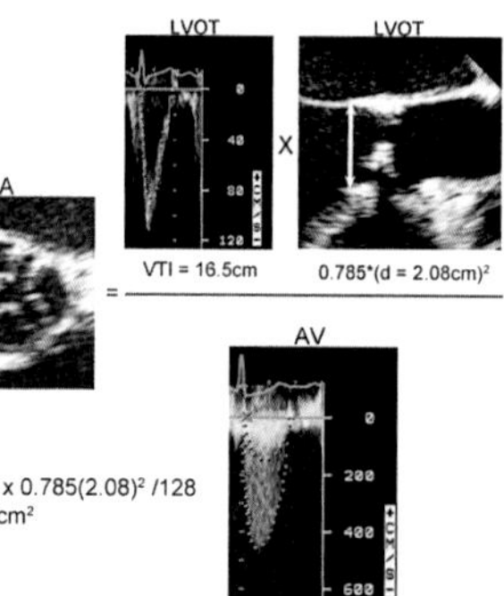

Aortic Valve Pressure Half-Time (PHT, PT1/2)

- The rate of AI velocity decline is determined by the pressure gradient between the aorta and the LV. Worse regurgitation (wider orifice) has a more rapid decline of aortic and a rise in LV pressures which results in a steeper slope of regurgitant velocity decline.
- Diastolic decay slope is measured as the deceleration slope (m/s) or time in milliseconds (ms) for the pressure gradient to fall to half of its initial value, the pressure half-time (PT1/2 or PHT).
- Deceleration time (DT) is time for Vmax to fall to zero. By the Bernoulli equation, when pressure is halved, velocity equals the peak transvalvular velocity (Vmax) divided by the square root of 2 (= 1.4), or velocity drops by 0.7 Vmax.
- The rate of pressure decline is significantly affected by changes in LV compliance and pressure, afterload, aorta size, and compliance irrespective of regurgitant orifice size.

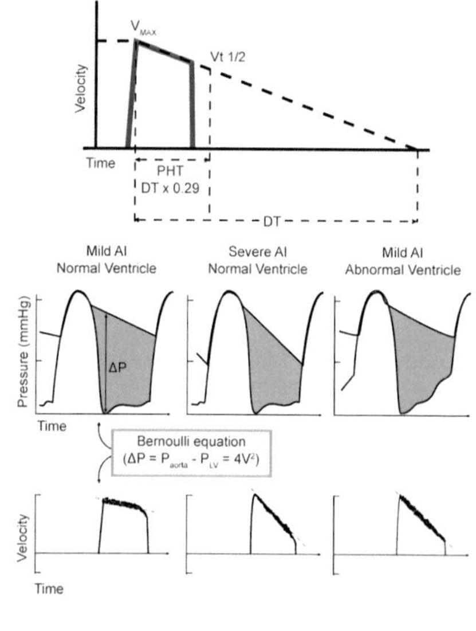

Low Slope	Steep Slope
Mild AI	Severe AI
High SVR	Low SVR
Dilated aorta	Elevated LVEDP

MVA Pressure Half-Time (PT1/2, PHT)

- In MS, LAP is elevated as LA empties slowly through the narrow MV. CW Doppler shows:
  - Decrease or flattening of deceleration slope (after the E wave).
  - Fusion of E and A waves as is an absence of diastasis from persistently elevated LAP.
- The time it takes for peak pressure to decrease in half is the PHT.
- By the Bernoulli equation, when pressure is halved, velocity equals the peak transvalvular velocity (Vmax) divided by the square root of 2 (=1.4), or for the velocity to drop by 0.7 Vmax.
- MVA in native valve MS is obtained from an empiric formula.

DT
PHT
Time
Velocity
E
A
$\frac{V_{max}}{\sqrt{2}}$
Vmax
E
A

$$MVA = \frac{220}{PHT}$$

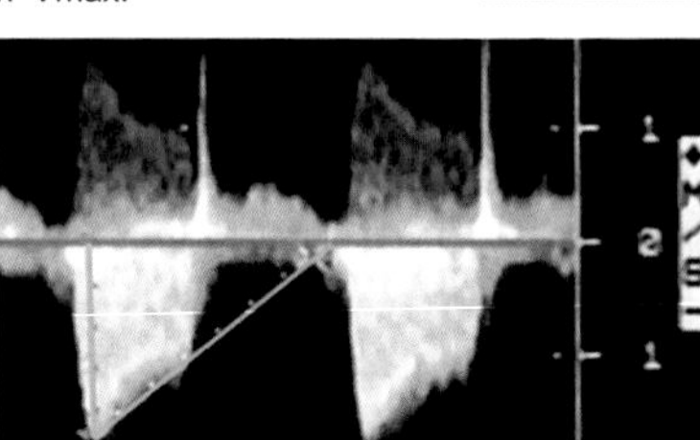

PT1/2, PHT Method

1. Optimize PW/CW MV inflow (sample at MV leaflet tips)
2. Increase sweep speed to 100 m/s
3. Press analysis → MVA $Pt_{1/2}$
   - Caliper button: place caliper at peak of E wave (+ enter)
   - Caliper at baseline on the slope of E wave (+ enter)
   - Displays a calculated MVA

Max velocity (m/s)
Time (s)
Max pressure (mmHg)
PHT (ms)
MVA (cm^2)

In a normal native MV, the PHT is primarily a function of LV compliance and is not useful for estimation of MVA.
Limitations of PHT for MVA in MS:

- Underestimate: post balloon valvuloplasty, LV impaired relaxation
- Overestimate: AI, high CO, MR, tachycardia, LV restrictive filling
- Unreliable: prosthetic valves, A-V block
- EROA is the gap in coaptation through which the regurgitant volume flows.

Proximal Isovelocity Surface Area (PISA) Method

The PISA method calculates mitral flow during diastole based on the hemispheric shape of the convergence zone seen with color Doppler in the left atrium. MVA is calculated by dividing the mitral flow rate by the maximum velocity of mitral flow.

$$\text{MV Area}\left(cm^2\right) = \frac{\text{Flow (cc/s)}}{V_{ms}\,(cm/s)}$$

- Flow Rate is calculated using measurements:

$$\text{Flow rate (cc/s)} = 2\pi r^2 \times \frac{\text{angle } \alpha}{180^\circ} \times V_{alias}$$

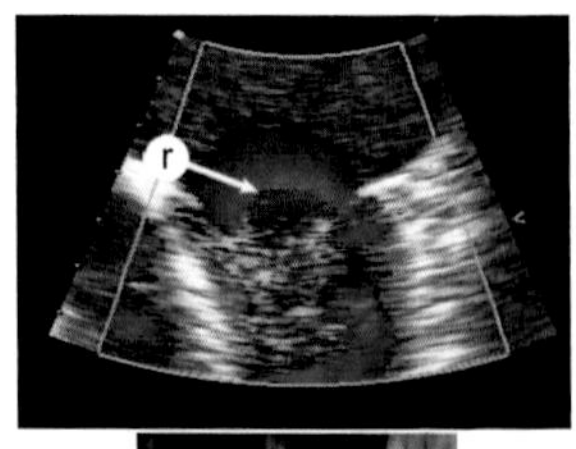

r (cm) = radius of flow convergence region
V_{alias} (cm/s) = aliasing velocity

$$\frac{\text{angle } \alpha}{180} = \text{correction angle}$$

The correction angle is measured if the hemisphere is <180°.

- V_{ms} is the peak PW/CW Doppler velocity of MV inflow in cm/s

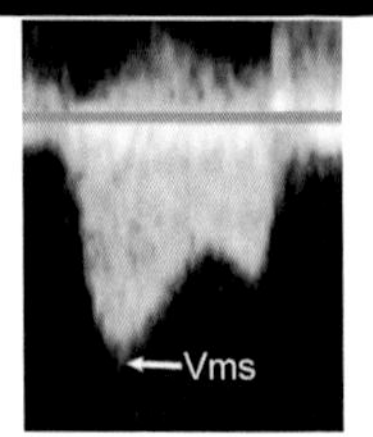

Advantages of PISA Method

Though a less validated method to estimate MVA, it is useful in the presence of AI, MR, prosthetic valve, or arrhythmia. It is less affected by LA and LV compliance.

- It corresponds to the vena contracta cross-sectional area, the narrowest portion of the regurgitant jet and is slightly smaller than the anatomic orifice.
- EROA represents unique information for valvular regurgitant lesions (aortic, mitral, tricuspid) and correlates with severity of regurgitation.
- Can calculate EROA by using the continuity or PISA methods, or directly measure using 3D color Doppler.
- EROA is:
  - More accurate central jets
  - Less useful eccentric jets
  - Not useful in multiple jets
  - Errors in "r" are squared

EROA (cm^2)	MR	TR	AI
Mild	<0.20	<0.2	<0.1
Moderate	0.20–0.39	0.20–0.40	0.1–0.29
Severe	≥0.4	>0.4	≥0.3

MR EROA by PISA Method

1. Optimize 2D image MV orifice (zoom)
2. Optimize color of convergence region
3. Shift color flow baseline up to ↑ the size of the MR hemispheric shell
4. Note lower alias velocity (Vr)
5. Measure "r" from aliased region to the orifice (cm), mid-systole
6. Measure peak regurgitant velocity (V_{MR}) of CW MR jet and trace for VTI
7. Calculate flow $_{MR}$

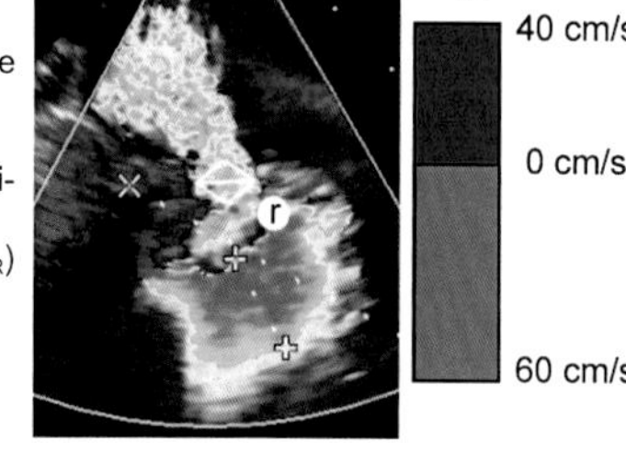

$$\text{Flow MR(cc/s)} = 6.28r^2 \times \text{Vr (cm/s)}$$

8. Calculate EROA $_{MR}$
9. Calculate regurgitant volume

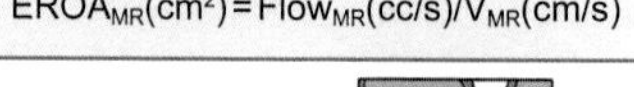

$$EROA_{MR}(cm^2) = Flow_{MR}(cc/s)/V_{MR}(cm/s)$$

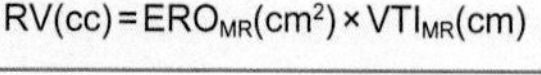

$$RV(cc) = ERO_{MR}(cm^2) \times VTI_{MR}(cm)$$

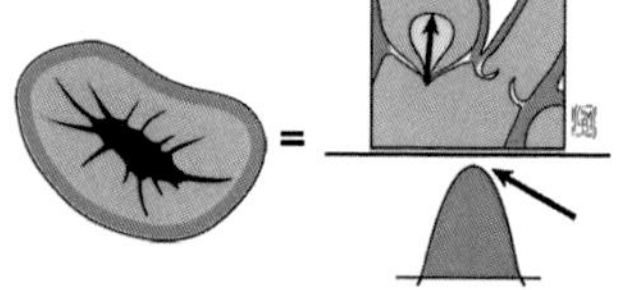

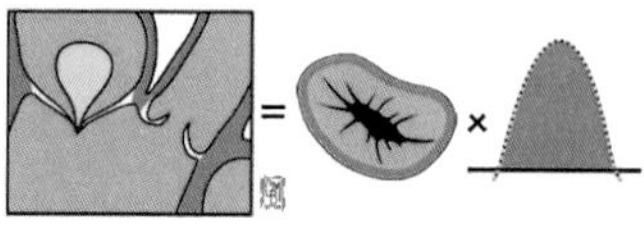

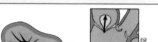

PISA for Pinheads		
EROA = $2\pi r^2 \times V_r \times \alpha/180$	Assume: MR peak velocity = 400 cm/s Vr at 40 cm/s	Simplify equation: EROA α $r^2/2$

Aortic Insufficiency (AI) EROA by PISA Method

1. Optimize color of convergence region (deep TG view)
2. Shift color flow baseline up to ↓ color flow aliasing velocity (Vr), ↑ hemisphere
3. Measure "r" from aliased region to orifice (cm), mid-diastole
4. Measure peak regurgitant velocity (V_{AI}) of CW jet and trace for VTI
5. Calculate Flow $_{AI}$ (cc/s) = $6.28r^2 \times$ Vr (cm/s)
6. Calculate ERO $_{AI}$ = Flow $_{AI}$ (cc/s)/V_{AI} (cm/s)

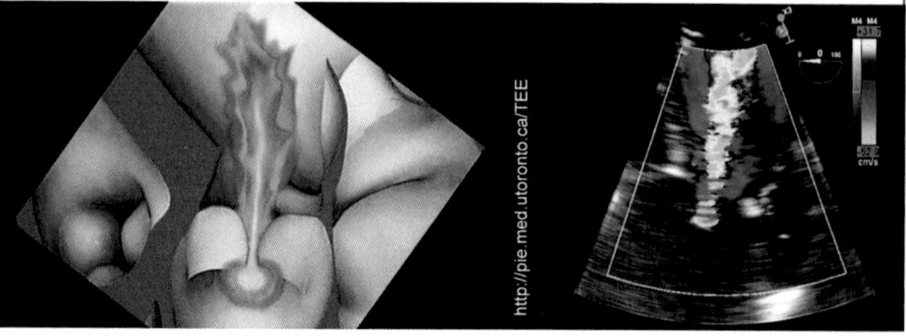

Regurgitant Volume (RegV) is the volume of blood that regurgitates through an incompetent valve. It is the difference between the stroke volume (SV) through an incompetent valve and a competent valve. It can be calculated by using the PISA (see previous page) or continuity (see below) methods.

$$\mathbf{Reg_V\left(cc\right) = SV_{MV} - SV_{AV}\left(cc\right)}$$

Mild <40 cc
Moderate 40–60 cc
Severe >60 cc

Regurgitant Fraction (RF) is the fraction or percentage of total stroke volume that regurgitates through an incompetent valve.

$$\mathbf{RF\left(\%\right) = \frac{SV_{MV} - SV_{AV}}{SV_{MV}} = \frac{RegV_{MV}}{SV_{MV}}}$$

Normal/trivial <20%
Mild 20–30%
Moderate 30–50%
Severe >50%

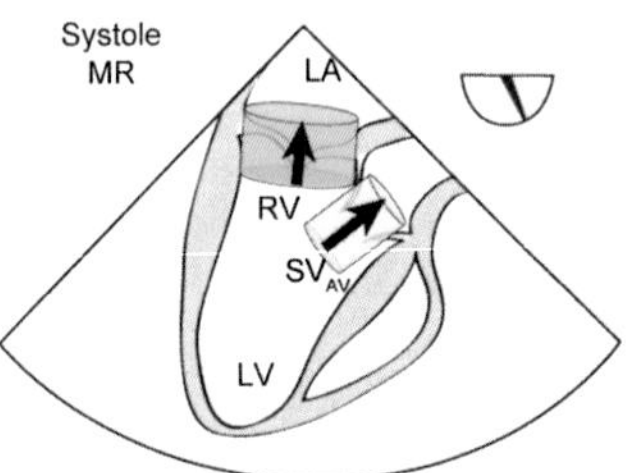

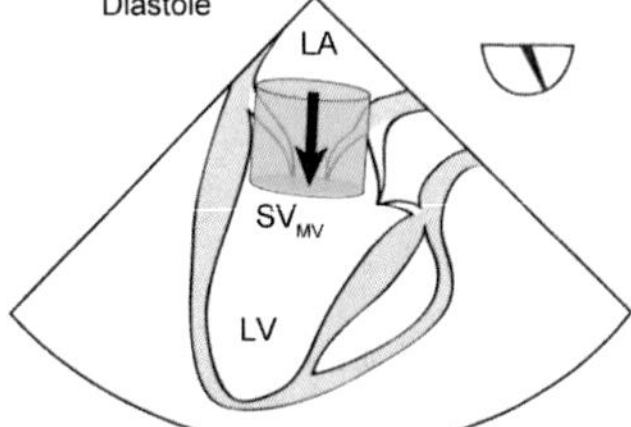

SV_{AV} (cc) = VTI_{AV} (cm) × CSA(cm^2)

1. CSA AV = $\pi r^2 = 0.785d^2$ measure diameter AV annulus (cm) in ME AV LAX (120°) or planimeter area in AV SAX, normal AV_d 1.8–2.2 cm
2. VTI AV from a CW trace through the aortic outflow (TG views) and trace for stroke distance (cm), normal VTI 18–22 cm
3. Multiplying the two together will give the stroke volume through the AV

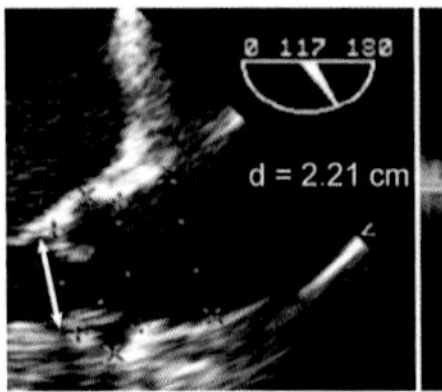

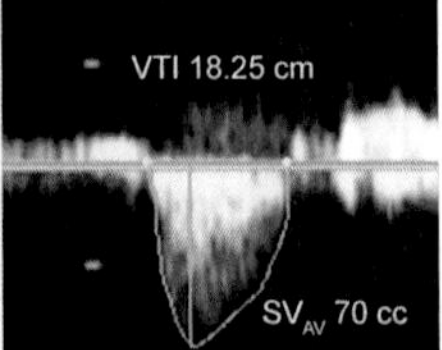

SV_{MV} (cc) = VTI_{MV} (cm) × CSA (cm^2)

1. CSA MV = $\pi r^2 = 0.785d^2$ measure diameter MV annulus (cm) at mid-diastole in ME 2C/4C/LAX, normal MV_d 3.0–3.5 cm.
2. VTI MV from a PW trace at mitral annulus (ME views) and trace for stroke distance (cm), normal VTI 10–13 cm.
3. Multiplying the two together will give the stroke volume through the MV

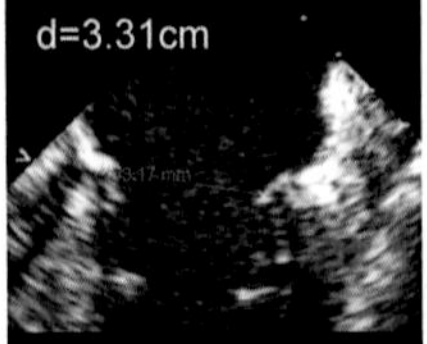

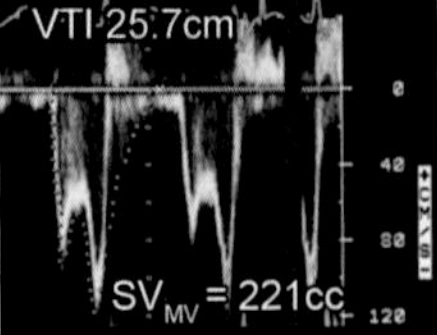

$$\mathbf{RegV_{MR}\left(cc\right) = 221 - 70 = 151cc}$$

$$\mathbf{RF_{MR}\left(\%\right) = 151 / 221 = 68\%}$$

Pitfalls using the volumetric method:

- PW sample volume location: MV annulus not at leaflet tips/LVOT
- Diameter measurements: location, timing, any measurement error is squared
- Arrhythmias: average over 5 beats
- Multi-valve lesions/shunts: formulas invalid if significant shunt or more than mild regurgitation of normal valve

- Calculation of intra-cardiac shunt fraction compares the stroke volume (SV) at two intra-cardiac sites that reflect total pulmonic blood flow (Qp) and total systemic blood flow (Qs).
- Measure blood flow proximal and distal to the shunt, at the sample sites listed.
- Shunt size is determined by the defect location and size, and relative resistance to blood flow on either side of the defect.
  Qp: Qs normal is 1
  Qp: Qs > 1 is L to R shunt
  Qp: Qs < 1 is R to L shunt

Significant shunt Qp:Qs >1.5:1

Sample sites for shunts

Shunts	Qp	Qs	Shunt flow
	Site distal to shunt inflow	Site distal to shunt outflow	Direction of flow determinants
ASD: LA → RA	TV annulus RVOT Main PA	MV annulus LVOT Asc Aorta	RAP, LAP RV/LV compliance Valsalva
VSD: LV → RV	RVOT Main PA MV annulus	LVOT Asc Aorta TV annulus	RVSP, LVSP PVR, SVR
PDA: Aorta → PA	MV annulus LVOT Asc Aorta	TV annulus RVOT Main PA	AoP, PAP SVR, PVR

- Pitfalls calculating stroke volume:
  - Need accurate x-sectional area measurement, difficult if not circular orifice
  - Assumes laminar flow, with a spatially "flat" flow velocity profile
  - Doppler alignment is parallel to flow for an optimal spectral trace
  - Velocity and diameter measurement are made at the same anatomic site.

Shunt Fraction (ASD)

Qp = trans-pulmonic volume flow = CSA × VTI PA

Qs = LVOT volume flow = CSA × VTI LVOT

$SV_{LVOT} = VTI_{LVOT}$ (cm) × CSA (cm^2)

1. CSA LVOT = $\pi r^2 = 0.785d^2$ measure diameter LVOT (cm) in ME AV LAX (120°) within 1 cm of AV annulus
2. VTI LVOT by obtaining a PW trace at the aortic outflow (TG views) and trace for (VTI) stroke distance (cm)
3. Multiplying the two together will give the stroke volume through the LVOT

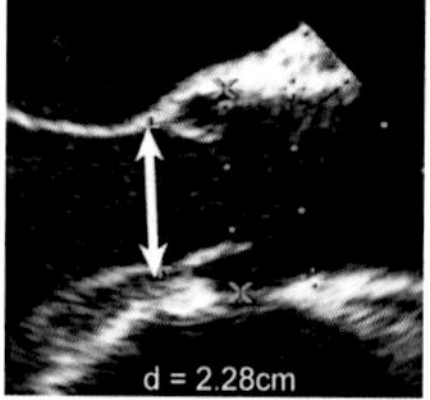

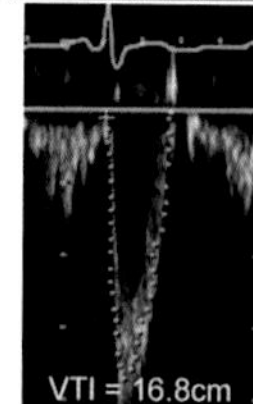

$SV_{LVOT} = (2.28)^2 \times 0.785 \times 16.8 = 68.5$cc

$SV_{PA} = VTI_{PA}$ (cm) × CSA (cm^2)

1. CSA PA = $\pi r^2 = 0.785d^2$ measure PA diameter in ME RVOT view
2. VTI PA by obtaining a PW trace through the PA and trace for (VTI) stroke distance (cm)
3. Multiplying the two together will give the stroke volume through the PA

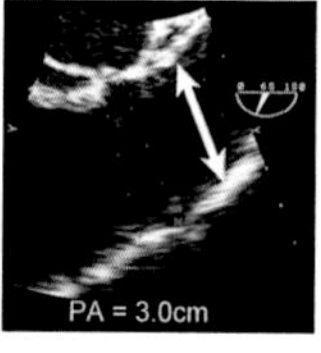

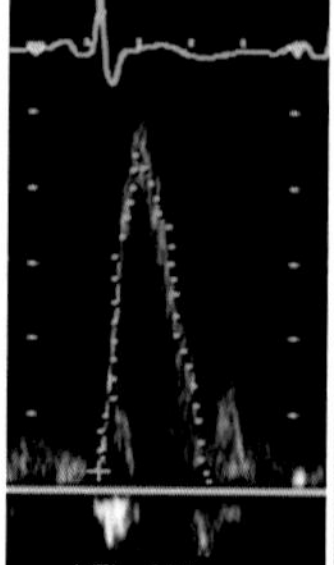

$SV_{PA} = (3.0)^2 \times 0.785 \times 22.3$
$= 157.5$cc

Shunt fraction (Qp/Qs) = 157.5/68.5
= 2.3:1

3
Left Ventricle

A. Vegas, *Perioperative Two-Dimensional Transesophageal Echocardiography*, https://doi.org/10.1007/978-3-319-60902-7_3

- The left ventricle (LV) is the largest chamber in a normal heart.
- Determining LV size and function is often the focus of an echocardiographic exam
- The LV is assessed for size (cavity dimensions, volume), mass (wall thickness), and function in systole and diastole using different echocardiographic parameters.

LV Anatomy

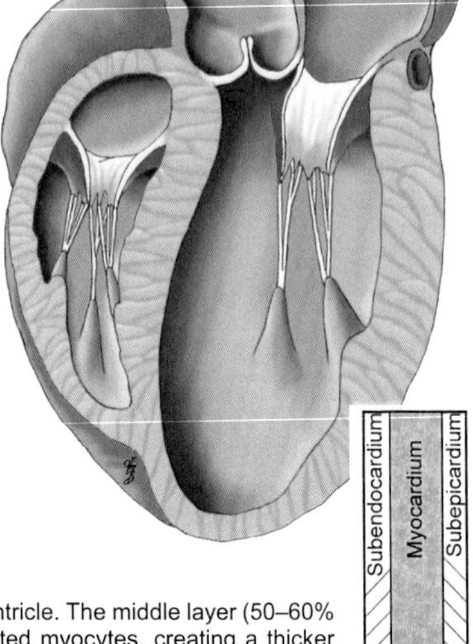

- The normal LV is a bullet-shaped structure with a wide inlet (mitral valve), trabecular apex, and narrow outlet (outflow tract).
- The LV wall comprises 3 layers: epicardium (outer), myocardium (middle), and endocardium (inner). The epicardium is the visceral layer of serous pericardium. The endocardium is composed of endothelial cells and is trabeculated with muscle bundles in all parts except the outflow tract. The myocardium is the thickest layer and is composed of myocytes with a complex arrangement of fibers that contribute to LV mechanics.
- Subepicardium (25% thickness) has oblique myocardial fiber strands arranged in a left helical pattern which extend onto the right ventricle. The middle layer (50–60% thickness) has circumferential orientated myocytes, creating a thicker base and thin apex. The subendocardium (20% thickness) has a right helical fiber orientation. Two major papillary muscles that support the mitral valve are integral components of the LV wall in the antero-lateral and posteromedial aspects.
- The blood supply to the LV is described in Chap. 5.
- Normal LV shape is symmetric with short circumferential axes and a greater long axis from base to apex. The apex is rounded and best represented by a hemiellipse; the base is circular and more like a cylinder. Various simplified formulas can describe ventricular geometry.

LV Mechanics

- Adequate function of the LV relies on contraction during systole and relaxation during diastole (see Chap. 6). Dysfunction during any part of the cardiac cycle impairs LV function. The fiber arrangement of the different myocardial layers creates a complex vortex of blood during filling and ejection. To efficiently eject blood, the normal heart contracts in systole using 3 movements:
  1) Longitudinal shortening of 15–20 mm (10–15% shortening) from base to apex involving the subendocardium
  2) Radial thickening of the myocardium moving inward around the long axis (25% circumferential shortening)
  3) Circumferential torsion (rotation or twisting) of the base (subepicardial) clockwise and the apex (subendocardial) counter-clockwise.

  The opposite movements occur during diastole to help the heart relax.

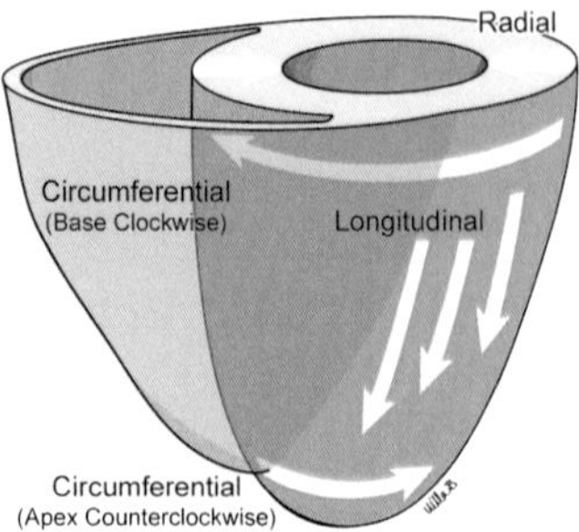

- It is now possible to assess each of these components of myocardial mechanics by echocardiography.
- LV systolic function is influenced by loading conditions (preload, afterload).

- Left ventricular models arbitrarily divide the LV into segments that more accurately describe regional wall motion abnormalities (RWMA) with correlation to coronary artery anatomy. Most models divide the chamber into three equal regions along the long axis: basal, mid, and apical.
- The 16 segment LV model (ASE 1989) does not include a true apical segment devoid of cavity. The **17 segment LV model** was created in a consensus guideline (AHA 2002) to describe LV segmental anatomy for all cardiac imaging modalities including echocardiography, CT, and MRI. The LV is divided at the basal and mid-levels each into six segments, and the apex into four segments with an apical cap that is devoid of LV cavity as the 17th segment.

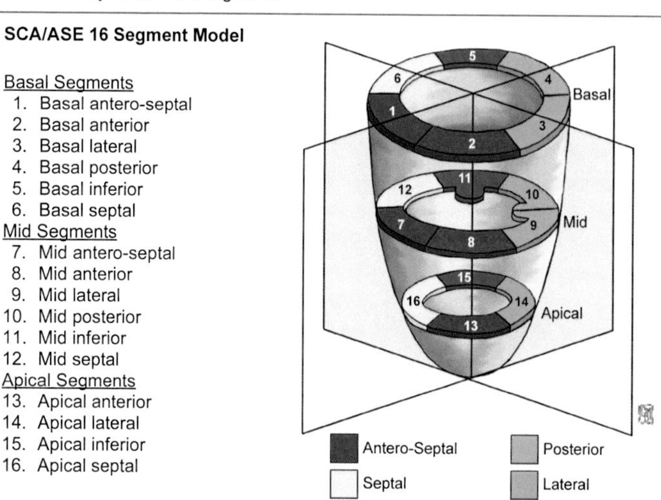

SCA/ASE 16 Segment Model

Basal Segments
1. Basal antero-septal
2. Basal anterior
3. Basal lateral
4. Basal posterior
5. Basal inferior
6. Basal septal

Mid Segments
7. Mid antero-septal
8. Mid anterior
9. Mid lateral
10. Mid posterior
11. Mid inferior
12. Mid septal

Apical Segments
13. Apical anterior
14. Apical lateral
15. Apical inferior
16. Apical septal

Source: Schiller NB, et al. J Am Soc Echocardiogr 1989; 2:358–87

SCA/ASE 17 Segment Model

Basal Segments
1. basal anterior
2. basal antero-septal
3. basal infero-septal
4. basal inferior
5. basal infero-lateral
6. basal antero-lateral

Mid Segments
7. mid anterior
8. mid antero-septal
9. mid infero-septal
10. mid inferior
11. mid infero-lateral
12. mid antero-lateral

Apical Segments
13. apical anterior
14. apical septal
15. apical inferior
16. apical lateral
17. apex

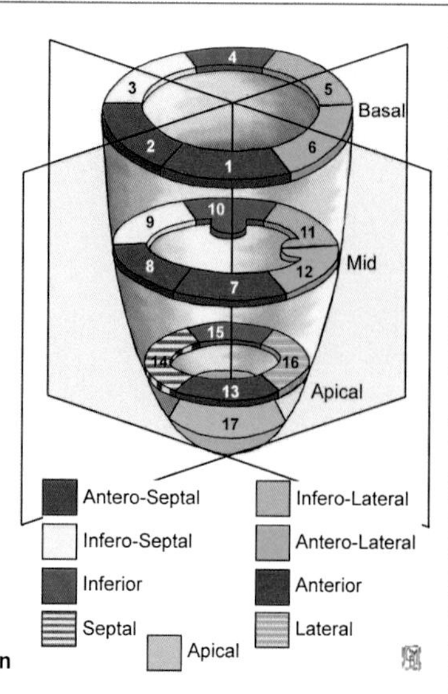

Source: Cerqueira M, et al. Circulation 2002;105:539–42

- The LV is examined by TEE in long axis (LAX) and short axis (SAX) from standard mid-esophageal (ME 4C, 2C and LAX) and transgastric views (TG basal SAX, TG mid-SAX, TG apical SAX, TG 2C, TG LAX). All views provide complimentary information when it is difficult to obtain either TG or ME views due to artifacts (dropout, shadowing) and poor patient anatomy (dilated LV, hiatal hernia).
- Individual LV wall segments should be identified and examined.

Mid-Esophageal Views

- In the ME views, the LV is shown without moving the probe by simply rotating the transducer angle from 0 to 160° beginning in the ME 4C view. Probe tip retroflexion avoids foreshortening the LV and with depth adjustment that best images the LV apex in the ME 2C view. Dropout from the ultrasound beam imaging parallel to the LV wall may poorly visualize the endocardium. Overall gain is adjusted to ensure the entire LV wall is well seen with good blood to endocardial border definition.

Transgastric Views

- The TG SAX views show one LV level at a time from base to apex. To avoid an oblique cut of the LV walls in the mid-SAX view, compare it to a TG 2C view in which the walls should appear horizontal on the screen. A perpendicular imaging plane best shows LV endocardium for accurate measurements of LV dimensions.
- SAX views are particularly valuable as segments of all 6 LV walls are displayed at once. The LAX views best demonstrate the subvalvular mitral apparatus including the chordae and papillary muscles of the LV. The LAX view allows Doppler placement to measure left ventricular outflow tract (LVOT) and AV velocities.

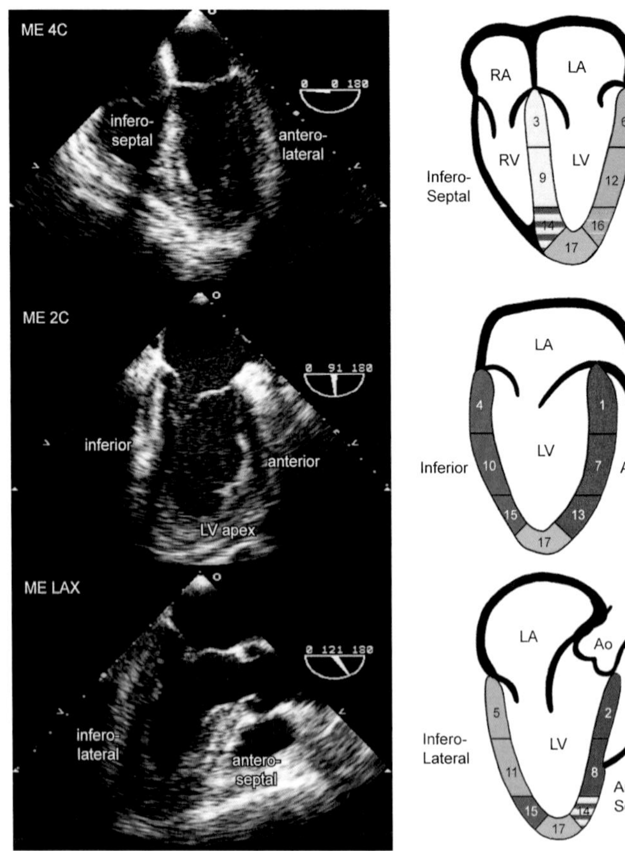

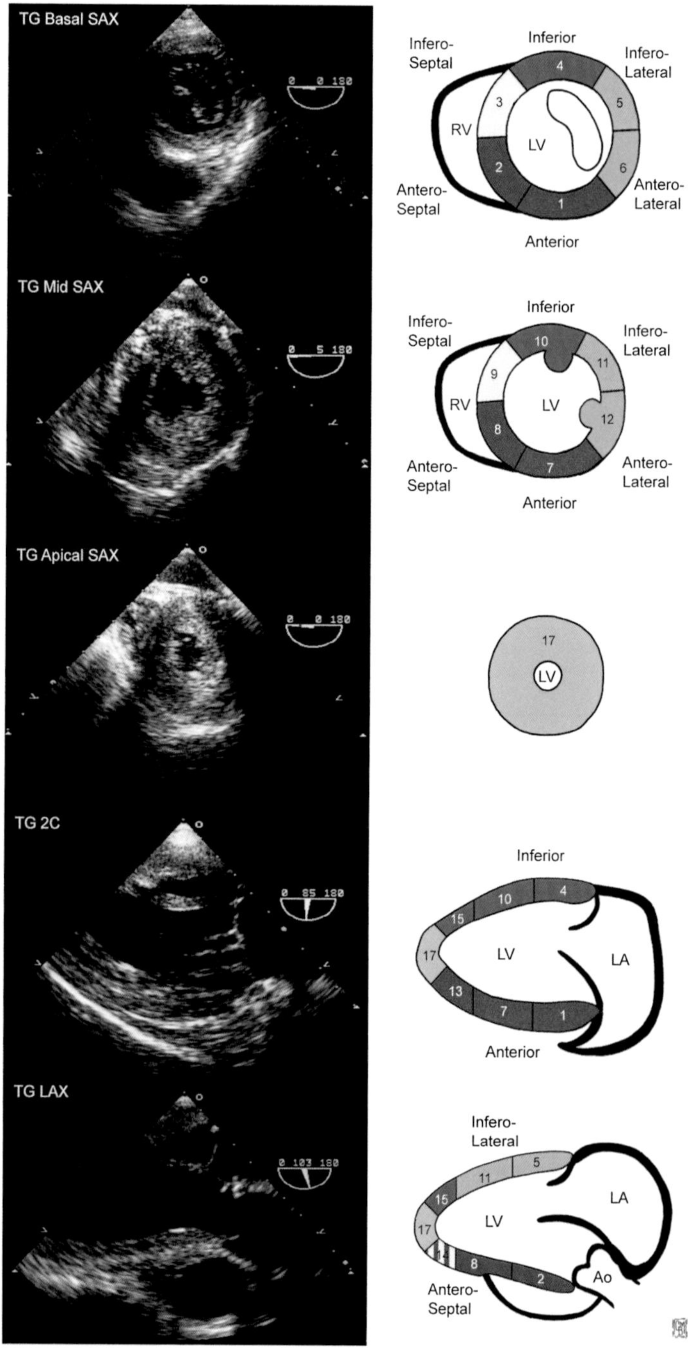

TG Basal SAX

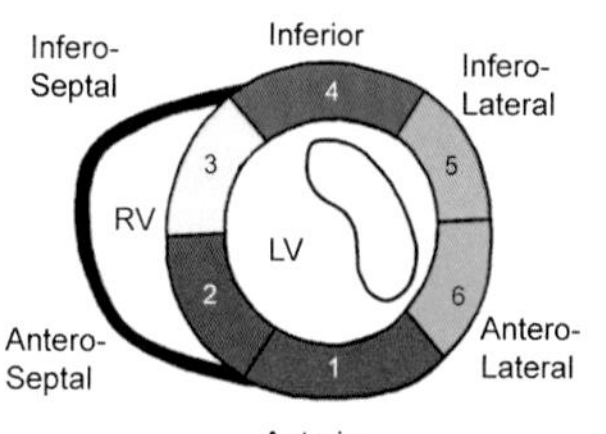

TG Mid SAX

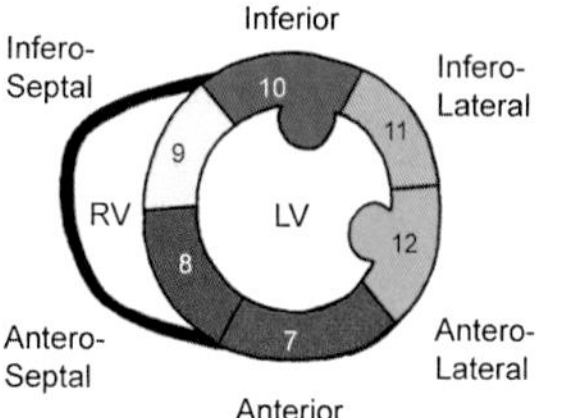

TG Apical SAX

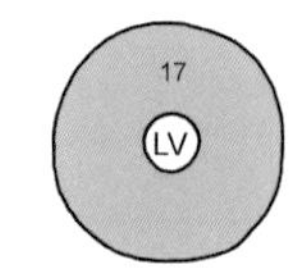

TG 2C

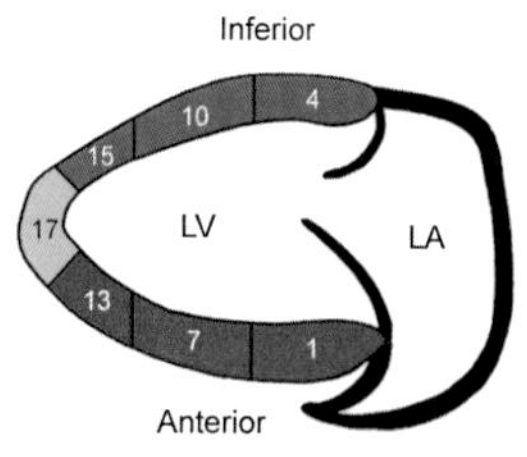

TG LAX

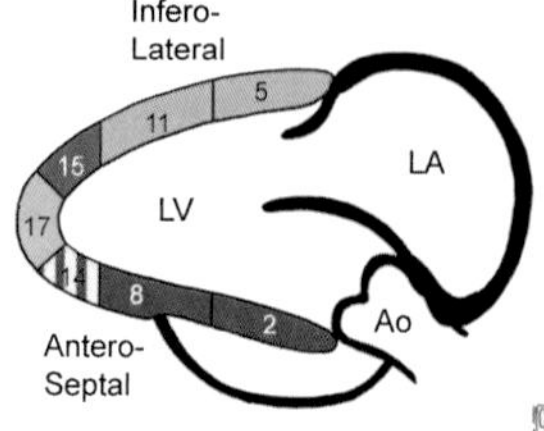

- LV size is assessed by using linear and volume measurements obtained at end-diastole and end-systole. These vary by gender and are indexed to body surface area (BSA). The stated values obtained for TTE are almost identical to TEE.

Normal Left Ventricle Size	Male		Female	
	Mean ± SD	2-SD range	Mean ± SD	2-SD range
LV Diameter (LVD)				
Diastole, mm	50.2 ± 4.1	42.0–58.4	45.0 ± 3.6	37.8–52.2
Systole, mm	32.4 ± 3.7	25.0–39.8	28.2 ± 3.3	21.6–34.8
LV Volume				
Diastolic volume, mL	106 ± 22	62–150	76 ± 15	46–106
Diastolic volume/BSA, mL/m²	54 ± 10	34–74	45 ± 8	29–16
Systolic volume, mL	41 ± 10	21–61	28 ± 7	14–42
Systolic volume/BSA, mL/m²	21 ± 5	11–31	16 ± 4	8–24
Adapted from: Lang R, et al. J Am Soc Echocardiogr 2015;28:1–39				

- The recommended TEE views used to measure LV size are controversial.
- Transgastric views (TG 2C, TG LAX) are preferred to mid-esophageal views (ME 2C) in which lateral dropout may sacrifice accurate imaging of LV endocardium.
- Diameter measurements are made perpendicular to the LV long axis. To use the TG SAX view first ensure the measurement is on-axis and perpendicular to the LV long axis by checking a TG 2C or using simultaneous multiplane imaging.
- Measurements of the LV length (L) and minor diameter (LVD) are made at end-diastole. The LVD is measured in 2D from the endocardium of the anterior and inferior walls at the junction of the basal and mid portions of the LV.

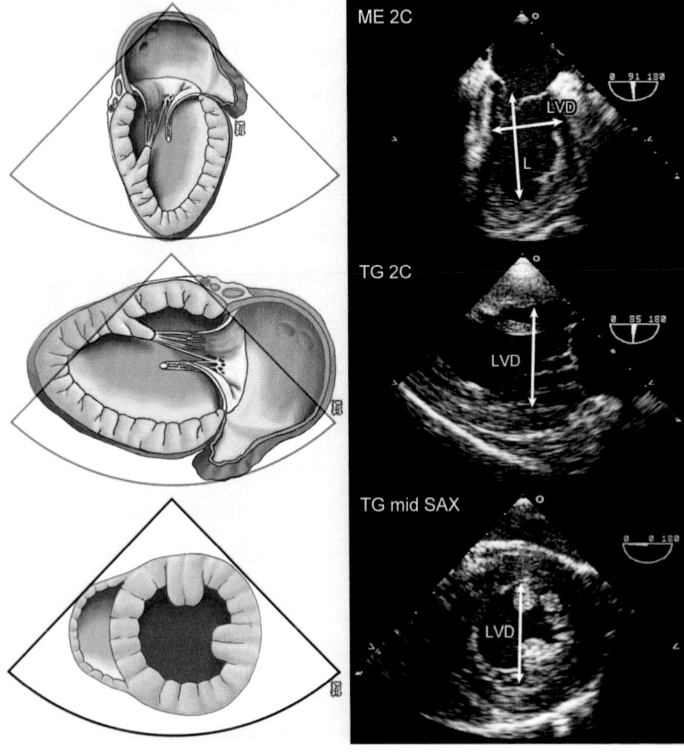

Left Ventricle Size	Female				Male			
LV Dimensions (LVD)	Refer. Range	Mild	Moderate	Severe	Refer. Range	Mild	Moderate	Severe
Diastole diameter, cm	3.8–5.2	5.3–5.6	5.7–6.1	**>6.2**	4.2–5.8	5.9–6.3	6.4–6.8	**>6.8**
Diastole Diameter/BSA, cm/m²	2.2–3.1	3.2–3.4	3.5–3.7	**>3.7**	2.2–3.0	3.1–3.3	3.4–3.6	**>3.6**
Systole diameter, cm	2.2–3.5	3.6–3.8	3.9–4.1	**>4.1**	2.5–4.0	4.1–4.3	4.4–4.5	**>4.5**
Systole diameter/BSA, cm/m²	1.3–2.1	2.2–2.3	2.4–2.6	**>2.6**	1.3–2.1	2.2–2.3	2.4–2.5	**>2.5**
LV Volume								
Diastolic volume, mL	46–106	107–120	121–130	**>130**	62–150	151–174	175–200	**>200**
Diastolic volume/BSA, mL/m²	29–61	62–70	71–80	**>80**	34–74	75–89	90–100	**>100**
Systolic volume, mL	14–42	43–55	56–67	**>67**	21–61	62–73	74–85	**>85**
Systolic volume/BSA, mL/m²	8–24	25–32	33–40	**>40**	11–31	32–38	39–45	**>45**

BSA, body surface area; LV, left ventricle
Adapted from: Lang R, et al. J Am Soc Echocardiogr 2015;28:1–39

Global LV Dilatation

- This refers to LV chamber enlargement often with thinning of the myocardium and systolic dysfunction from various causes (see below).
- The LV must accommodate more blood resulting in papillary muscle dysfunction and dilation of mitral and tricuspid annuli causing functional valvular regurgitation.
- Stagnated blood in the LV is seen as spontaneous echo contrast and has the potential for thrombus formation.

LV Dilatation Causes

Ischemic
Valvular (MR, AI, AS)
Cardiomyopathy (idiopathic)
Toxic (alcohol, cocaine)
Drugs (doxorubicin, Trastuzumab)
Metabolic (Beriberi, thyrotoxicosis, acromegaly, pheochromocytoma)
Metals (iron, cobalt, lead, mercury)
Infectious (HIV, HCV, Chagas)
Pregnancy

LV Dysfunction TEE Findings

LV enlarged
LA enlarged
Segmental myocardial thinning
Reduced systolic function
Spontaneous echo contrast
Reduced MV and AV VTIs
± Regurgitant valves MV/TV

(A) TG 2C and (B) TG mid SAX views show a dilated LV, at end-diastole with EDD measurements of >70 mm. Note in the TG 2C view, this measurement is made perpendicular to the LV walls to avoid an oblique measure which would overestimate the LV size. The TG SAX view shows thinned myocardium and spontaneous echo contrast ("smoke") in the LV. (C) The ME 4C view shows a dilated LV, at EDD, with poor MV leaflet coaptation.

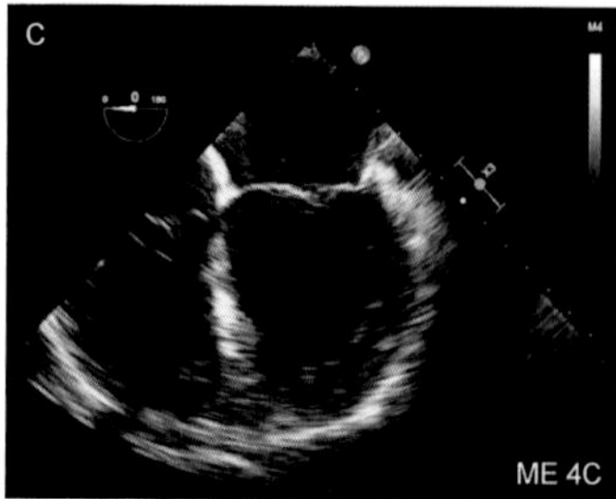

Left Ventricle Wall Thickness

- TEE measurements of LV septal wall thickness (SWT) and posterior wall thickness (PWT) is performed in the TG mid-SAX view (0–30°) at end-diastole (ED) excluding the papillary muscles.
- LV wall thickness (at ED)
  - Normal LV wall thickness <12 mm
  - LV Hypertrophy (LVH) >12 mm

Differential Symmetric LVH
Hypertension
Aortic Stenosis
Infiltration (amyloid, sarcoid, Fabry's)
Metabolic (Cushing, diabetes)
Renal disease
Athletic heart, obesity
Congenital (Noonan, Friedrich's Ataxia)

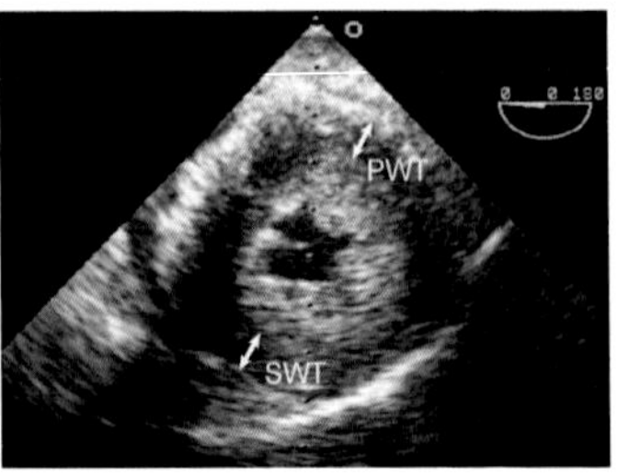

LV Wall Mass (LVM)

- LVM is the total weight of myocardium, as calculated from estimating myocardial volume and multiplying by the specific density of cardiac muscle.
- Measure thickness of septal + posterior myocardial walls and LV internal diameter (LVID) at ED and add a correction factor to the formula. Index to body size.

LV Mass =	$0.8 \times \{1.04[(LVIDd + PWTd + SWTd)^3 - (LVIDd)^3]\} + 0.6$ g
Normal mass: Male 88–224 g (49–115 g/m²), female 67–162 g (43–95 g/m²)	
RWT =	$(2 \times PWTd)/LVIDd$

LV Remodelling

- LV remodelling describes how the LV changes in size, geometry, and function over time. LV wall mass (LVM) and relative wall thickness (RWT) measures can help categorize an increased LVM as concentric or eccentric.
- **Concentric hypertrophy** is ↑ LVM and ↑ RWT with no LV cavity enlargement and preserved LV function from pressure overload (hypertension, AS).
- **Eccentric hypertrophy** is ↑ LVM and normal RWT with LV cavity enlargement but preserved LV function (MR, AI).
- **Concentric remodelling** is normal LVM with ↑ RWT from high peripheral resistance, low cardiac index, and increased arterial stiffness and is often an early response to pressure overload (hypertension, AS).

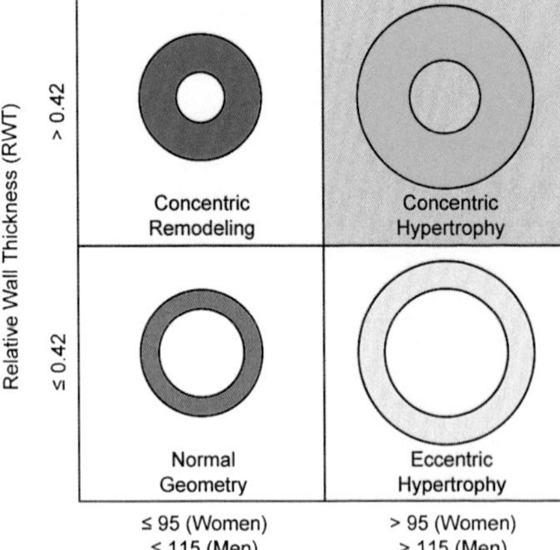

Wall Stress

- Wall stress is the force/unit area exerted on myocardium and depends on cavity dimensions, pressure, and wall thickness.
- Measures of wall stress are most useful in ventricular pressure and volume overload states (hypertension, AS, AI, MR) to evaluate systolic function. The benefit of calculating wall stress is that it is theoretically less load-dependent than other indices of systolic ejection (EF, FAC). Typically, end-systolic calculations of circumferential and longitudinal stress are used clinically.

Global Systolic Function

- Assessment of LV systolic function is a common indication for echocardiography.
- Qualitative assessment is easier to perform and is often used to "eyeball" the ejection fraction (EF). Quantitative assessment of LV systolic function may vary from simple to more complex methods. This involves determining changes in LV volume by measuring stroke volume (SV) and calculating EF. It is challenging to make accurate LV volume calculations using TEE as there may be inadequate endocardial border definition and LV foreshortening.
- Simple linear and area measures are converted to indices that assess LV systolic performance, but should not be confused with measurements of EF. Limitations for many of these systolic indices are the assumptions of: (a) uniform global LV function without regional wall motion abnormalities (RWMA), (b) symmetric LV shape, and (c) load dependence (preload and afterload).
- There are no normative values for TEE, the values listed below refer to TTE data.

LV Systolic Indices

Dimensions

- Linear Measurements
  - Fractional Shortening (FS)
- Area Measurements
  - Fractional Area Change (FAC)
- Volume Calculations, Ejection Fraction
  - Teicholz
  - Quinones
  - Area-Length
  - Method of Discs (MOD)
  - 3-Dimensional Volume
- Mitral Annular Motion
  - Mitral Annular Planar Systolic Excursion (MAPSE)

Spectral Doppler

- Stroke Volume (SV)/Cardiac Output (CO)
- Myocardial Performance Index (MPI)
- Rate of Pressure Rise (dP/dt)
- Velocity Circumferential Shortening (Vcf)

Tissue Doppler

- Systolic Mitral Annular Velocity (Sm)
- Strain
  - Global Longitudinal Peak Systolic Strain (GLPSS)
- Strain Rate

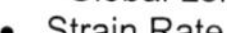

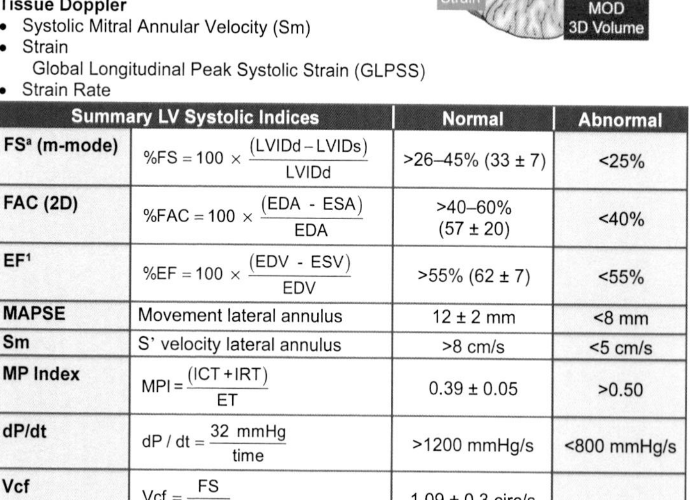

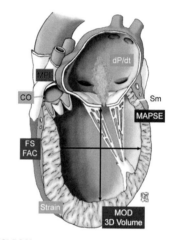

Summary LV Systolic Indices		Normal	Abnormal
FS[a] (m-mode)	$\%FS = 100 \times \frac{(LVIDd - LVIDs)}{LVIDd}$	>26–45% (33 ± 7)	<25%
FAC (2D)	$\%FAC = 100 \times \frac{(EDA - ESA)}{EDA}$	>40–60% (57 ± 20)	<40%
EF[1]	$\%EF = 100 \times \frac{(EDV - ESV)}{EDV}$	>55% (62 ± 7)	<55%
MAPSE	Movement lateral annulus	12 ± 2 mm	<8 mm
Sm	S' velocity lateral annulus	>8 cm/s	<5 cm/s
MP Index	$MPI = \frac{(ICT + IRT)}{ET}$	0.39 ± 0.05	>0.50
dP/dt	$dP/dt = \frac{32\ mmHg}{time}$	>1200 mmHg/s	<800 mmHg/s
Vcf	$Vcf = \frac{FS}{LVET}$	1.09 ± 0.3 circ/s	–
GLPSS[b]	Speckle tracking vendor-dependent	>–20 (more negative)	<–20 (more positive)

[a]Lang R, et al. J Am Soc Echocardiogr 2005;18:1440–63
[b]Lang R, et al. J Am Soc Echocardiogr 2015;28:1–39

Fractional Shortening (FS)

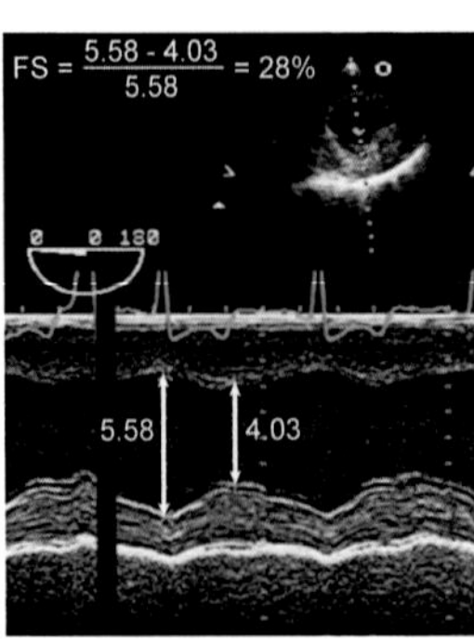

- FS estimates LV systolic function using linear measurements of LV internal diameters at end-diastole (LVIDd) and end-systole (LVIDs). These measures may be obtained from a TG mid-SAX view using 2D or m-mode.
- FS only assesses mid or basal segments and poorly reflects the overall LV function particularly with RWMA and an abnormal chamber shape.
- Not a recommended method (ASE) to assess LV

$$FS(\%) = \frac{LVID_d - LVID_s}{LVID_d} \times 100\%$$

Normal FS > 26 – 45% (Lang 2005)
Male: 25 – 43%, Female: 27 – 45%

Fractional Area Change (FAC)

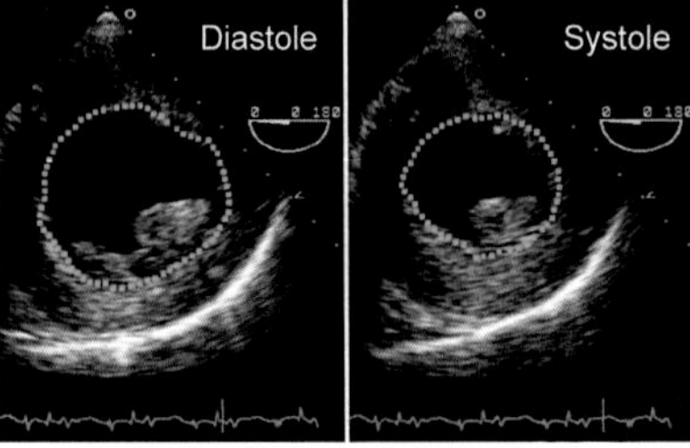

- FAC estimates LV systolic function using area measurements. This is not the ejection fraction as it is not a volume measurement. Endocardium is traced, excluding the papillary muscles, in a TG mid-SAX view at end-diastole (EDA) for the largest and in end-systole (ESA) for the smallest areas. The FAC varies slightly depending on the LV level, increasing from base to apex.
- Like FS, it assumes global dysfunction without RWMA. A high FAC (>80%) is associated with significant pathology (low SVR, AI, MR, VSD) that has a normal EDA and small ESA which helps distinguish these from hypovolemia with a small EDA and ESA.

$$FAC(\%) = \frac{LVD\,area \quad LVS\,area \times 100\%}{LVD\,area}$$

Normal FAC 45–80%
Base: >40%, Mid: >50%, Apex >60%
Male: 56–62%, Female: 59–65%

FAC <20%: LV failure
FAC >80%: hypovolemia, low SVR, AI, MR

---

dP/dt

- Rate of rise of intra-ventricular pressure (dP/dt) during systole can be estimated from the mitral regurgitation (MR) CW Doppler trace. It represents an isovolumic phase index of LV contractility that may be less load-dependent than FAC or EF.
- Measure the time (dt) taken for velocity to increase from 1 to 3 m/s. Calculate dP as 36 mmHg (3 m/s) –4 mmHg (1 m/s) = 32 mmHg and divide by the measured dt to obtain a value. This is a useful method for patients with significant MR to assess LV function, but is not useful if there is trivial MR, eccentric MR, or RWMA.
- Place caliper on the upslope of the MR jet at 1 and 3 m/s, and measure time. The calculation is automatically made by the ultrasound machine.

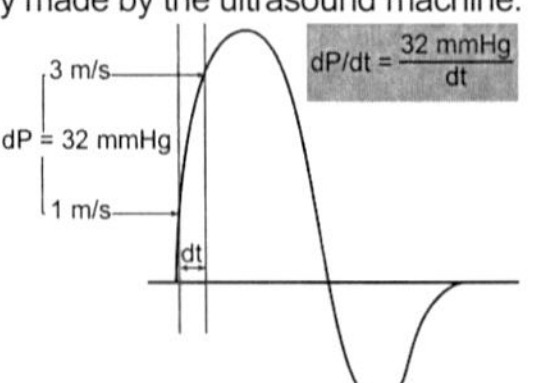

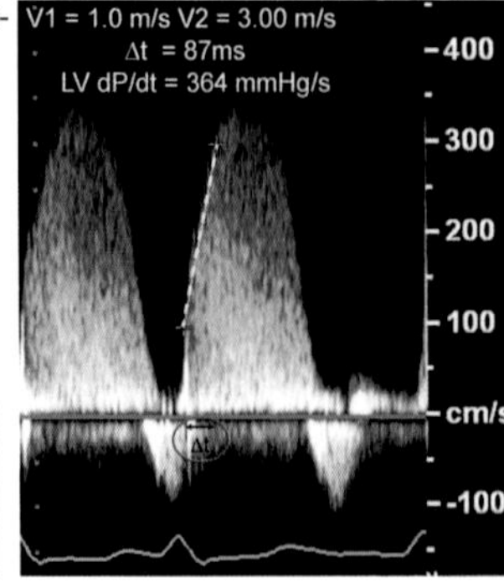

Normal >1200 mmHg/s (dt <26 ms)
Borderline: 800–1200 mmHg/s
Reduced LV: <800 mmHg/s (dt > 40 ms)
Severe LV: <500 mmHg/s (dt >64 ms)

Myocardial Performance Index (MPI) or Tei Index

- The right and left ventricular MPI incorporates both systolic and diastolic time intervals, as measured by Doppler, to assess systolic and diastolic function.
- The sum of the isovolumic contraction time (ICT) and the isovolumic relaxation time (IRT) is divided by the ejection time (ET).
- Value is independent of arterial pressure, HR, ventricular geometry, atrioventricular valve regurgitation, afterload, and preload. Systolic dysfunction manifests as an ↑ ICT, ↑ IRT, and ↓ ET, resulting in MPI >0.50.
- Obtain TEI Index time measures from PW Doppler spectral traces of MV inflow and LVOT outflow.

LV MPI normal: 0.39 ± 0.05
Abnormal LV MPI >0.50

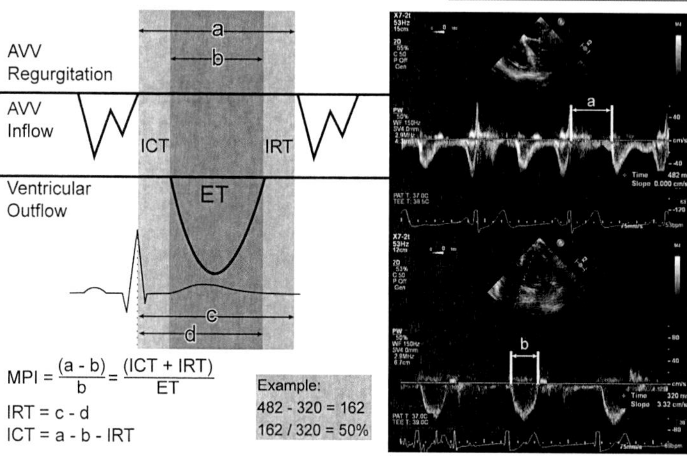

Circumferential Fiber Shortening (Vcf)

- This index of systolic function reflects the mean velocity of ventricular circumferential shortening of the LV minor axis over time (LVET, left ventricular ejection time) and is described by this equation.
- LV fractional shortening is calculated and divided by LV ejection time obtained from a LVOT spectral Doppler trace. The value is less preload-dependent than EF.

$\text{Mean Vcf} = \frac{FS}{LVET} = \frac{LVID_d^2 - LVID_s^2}{LVID_d \times LVET}$	**Normal** 1.09 ± 0.3 circ/s

Mitral Annulus Velocity (S′)

- Longitudinal myocardial velocity of the LV can be assessed using tissue Doppler imaging (TDI) at the lateral MV annulus (see pp. 54–55). This measure is limited by mitral annular calcification (MAC), RWMA, and poor Doppler alignment.
- The S′ wave estimates global EF, but is not a surrogate measure of contractility.

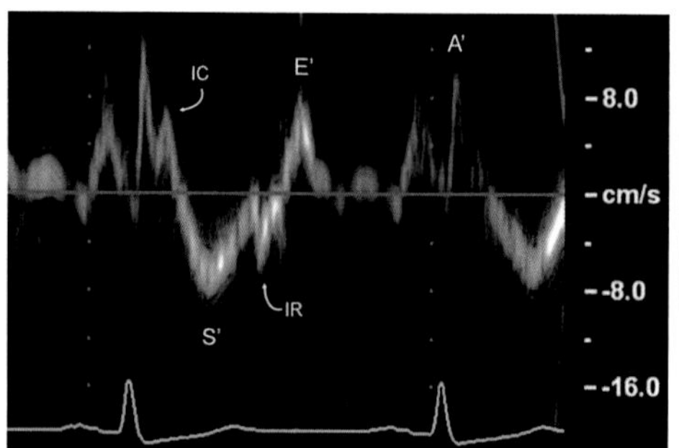

Mitral Annulus S'
Normal value:
S′ > 8 cm/s
S′ < 5 cm/s estimates an EF < 50%

Ventricular Volumes

- The LV has a relatively symmetric geometry, so various mathematical models using 2D imaging and m-mode measurements can be used to calculate ventricular volumes in systole and diastole.
- Use of these models is based on assumptions: (a) LV is a prolate ellipse with (b) equal short axis and a long axis twice the short axis, and (c) uniform wall motion.

Ejection Fraction (EF)

- This is the percent of LV diastolic volume ejected during systole and can be obtained by calculating the stroke volume (SV) and dividing by the end diastolic volume (EDV). The SV is the EDV–ESV.
- EF is not significantly related to age, sex, or body size. EF is not the same as cardiac output (CO) which is also calculated from SV.

$$EF\% = \frac{EDV - ESV}{EDV} \times 100\%$$

EF (%)	Normal	Mild	Mod	Severe
Male	52–72	41–51	30–40	<30
Female	54–74	41–53	30–40	<30
Lang R, et al. J Am Soc Echocardiogr 2015; 28:1–39				

Teicholz Method

- TG mid-SAX view
- M-mode through the center, measure EDD, ESD diameters
- Calculate EDV and ESV, then EF

$$EF\% = \frac{EDD^3 - ESD^3}{EDD^3} \times 100\%$$

- Volume = D^3, this assumes the LV length is twice the diameter

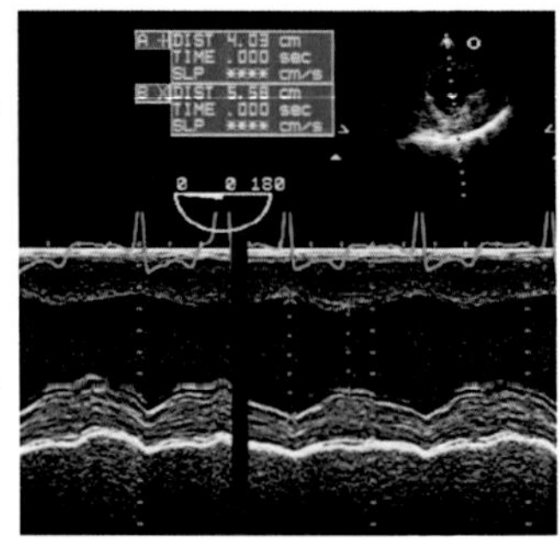

Modified Teicholz

Use if LV shape changes to be spherical

$$LV\ Vol = \frac{(7)}{2.4 + EDD} \times EDD^3$$

For all linear techniques:

- None are recommended by the ASE
- Assume: normal global function
  normal LV shape
- Limitations:
  poor endocardial definition, RWMA

Quinones

- Calculate radial EF%, estimate overall EF%, but correct for longitudinal EF%
- Longitudinal correction factor (EF%) = constant × (100-radial EF%)

$$Radial\ EF\% = \frac{EDD^2 - ESD^2}{EDD^2} \times 100\%$$

Quinones Constant
Normal 0.1
Hypokinetic 0.05
Akinetic 0
Dyskinetic –0.05

Area-Length

- Trace endocardial border at ES and ED using a single view (ME 4C or ME 2C)
- Start and end at the MV annulus which automatically closes the area loop
- Determine the LV apex (avoid foreshortening of LV)
- Calculate

$$SV = \frac{0.85\ (area\ LV\ SAX)^2}{LV\ LAX\ length}$$

- Normal SV = EDV—ESV
  ME 4C = 57 ± 13 (37–94) cc/m^2
  ME 2C = 63 ± 13 (37–101) cc/m^2

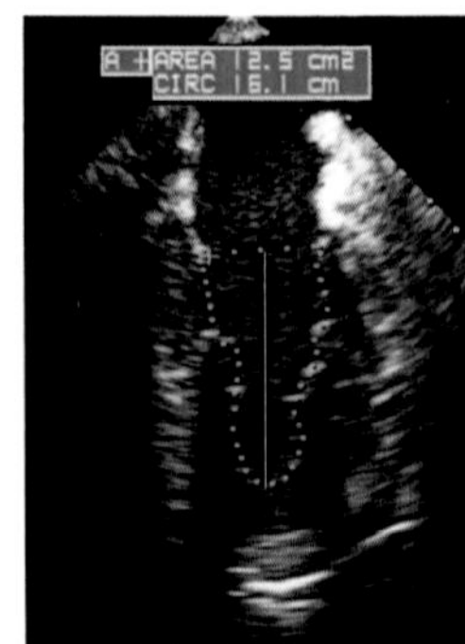

Method of Discs (MOD) or Modified Simpson's Method

- This method divides the ventricle into 20 discs and measures and sums the volume of each of the discs at end-diastole (EDV) and end-systole (ESV).
- The endocardial border is traced at ED, ES in ME 4C and 2C views. Depending on the software used, the border is manually traced beginning and ending at the MV annulus which closes the volume loop. The apex is identified and the volume is displayed. Alternatively, points are identified at the edges of the MV annulus and LV apex. The endocardial border is tracked (and modified) to produce a volume.
- Calculate: SV = EDV – ESV
- Calculate EF(%) = SV/EDV
- This method is recommended by the ASE
- It is useful if LV shape is distorted or RWMA

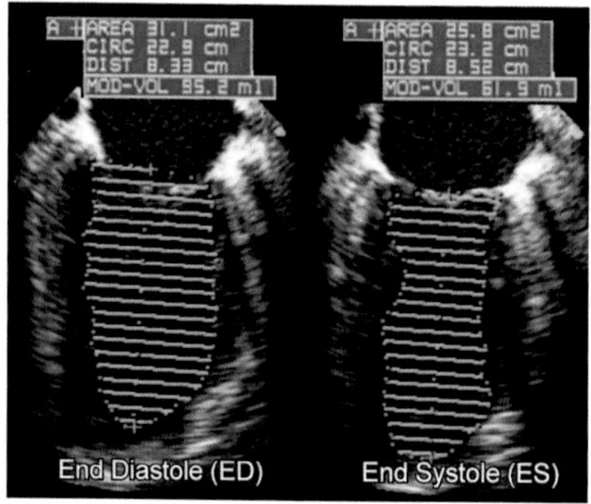

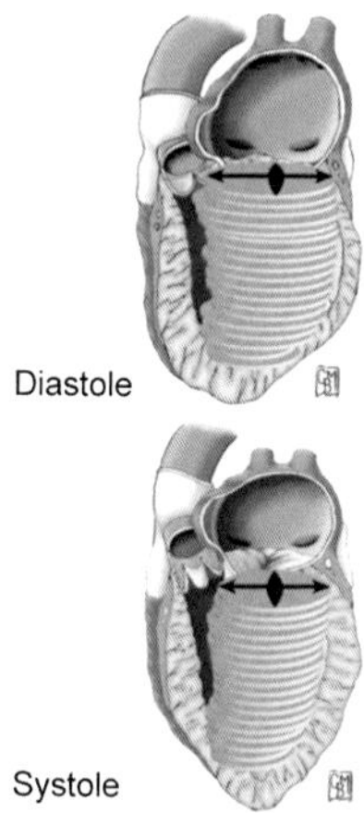

Automated Ejection Fraction (EF)

- Automated 2D Cardiac Quantification (a2DQ) with Anatomical Intelligence software using the Epiq 7 ultrasound machine (Philips Healthcare, Andover, MA) employs a semi-automated technique of speckle tracking to rapidly determine LV volumes, EF, ejection time, and early filling fraction.
- (a) Use a standard 2D ME 4C or 2C view, to identify a region of interest (ROI) by placing points at the MV annulus and cardiac apex. (b) Without manual tracing, the endocardial border is automatically defined by speckle tracking for each frame of the cardiac cycle. For better agreement, the endocardial border can be manually edited by adjusting points along the border.
- The LV volume in each frame is calculated by Simpson's MOD to produce a volume curve over the cardiac cycle. The maximum volume at ED and minimum volume at end-systole are measured and the EF is calculated and displayed.

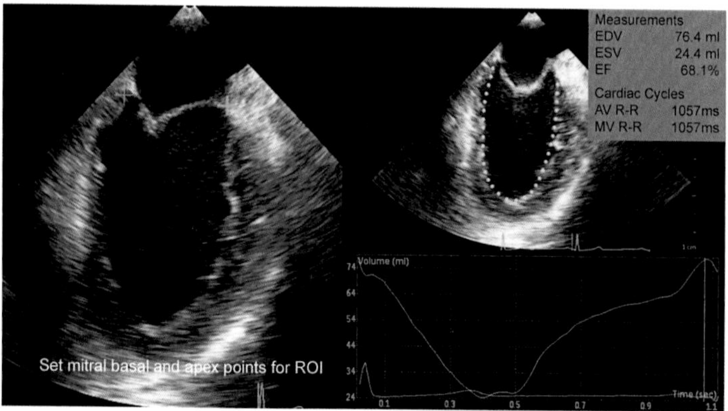

3D Ventricular Volumes

LV volumes are measured with RT 3D TEE using 2 methods: 3D–guided biplanes or direct volumetric analysis. Both methods use a LV full volume (FV) dataset exported for analysis into a quantification software (3DQ QLab, Philips Medical Systems).

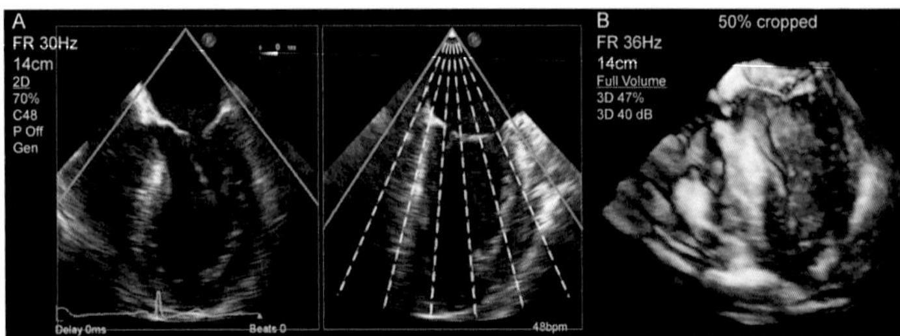

3D–Guided Biplanes

(A) In this software, the FV 3D dataset is displayed on three MPRs (multiplanar reconstructions **G**reen, **R**ed, **B**lue). (B) Red and green planes are adjusted to cut along the LV long axis at the true apex. Ideal (C) ME 4C and (D) ME 2C views are created that minimize LV foreshortening. The endocardium and the epicardium are manually traced in diastole and systole. Automated measurements and calculations include: Stroke Volume, Ejection Fraction, End-Diastolic and End-Systolic Volumes, LV Mass.

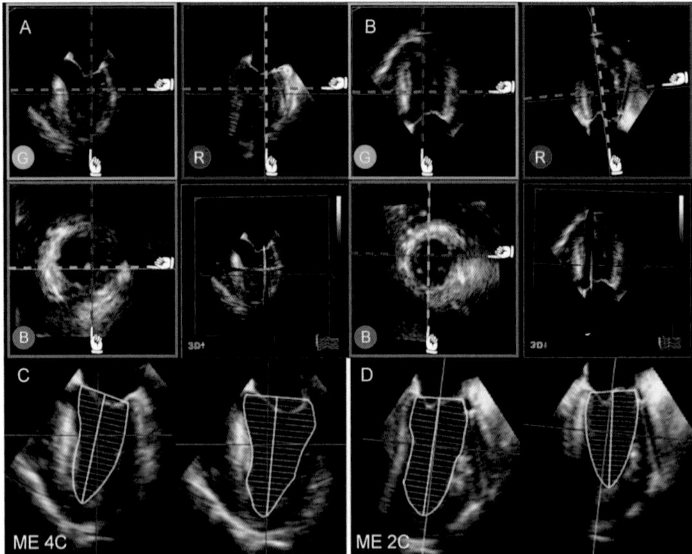

3D Direct Volumetric Analysis

- This can assess global systolic function by using a semi-automated method for direct LV volume measurement.
- Following sequence analysis, a 3D endocardial shell is surface-rendered with a graph of LV volume over time for each frame of the cardiac loop (see next page).
- EDV and ESV are measured and SV and EF are automatically calculated and shown. Maximum (blue) and minimum (red) ventricular volumes are shown by the dots. EDV and ESV are determined using the voxel count and thus differs from the single frame method of discs (see p. 75).
- This technique slightly overestimates ventricular volumes, but it is currently the ASE preferred method for LV volume assessment.

To generate a dynamic LV endocardial cast, the 3D FV dataset is imported into analytical software (3DQA, QLab, Philips Medical Systems) and analyzed as follows:

1. Identify the end-diastolic frame
2. Align MPR axis (red and green lines) through the LV apex in 2C and 4C views
3. Identify the middle of the IVS in the blue pane using the yellow arrow
4. Add reference points to the LV walls (4C S + L, 2C I + A) and apex
5. Repeat procedure for the end-systolic frame

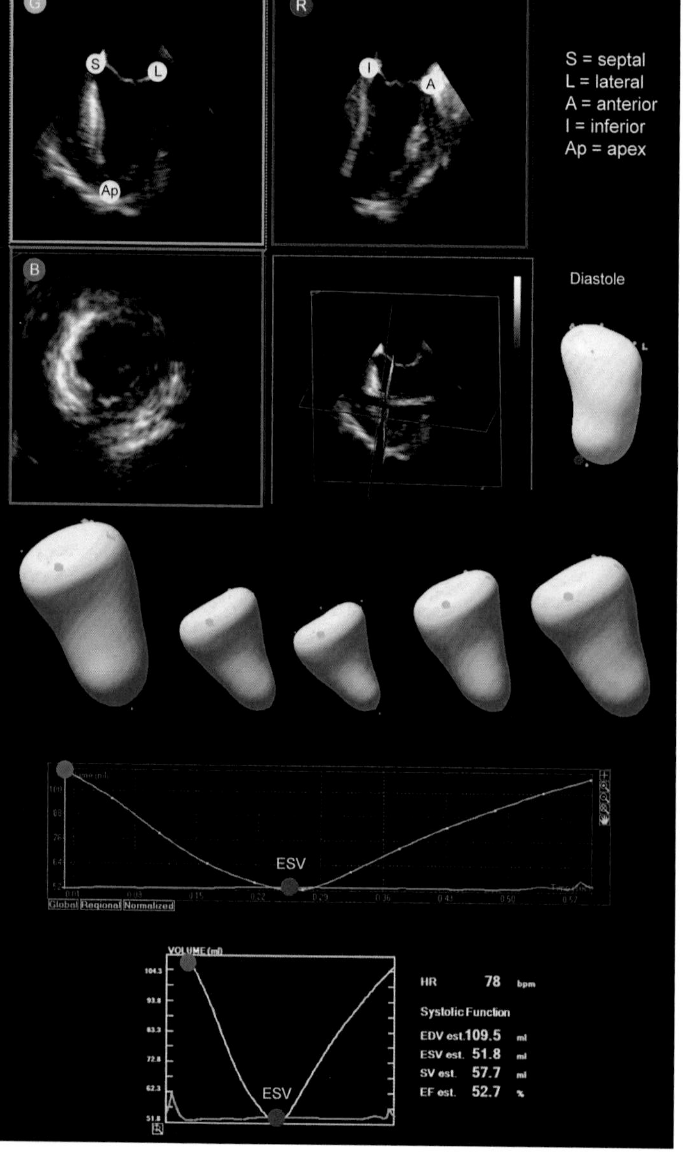

Doppler Method

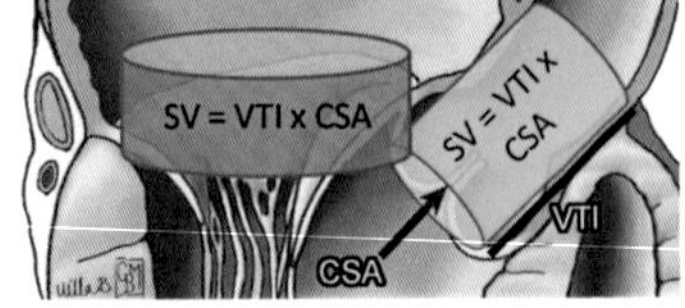

- Stroke volume (SV) across the valves, either during systole or diastole, can be calculated using spectral Doppler by measuring the annular diameter and the velocity time integral (VTI).
- Cross-sectional area (CSA) is calculated using the formula of a circle as CSA = $\pi r^2 = 0.785d^2$.
- The VTI is the cumulative distance (stroke distance in cm) that rbcs travel and is obtained by tracing the spectral Doppler profile.
- SV is the total amount of blood leaving the ventricle during systole and includes both antegrade and retrograde flow. SV estimates obtained by Doppler do not rely on any geometric assumptions about the LV cavity, and thus may better assess LV function with abnormal geometry.

$$SV = CSA \times VTI$$
$$(cm^3) = (cm^2) \times (cm)$$

- The cardiac output (CO) is the amount of blood through the systemic circulation over time (L/min) and can be calculated as:

$$\text{Cardiac output (CO)} = \text{Stroke volume (SV)} \times \text{Heart rate (HR)}$$

- Cardiac output is not the LVEF as the two may have different values depending on the disease state. In mitral regurgitation and hypovolemia, EF is excellent as the LV ejects nearly all the volume that fills it, but CO is reduced as not all the blood flows into the peripheral circulation. In aortic insufficiency, CO is high as blood continues to fill the LV during diastole, but EF is low as not all the end-diastolic volume is ejected.

Right Ventricle Stroke Volume

VTI = pulmonary artery PW/CW × CSA = $0.785d^2$ (d = PA or PV) = SV_{RV}

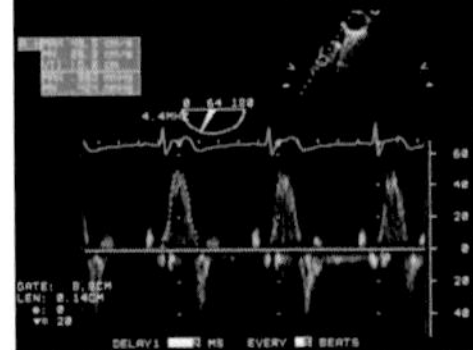

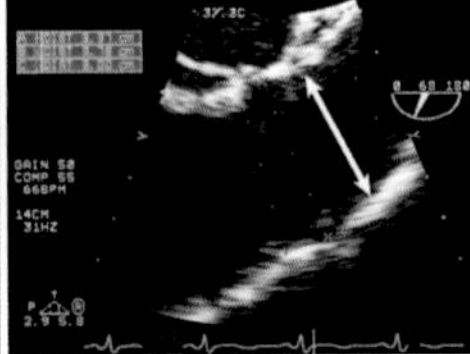

VTI = 10.8cm
CSA = 0.785 $(3cm)^2$
SV = 10.8 x 9
= 97cc

Transaortic Stroke Volume

VTI = aortic valve CW × CSA = $0.785d^2$ (d = AV LAX) = $SV_{transaortic}$

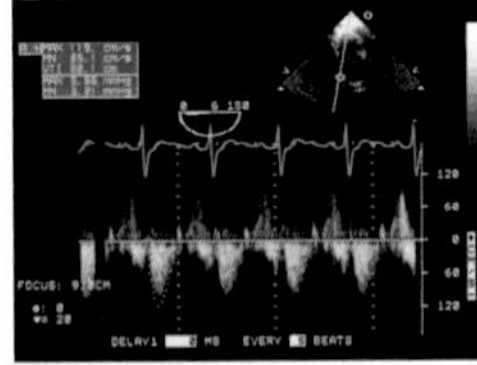

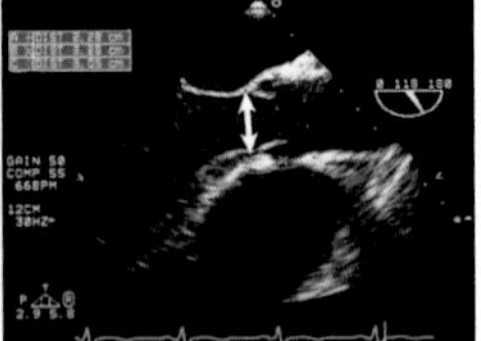

VTI = 22.1cm
CSA = 0.785 $(2.3cm)^2$
SV = 22.1 x 4.15
= 92cc

LVOT Stroke Volume

VTI = PW at LVOT × CSA = $0.785d^2$ (d = TG LVOT) = SV_{LVOT}

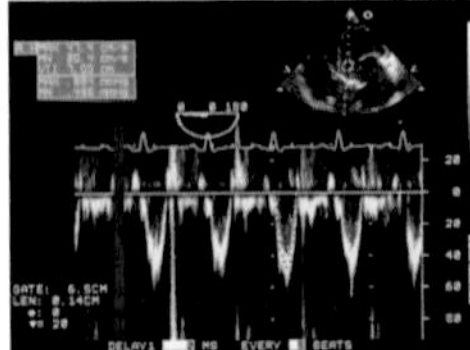

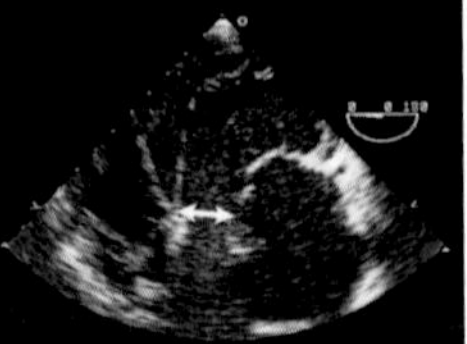

VTI = 16.8cm
CSA = 0.785 $(2cm)^2$
SV = 16.8 x 3.14
= 53cc

Mitral Annular Plane Systolic Excursion (MAPSE)

- MAPSE is similar to TAPSE and is measured using m-mode at the lateral MV annulus.
- MAPSE evaluates only LV longitudinal motion and has a strong association with systolic EF only if the LV is normal or dilated.
- The technique has high temporal resolution and relies less on 2D image quality. Measurement is limited by angle dependency (inadequate m-mode alignment), pre/afterload, and RWMA.
- Despite limitations, MAPSE may detect early reduction in longitudinal motion with a normal EF that occurs in certain cardiac pathologies (hypertension, acute MI, aortic stenosis).

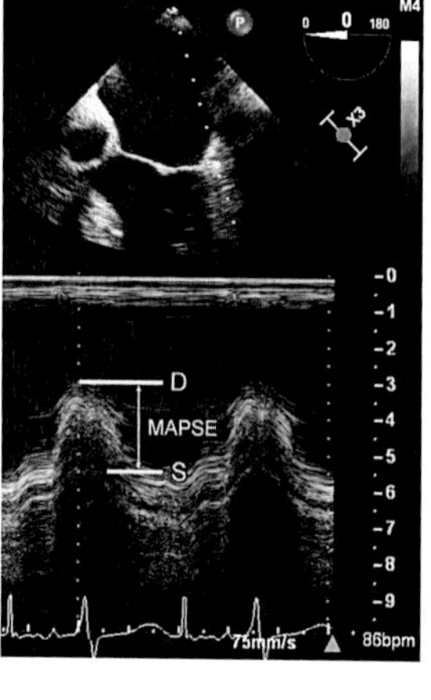

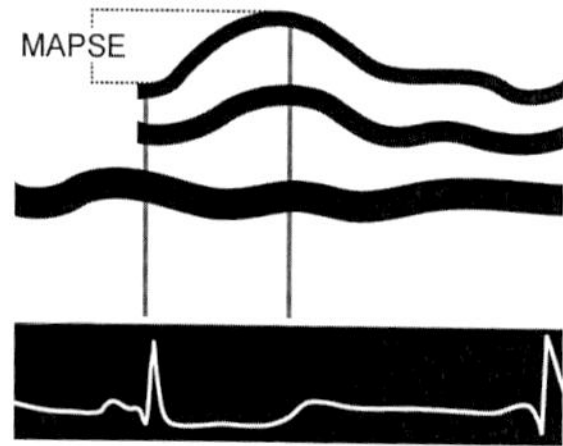

Normal MAPSE: 12 ± 2 mm
MAPSE < 8 mm → EF < 50%

Tissue Mitral Annular Displacement (TMAD)

- Mitral annulus displacement (MAD) during the cardiac cycle can be determined by different echocardiographic techniques, M-mode (see above), color TDI, and 2D speckle tracking echocardiography (STE), which are not interchangeable.
- Assessment of global LV longitudinal systolic function using MAD can give incremental information to LVEF. A reduced TMAD with ischemic, valvular, and HCM may indicate early subclinical longitudinal systolic dysfunction despite preserved LVEF.
- TMAD by 2D STE is a simple option to measure MAD from any angle using standard ME 2C, 4C views. Automated 2D Cardiac Quantification software (Philips Medical Systems) 3 regions of interest are identified by placing points at the mitral annulus (leaflet/LV level) and cardiac apex (use epicardium). MAD (in mm) towards the apex is displayed for the cardiac cycle:
  - TMAD MV 1 (inferior)
  - TMAD MV 2 (anterior)
  - TMAD MV midpoint
- TMAD MV midpoint normalizes for LV length, as the ratio of chamber length (EDL-ESL/EDL)
- By using a quadratic formula, TMAD midpoint can estimate the LVEF with good correlation to MRI.

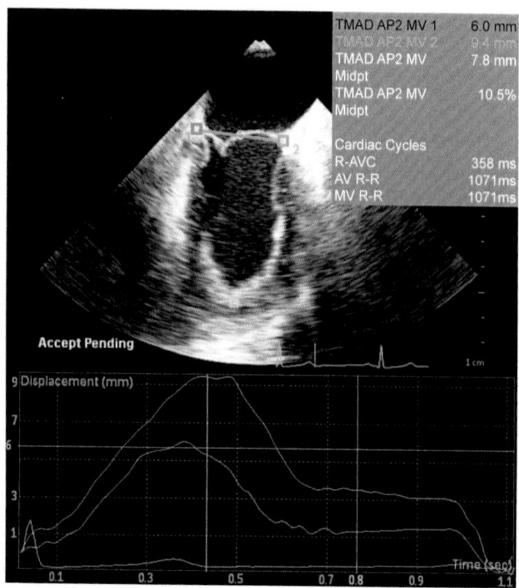

Myocardial Deformation

- Ventricular contraction involves complex movements during the cardiac cycle. The actual volume of myocardial tissue remains unchanged, but the myocardium changes shape or deforms in 3 dimensions: longitudinal, radial, and circumferential (see p. 64). Strain and Strain Rate can analyze ventricular deformation to more accurately quantify global and regional ventricular function.
- **Strain (ε)** looks at the motion-deformation between two points in the myocardial wall. Strain importantly discriminates passive movement (tethering or translational) from true contraction as it is unrelated to motion towards the transducer. The total deformation in all dimensions is related to a % change from the initial length (L0): **Strain (ε) = (L−L0)/L.** It is a single dimensionless (%) parameter. Negative strain occurs when fibers shorten (circumferential + longitudinal) or thin (radial). Positive strain occurs when fibers thicken (radial) or lengthen (circumferential + longitudinal). Measurement of end-systolic strain estimates ejection fraction.
- **Strain rate (SR)** is the speed of deformation or the change in strain over time (1/s), **SR = Δ strain/Δ time** = **Δ velocity/L** (where L is the initial distance between given tissue area). Peak systolic SR is a measure of contractility.

Myocardial Deformation Imaging

- Two methods can assess myocardial deformation:
  - (A) **Tissue Doppler Imaging (TDI)** uses offline analysis of tissue Doppler velocities from different myocardial regions for strain and strain rate traces. TDI is limited by incomplete dataset (reverberations, dropout) and poor Doppler alignment.
  - (B) **2D speckle tracking echocardiography (STE)** tracks the speckles of different brightness and shape that comprise the grey-scale myocardial image. STE involves frame by frame analysis of the movement of a region of speckles (not individual speckles) to derive their direction and velocity (shift over time) of tissue movement relative to each other. Frame rate (FR) is important to speckle tracking; the best compromise is FR 60–100/s. If the FR is too high, the speckles move short distances making them difficult to analyze, if the FR is too low movements may be missed. STE is angle-independent and is less influenced by artifacts, though reverberations and dropout are problematic.

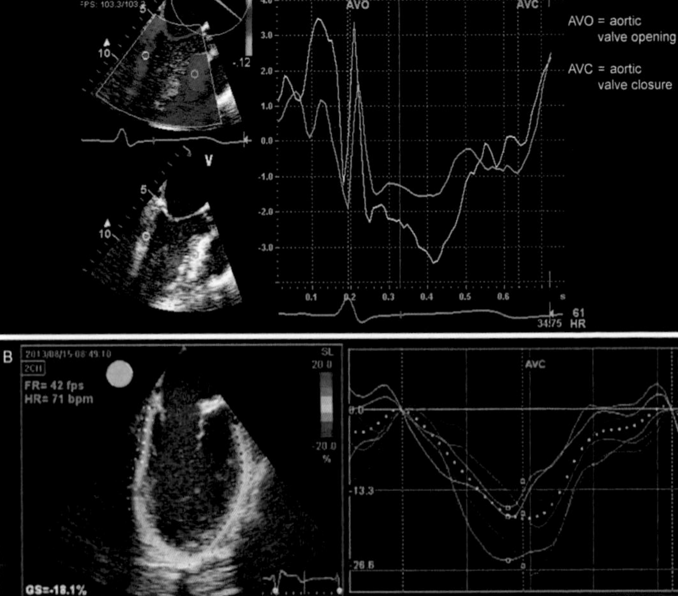

STE Technical Considerations

- Strain and strain rate determination by speckle tracking is currently available as machine software from different vendors for analysis of stored 2D images. The process begins by acquiring quality 2D images ME (4C, 2C, LAX), TG SAX (basal, mid, apical), followed by analysis + display using semi-automated software.
- **Quality 2D images** are required with (a) an appropriate depth to encompass the entire LV including the apex without foreshortening, (b) good endocardial definition by use of gain settings, (c) similar heart rate (<10% variation), and (d) an adequate FR 70–100/s. In the OR, it is best to obtain these optimized views early to avoid cautery artifact and consecutively for a similar FR and HR.
- **Analysis** of each view is semi-automated and only requires identification of the MV leaflet insertion points and LV apex to define the region of interest, the myocardial wall. (A) The entire myocardial wall is automatically segmented, labelled, and tracked during the cardiac cycle. Manual adjustment can be made to ensure the entire LV wall is included and tracked appropriately over the cardiac cycle. While any view can be analyzed, it is best to begin with the ME LAX view to identify the timing of aortic valve closure.
- **Display** is as (1) parametric transparent overlay over each wall using a color map (red/blue, red/green) for (C) strain and (D) SR, (2) graph of (C) strain and (D) SR for each wall segment over time, (3) a parametric bull's eye of (B) peak strain or time to peak strain of each LV wall segment. The graph has a white dotted line that indicates global function. The aortic valve closure (AVC) is indicated to determine time to peak strain and post-systolic strain index (see p. 104).

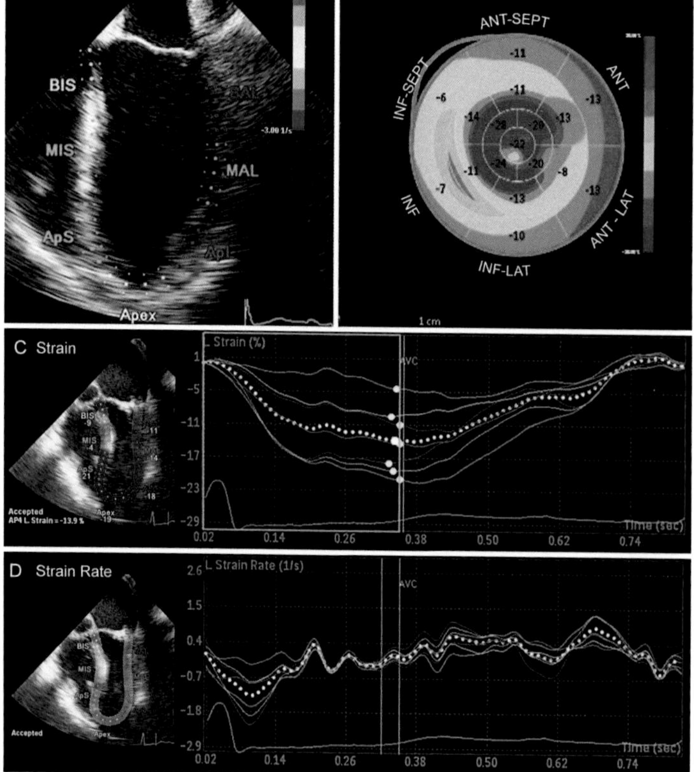

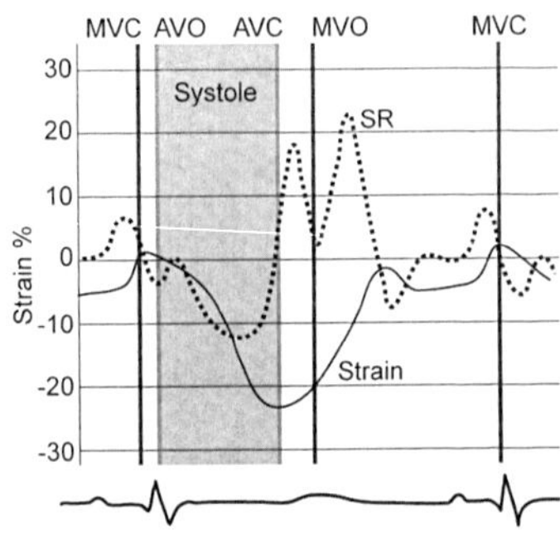

Myocardial strain plotted against time.

- **Strain** is negative for the entire cardiac cycle and is least (shortest myocardial length) in systole at the time of aortic valve closure (AVC). During diastole, strain is less negative, returns to 0 in 3 phases, plateaus with diastasis, and is at baseline with atrial contraction.
- **Strain Rate** is negative and positive during the cardiac cycle. In systole, SR peaks after aortic valve opening (AVO), then reduces before AVC. In diastole, there are 2 positive peaks.
- Timing is critical for proper curve analysis.
  - Normal systolic contraction ends with AVC.
  - Relaxation starts with mitral valve opening (MVO).

LV Systolic Function

- Longitudinal (ME views), circumferential (TG views), and rotational strain (TG views) can be assessed using vendor-specific ultrasound machine software.

(A) Analysis of circumferential strain includes: peak strain (systolic, post-systolic), peak strain rate, and time to peak strain recorded from multiple TG views (SAX B, basal; SAX M, mid; SAX A, apical). (B) Analysis of rotational strain from similar TG views refers to peak rotation (°), speed of rotation as peak rotation rate (°/s), and peak torsion (°/s) which is the difference between apical and basal rotation.

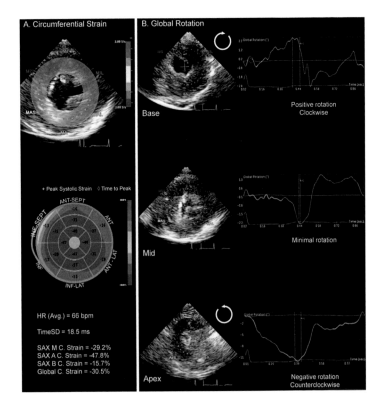

A. Circumferential Strain

+ Peak Systolic Strain ◊ Time to Peak

ANT-SEPT, ANT, ANT-LAT, INF-LAT, INF, INF-SEPT

HR (Avg.) = 66 bpm

TimeSD = 18.5 ms

SAX M C. Strain = -29.2%
SAX A C. Strain = -47.8%
SAX B C. Strain = -15.7%
Global C. Strain = -30.5%

B. Global Rotation

Base — Positive rotation Clockwise

Mid — Minimal rotation

Apex — Negative rotation Counterclockwise

- **Global Longitudinal Peak Systolic Strain (GLPSS)** assesses global systolic function. Obtain GLPSS values from all 6 LV walls in 3 ME views: 4C, 2C, LAX.
- Analysis by speckle tracking displays peak systolic strain (PSS) as an average of values for each wall. Often displayed as a colorized bulls eye with distribution of regional PSS, GLPSS is obtained by averaging all PSS values from each wall.
- Measurements of peak GLPSS vary among vendors and software versions.
- According to current guidelines, a GLPSS of −20% is normal and the lower the absolute strain value is below this value, the more likely it is abnormal.
- During ischemia, contraction is delayed and prolonged beyond AVC with a characteristic post-systolic peak. Detection of post-systolic shortening is a powerful tool to detect ongoing ischemia. This can be displayed on strain-curves, or in a colorized bulls eye view with regional distribution (see p. 105).
- Normal strain bull's eye shows all LV segments as deep red and −20 or below.

Examples of abnormal bull's eyes are shown. (A) A patient with hypertension and left ventricular hypertrophy shows pink basal segments and red apical segments, but normal GLPSS of −20.7 and an EF 62%. (B) A patient with coronary artery disease and a large anterior infarction from obstruction of the LAD artery shows lower strain in the anterior and antero-septal regions. GLPSS is low at −16.7 and an EF 52.8%. (C) A patient with non-ischemic cardiomyopathy shows diffusely abnormal segments without correlation to coronary anatomy. GLPSS is low at −16.9 and an EF 47.9%.

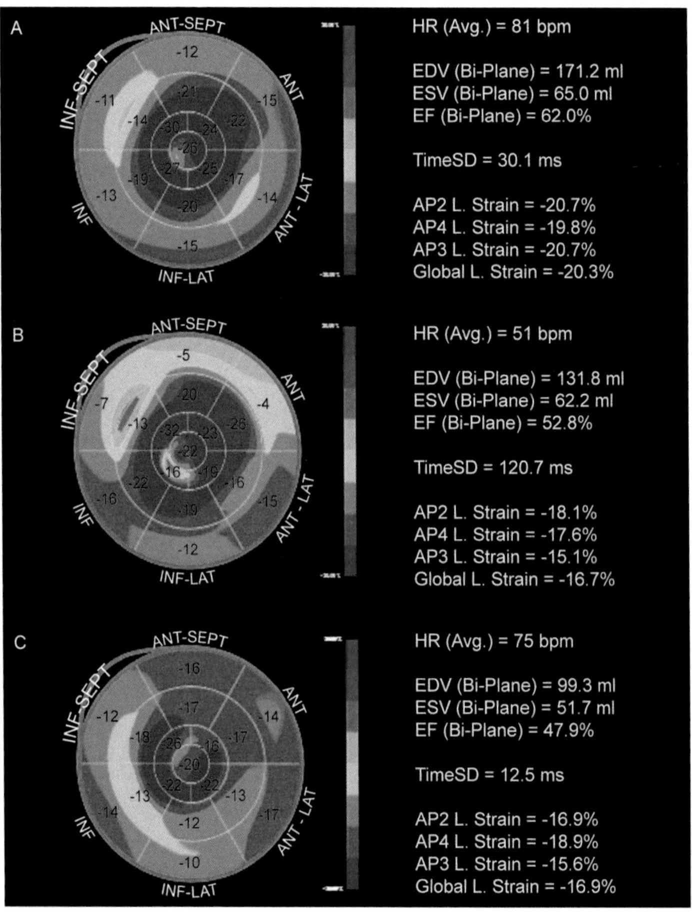

4
Right Ventricle

A. Vegas, *Perioperative Two-Dimensional Transesophageal Echocardiography*, https://doi.org/10.1007/978-3-319-60902-7_4

Right Ventricle Anatomy

- The normal RV is a crescent-shaped chamber that curves over the LV.
- The RV may be described by its inflow (sinus), outflow (conus) tract, and apical portions that relate to their separate embryologic origins. The heavily trabeculated RV inflow portion begins inferoposterior to the TV. The smooth-walled outflow portion is antero-superior and is the RV infundibulum (conus arteriosus) that ends at the pulmonic valve (PV).

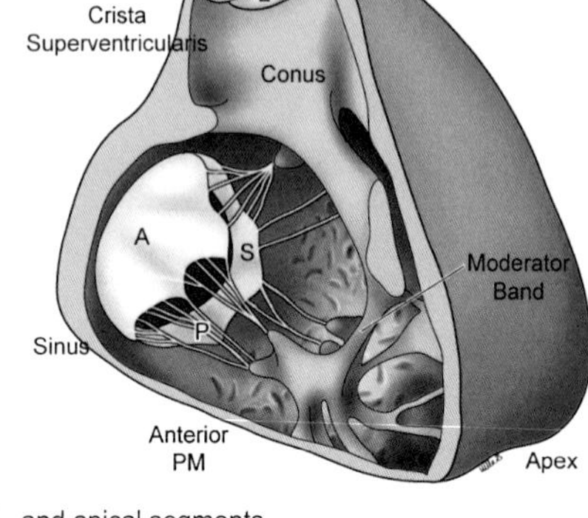

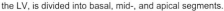

- An encircling muscular band of four distinct structures (parietal band, crista supraventricularis, septal band, moderator band) separates the RV regions. The moderator band between the anterior papillary muscle and septal wall is a prominent echodense structure that helps distinguish the RV from the LV.
- RV is composed of a free wall, interventricular septum (IVS), and apex. The RV free wall is described as lateral, anterior, and inferior portions and, like the LV, is divided into basal, mid-, and apical segments.
- There are three papillary muscles (PM), anterior PM (from anterior wall), posterior PM (from posterior wall), and a series of smaller septal papillae from the septal wall. Chordae tendinae pass from PM tips and septal wall to free margins and ventricular surfaces of all TV leaflets.

Coronary Blood Flow

- Acute marginal branch of the right coronary artery (RCA) supplies most coronary blood flow to the RV (see p. 100). In a left dominant circulation (10%), posterior descending artery from left anterior descending artery supplies RV inferior wall.
- The first septal perforator supplies the moderator band and the posterior septal perforators from the RCA supply the inferior (posterior) 1/3 of the IVS. In 30% of patients, a separate conus artery branch supplies the infundibulum.

RV Function

- RV contraction involves sequential peristaltic movement from the inlet to the apex then to the infundibulum. Shortening of the RV base towards the apex by contraction of the inner longitudinal configured myocardial fibers is a major contributor to RV ejection. There is also radial shortening by transverse myocardial fibers that creates a bellows-type motion of the RV free wall against the IVS. Unlike the LV, twisting and rotational movements contribute less to RV systolic pressure.

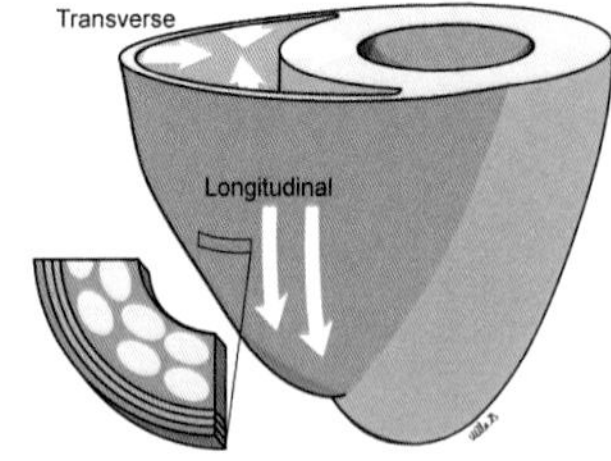

- The RV is structurally and mechanically distinct from the LV and responds differently in diseased states. The RV and LV are connected in series; the output of one ventricle is the input for the other. The RV is designed to function as a volume pump, while the LV is a pressure pump.
- RV ejection is coupled to a highly compliant pulmonary vasculature, with an inverse relationship of RVEF (↓) and pulmonary artery pressure (↑). Stroke volume is significantly reduced for the RV compared to the LV with a similar change in afterload. In contrast, the RV tolerates and adapts easily to volume overload.
- RV shape and function is significantly influenced by IVS position, particularly when either ventricle is affected by abnormal loading conditions. Over time, progressive contractile dysfunction causes RV dilatation. RV free wall works harder and eventually fatigues. RV failure worsens tricuspid regurgitation (TR) causing hepatic venous hypertension, which contributes to hepatic hypoxia and liver dysfunction.

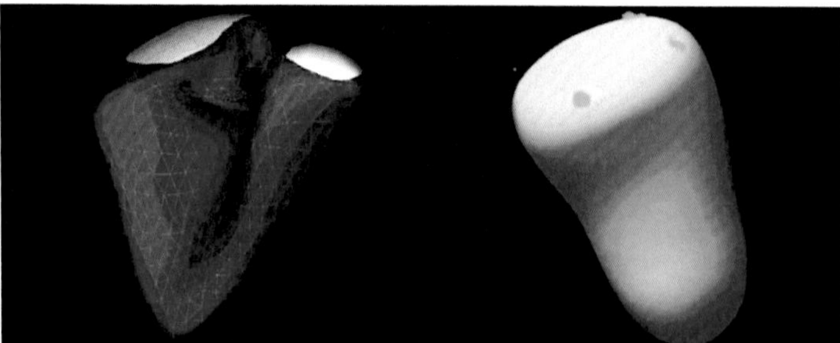

Normal Parameters	Right Ventricle	Left Ventricle
EDV, mL/m^2	75 ± 13	65 ± 12
Mass, g/m^2	26 ± 5	87 ± 12
Wall thickness, mm	2–5	7–11
Ventricular pressure, mmHg	25/4	130/8
PVR versus SVR, dynes.s.cm^{-5}	70	1100
Ejection fraction, %	40–45	50–55

EDV end-diastolic volume, *PVR* pulmonary vascular resistance, *SVR* systemic vascular resistance	RV volume larger than LV RV mass 1/6 of LV RVEF lower than LV

Ventricular Interdependence

- This is the direct mechanical effect of each ventricle on the other through changes in shape, size, and compliance. Interdependence in systole is mediated by the IVS, while in diastole it is mainly by the pericardium.
- Normally, the IVS functions as part of the LV as its motion is controlled by the center of greater cardiac mass located in the LV. RV dysfunction often occurs from problems with pressure overload, volume overload, or ischemia. The presence of distinctive patterns of abnormal septal motion is often the first clue to RV pressure or volume overload.
- **RV pressure overload,** there is leftward IVS shift throughout the cardiac cycle with most marked LV distortion at end-systole, at the time of peak RV afterload.
- **RV volume overload**, the IVS shift and flattening occurs mainly in mid-late diastole during peak RV filling. This reverses during systole, sparing LV deformation at end-systole, but causing paradoxical systolic septal motion toward the RV cavity.

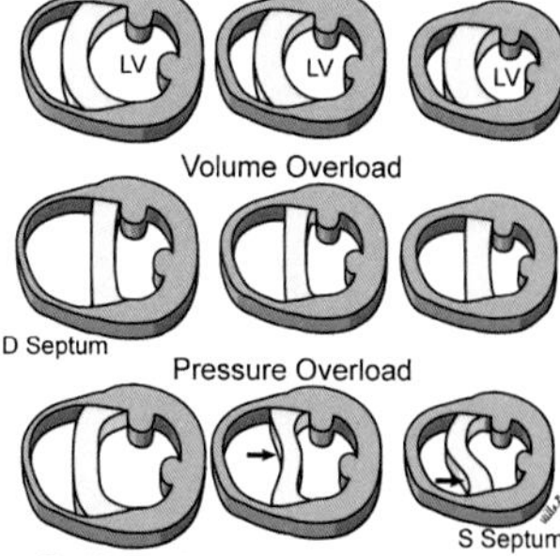

- Increased ventricular interdependence (tamponade and constrictive pericarditis) results in more exaggerated changes with respiration of TV and MV inflow velocities, and RV and LV size.

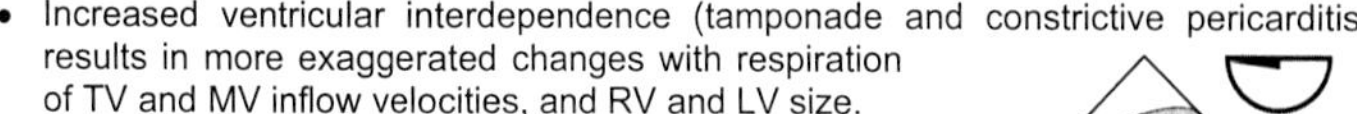

Eccentricity Index (EI)

- The EI is a measure of LV shape during different parts of the cardiac cycle and reflects abnormal IVS motion depending on the type of RV overload.
- To calculate EI, measure the (A) anterior-posterior and (B) lateral-septal internal LV diameters at end-diastole (ED) and end-systole (ES).
- A normal heart has an EI ratio of 1.
- RV volume overload, the septum shifts left at end-diastole, so EI > 1.
- RV pressure overload, the septum shifts left during end-systole and end-diastole, EI > 1.

RV B LV A

Eccentricity Index (EI) = A/B

Eccentricity Index = A/B
Normal = 1 at ED and ES
RV volume overload (ED) EI > 1
RV pressure overload (ES) EI > 1

Multiple TG and ME TEE views can assess the RV. Many views are modified from the standard TEE planes which often transect the RV, obliquely making even qualitative assessment of the RV challenging. Other TEE views are used to determine RV inflow (hepatic vein, right atrium), RV outflow (pulmonic valve, pulmonary artery), and estimate RV systolic pressure (RVSP) from TR (see p. 56). Distinguishing the RV from the LV is an important initial step in evaluating the RV. This relies on identifying anatomic features of the RV and not by measuring chamber size and wall thickness, both of which may become increased in pathological states.

Anatomic Features RV
1. Apical displacement of septal A-V valve leaflet
2. Moderator band
3. >2 papillary muscles
4. 3 leaflets of A-V valve
5. Separation inflow/outflow

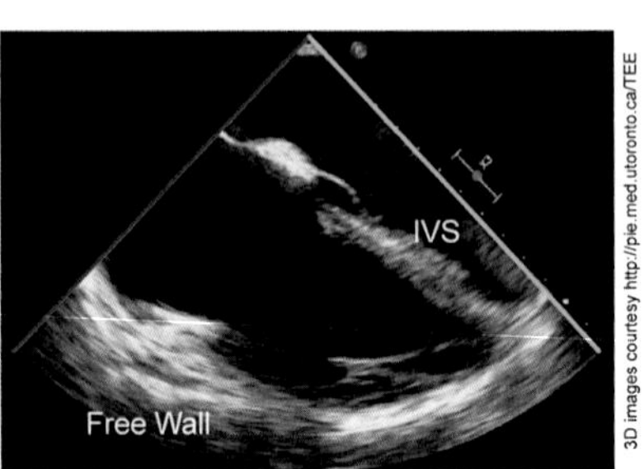

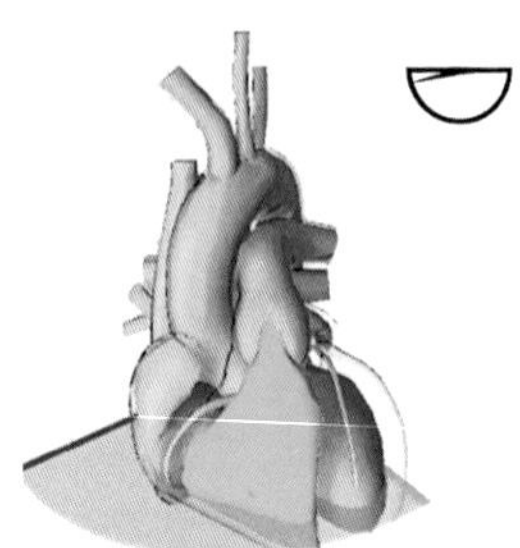

The modified **ME 4C view at 0°** (p. 7) is obtained by slightly turning the probe to the right, thus placing the RV in the display center. This view shows the RV free wall and interventricular septum (IVS) and is important for identifying the anatomic features of the RV, determining RV size and RV function (TAPSE or FAC).

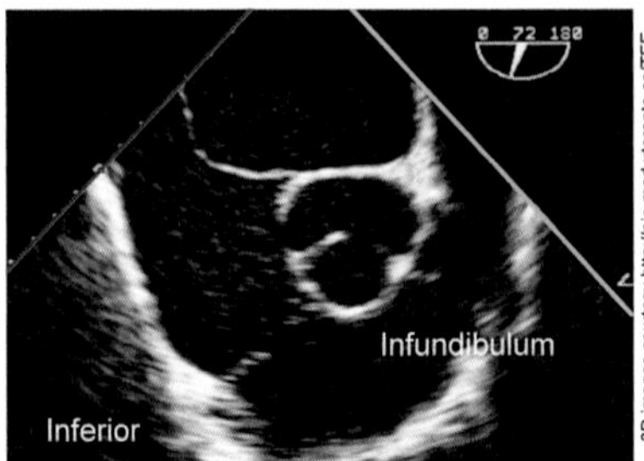

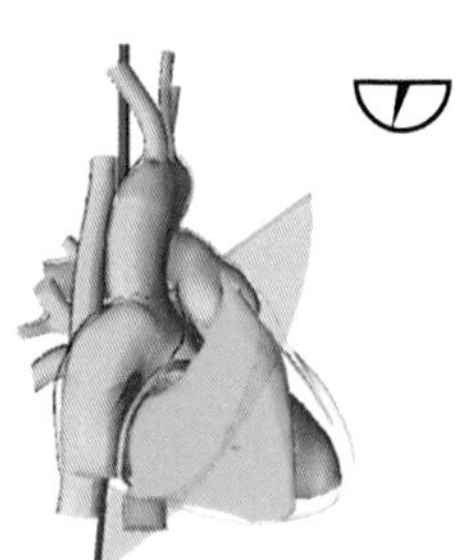

The standard **ME RV inflow-outflow view at 60–80°** (p. 16) shows the RV infundibulum, TV, pulmonic valve, and inferior RV wall. RV outflow tract (RVOT) and pulmonary artery (PA) size (p. 90) can be measured and RVOT wall motion assessed.

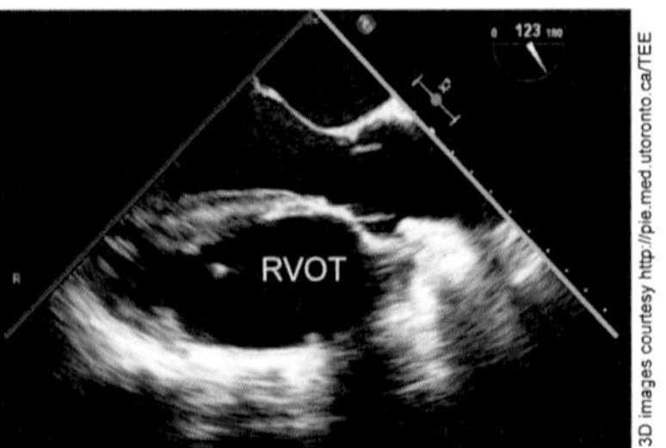

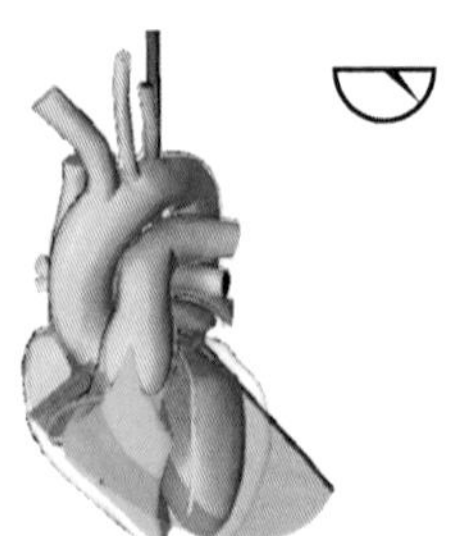

The standard **ME LAX view at 120°** (p.10) shows a portion of the RVOT and occasionally the pulmonic valve (PV) in short axis. RV dilatation, as show here, may displace the IVS into the LV outflow tract.

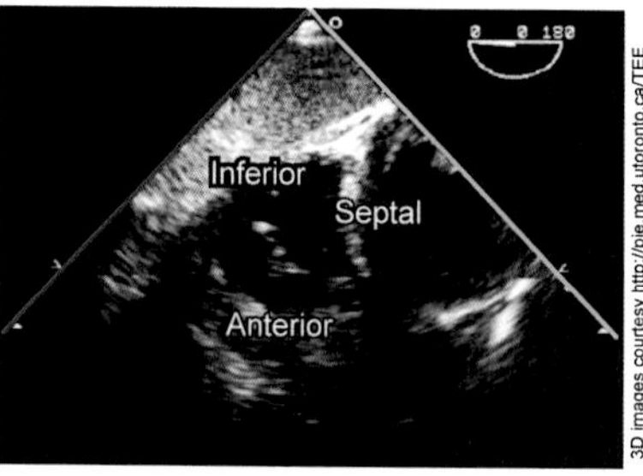

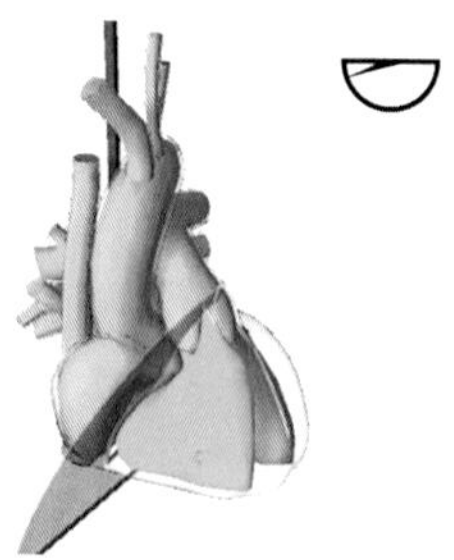

The modified **TG basal SAX view (0°)** is obtained by turning the probe right to center the TV in SAX and RV basal walls in the display. The septal wall abuts the LV, the inferior wall is closest, and the anterior-free wall furthest from the probe.

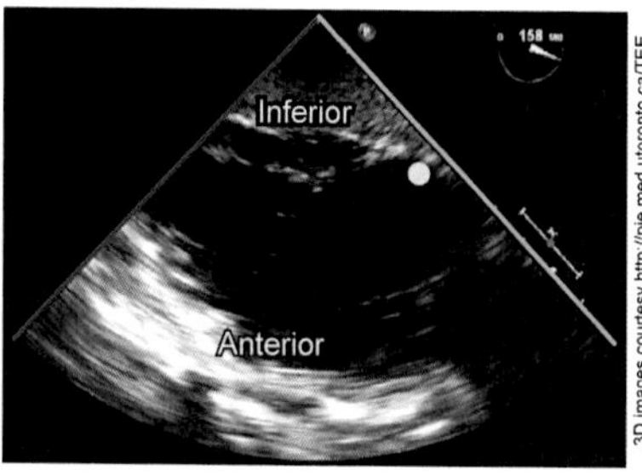

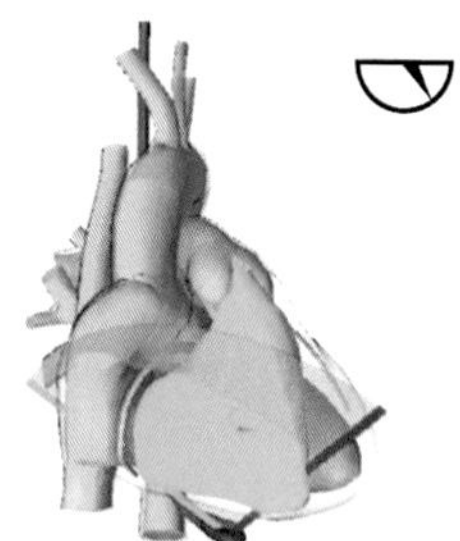

The standard **TG RV Inflow view at 120–150°** (p. 23) shows the anterior and inferior walls of the RV. This view permits good alignment along the basal inferior wall for m-mode (TAPSE) and TDI of S′ velocity at the lateral TV annulus (*yellow dot*).

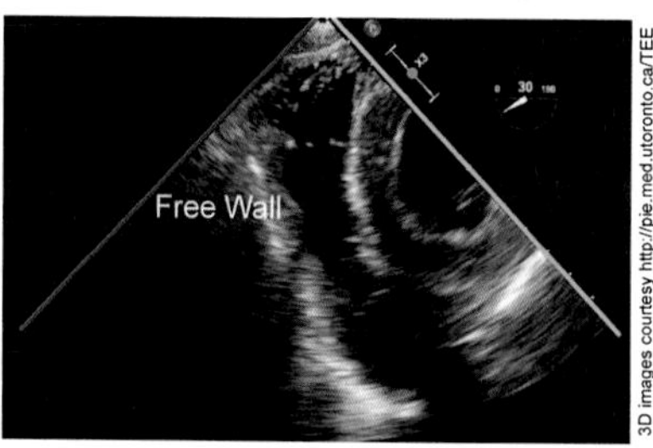

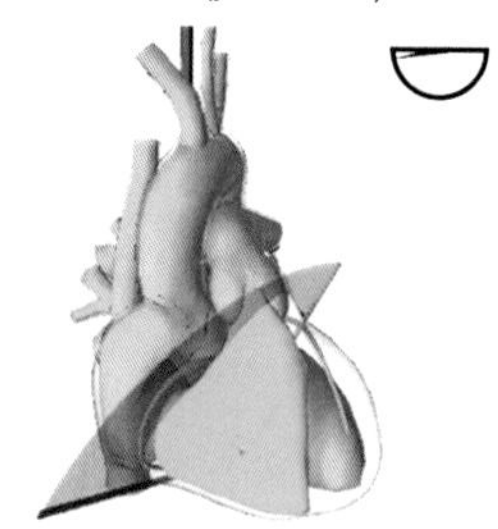

The standard **TG RV basal view at 0–30°** (p. 25) is obtained from the modified TG basal SAX by manipulating the probe to show both the TV and PV.

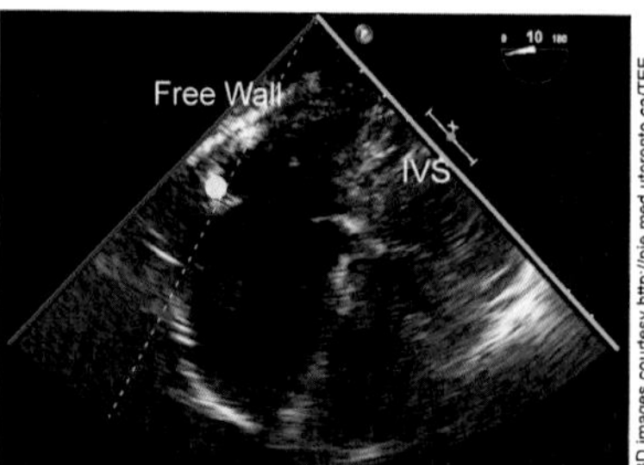

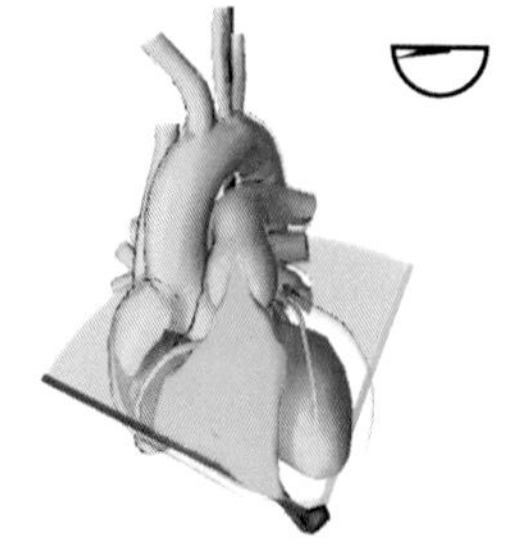

The modified **deep TG view at 0–10°** requires probe manipulation that better images the RV in long axis and allows TDI assessment of the lateral TV annulus (S′ velocity).

- RV size can be assessed using linear, area, and volume measurements.
- In the ME 4C view, the RV shape is triangular compared to the elliptical LV and is 2/3 the LV length. In a normal heart, the cardiac apex is formed by the LV, not RV.
- Measurements of RV dimensions are made from ME 4C and ME RVOT views during end-diastole when the ventricle is largest. RV size also changes with respiration, so make the measurements at end-expiration.
- Despite the RV appearing smaller in size than the LV, RVED volume (75 ± 13 mL/m^2) is actually more than LVED volume (65 ± 13 mL/m^2) due to its unusual shape.

RV and Pulmonary Artery Size						
All measures in mm at end-diastole	Ref range[a]	Mild[a]	Mod[a]	Severe[a]	Mean[b]	Normal range[b]
RV dimensions	Fig. 1					
Basal RV diameter (RVD 1)	20–28	29–33	34–38	**≥39**	33 ± 4	25–41
Mid-RV diameter (RVD 2)	27–33	34–37	38–41	**≥42**	27 ± 4	19–35
Base-apex length (RVD 3)	71–79	80–85	86–91	**≥92**	71 ± 6	59–83
RVOT diameters	Fig. 2					
Below PV (RVOT 1)	25–29	30–32	33–35	**≥36**	28 ± 3.5	21–35
Above PV (RVOT 2)	17–23	24–27	28–31	**≥32**	22 ± 2.5	17–27
PA diameter	Fig. 2					
Above PV (PA 1)	15–21	22–25	26–29	**≥30**	–	–

RVOT right ventricular outflow tract, *PA* pulmonary artery, *PV* pulmonic valve
[a]Adapted from: Lang RM, et al. J Am Soc Echocardiogr 2005;18:1440-63
[b]Source: Lang RM, et al. J Am Soc Echocardiogr 2015;28:1-39

Fig. 1 TEE measurements of RV diameters from the ME 4C view are best imaged after optimizing the maximum obtainable RV size by varying angles from 0–20°. The RVD1 is determined at the base (1 cm below TV), while RVD2 is at half way between the RV base and apex at end-diastole and end-expiration. RV dilatation is present if RVD1 > 41 mm and RVD2 > 35 mm.

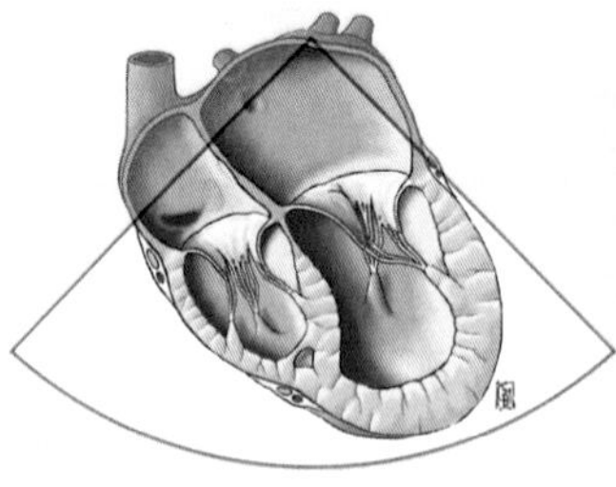

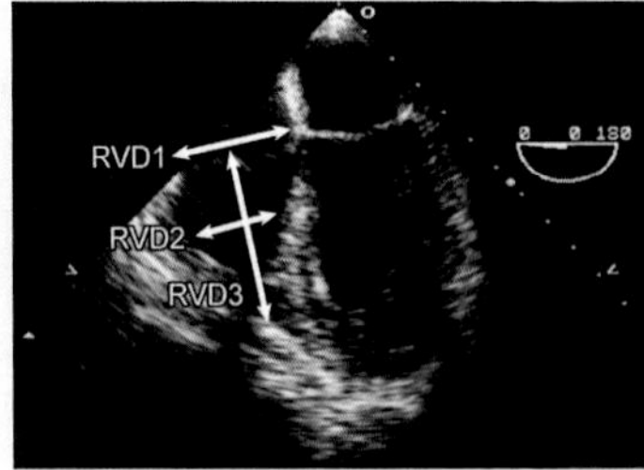

Fig. 2 Measurement of right ventricular outflow tract (RVOT1) at the PV annulus (RVOT2) and main pulmonary artery (PA1) from ME RV Inflow-Outflow view.

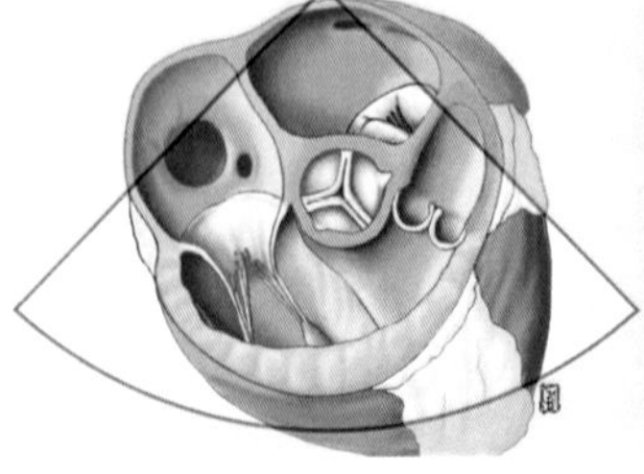

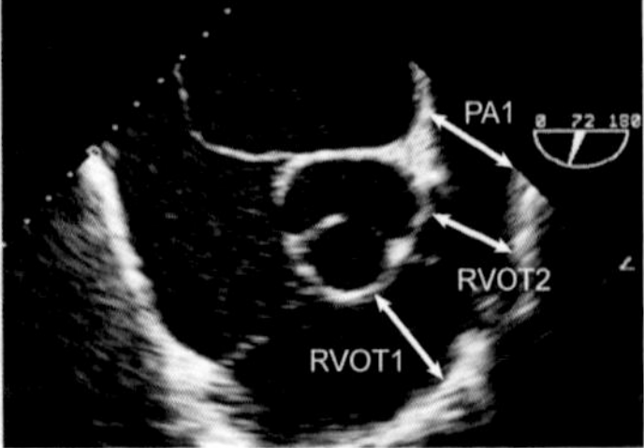

Global RV Dilatation

- As the RV dilates, it assumes a rounder shape that forms the cardiac apex. Qualitative RV assessment is usually performed as depending upon the cut planes; there can be significant variation in measured linear dimensions which can over/underestimate size. RV area can be traced at end-diastole and end-systole.
- RV enlargement occurs in response to (1) volume overload, (2) pressure overload, or (3) cardiac disease and mandates evaluation of the entire right heart. This includes assessment of (a) the RA which is often enlarged, (b) tricuspid regurgitation (TR) severity, (c) estimate of PAP from TR jet (see p. 56), and (d) color Doppler of the inter-atrial septum (ASD), interventricular septum (VSD), mitral valve (MR), and pulmonic valve (PS, PI).

In the ME 4C, the apex is formed by the RV
Mild: RV area 60% of LV area
Moderate: RV area = LV area
Severe: RV area > LV area

Normal values	RV End-Diastolic Area		RV End-Systolic Area	
	cm^2	cm^2/m^2	cm^2	cm^2/m^2
Men	17 ± 3.5	8.8 ± 1.9	9 ± 3.0	4.7 ± 1.35
Women	14 ± 3.0	8.0	7 ± 2.0	4.0 ± 1.20

Lang RM, et al. J Am Soc Echocardiogr 2015;28:1-39.

RV Dilatation Causes
Volume overload
- ASD/VSD
- Pulmonic Insufficiency
- TR (1 or 2°)
- Congenital

Pressure overload
- Pulmonary hypertension
- Pulmonary embolism
- Hypoxia (cor pulmonale)
- Left heart disease

Cardiac disease
- CAD (MI)
- Cardiomyopathy (ARVD)

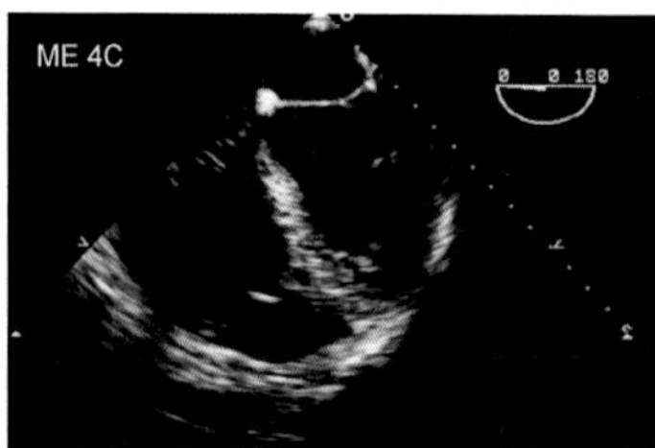

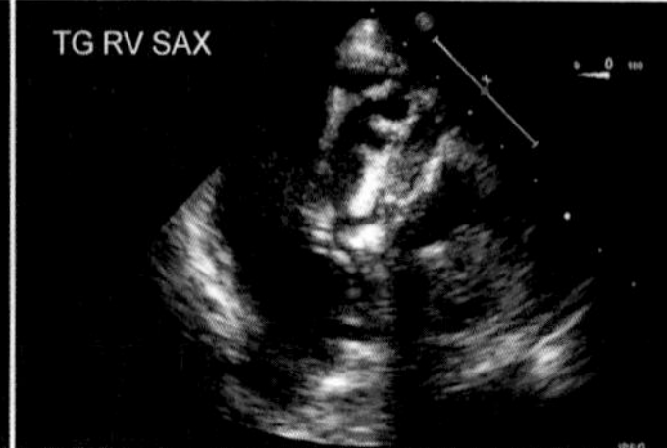

Right Ventricle Wall Hypertrophy

- Normal RV free wall thickness of <5 mm is half of the LV at end-diastole as measured in the inferior or posterior free walls. Measurement of the anterior free wall should be avoided as there is more epicardial fat.
- RV hypertrophy (RVH) is present when wall thickness is >6 mm and severe >10 mm. In RVH, the intra-cavitary trabecular pattern is more prominent particularly at the apex. RVH occurs from pressure overload or infiltration.
- In the TG mid-SAX view, the septum appears D-shaped throughout the cardiac cycle from pressure overload.

RV Hypertrophy
TG view (EDD)
Normal: <5 mm
Moderate: >6 mm
Severe: >10 mm

RV Hypertrophy Causes
Pressure overload
- Pulmonary hypertension
- Pulmonary embolism
- Hypoxia (cor pulmonale)
- Left heart disease
- RVOT obstruction
  - Subvalvular (TOF)
  - Valvular (PS)
  - Supravalvular

Cardiac
- Infiltrates (amyloid)

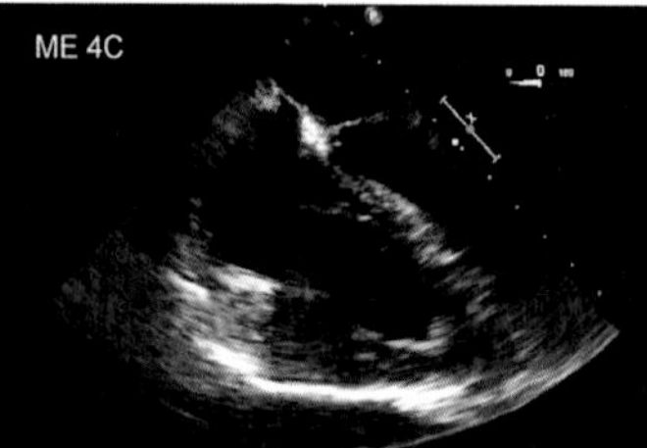

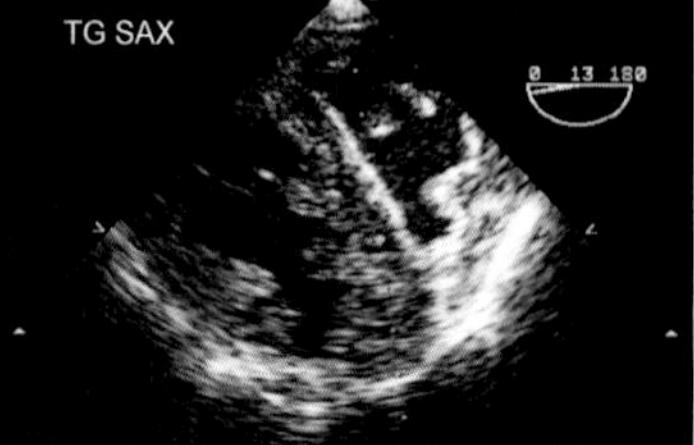

Global RV Systolic Function

- Right heart function is not always assessed as thoroughly as the LV, despite the RV having a prominent role in morbidity and mortality of patients with cardiopulmonary disease. Complex shape with less muscle mass and sequential contraction confounds simple quantitative assessment of RV global and regional wall motion by echocardiography. Nevertheless, all TEE studies should examine RV size and function using multiple views and different quantitative parameters.
- Current ASE guidelines suggest that visual RV assessment is insufficient. Quantification of RV systolic function is challenging because of its non-geometric shape, changes in shape with loading conditions, and absence of a geometric model.
- Different options exist for evaluating RV systolic function. TAPSE, 2D FAC, S′, and RIMP have the most clinical utility and value. 3D EF seems more reliable, but is time-consuming requiring off-line analysis of 3D datasets. Few of these indices have been validated using TEE or in ventilated or anesthetized patients.
- In the presence of RV dysfunction, additional assessment is required of (a) RA size, (b) tricuspid regurgitation (and RVSP), (c) IAS position, bows to the left from high RA pressure, (d) IVS position, and (e) hepatic vein flow.

Indices of RV Systolic Function

Geometric
- Fractional area change (FAC)
- Ejection fraction (EF)
- Tricuspid annular plane systolic excursion (TAPSE)

Myocardial Velocity
- Tissue Doppler annular velocity (TDI S′)
- Isovolumic acceleration

Hemodynamic
- dP/dt

Time Intervals
- RV Myocardial Index (RIMP)

Myocardial Deformation
- Strain
- Strain rate

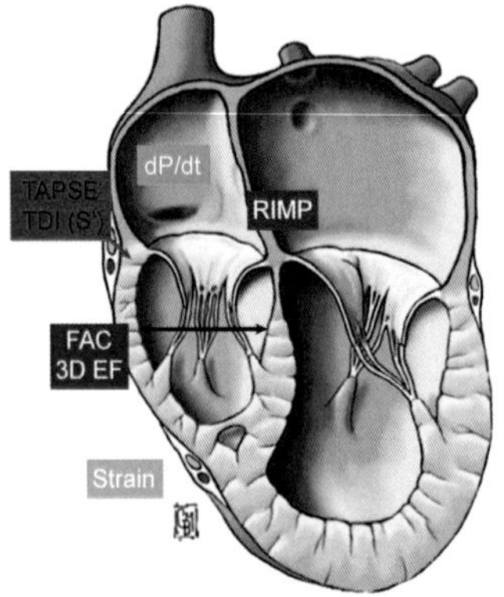

The values listed in the table differ from previous recommended values. These values are obtained from larger populations/pooled results of normal individuals without heart disease. Patients with congenital heart disease are excluded. These values are not indexed to BSA/height, so patients at extremes may be misclassified. There is insufficient data to classify some methods into abnormal categories.

	Summary RV Systolic Indices	Normal	Abnormal
FAC[a] (2D)	$\%FAC = 100 \times \frac{(EDA - ESA)}{EDA}$	>42–56% 49 ± 7	<35%
EF[a] (3D)	$\%EF = 100 \times \frac{(EDV - ESV)}{EDV}$	>51.5–64.5% 58 ± 6.5	<45%
TAPSE[a] (m-mode)	Movement lateral annulus	21–27 mm 24 ± 3.5	>17 mm
S′[a] (TDI)	S′ velocity lateral annulus	>9.8–16.4 14.1 ± 2.3	<9.5 cm/s
IVA	Isovolumic Acceleration	1.4 ± 0.5 m/s	
RIMP[a]	$MPI = \frac{(IVRT + IVCT)}{ET}$	0.26 ± 0.085 (PW) 0.38 ± 0.08 (TDI)	>0.43 >0.54
dP/dt	$dP/dt = \frac{12\ mmHg}{time}$	>400 mmHg/s	<400 mmHg/s
GLPSS[a]	Speckle tracking Free wall 2D strain	> −29 ± 4.5 (more negative)	< −20 (more positive)

PW pulse wave, *TDI* tissue Doppler imaging.
[a]**Adapted from: Lang RM, et al. J Am Soc Echocardiogr 2015;28:1-39.**

Fractional Area Change (FAC)

- ME 4C view the RV endocardial border is traced including TV leaflets, trabeculae, and papillary muscles in systole and diastole.
- RVFAC correlates with RVEF if there is no regional dysfunction.
- This method is recommended (ASE) to assess RV systolic function.

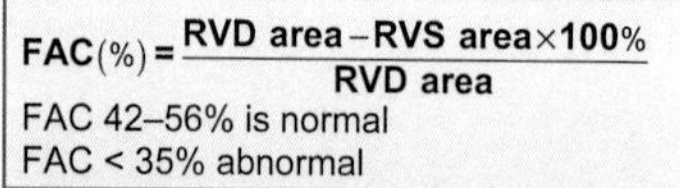

$$\text{FAC}(\%) = \frac{\text{RVD area} - \text{RVS area} \times 100\%}{\text{RVD area}}$$

FAC 42–56% is normal
FAC < 35% abnormal

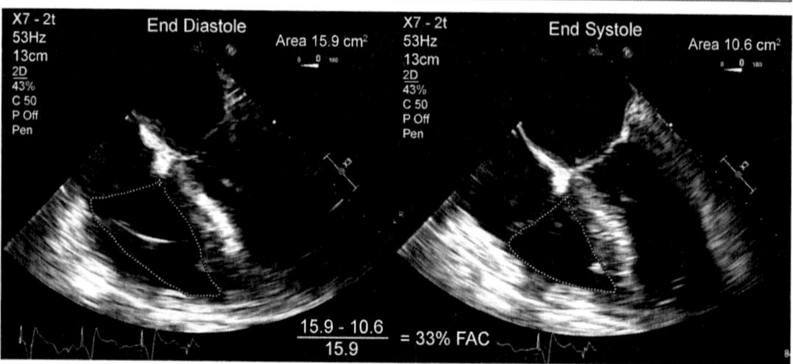

Ejection Fraction (EF)

- This uses volume measurements obtained during end-diastole and end-systole by tracing the endocardial border using the method of discs similar to the LV.
- This assesses the RV body, but does not include the infundibulum. 2D assessment of RVEF is not a method recommended to assess RV systolic function.
- 3D models of the RV better estimate RV volumes and EF (see p. 96).

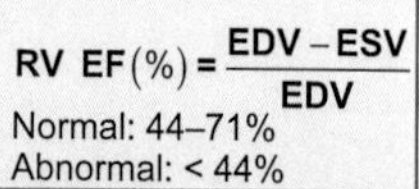

$$\text{RV EF}(\%) = \frac{\text{EDV} - \text{ESV}}{\text{EDV}}$$

Normal: 44–71%
Abnormal: < 44%

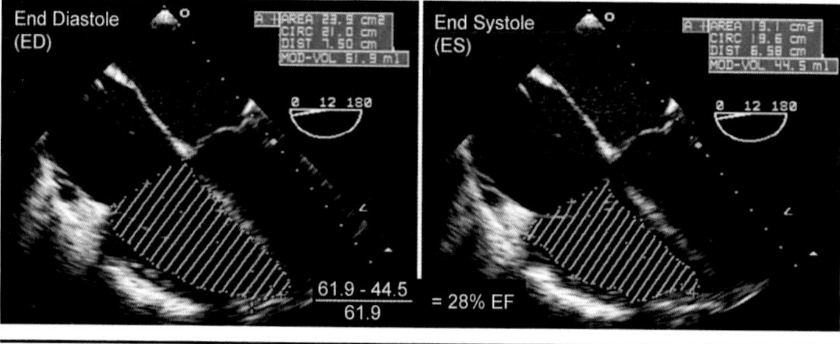

dP/dt

- Rate of rise of intra-ventricular pressure (dP/dt) during systole can be estimated from the tricuspid regurgitation (TR) CW Doppler trace. Measure the time (dt) for velocity to increase from 1 to 2 m/s. Calculate dP as 16 mmHg (2 m/s) – 4 mmHg (1 m/s) = 12 mmHg and divided by the measured dt to obtain a value.
- Better correlation between echo and invasive pressures when time measured from 0.5 to 2 m/s represents a 15 mmHg change.
- dP/dt is not useful if trivial or severe TR, eccentric TR jet, or RWMA is present.
- There is limited data to recommend its routine use to assess RV function.

$$\text{dP / dt} = \frac{15\ \text{mmHg}}{\text{dt}}$$

Normal > 400 mmHg/s (dt ≤ 37.5 ms)
Reduced RV: <400 mmHg/s (dt > 37.5 ms)

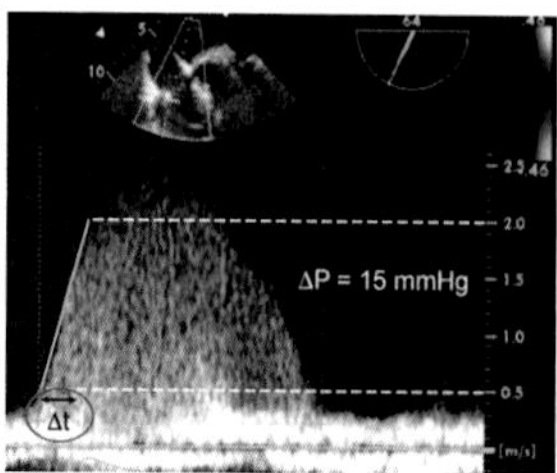

Tricuspid Annular Plane Systolic Excursion (TAPSE)

- This is the distance of systolic excursion of the lateral TV annulus measured in a longitudinal plane. TAPSE is a simple easily reproducible surrogate measure of global RV function that correlates with angiography, biplane method of disc, and FAC. It assumes that basal segment displacement represents the function of the entire RV and is invalid in the presence of RV RWMA as may occur with RV infarction or pulmonary embolism.
- Measurement of the lateral TV annulus motion by m-mode is angle-dependent.

Alignment using m-mode is difficult in the (**A**) ME 4C view compared with TTE views ❶. (**B**) The ME RVOT and the (**C**) TG RV inflow views may improve alignment for m-mode. (**D**) Anatomical m-mode, a feature on some US machines, adjusts the position of the m-mode cursor to any angle, ❷ including parallel to the motion of the annulus improving alignment.

TAPSE
Normal: 17–30 mm (23 mm)
Abnormal TAPSE <17 mm

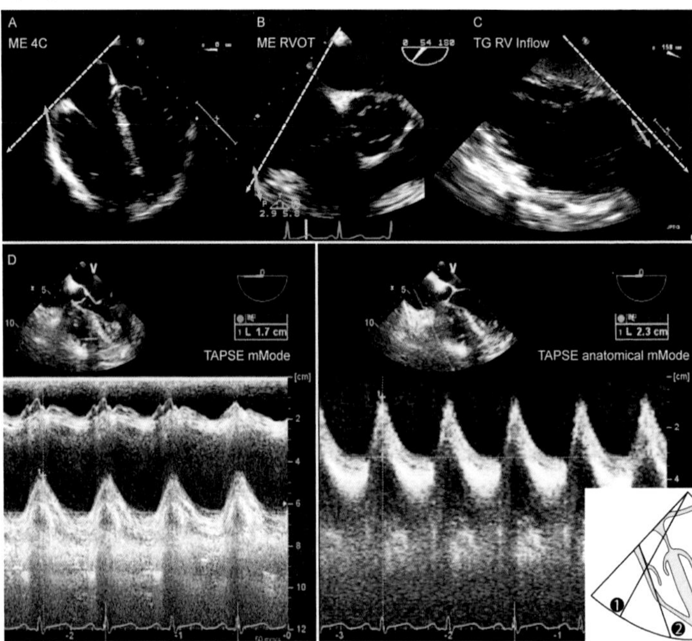

Tricuspid Annulus Velocity (S′)

- Longitudinal myocardial velocity of the RV can be assessed using tissue Doppler imaging (TDI) at the lateral TV annulus. This is easy to measure and reproducible using basal segments (or RV free wall) but is less reliable for mid and apical segments. The IVS is not used as it does not exclusively reflect RV function.
- The S′ wave velocity estimates global systolic function and is not a surrogate of contractility. It is validated against radionuclide RVEF.
- This measure is limited by mitral annular calcification (MAC), RWMA (from ischemia or pulmonary embolism), and poor Doppler alignment. It is also less reliable after thoracotomy, pulmonary thromboendarterectomy, or heart transplantation.
- This measure is performed using the TV annulus in the TG LAX view (posterior TV annulus) or ME RVOT view (inferior TV annulus). TDI mode is activated and the Doppler sample volume is positioned at the lateral annulus to give a clean spectral trace (see p. 95). The peak S′ velocity is measured. Note the S′ wave appears above or below the baseline depending in which view is used.

Normal S′ > 9.8–16.4 cm/s
Abnormal S′ < 9.5 cm/s

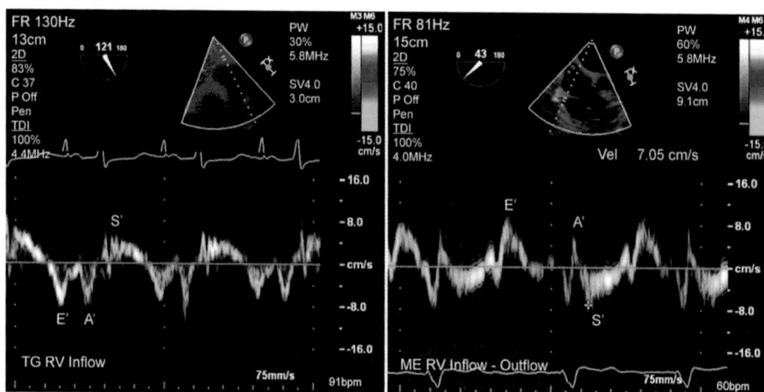

Right Index of Myocardial Performance (RIMP) or Tei Index

- Right ventricular MPI incorporates systolic and diastolic time intervals, measured by Doppler, to provide a global assessment of RV systolic and diastolic function.
- The sum of the isovolumic contraction time (IVCT) and isovolumic relaxation time (IVRT) is divided by the ejection time (ET).
- Value is independent of arterial pressure, HR, ventricular geometry, atrioventricular valve regurgitation, afterload, and preload. It is unreliable with elevated RAP (rapid pressure equilibration shortens IVRT, small MPI), arrhythmias, or A-V block.
- RIMP is well-validated in normal subjects and different pathological states.
- RIMP can be determined using spectral Doppler or tissue Doppler.

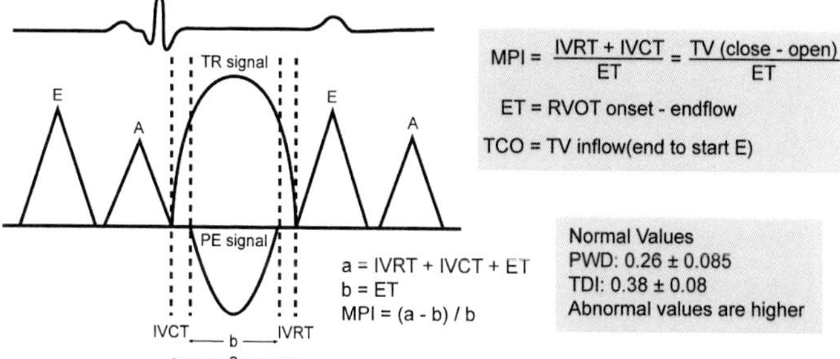

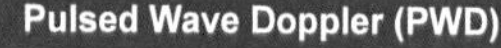

Obtain tricuspid valve (TV) and pulmonic valve (PV) ejection Doppler traces with similar RR intervals. Measure these time intervals:

1. ET: flow through PV
2. TCO: TV from end A wave to start E wave or the duration of TR

Tissue Doppler Imaging (TDI)

Obtain TDI lateral TV annulus, measure

1. ET
2. TCO

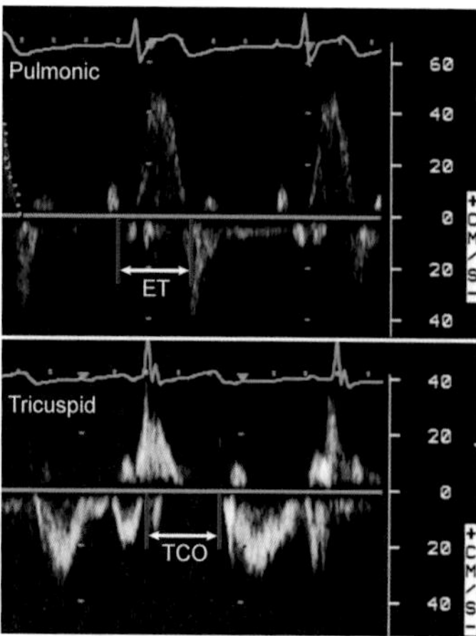

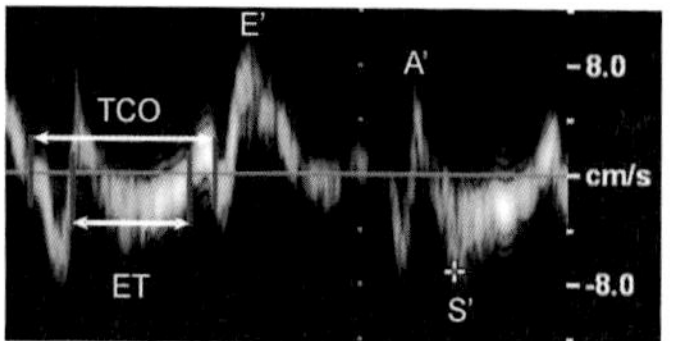

- 3D volume estimation requires an adequate 3D dataset of the entire RV at 20–25vol/s and off-line analysis by third party software (TomTec, Munich, Germany). The software tracks the endocardial border and gives measures of RV volumes and a calculated ejection fraction (RVEF).
- The advantage of this technique is the measuring of global RV size is independent of geometric assumptions. It is valid against MRI, the current gold standard for estimating RV volume.
- The major disadvantage of 3D RVEF is the need for off-line analysis by specialized software using a high-quality 3D dataset.
- TTE 3D volumes and RVEF are slightly underestimated compared with MRI, slightly higher in women, and decrease with age.

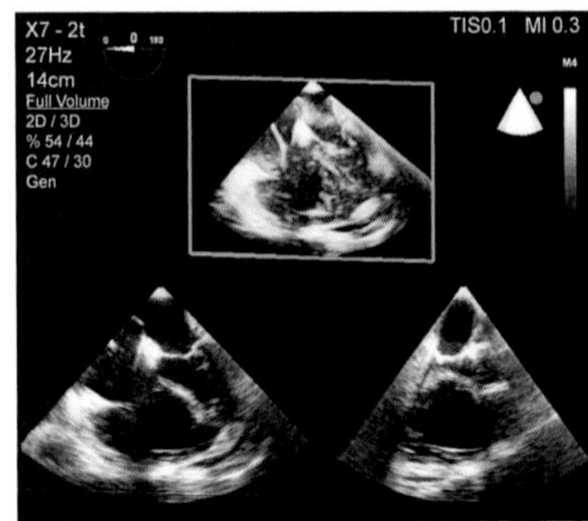

3D RVEF
Normal > 51.5–64.5% (58 ± 6.5)
Age and sex dependent
Female: 60–71%
Male: 56–65%
Reduced RV: <45%

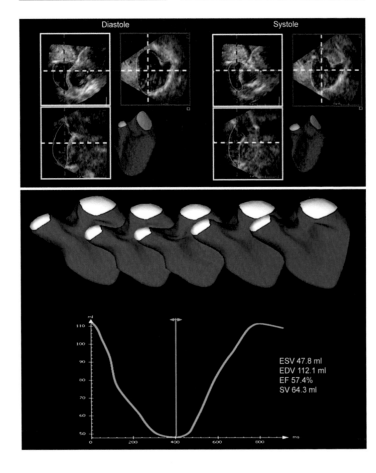

- RV strain can be easily assessed and displayed on the ultrasound machine using speckle tracking software. Similar to the LV, strain is the percentage change in myocardial deformation and stain rate is the rate of deformation of myocardium/time. These are estimates of global and regional RV function.
- Strain information for segments can be displayed as an overlay or as a spectral trace. Typically, global longitudinal peak systolic strain (GLPSS) is determined in the ME 4C view as an average of RV-free wall segments (basal/mid +/– apical) alone or as an average of free wall and septum.
- Abnormal RV free wall GLPSS is < –20%, but is vendor-dependent. RV free wall GLPSS is significantly higher (as an absolute value) than the strain averaged from both septal and free wall segments.

RV Free Wall GLS
Normal > –29 ± 4.5
Reduced RV: < –20

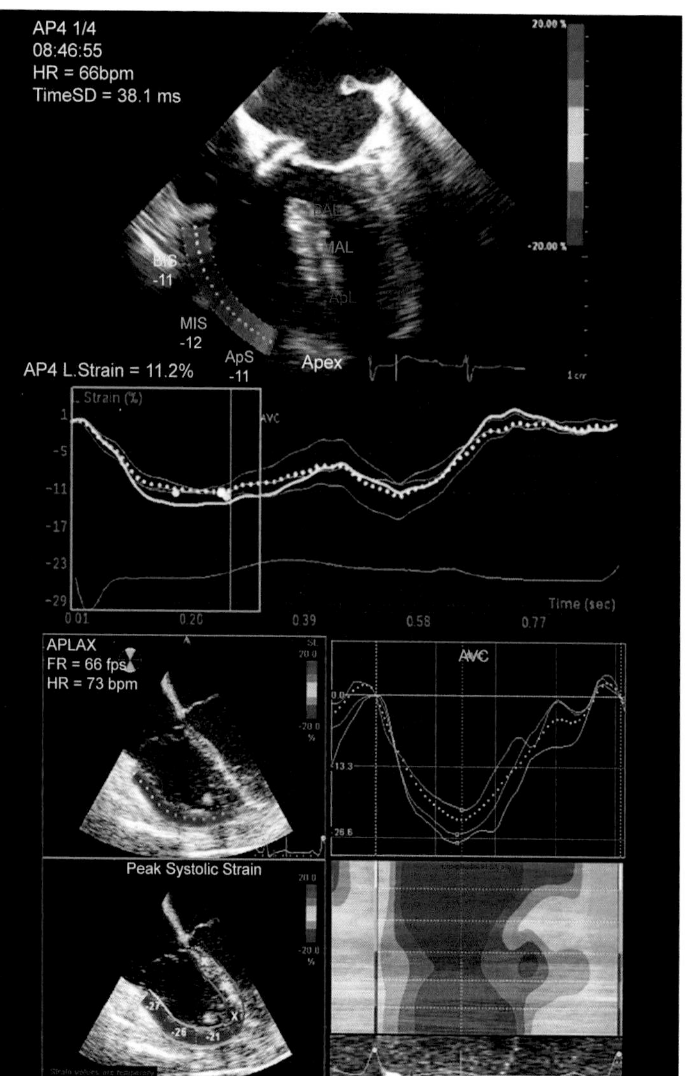

5
Coronary Artery Disease

A. Vegas, *Perioperative Two-Dimensional Transesophageal Echocardiography*, https://doi.org/10.1007/978-3-319-60902-7_5

Coronary Artery Distribution

- The coronary circulation is formed by the right coronary artery (RCA), left coronary artery (LCA) and various branches. Coronary dominance refers to which vessel (RCA, circumflex) supplies the posterior interventricular (PIV) or posterior descending artery (PDA) branch to the inferior septum. Majority of hearts are right dominant (85% RCA) with the remainder either circumflex 8% or co-dominant 7%.
- The LCA supplies blood to the left heart, including the LA and LV. The left main coronary artery divides early into the left anterior descending (LAD), circumflex (Cx) and intermediate (15%) arteries. The LAD runs in the anterior interventricular groove and supplies the anterior and lateral LV walls (diagonal branches), anterior septum (septal perforators) and atrioventricular (A-V) bundle. The Cx artery runs in the left A-V groove around the posterior heart to supply the infero-lateral LV wall (obtuse marginal branches). In 10–15% of patients the Cx continues as the PIV.
- Most of the coronary blood flow to the RV is from the acute marginal branch of the RCA. The first septal perforator supplies the moderator band and the posterior septal perforators from the RCA supply the inferior (posterior) 1/3 of the IVS. In 30% of patients a separate conus artery branch supplies the infundibulum. Under normal conditions the RV is well perfused during both systole and diastole.

Left Coronary Circulation	Right Coronary Circulation
Left Coronary Artery (LCA) • Left Anterior Descending (LAD) artery – Septal perforators (S1, S2): ant septum – Diagonal branches (D1, D2): ant wall LV – ± Conus branch: RV free wall • Intermediate Artery • Circumflex (Cx) Artery – Obtuse Marginal (OM) branches: anterior/inferior-lateral walls LV, LA walls – Posterior Descending Artery (PDA) 15%: Inferior LV, IVS, posterior PM	Right Coronary Artery (RCA) – Conus branch (50–60%): RVOT – Sinus node (60%) – Acute Marginal (AM): lateral RV – Diagonals: anterior RV – Posterior Descending Artery (PDA) 85%: Infero-lateral, inferior LV Papillary Muscles blood supply: – AL by 2 arteries (obtuse + diagonal) – PM by 1 artery (RCA or obtuse)

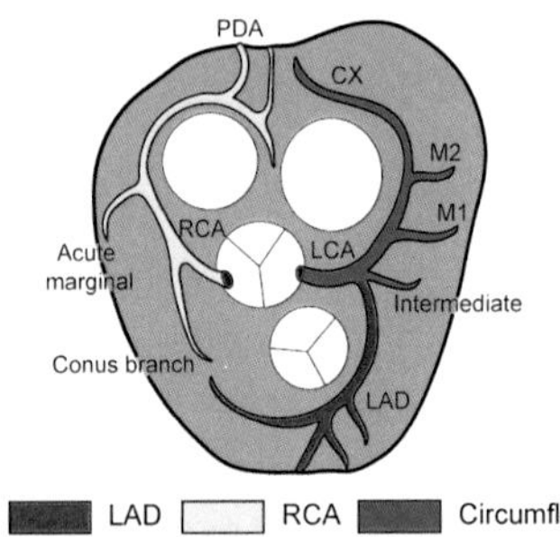

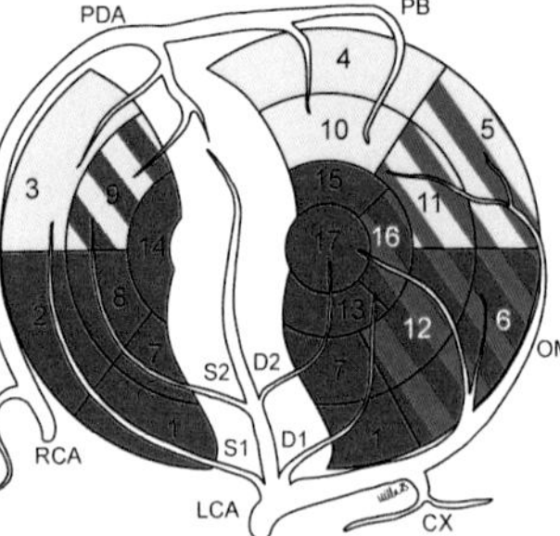

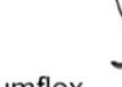

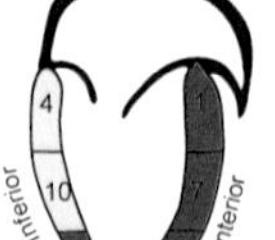

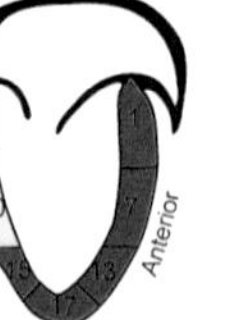

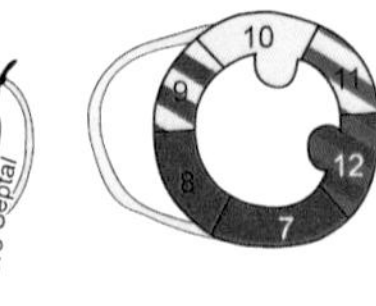

17 Segment Model					
Basal Segments		**Mid Segments**		**Apical Segments**	
1	Basal anterior (D1)	7	Mid anterior (D1)	13	Apical anterior (D2)
2	Basal antero-septal (S1)	8	Mid antero-septal (S1)	14	Apical septal (S1)
3	Basal infero-septal (PDA)	9	Mid infero-septal (PDA)	15	Apical inferior (PDA)
4	Basal inferior (PB)	10	Mid inferior (PB)	16	Apical lateral (OM)
5	Basal infero-lateral (OM)	11	Mid infero-lateral (OM)	17	Apex (D2)
6	Basal antero-lateral (OM)	12	Mid antero-lateral (OM)		

Coronary Artery Imaging

- Although TEE can image the coronary arteries it is suboptimal as because of their curved nature only the short proximal length is well visualized.
- The proximal LCA is followed to its bifurcation into the LAD + Cx arteries; with the posterior directed Cx closest to the probe in the ME AV SAX. The Cx artery is seen in SAX near the LAA in the ME 2C view. The anterior positioned RCA is seen at 6 o'clock in the ME AV SAX and AV LAX views.
- Coronary artery size (5 mm) can be measured.
- Color Doppler at a low Nyquist (30 cm/s) demonstrates coronary flow. It is difficult to assess coronary obstruction by echocardiography. Rarely is flow acceleration proximal to an obstructing lesion seen with an increased peak diastolic flow.
- PWD shows continuous biphasic flow with higher velocity signals during diastole.

D

Coronary Flow (cm/s)
LMCA (D) 71+19 (S) 39+11
RCA (D) 39+12 (S) 25+9

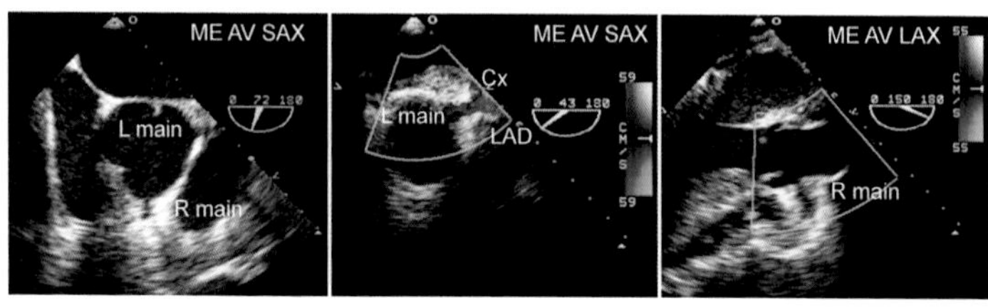

The course of the circumflex artery can be followed from a modified ME AV LAX view (110°). (A) Start by slowly turning the probe left (counterclockwise) to identify the left main coronary artery (LMCA) origin from the aorta. (B) Further left turning of the probe identifies the LMCA bifurcation into the LAD and Cx arteries. (C) The crossover point (intersection) of the Cx which is above and the coronary sinus (CS) is identified in SAX. (D) The distal Cx and CS run in parallel along the A-V groove.

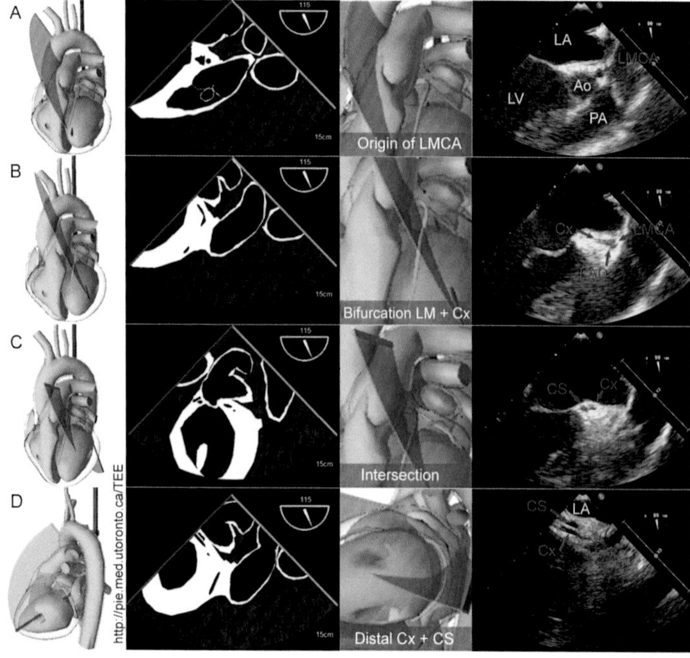

Coronary Artery Anomalies

- Coronary anomalies are uncommon with a prevalence of 1%.
- There is no universally agreed upon classification, but they can be differentiated into anomalies of (1) origin, (2) course and (3) termination.
- The commonest and potentially most lethal from sudden cardiac death are associated with anomalous coronary origin. A single coronary artery is particularly vulnerable to compression if it lies between the aorta and PA.
- A muscle bridge is defined as muscle that overlies an intramural segment of an epicardial artery which during systole may cause dynamic arterial compression.
- Congenital arterial fistulae (CAF) are direct connections between a coronary artery branch and a cardiac chamber, coronary sinus, SVC, PA, or pulmonary veins. This condition results in chronic volume overload.

Coronary Anomalies
Anomalous Origin
- Pulmonary artery
- Single coronary artery
- Non-coronary cusp

Anomalous course
- Myocardial bridging
- Duplication

Anomalous Termination
- Coronary artery fistula

Anomalous Left Coronary Artery From the Pulmonary Artery (ALCAPA)

- This condition in adults is referred to as Bland Garland White Syndrome.
- Patients often die in infancy but may survive to adulthood by developing collateral flow between the right and left coronary circulation. There is retrograde flow in the left coronary circulation (arrows inset) into the PA causing anterior wall ischemia.
- The origin of the left main coronary artery (LMCA) is from the main PA.
- Large RCA seen in ME AV LAX and SAX views.
- Collateral flow results in multiple intramyocardial flow turbulences which makes the myocardium appear to be "on fire".
- LMCA origin is absent in left sinus of Valsalva but may be identified originating from main PA.
- PW Doppler LCA flow shows systolic predominance, while normal has diastolic predominance. Diastolic retrograde flow from LMCA to the PA is identified by color/PW spectral Doppler.

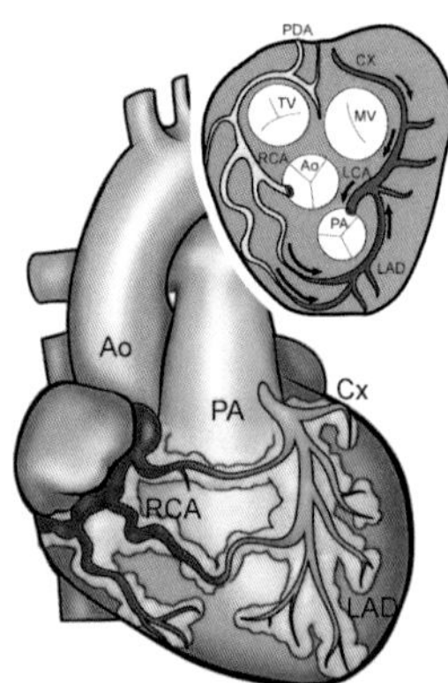

(A) ME AV LAX views with color Doppler shows a large RCA (arrows) with coronary perfusion during systole and diastole. (B) TTE parasternal SAX view showing intramyocardial collateral blood flow, the "heart on fire". (C) TTE parasternal inflow outflow view shows coronary flow originating from the main PA (arrow) and coursing between the PA and aorta.

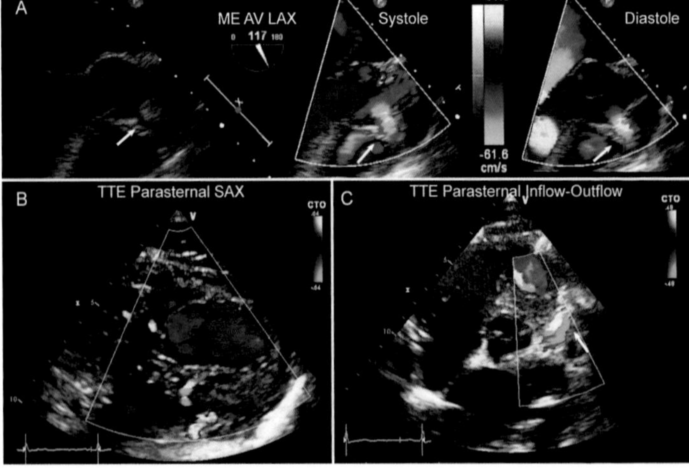

- The 17 segment model divides the LV into segments to better convey information about regional wall motion abnormalities (RWMA).
- Detection of RWMA is often based on qualitative visual assessment and a grading scale for motion and/or thickening of a segment during systole. Hypokinesis refers to a reduced wall thickening with inwards motion, akinesis has no wall thickening or movement and dyskinesis has systolic thinning and moves paradoxically outwards during systole (e.g. aneurysm).
- The presence of RWMA suggests myocardial ischemia. Following vessel occlusion, TEE detects myocardial ischemia within seconds even before ECG ST or hemodynamic changes occur. The first change is impaired diastolic relaxation followed by reduced contractility (wall thickening is more sensitive). Regional function may deteriorate with just 20% reduction in transmural flow.

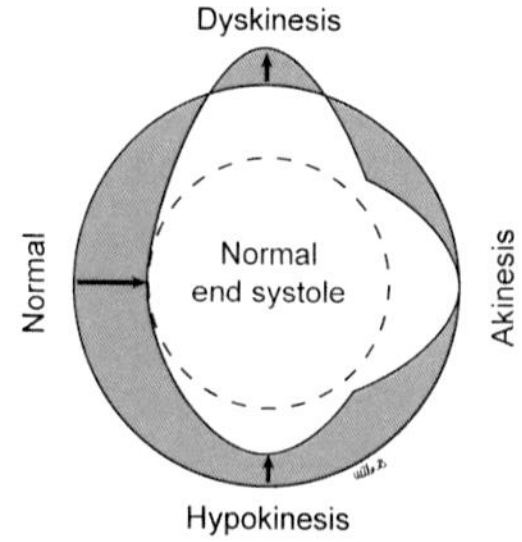

- However not all RWMAs are due to acute myocardial ischemia as different factors may confound RWMA assessment. These factors reduce the specificity of abnormal endocardial thickening as an ischemic marker.
  - Foreshortening from imaging plane misalignment reduces the true LV length in the ME LV views which can often distort the apical segments.
  - Pseudothickening occurs from normal side to side heart motion (translation) creating the illusion of changes in wall thickness.
  - Conduction (LBBB but not RBBB) or pacing abnormalities result in disco-ordinate IVS movement, with paradoxical septal motion outwards in systole.
  - RWMA may occur with other pathologies such as myocarditis, sarcoidosis, and stress-induced (Takotsubo) cardiomyopathy.
- A semiquantitative wall motion score can be assigned to each segment to calculate the LV wall motion score index as the average of the scores of all of the segments visualized. Current ASE guidelines include 4 wall scores as opposed to the previous 5 by not assigning a separate score for an aneurysm.

Wall Score		Wall Motion	% Radius Change	Wall Thickening	
1	Normal/hperkinesis	Inward	>30%	+++	30–50%
2	Hypokinesis	Inward	10–30%	++	30–50%
3	Akinesis	None	None	0	<10%
4	Dyskinesis	Outward	None	0	None

Source: Lang R, et al. J Am Soc Echocardiogr 2015;28:1–39

$$\text{Wall Montion Score Index (WMSI)} = \frac{\text{sum of wall motion scores}}{\text{number of visualized segments}}$$

Normal WMSI = 1, WMSI > 1.7 indicates perfusion defect >20%

Chronic Segmental Dysfunction

- Myocardial infarction (MI) is an irreversible injury to the myocardium from a prolonged reduction in coronary blood flow. The myocardium is initially akinetic with normal wall thickness, that becomes thinned and echogenic over 4–6 weeks. A transmural MI has a definite area of akinesis and wall thinning. A non-transmural MI has hypokinesis and less wall thinning.
- Echocardiography cannot distinguish an acute MI from ongoing ischemia. The amount of ischemic myocardium is overestimated, as the wall motion of adjacent regions may be affected by tethering, regional loading conditions, and stunning.
- Stunned myocardium is viable myocardium with reversible post-ischemic dysfunction that is typically seen after restoring normal coronary blood flow during cardiac surgery or percutaneous coronary intervention.
- Hibernating myocardium is persistently impaired segmental myocardial dysfunction from reduced coronary perfusion that can be improved by restoring coronary perfusion. This can be assessed by using Dobutamine Stress Echocardiography (DSE) which shows a biphasic response to dobutamine, initially have improved wall motion with low dose that worsens with high dose dobutamine.

- Myocardial contractility is reduced and myocardial deformation is altered during ischemia in both the ischemic and adjacent myocardium. Tissue velocities, strain, and strain rates are reduced in ischemia and infarction. Early within 5 seconds S′ velocity is reduced in affected segments but this finding cannot separate active ischemia from reperfusion-induced contractile dysfunction. Tissue velocities may not accurately reflect regional function due to tethering.
- In comparison to non ischemic regions, three characteristics can identify an ischemic myocardial systolic velocity pattern:
  - (1) Early peak positive strain (PPS)
  - (2) Reduced peak systolic strain (PS)
  - (3) Postsystolic shortening (PSS)
- By definition PSS is myocardial shortening from delayed regional relaxation that occurs after end-systole (AV closure), and is seen in myocardium with regional contractile dysfunction.
- Postsystolic strain (PSS) is superior to peak systolic strain or wall thickening in detecting acute ischemia and diagnosing CAD. PSS persists after recovery from brief ischemia despite the rapid recovery of peak systolic strain. PSS may be seen in normal patients so it does not always indicate myocardial ischemia.

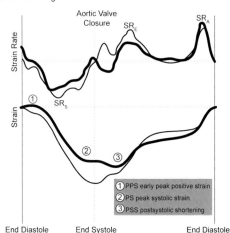

Shown below is an example of an anterior basal RWMA (red curve) from ischemia with features of (1) PPS, (2) PS (at −12) and (3) PSS.

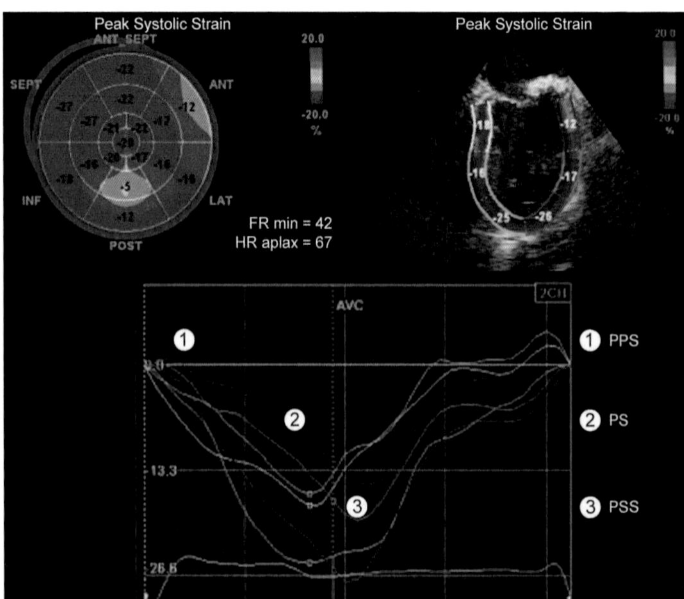

- Bull's eye patterns for strain can help identify regional involvement with coronary artery disease by the presence of pink or blue segments. Extremely low strain values (less negative or positive) suggest the non-viability of those segments.

(A) The bull's eye can be overlayed with the coronary artery distribution. Abnormal bull's eye are shown for (B) LAD disease, (C) RCA disease and (D) combined LAD and circumflex artery disease.

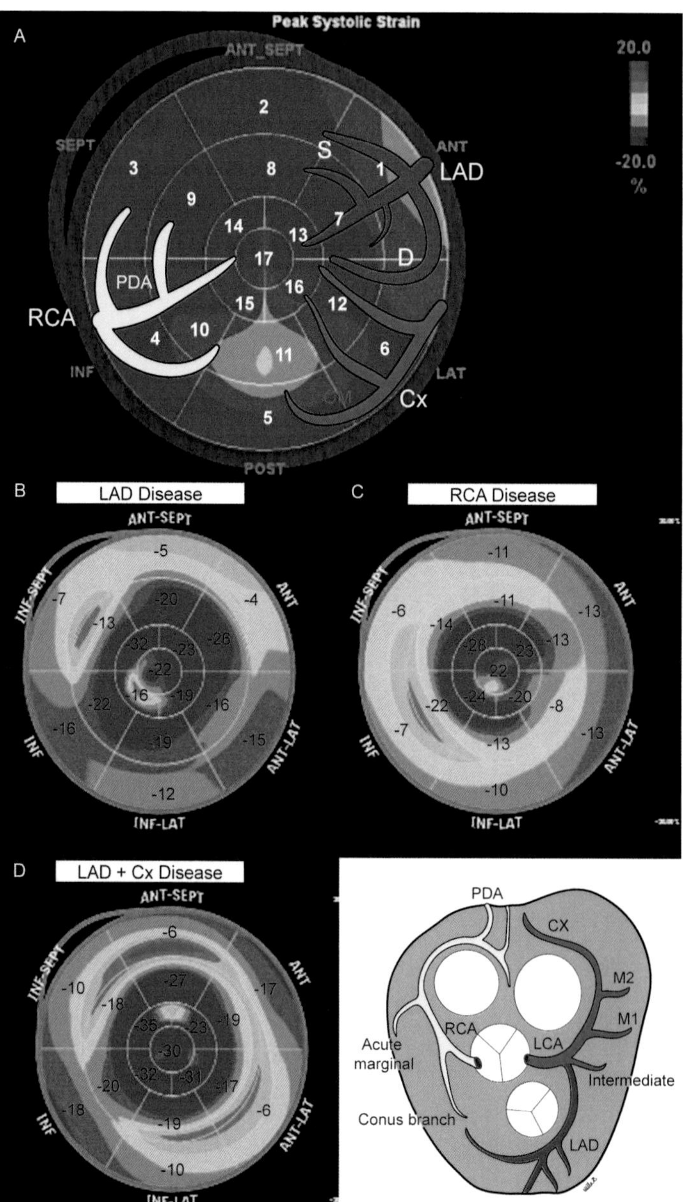

- Echocardiography can diagnose myocardial infarction (MI) with high sensitivity, but it is more valuable as a prognostic and risk stratification tool.
- The perioperative presence of RWMA post-ACB increases morbidity and mortality.
- The most important predictors of post-MI mortality, LV dysfunction and cardiogenic shock, are easily assessed by echo.
- Cardiogenic shock may occur acutely within 1–7 days post-MI as a result of poor myocardial function and uncommon acute mechanical complications such as ventricular septal rupture, free wall rupture, acute MR and dynamic LVOT obstruction.
- Chronic mechanical complications such as aneurysms or thrombus worsen prognosis.

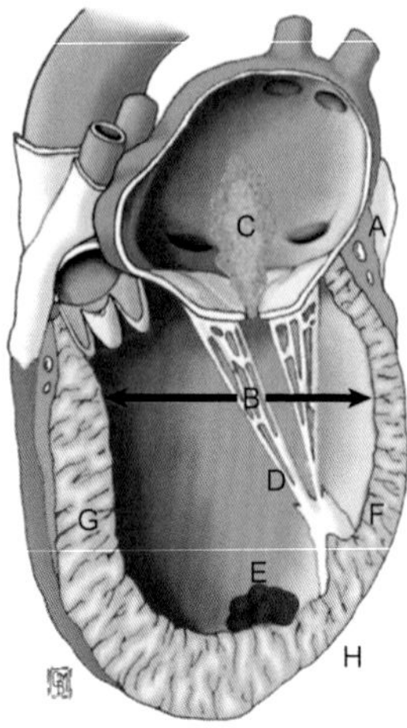

Ischemic Complications
A. Chronic segmental dysfunction
B. Ventricular dilatation
C. Mitral regurgitation (MR)
D. Papillary muscle dysfunction or rupture
E. Thrombus
F. Aneurysm
G. Ventricular septal rupture
H. Pericardial effusion

Chronic Segmental Dysfunction

- RWMA occurs as a result of myocardial ischemia (see p. 103). Transmural myocardial infarction (MI) creates myocardial scar which appears as echogenic thin akinetic segments. Non transmural MI has hypokinesis and less wall thinning.
- Echocardiography cannot distinguish an acute MI from ongoing ischemia, stunned or hibernating myocardium as all cause RWMA.
- TG mid-SAX view is the classic doughnut image used to assess the mid LV wall segments and LV cavity size. Check during diastole and systole for RWMA and systolic thickening.

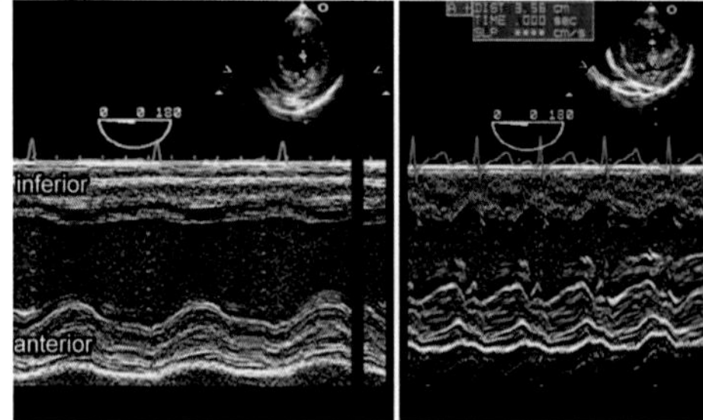

M-mode TG SAX views of anterior (hypokinesis) + inferior (akinetic) RWMA, compare with normal.

LV Ventricular Dilatation

- Myocardial ischemia involving multiple coronary arteries can result in a dilated hypofunctioning ventricle, termed ischemic cardiomyopathy. The LV walls appear thinned in diastole with displaced papillary muscles. Low flow in the cardiac chamber causes smoke.
- The IVS is bowed to the right making the LV spherical. The altered LV geometry is described by the sphericity index, determined by measuring LV size in the ME or TG views at ED or ES.

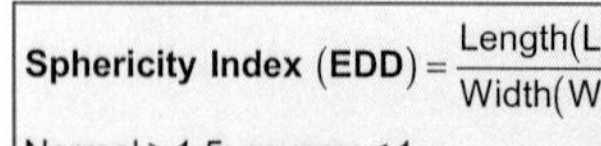

$$\textbf{Sphericity Index (EDD)} = \frac{\text{Length(L)}}{\text{Width(W)}}$$

Normal ≥ 1.5; severe: ≤ 1

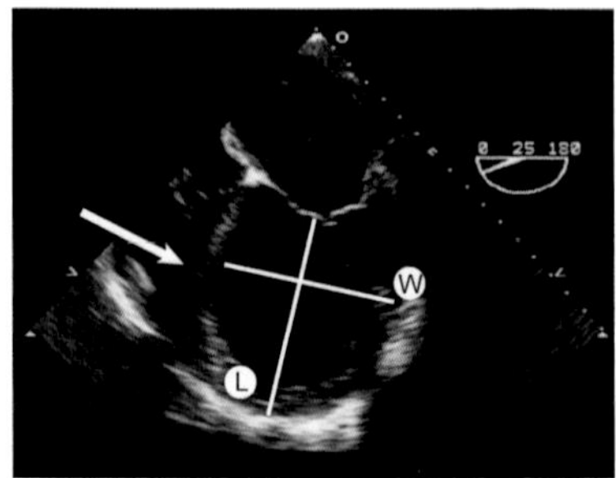

Right Ventricular Dysfunction

- RV dysfunction is mostly independent of overall LV function and is more dependent on the location and extent of the LV infarction. Mild (40%) to severe (10%) RV dysfunction may occur after an inferior or infero-lateral MI, but is unusual with an anterior MI of the LV.
- Isolated RV infarction rarely occurs (prevalence 3%) unless there is proximal RCA occlusion before the acute marginal branch.
- The RV is protected from ischemia by a number of factors including: (1) lower O_2 requirements as there is less RV muscle mass, (2) coronary perfusion during the entire cardiac cycle, and (3) diffusion of O_2.
- RV function is an independent predictor of death and the development of heart failure (HF) in patients after MI.

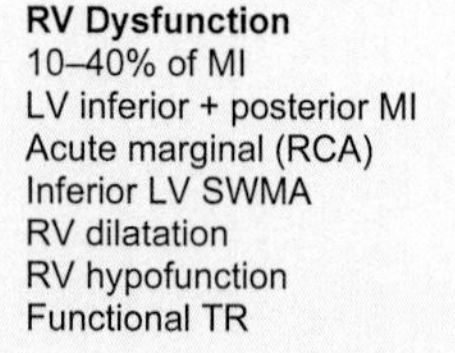

RV Dysfunction
10–40% of MI
LV inferior + posterior MI
Acute marginal (RCA)
Inferior LV SWMA
RV dilatation
RV hypofunction
Functional TR

TEE of the RV in the (A) ME 4C, (B) ME inflow-outflow or TG views show regional or global dysfunction with a dilated RV. Assessment of systolic RV function is described in Chap. 4. An inferior LV RWMA may be present. Rarely a papillary muscle may rupture producing severe tricuspid regurgitation (TR) by color Doppler.

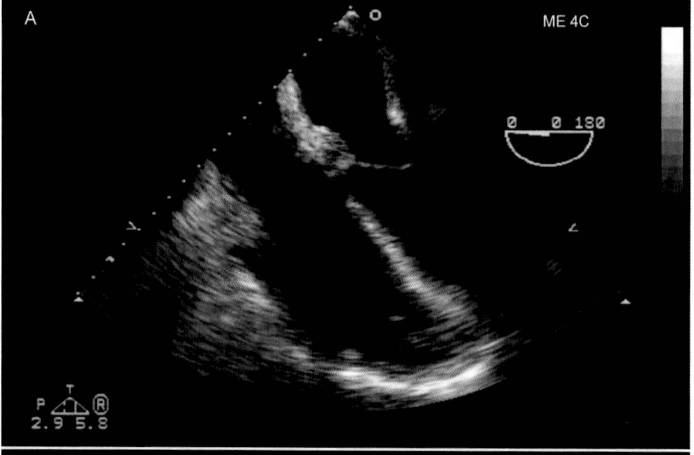

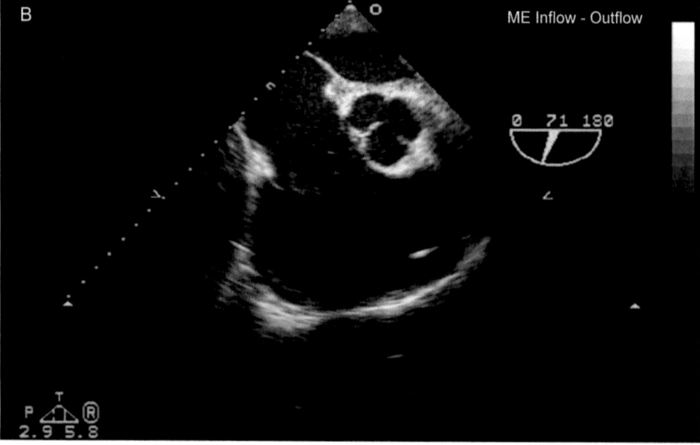

- Mild to moderate MR occurs in up to 45% of patients (anterior MI 15%, inferior MI 40%) following an acute MI and predicts a worse prognosis.
- Acute MR may result from papillary muscle ischemia or rupture (posterior medial PM has single blood supply) or high diastolic pressures from LV dysfunction.
- Chronic ischemic MR (CIMR) occurs from LV remodelling with changes in LV geometry that distort the mitral apparatus. Annular dilatation with loss of annular height and outward displacement of the papillary muscles stretches the chordae tendinae and pulls the body of the MV leaflets towards the LV apex which is called tenting. Leaflet tenting is quantified by distance, area and volume measures.
- There is incomplete leaflet coaptation from tethering of the MV leaflets. Symmetric tethering involves both MV leaflets and results in central MR. Asymmetric tethering involves greater restriction of one leaflet, often the posterior as shown below, causing an eccentric MR jet and typically more significant MR
- CIMR represents functional MR (Type IIIB Carpentier Classification, see p. 152) as this is a problem of LV muscle with structurally normal but restricted MV leaflets.

TEE Findings CIMR

A. MR: central, eccentric, severity
B. LV: dilated, RWMA, sphericity index
C. MV: annulus diameter, flattened
D. Posterior and apical displaced PM
E. Tethering angle between mitral leaflet and annulus
F. Tethering MV leaflet (mid systole): height, area, volume

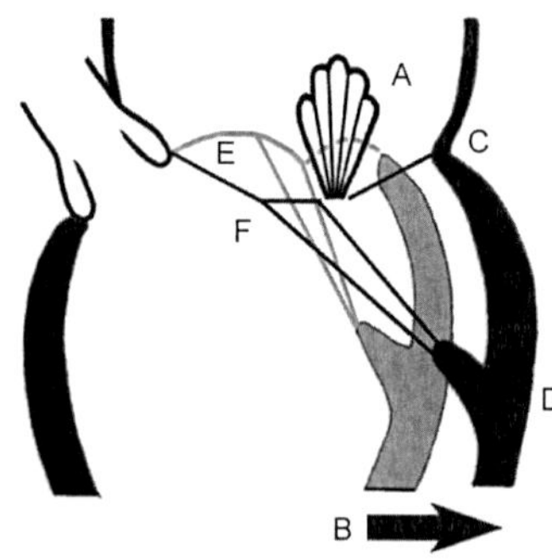

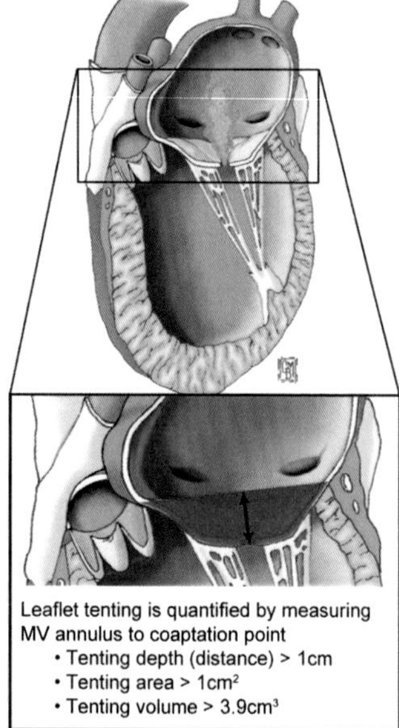

Leaflet tenting is quantified by measuring MV annulus to coaptation point
- Tenting depth (distance) > 1cm
- Tenting area > $1cm^2$
- Tenting volume > $3.9cm^3$

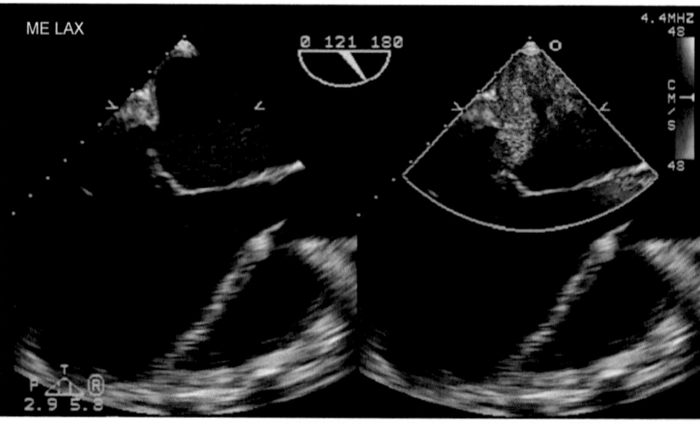

- Recent 2014 ACC/AHA guidelines (see below) endorse lower cut-off values for EROA and regurgitant volume in functional MR compared with primary organic MR (see p. 153). This relates to the elongated shape of the central MR jet along the line of leaflet malcoaptation. The 2017 ASE guidelines do not distinguish between 1° and 2° MR for using EROA to establish MR severity.
- EROA is lower 0.2cm^2 for severe CIMR compared with 1° MR 0.4cm^2.
- There is a difference in prognostic values for regurgitant volume based on 1° organic (>60 cc) versus 2° functional (>30 cc) disease.

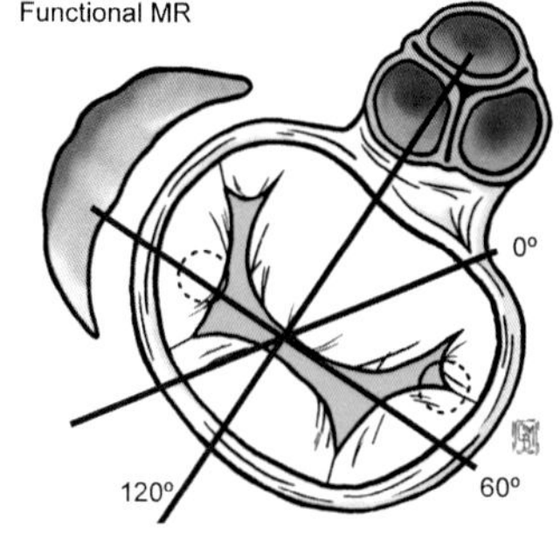

- PISA radius changes during systole in CIMR with early + late peaks, and a decrease in mid-systole. Care should be taken when using PISA to calculate EROA.
- Vena contracta width (VCW) is the MR jet diameter measured above the flow acceleration region at a Nyquist 50–60 cm/s from the ME AV LAX or ME 4C views which are perpendicular to the line of leaflet coaptation.
- Early revascularization helps prevent CIMR. Despite various surgical procedures on the MV none have proven superior to medical management of chronic heart failure for long term prognosis. Predictors of failed MV repair are listed below and in the presence of severe CIMR may suggest the need for MV replacement.

Ischemic Mitral Regurgitation Severity

	Stage A	Stage B	Stage C	Stage D
Parameter	At risk	Progressive	Asymptomatic	Symptomatic
EROA (cm^2)	<0.2	<0.2	≥0.2	≥0.2
VC width (cm)	<0.3		≥0.7	≥0.7
RegFr (%)		<50	≥50	≥50
RegVol (cc)		<30	≥30	≥30

EROA, effective regurgitant orifice area; VC, vena contracta; RegFr, regurgitant fraction; RegVol, regurgitant volume
Source: Nishimura RA, et al. AHA/ACC Guidelines. JACC 2014; 63 (22): e57–188

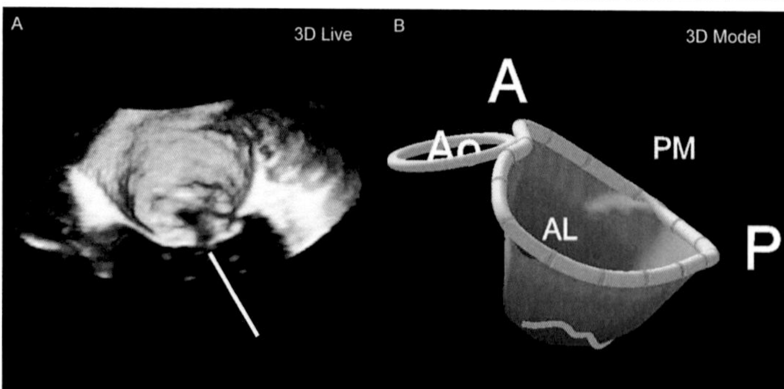

Predictors Failed MV Repair in CIMR
Complex MR jet
Lateral wall motion abnormality
Increased tenting height ≥ 11 mm
Mitral annulus diameter (ME 4C) ≥ 3.7 cm
Tenting area (ME LAX) ≥ 1.6 cm^2
MR grade of >3.5

(A) Patient with restricted MV leaflet motion and central malcoaptation (arrow) from ischemic dilated cardiomyopathy shown during systole using real time 3D TEE from the LA side in 3D Live. (B) Reconstructed static MV 3D model shows severe bileaflet restriction and tenting.

Papillary Muscle Rupture (PMR)

- PMR is rare (1%) post-thrombolysis but may occur early (2–7 days) with a 50% mortality rate. Patients with PMR are surgical emergencies as the prognosis is dismal in medically treated patients.
- The posteromedial papillary muscle is most often involved because of its single blood supply from the posterior descending artery (RCA > Circumflex artery). Since both MV leaflets attach to the posterior PM, either anterior or posterior leaflet could be flail with severe eccentric directed MR (opposite to flail).
- There may be an accompanying small inferior MI with inferior RWMA with surrounding hyper-contractility of normal myocardium.
- Characteristic 2D image findings of PMR are a flail or prolapsing MV leaflet and attached mass (arrow) in the LA as seen in systole in the (A) ME and (B) TG views. (C) Color Doppler shows severe MR that fills the LA. The color jet area may appear small in size as the LAP is raised acutely creating a lower gradient between LA and LV.

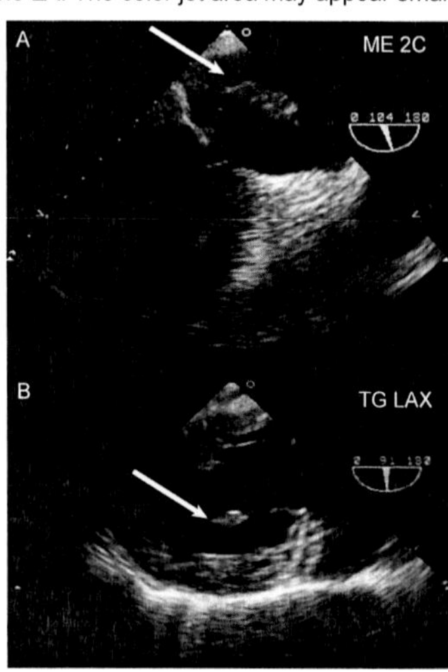

TEE Papillary Muscle Rupture
ME and TG views
Posterior PMR (Cx) > Anterior PMR
Mobile mass thru MV
Inferior RWMA
Hyperdynamic LV

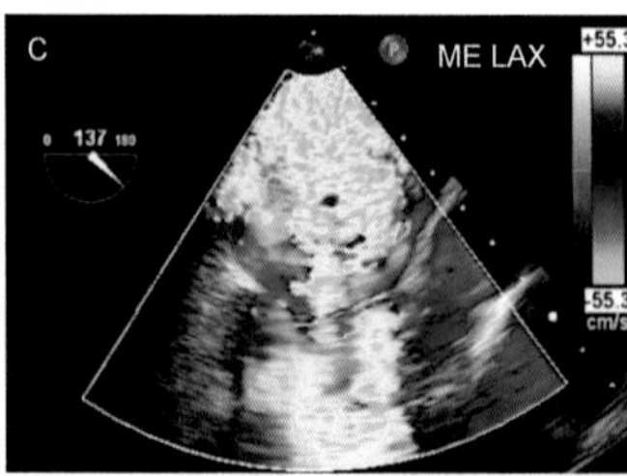

Free Wall Rupture

- This occurs in 1–3% of MI patients within 5 days (50%) to 2 weeks (90%) and accounts for 10% of post MI mortality. Rupture only occurs among patients with a transmural MI and most often involves the lateral wall (circumflex artery).
- Three pathologic subsets are described:
  - Type I (first 24 h) full-thickness rupture from the use of thrombolytics.
  - Type II (1–3 days) from erosion of the myocardium at the infarct site.
  - Type III (late) at the border zone of the MI and normal myocardium.
- 2D imaging of the ME or TG views may show a diffuse or localized pericardial effusion containing thrombus. A RWMA may be seen. Color Doppler rarely shows flow from the ventricle into the pericardial space.
- Although hemopericardium may result from thrombolytic therapy, contrast enhanced echocardiography, while highly sensitive, is not 100% specific for diagnosing cardiac rupture.

Shown here in this ME 4C view is a pericardial effusion (arrow) in a patient 1 week post MI.

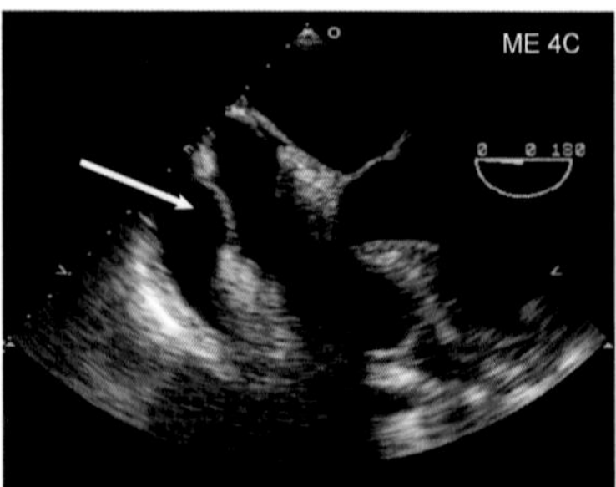

TEE Free Wall Rupture
ME and TG views Transmural MI
RWMA lateral (Cx)
Pericardial effusion
Tamponade

- There has been a decreased incidence (0.2%) of ventricular septal rupture (VSR) in the post-thrombolytic era, occurs 2–5 days post acute MI, with 50% mortality.
- A defect in the IVS occurs at the junction of preserved and transmural infarcted myocardium, that results in communication between the ventricles
  - apical (anterior MI, LAD) >> basal posterior (inferior MI, RCA + Cx) septum
  - simple single gap; or in 30–40% a complex meshwork of serpiginous channels
- Results in L to R shunt, RV volume overload, increased pulmonary blood flow, and secondary LA and LV volume overload.
- Color Doppler imaging is the best method for diagnosing VSR showing systolic turbulent flow on the RV side, with single or multiple holes. An apical/anterior VSR is seen in the ME AV LAX/4C or deep TG views, a basal/infero-posterior VSR in the ME 4C and TG basal or mid SAX view.
- 2D imaging shows thinned myocardium, RWMA with surrounding LV hypercontractility of normal myocardium. Measure the defect size in mm or cm.
- CW spectral Doppler trace has high velocity L to R flow between the ventricles. The shunt fraction (Qp/Qs) is calculated by measuring flow thru the pulmonic and aortic valves.

(A) A small serpiginous apical antero-septal VSD with color flow into the RV is seen in ME 4C and TG views. (B) Post ventricular patch repair flow is seen on the LV side but not thru the septum. (C) In this patient, a large gap is seen in the infero-septal region with turbulent color Doppler flow (Nyquist 59 cm/s) in the mid TG views.

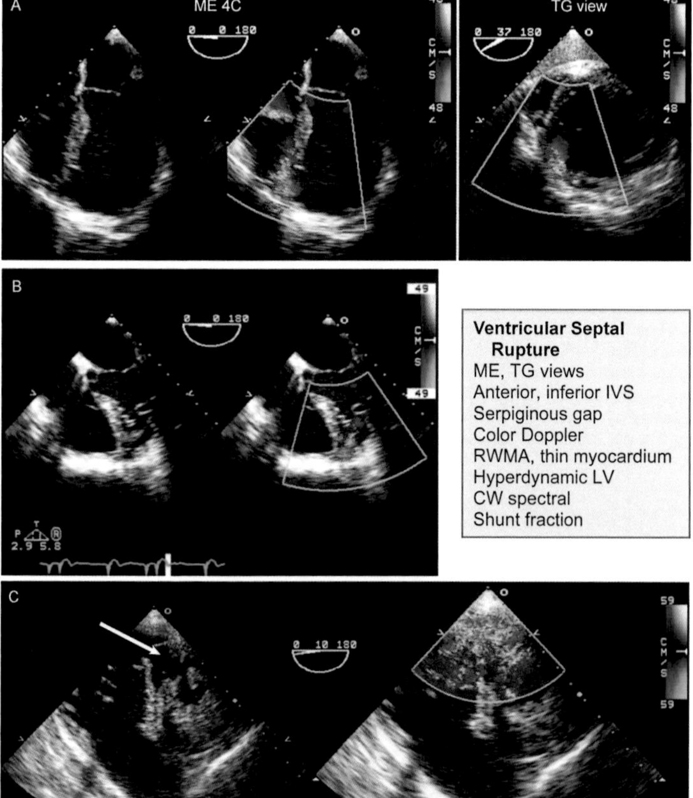

Ventricular Aneurysm

- An aneurysm wall contains all 3 cardiac muscle layers and is connected to the ventricle by a wide neck. This complication occurs in 12–15% of transmural infarctions with (A) anterior and (B) apical infarcts (LAD) at highest risk, followed by (C) inferior basal infarcts. Mural thrombus may be present (40–50%) and is an indication for anticoagulation.
- Refractory heart failure, recurrent emboli and malignant ventricular arrhythmias are all indications for surgical resection.
- 2D image findings include RWMA, thinned or bulging LV wall with a wide mouth opening. The aneurysmal wall may appear thickened from the presence of layered thrombus.

TEE Aneurysm
ME 2C, TG SAX, TG LAX.
Anterior + LV apex (LAD), infero-basal (Cx)
Smooth transition to thinned aneurysm wall
Wide mouth, ratio of neck: aneurysm >0.5
LV wall distortion systole + diastole
Non-contractile RWMA
Thrombus

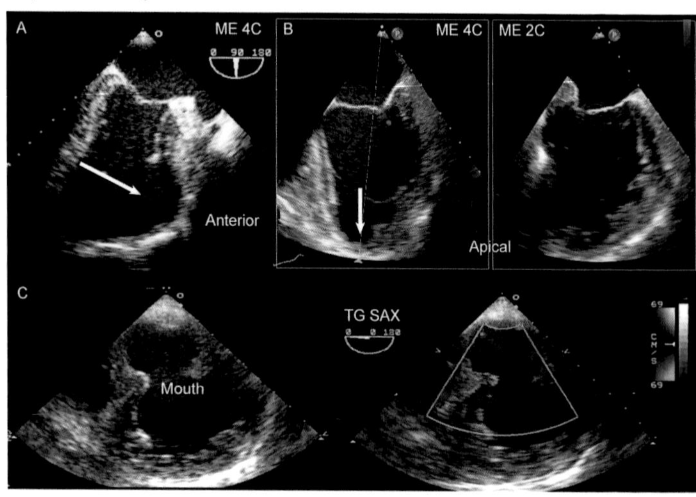

Pseudoaneurysm

- Pseudoaneurysm is a contained rupture of the LV free wall with the outer aneurysm wall formed by pericardium and mural thrombus. There is a narrow neck into the LV, the diameter of which is by definition <50% of the aneurysm diameter.
- The aneurysm may remain small or progressively enlarge. Surgical intervention to prevent sudden death is recommended for all patients regardless of symptoms or aneurysm size.
- 2D imaging can demonstrate the pseudoaneurysm in ME or TG views. RWMA with an abrupt transition from normal myocardium to thin aneurysm wall (acute angle). Narrow neck with a ratio of neck/aneurysm diameter <0.5. The pseudoaneurysm may be partially filled with thrombus.
- Color Doppler shows low velocity bidirectional flow.

Pseudoaneurysm
TEE ME, TG views
Pericardium + clot
Narrow neck
Expands in systole
Color Doppler in/out

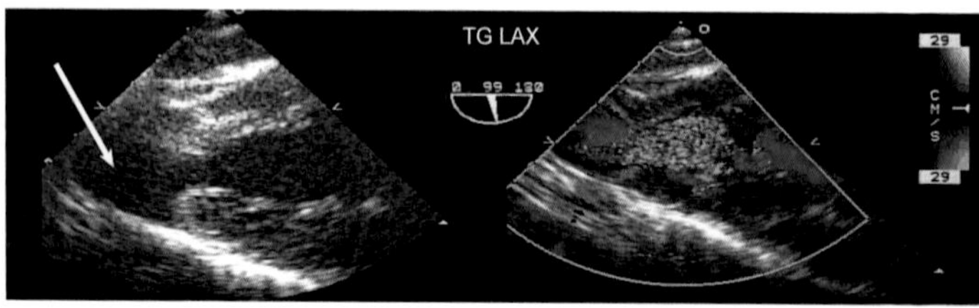

Thrombus and Embolus

- Overall incidence of mural thrombus after MI is 15–60%, reduced with reperfusion.
- LV thrombus occurs from blood stasis in the presence of RWMA (related to size), an aneurysm and severe global dysfunction. Common in large anterior MI and occurs less often in an inferior or lateral MI.
- Clinically evident systemic embolism results in stroke, limb ischemia, renal infarction, or intestinal ischemia is uncommon (<2%) in the first 10 days after acute MI. Anticoagulation should be started immediately and continued for 3–6 months.
- Echocardiography is the diagnostic test of choice and accurately depicts thrombus. The diagnosis of thrombus is best made by TTE as the LV apex is closest to the TTE probe. ME and TG views can show 2D findings of laminated thrombus as a thickening of the LV apex (compared with the IVS) and an underlying RWMA. Early thrombus may be pedunculated and mobile with a higher risk of embolization (35%). Color Doppler shows no flow in the thrombus.

(A) TTE apical 4C view zoomed to show thickening of the LV apex consistent with thrombus. (B, C) A large apical thrombus is seen in the ME 4C and a zoomed view of the LV apex. The echogenicity of thrombus is similar to the underlying myocardium. (D, E) Patient with a large anterior MI shows significant thrombus formation along the LV walls in both the modified deep TG and ME LAX views.

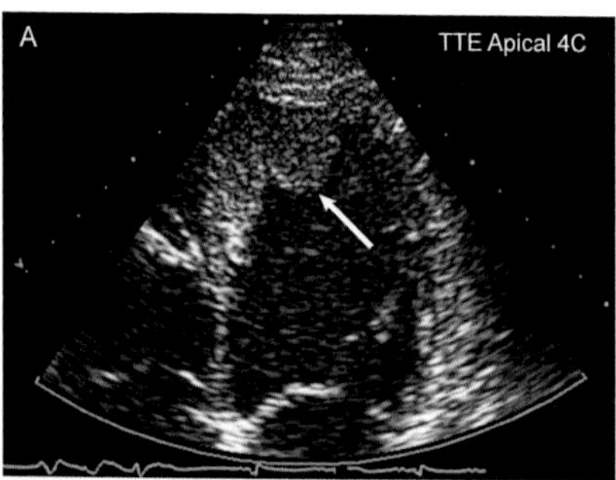

LV Thrombus Echo
TTE gold standard
TEE ME, TG views
Anterior, apical, inferior
RWMA (akinesis/dyskinesis)
Thick myocardium
Pedunculated early
Laminated late.
Spontaneous echo contrast
Color Doppler no flow

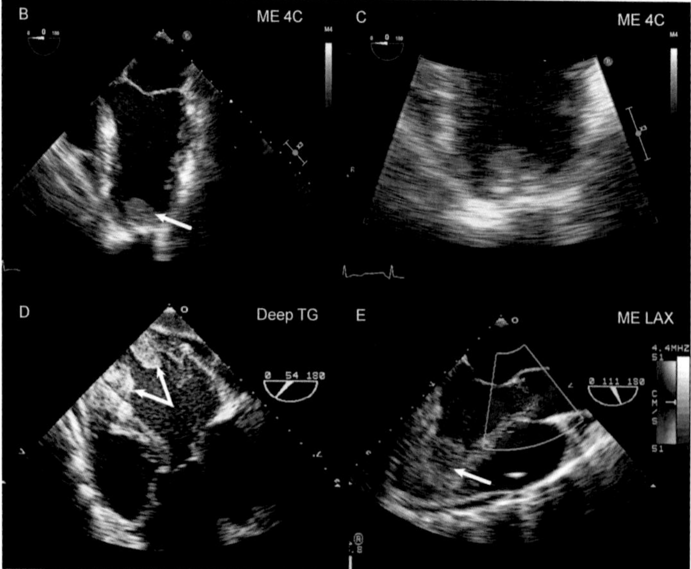

6 Diastology

A. Vegas, *Perioperative Two-Dimensional Transesophageal Echocardiography*, https://doi.org/10.1007/978-3-319-60902-7_6

Normal Physiology of Diastole

- Diastole is the period of ventricular filling after contraction. It is defined clinically from aortic valve (AV) closure to mitral valve (MV) closure or, physiologically, as the duration of myocardial relaxation (although this actually begins in late systole).
- Diastole involves energy-dependent interrelated cellular and mechanical processes that allow the heart to relax and fill. Adequate diastolic filling is essential for normal systolic ventricular function. Diastole forms 2/3 of the cardiac cycle at resting heart rates (HR), but shortens at faster rates.
- Diastole is divided into 4 phases.

Phases of Ventricular Diastole

❶ **Isovolumic Relaxation (IVRT)**: begins at AV closure when aortic pressure exceeds LVP and ends as LVP falls rapidly to below LAP, opening the MV.

❷ **Rapid Filling (E wave velocity)**: begins with MV opening as LAP exceeds LVP; with further LV relaxation, blood is rapidly "sucked" into the LV, increasing LVP.

❸ **Diastasis (slope of filling)**: LV relaxation ends during the first 1/3 of diastole. LV compliance slows ventricular filling as LVP rises to equal LAP. When LAP = LVP, there is no flow across the open MV, a period called diastasis.

❹ **Atrial Contraction (A wave velocity)**: occurs at end-diastole to complete LV preload. LAP exceeds LVP allowing the MV to reopen wider to fill the LV. This normally contributes 15–20% of LV preload, but may contribute 50% in diastolic dysfunction. It is absent in atrial fibrillation.

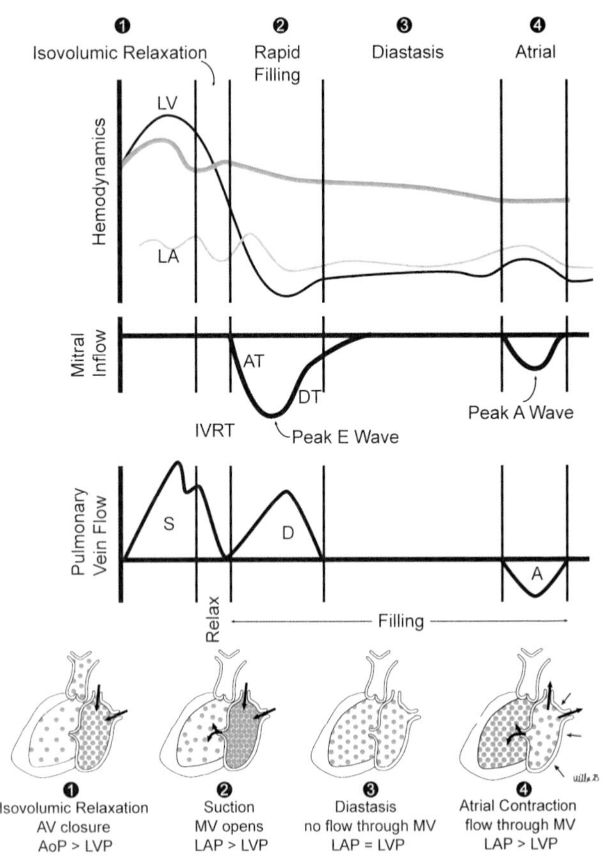

Determinants of Diastolic Function

- As the cavity volume increases, the myocardial fibers stretch in a nonlinear fashion; pressure increases geometrically in a relationship termed LV stiffness (compliance). The curvilinear slope of LV stiffness varies according to myocardial fiber distensibility, connective tissue elasticity, cavity diameter, wall thickness, and the pericardial constraining effect. In normal ventricles, diastolic stiffness is low (high compliance) as large volumes only cause small pressure increases.
- The LA is a key determinant of LV diastolic function as it acts as a blood reservoir, conduit, and an active pump at end-diastole. There are a number of determinants of normal diastolic function as listed here.
- The gold standard for the assessment of diastolic function uses specialized high fidelity pressure catheters to simultaneously measure LV volumes, LV pressures, and determine stiffness.
- Invasive measures of diastolic function include the peak instantaneous rate of LV pressure decline (−dP/dt), time constant of LV relaxation (tau, t), and the stiffness modulus. A small value of t indicates rapid relaxation.

Determinants of Diastolic Function
Myocardial relaxation
Myocardial stiffness
Left atrial function
Pericardial constraint
RV size and function
Intra-thoracic pressure
HR, AV conduction
MV function
Neurohormones
Preload
Afterload

Normal Diastole Values	
- dP/dt	- 2000 mmHg/s
tau, t	25 - 40 ms
IVRT	60 - 90 ms

Diastolic Function by Echocardiography

- This begins with an examination of the heart for structural abnormalities. Abnormal LV size, wall thickness and reduced function, and an increased LA size suggest the possible presence of diastolic dysfunction (DD).
  - DD is unlikely to occur in a normal heart.
  - DD may occur with normal systolic function.
- It is important to exclude the presence of mitral valve disease and rhythm disorders such as atrial fibrillation, heart block, or ventricular pacing, which invalidates some of the Doppler parameters used to assess diastolic function.
- Doppler echocardiography can noninvasively assess DD, by determining the diagnosis, prognosis, and treatment. Doppler evaluation of LV diastolic function involves examining parameters related to: (1) Ventricular relaxation, (2) Chamber compliance, and (3) Filling pressures.
- Guidelines suggest that multiple parameters be used to assess diastolic function.
  - There is overlap between normal values and those associated with DD.
  - No one parameter is superior.
  - Doppler parameters may be discordant; the more concordant the measures, the more likely DD is present.
  - Many of these indices are preload, afterload, HR, and rhythm-dependent, making assessment difficult in the perioperative setting.

Initial Assessment
Structural heart disease
LV size, thickness, function
LA size
Exclude
Arrhythmias
MV disease
Measure
MV inflow (PW)
TDI mitral annulus
Pulmonary vein flow (PW)

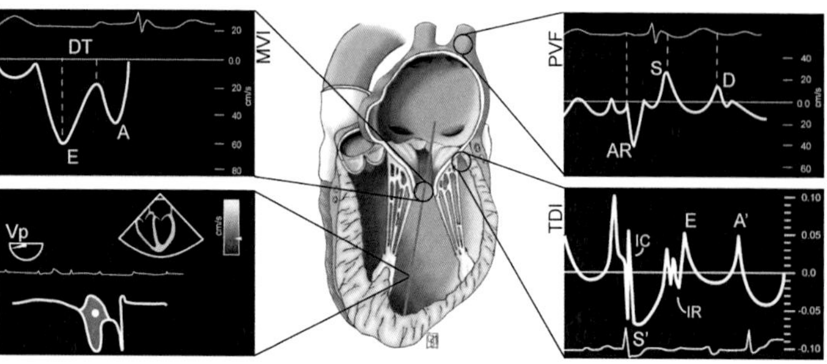

Mitral Valve Inflow (MVI)	
• PW Doppler ME 4C/AV LAX view use 1–3 mm sample volume between MV leaflet tips (not at annulus). • Sweep speed 50–100 mm/s during apnea, adjust baseline and scale so spectral trace fills the space • Measure peak E and A wave velocities and DT from E wave peak to baseline. • Reflects LA to LV pressure gradient and LV filling through MV	• Affected by changes in relaxation (E wave) and compliance • Unreliable in normal systolic function • Very preload dependent – ↓ Preload or IPPV → ↓ E, ↑ DT • Rhythm + conduction – ↑ HR, 1st HB, paced: fused E + A – ↓ HR: small “L” wave of diastasis – AF: loss of A wave • Not used in diastolic assessment if: a fib, MV disease, LVAD, LBBB, V pace

Assess LV Filling	Normal
Peak early velocity (E wave)	50–80 cm/s
Peak late velocity (A wave)	30–50 cm/s
E/A ratio	1–2: 1
Deceleration time (DT) of E wave	140–240 ms
Isovolumic relaxation time (IVRT)	60–90 ms

Normal

- Early suction from adequate LV relaxation gives high peak E wave
  - E/A > 0.8–1.2
  - Normal DT, IVRT
- Age-related (↓ E/A, ↑ DT)

Impaired Relaxation

- Inadequate diastolic suction delays MV opening and reduces early MV inflow, but increases LA volume later in cardiac cycle from atrium
  - ↓ E wave velocity
  - E/A < 1
  - ↑ DT
  - ↑ IVRT
  - ↑ A wave

Pseudonormal

- ↑ LAP compensates for impaired filling returns MVI trace to normal
- MVI alone can’t distinguish normal from pseudonormal DD
- Valsalva ↓ E/A ratio by 50% to give impaired relaxation, so A > E wave

Restrictive

- Reduced LV compliance leads to ↑ LAP required to fill LV
  - ↑↑ E wave velocity
  - E/A >> 2
  - ↓ DT
  - ↓ IVRT

L Wave

- Mid-diastolic wave represents continuous PVF through the LA and open MV into the LV.
- It is found in bradycardiac patients with impaired relaxation and ↑ LAP.
- Correlates with prognosis

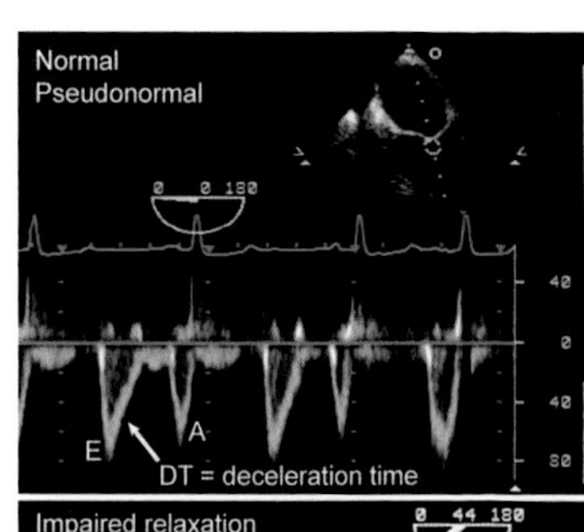

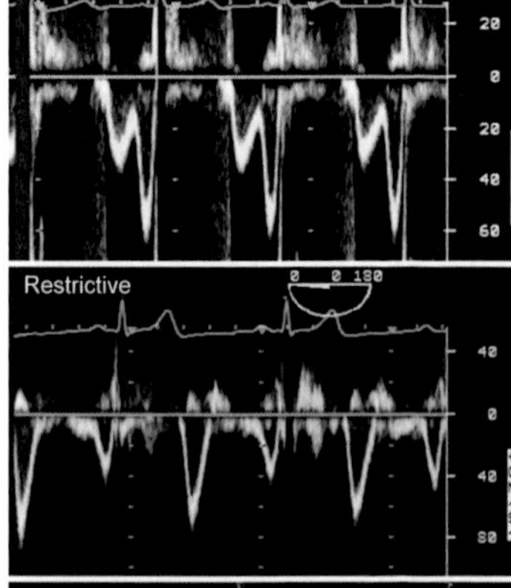

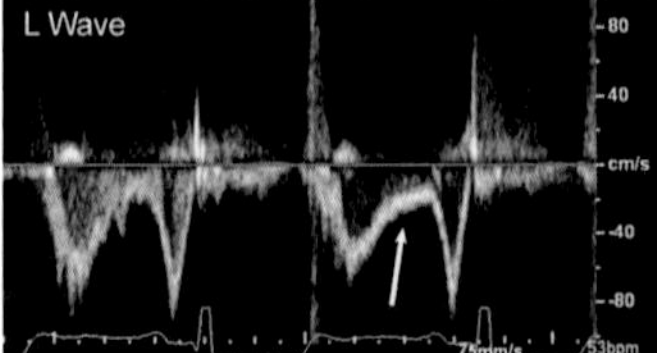

Mitral Annular Tissue Doppler Imaging (TDI)	
• PW TDI ME 4C view uses 5–10 mm sample volume placed 1 cm at lateral or septal insertion of MV leaflet. Minimize angulation • Sweep speed 50–100 mm/s at end-expiration • Identify: S′, E′, A′ waves • Assess myocardial velocities during contraction and relaxation	• Reflects intrinsic speed of myocardial relaxation • Inverse relation of E′ and relaxation • E' is influenced by – Regional function (septal, lateral) – Age – Location (lateral or septal) – Relatively preload-independent • Inaccurate if MAC, MV disease • Distinguish normal/pseudonormal DD
Assess LA Filling	**Normal**
Early (e′, Ea, Em, E′) wave	10–15 cm/s (septal), 13–20 cm/s (lateral)
Relates only to relaxation not compliance	<8 cm/s is abnormal relaxation
Late (a′, A′) wave	11.3 ± 2.9 cm/s ↑ If ↑ LA contractility, ↓ if ↑ LVEDP
Assess LV Filling Pressure	**Normal and Abnormal**
Mitral E/E′ ratio	<8 normal LAP
Relates to LV filling pressures	>15 → ↑ LAP and LVEDP
E′/A′ during Valsalva	0.9–3.1 cm/s (lateral) Persisting abnormality is pseudonormal

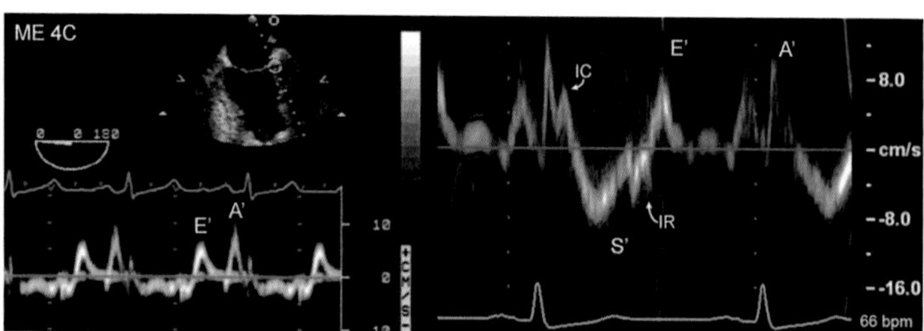

Isovolumic Relaxation Time (IVRT)	Normal 60–90 ms
• Interval from AV closure to MV open. • Assess using PWD or TDI • TG LAX view with PW sample volume placed between the MV inflow and LVOT. Arrow indicates the points of AV closure and MV opening representing IVRT. • TDI from lateral mitral annulus identifies duration of dip between systole (S′) and E′ wave.	• Affected by aortic diastolic pressure and LAP • Varies with age • Impaired relaxation: prolonged IVRT • Restrictive filling: shorten IVRT

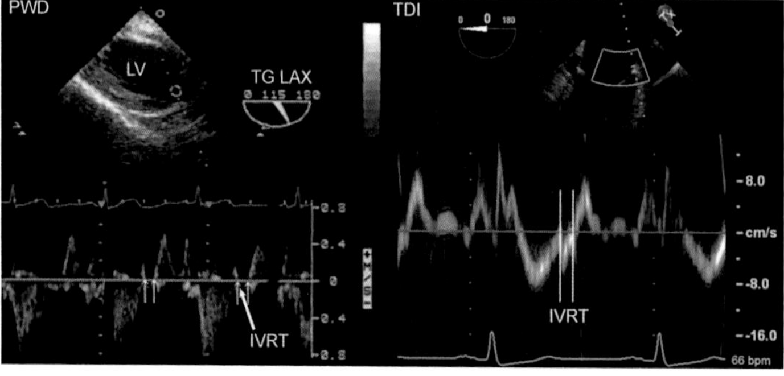

Pulmonary Vein Flow (PVF)	
• Represents LA filling as the pressure difference between PV and LA. • There are no valves in the PV; with LA contraction, there is forward flow into LV (MVI A wave) and retrograde flow into pulmonary veins (A wave). • PW Doppler ME 2C view uses 2–3 mm sample volume placed 0.5 cm into left upper pulmonary vein.	• Anything that ↑ LAP will ↓ PVF into LA, converse is also true • Load-dependent • Large PV A wave is seen with MS and complete heart block (CHB) • Reduced S wave (<40%) relates to ↓ LA compliance, ↑ mean LAP • Worsening DD has longer A wave duration
Assess LA Filling	**Normal**
Systolic Wave (S)	28–82 cm/s
Diastolic wave (D)	27–72 cm/s
S/D ratio	S > D
Atrial reversal wave peak (PV AR)	A velocity 15–35 cm/s
Atrial reversal wave duration (ARdur)	A dur 60–120 ms
Time difference AR and MV A wave	<20 ms
D velocity Deceleration Time	>275 ms

Normal (S > D)

- Normal PVF pattern (S.D) is found with normal diastolic function.

Pseudonormal or Restrictive DD

- S < D, if <40% have ↑ LAP (15 mmHg)
- Time difference between PV AR and MV A wave duration (>30 ms)
  - greater Ar relates to ↑ LVEDP
- Restrictive DD; there may have small A wave from LA mechanical failure

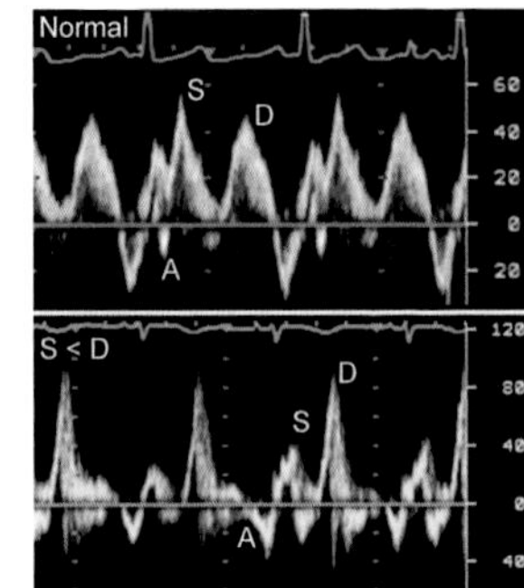

Velocity of Propagation (Vp)	
• ME 4C view color Doppler, position M-mode scan line through center of LV inflow blood column from MV to apex. Shift Nyquist limit <40 cm/s or 75% of E MVI velocity • Measure Vp as first aliasing velocity slope in early filling, from MV to 4 cm into LV, or the transition slope from no color to color	• Preload positively affects Vp, though less with DD • Normal LV volumes and EFs, but elevated filling pressures can have misleadingly normal Vp • Vp is reduced with ↓ EF
Assess LV Relaxation	**Normal and Abnormal**
Velocity of propagation (Vp)	>50 cm/s
Ratio of MVI peak E/Vp LV filling pressure with ↓ EF	E/Vp > 2.5 → PCWP >15 mmHg

Color M-mode Transmitral Flow (Vp)

- LV relaxes at the base before the apex, creating a wavefront of flow from LA to LV.
- Vp assesses LV suction during early diastole and better evaluates LV relaxation compared to the single point measures of MVI.
- Slowing of mitral-to-apical Vp is consistent with reduced apical suction, suggesting abnormal relaxation, but not its severity.

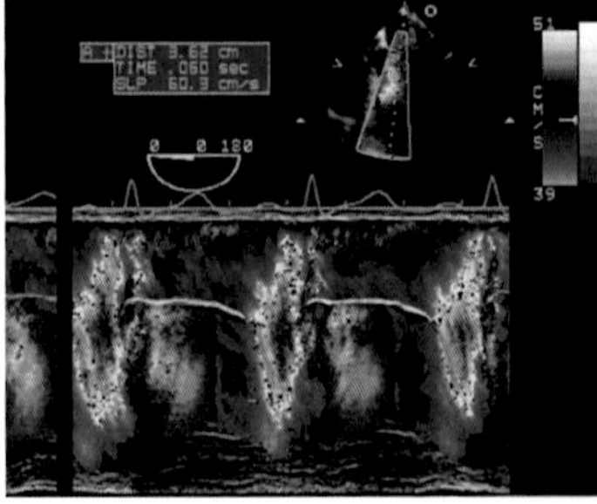

Algorithms for Elevated Pressures

- Echocardiography is unable to directly measure LAP and LVP, but these can be estimated by using different parameters.
- A normal LAP implies normal diastolic function.
- The following algorithm differs on choice of the initial diagnostic test based on the presence of ab/normal EF
  - Abnormal EF: MVI
  - Normal EF: TDI lateral E/E′

TTE Estimates	↑ LAP	↑ LVP
MV E/A	>2	>2
MV DT	<140 ms	<160 ms
E/e′ (lateral)	>15	>10
PFV S/D	<1	<40%
PFV A vel	>35 cm/s	>25 cm/s
PFV Adur-MV Adur	>20 ms	>30 ms
PASP	>35 mmHg	
Chamber	LAE	LAE, LVH

LAE, left atrial enlargement; LVH, left ventricular hypertrophy; PASP, pulmonary artery systolic pressure

Doppler Algorithm to Assess LAP

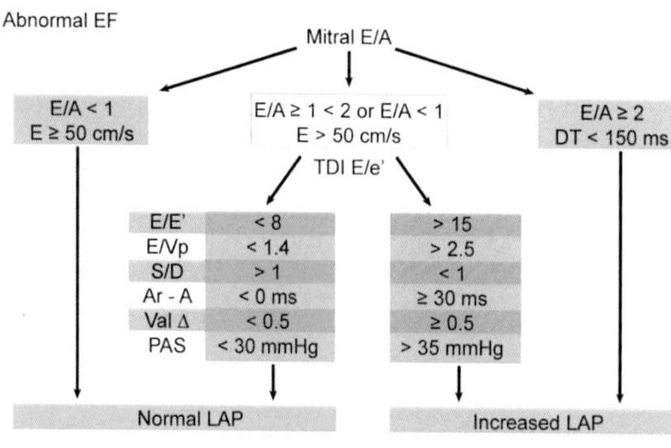

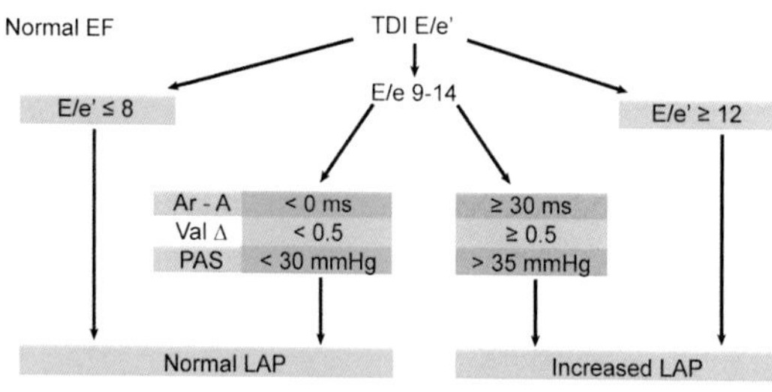

Algorithms for Diastolic Dysfunction

- Algorithms exist for the assessment of diastolic function and differ depending on the technique used (TTE or TEE) and ventricular function.
- TTE guidelines recommend the use of Doppler indices, assessment LA size, and TV velocity for the assessment of diastolic function.
- TEE does not specifically measure LA size as this is difficult.

Normal EF		TTE Assessment DD	
1. Average E/e′	>14	Normal Diastolic	<50% positive
2. Septal e′	<7 cm/s	Indeterminate	50% positive
Lateral e′	<10 cm/s	Abnormal	>50% positive
3. TR velocity	2.8 m/s	DD severity is determined by the number of positive findings (#/4)	
4. LA volume Index	>34 cc/m²		

Adapted from: Nagueh SF, et al. ASE Guidelines J Am Soc Echocardiogr 2016;29:277–314

Diastolic Dysfunction

- Diastolic Dysfunction (DD) is a limitation of the ventricle to fill to normal end-diastolic volume (EDV) without an abnormal increase in end-diastolic pressure (EDP) at rest or during exercise. DD can be defined as the need to inappropriately increase intracardiac pressures to achieve adequate LV filling to support CO. Early DD from impaired relaxation elevates LAP, while later DD increases LVEDP.
- DD occurs when LV filling is impeded from altered myocardial relaxation and compliance, as result of changes in the rhythm, myocardium, ventricular interaction, and pericardial restraint.

Grades of Diastolic Dysfunction

- Diastolic filling begins with a rapid influx of blood into the LV (MVI, E wave), which slows as LVP rises to exceed LAP (MVI DT time). During diastasis, there is no flow into the LV. Atrial contraction (MVI, A wave) completes LV filling.
- Normal subjects have rapid LV relaxation, low stiffness (normal compliance), and normal filling pressures with minimal atrial contribution to LV filling.

Normal	
MVI	High E (>0.8 m/s), E/A > 1, DT < 220 ms, IVRT <100 ms
TDI e′	>10 (young), >8 (old) cm/s
PVF	S/D > 1 (S/D < 1 in athletes)
Color M-mode Vp	>55 cm/s (young), >45 cm/s (old)

There is progression to different grades of DD.

(I) Impaired Relaxation	
MVI	↓ E wave, ↑ DT (>220 ms), ↑ A wave (high Peak A, greater VTI, prolonged A duration), E/A < 1.0
TDI e′	↓ e′ (<8 cm/s), E/e′ ratio > 1
PVF	Blunted D wave (S/D ≫ 1), Ap < Am duration

- This initial abnormality of DD results from a loss of elastic recoil such that the LV fails to generate suction. This prolongs the IVRT, leaving a longer time to open the MV. After the MV opens, the decreased suction causes a low peak E velocity and prolonged DT (longer time for early filling). LA is relatively full, so there is more filling late from atrial contraction (>30% of SV). There is impaired relaxation, but relatively normal compliance and filling pressures.
- These patients become symptomatic with exercise when diastolic filling time shortens. The pattern may be present in low preload, increased afterload, acute ischemia, LVH, HOCM, inhalation agents, and prolonged CPB.

(II) Pseudonormalization	
MVI	reverts to normal pattern, high E, E/A ratio 1:1.5, IVRT <100 ms, DT < 220 ms, Ap < Am duration
TDI e′	↓ e′ (<8 cm/s) with ↑ E/e′ ratio
PVF	blunted S wave (S/D < 1), Ap > Am duration

- Both compliance and relaxation abnormalities develop in this phase as LAP rises throughout diastole to “pseudonormalize” and maintain LV filling (reversible restrictive physiology). Blood is thus pushed rather than sucked across the MV.

(III-IV) Restriction	
MVI	Rapid early LV filling (high E wave, short DT < 150 ms, IVRT <60 ms). Atrial contribution diminishes from elevated LV stiffness and atrial mechanical failure (A wave small, short duration), ↑↑ E/A ratio (>1.5–2).
TDI e′	Shows persisting ↓ e′ wave with ↑ E/e′ ratio (abnormal > 15)
PVF	S/D < 1, ↑ A duration from prolonged flow in compliant pulmonary vasculature at atrial contraction. If $A_{PDF} > A_{MV}$ by 30 seconds, LVEDP is increased

- This occurs with end-stage cardiac disease
- As LV compliance worsens, DD deteriorates such that less volume causes a greater increase in LVP and a restrictive filling pattern develops. If it becomes irreversible despite manipulations (nitrates, diuretics, IPPV), it is grade IV. This pattern has abnormal relaxation and compliance with high filling pressure.
- Diseases causing restrictive diastolic pattern include: advanced ischemia heart disease, uncompensated congestive failure, or restrictive cardiomyopathy.

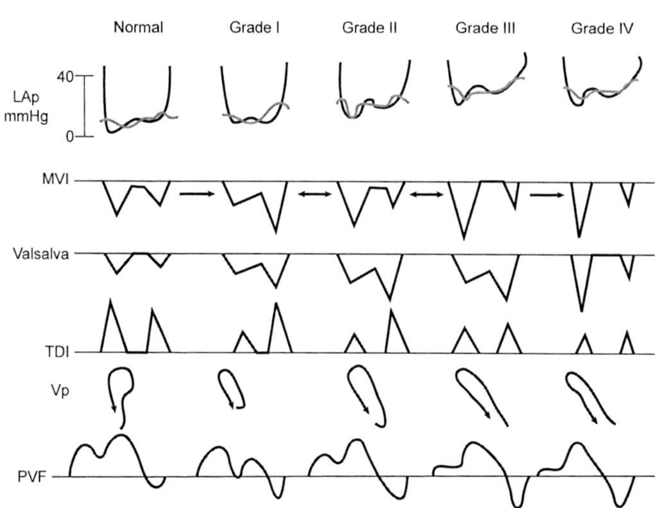

Stages of DD	Normal[a] Young	Normal[a] Adult[b]	Delayed Relax	Pseudo-normal	Restrict Filling
E/A	1.88 ± 0.45	1.5–0.96 ± 0.4	<0.75	0.75–1.5	>1.5
DT (ms)	142	166–200 ± 29	>220	150–200	<150
IVRT (ms)	50 ± 9	67–87 ± 7	>100	60–100	<60
S/D	1.8 ± 0.8	0.98–1.39 ± 0.47	1	<1	<1
Am: Ap Duration		Am ≥ Ap	Am > Ap	*Am < Ap*	Am ≪ Ap
PV AR (cm/s)	16 ± 10	21–25 ± 9	<35	*≥35*[a]	≥25[a]
Vp (cm/s)	>55	>45	<50	*<50*	<50
e′ (cm/s)	20.6 ± 3.8	19.8–12.9 ± 2.9	<8	*<8*	<8
E: e′		<10	<10	*≥10*	≥10
e′/a′		e′ > a′	e′ < a′	*e′ < a′*	e′ < a′

Italics differentiates normal from pseudonormal
MV inflow E/A: early-to-atrial ratio; DT: deceleration time; IVRT: isovolumic relaxation time;
Pulmonary vein S/D: systolic-to-diastolic ratio; AR: peak atrial contraction reversed velocity
Velocity of propagation (Vp) color M-mode
Tissue Doppler Imaging (TDI) e′: MV annular velocity
[a]ASE Guidelines 2009
[b]Adult increasing age

Doppler Algorithm of Diastolic Dysfunction

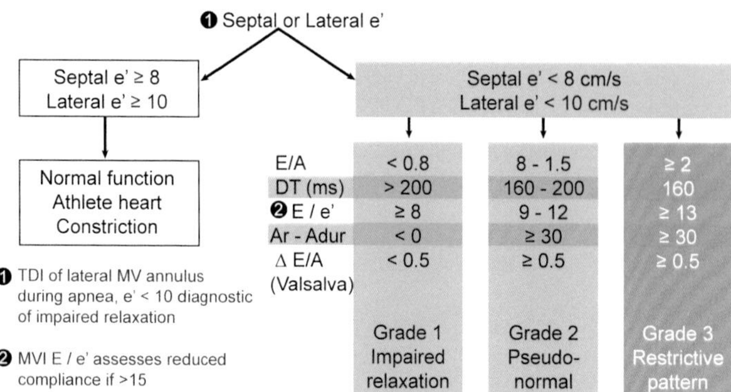

Clinical Application

- Common causes of DD include: hypertension, CAD, restrictive and dilated cardiomyopathies, constrictive pericarditis, and cardiac surgery patients (30–75%).
- DD is an independent cause of morbidity and mortality in many of these clinical settings.
- Diastolic heart failure includes symptoms of low cardiac output (CO) and elevated filling pressures, often with preserved LV systolic function but impaired diastolic function.
- Patients with DD usually do not have heart failure symptoms, but can become symptomatic with the loss of atrial function as with atrial fibrillation.
- Challenges exist in assessing DD in patients with arrhythmias and MV disease. Some additional validated parameters are listed.
- Anesthetic agents have a variable effect on diastolic function; some may impair relaxation (halothane, isoflurane, desflurane) and compliance (halothane).

Preload

- A moderate increase in preload does not affect normal relaxation.
- MVI, Vp, TDI are preload-dependent in patients with normal diastolic function, but Vp and TDI are preload-independent in patients with DD.

Afterload

- Normal systolic function with an increased afterload shortens DT (better relaxation), but with abnormal systolic function an increase in afterload lengthens DT.

Atrial Fibrillation	
E wave peak acceleration	≥1900 cm/s^2
IVRT	≤65 ms
PV DT diastolic velocity	≤220 ms
E/Vp ratio	≥1.4
Septal E/e′ ratio	≥11
Hypertrophic Cardiomyopathy	
Average E/e′	>14
Ar-A	≥30 ms
TR peak velocity	>2.8 m/s
LA volume	>34 cc/m^2
Restrictive Cardiomyopathy	
DT	<140 ms
Mitral E/A	>2.5
IVRT	<50 ms
Average E/e′	>14
Mitral Stenosis	
IVRT	<60 ms
IVRT/$T_{E\text{-}e'}$	<4.2
Mitral A velocity	>1.5 m/s
Mitral Regurgitation	
Ar-A	≥30 ms
IVRT	<60 ms
IVRT/$T_{E\text{-}e'}$	<5.6
Average E/e′	>14
Pulmonary Hypertension	
Lateral E/e′	>13 cardiac
Lateral E/e′	<8 noncardiac
Sinus Tachycardia	
MVI E wave	Prominent
IVRT	≤70 ms
PV systolic filling fraction	≤40%
Average E/e′	>14

Adapted from: Nagueh SF, et al. J Am Soc Echocardiogr 2016;29:277–314.

Specific Pathologies

Different patterns of DD are associated with different pathologies. Often a spectrum of diastolic dysfunction occurs in any single pathology. Many patients will start with impaired relaxation and progress onto restrictive filling.

Impaired Relaxation
Ischemia
Hypertrophy
Dilated
RV overload
↑ PAP
Reduced Compliance (Restrictive)
Infarction
Hypertrophy
Restrictive cardiomyopathy
Constrictive pericarditis
Tamponade

- **CAD** affects relaxation by limiting the availability of energy substrates. Acute ischemia impairs LV relaxation, while infarction increases stiffness from interstitial fibrosis and scar formation.
- **Restrictive cardiomyopathies** are a group of disorders (amyloidosis, post-radiation, glycogen storage disorders, muscular dystrophy) characterized by small LV cavity size, abnormal relaxation, and increased stiffness. Increased wall thickness is from infiltration or fibrosis and not myocyte hypertrophy; therefore, the ECG QRS voltage is normal or low.
- **Hypertrophic cardiomyopathy** is characterized by myocardial fiber disarray and global or segmental increase in LV wall thickness. LV chamber stiffness is increased and relaxation is impaired by the asynchronous deactivation of muscle fibers caused by abnormal electrical conduction.

- **Constrictive pericarditis** is a unique cause of DD characterized by increased LV stiffness from the constraining effects of a thickened rigid pericardium. Relaxation is normal in these patients and symptoms of right heart failure predominate. During respiration, the intra-thoracic pressures are not transmitted to the ventricular cavities causing extreme variations of blood flow into the heart. Consequently, despite similar Doppler indices at rest, there is profound respiratory variation.
- **Subacute cardiac tamponade** usually presents with signs and symptoms similar to those of constrictive pericarditis. There is impedance to diastolic flow due to compression of the more compliant right-sided chambers. MVI may identify exaggerated respiratory variation of peak "E" wave velocities (>30%) and should be taken in the context of the patient's clinical circumstance.
- **Aortic stenosis** pressure overload results in concentric hypertrophy which may result in impaired relaxation and progress to a restrictive pattern. The presence of concurrent MR (higher MVI E), MAC (lower e′), or fibrosis (altered compliance) confounds the assessment of DD.
- **Aortic regurgitation** results in eccentric hypertrophy which initially accommodates the increased volume (increased compliance, elevated volume with normal LV pressures). Over time, there is impaired relaxation and increased LV stiffness causing elevated LV pressures and pulmonary congestion.
- **Mitral stenosis** protects the LV and preserves systolic and diastolic function. LAP is increased (↑ A velocity > 1.5 m/s).
- **Mitral regurgitation** results in LA and LV enlargement from volume overload. The LV becomes stiffer over time. Assess DD as indicated in the Table (p. 124).

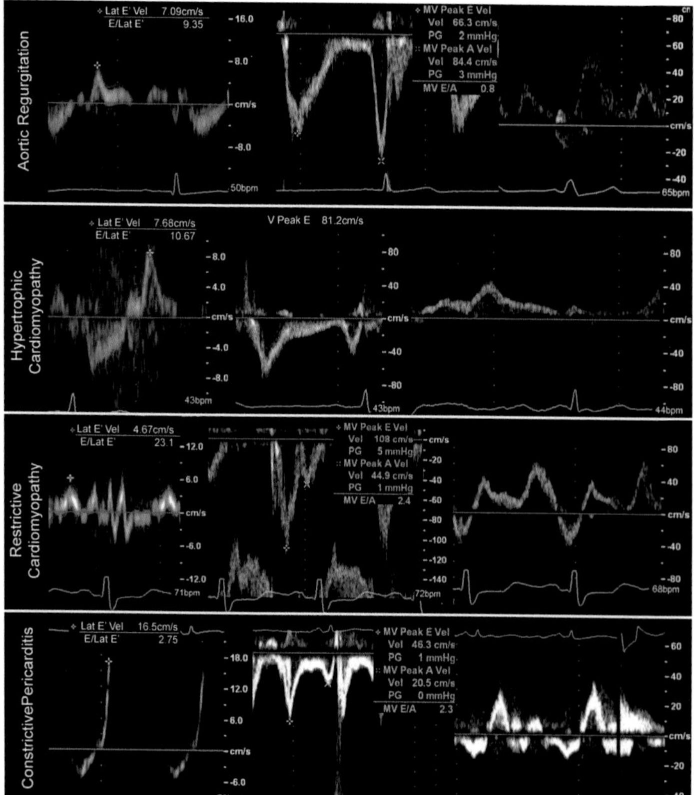

Echocardiographic Assessment

- Assessment of RV diastolic function should be made if there is RV systolic dysfunction. RV DD is a marker of poor prognosis in patients.
- Important measures of RV DD include:
  - Tricuspid valve inflow (TVI)
  - TDI of lateral TV annulus
  - Hepatic vein flow (HVF)
  - IVC size + collapsibility
- TVI E/A ratio, E/e′ ratio, deceleration time (DT), and RA size are the most validated measures of RV diastolic function.

RV Diastolic Indices TTE	Mean
TVI E	54 cm/s
TVI A	40 cm/s
TVI E/A	1.4
TVI DT E wave	174 ms
RV-IVRT	48 ms
TV e′	14 cm/s
TV a′	13 cm/s
E/e′ ratio	1.2
E′/a′ ratio	4

E velocity is lower in RV than LV
Deceleration time is longer in the RV
Source: Rudeski LG. J Am Soc Echocardiogr 2010;23:685–713

Tricuspid Valve Inflow (TVI)	Normal Values in Table Above
• PW Doppler in ME 4C/RVOT view use 1–3 mm sample volume between TV leaflet tips. • Sweep speed 50–100 mm/s baseline and scale, so spectral trace fills the space during end-expiration. • Measure peak E and A wave velocities and DT from peak of E wave • Reflects RA to RV pressure gradient and RV filling through TV	• Affected by HR, age, respiration • Tachycardia: reduced A wave and RA filling fraction, without any effect on peak E wave velocity • Age has little effect on peak A wave velocity, RA filling fraction, and E/A ratio, compared to mitral inflow • Respiratory variability: ↑ E with inspiration • Invalid if significant TR

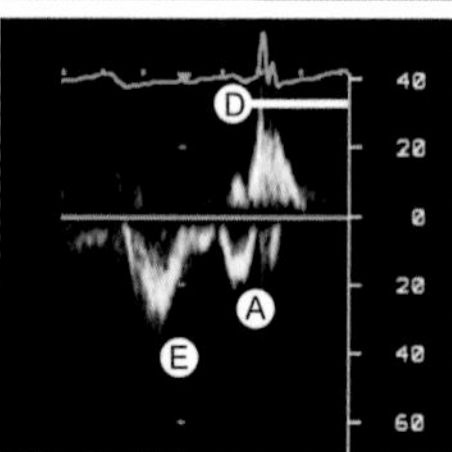

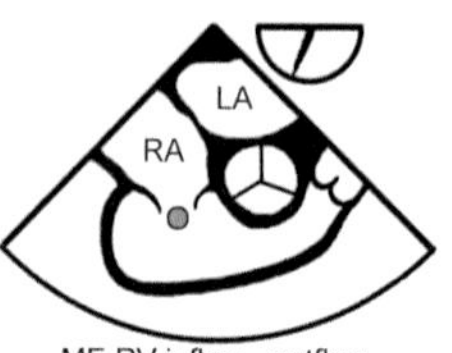

ME RV inflow - outflow

Tricuspid Annular TDI	Normal Values in Table Above
• PW TDI in TG LAX view use 5–10 mm sample volume placed 1 cm at lateral or septal insertion of TV leaflet • Minimize angulation • Sweep speed 50–100 mm/s at end-expiration • Identify: S′, E′, A′ waves	• Assess myocardial velocities during contraction and relaxation

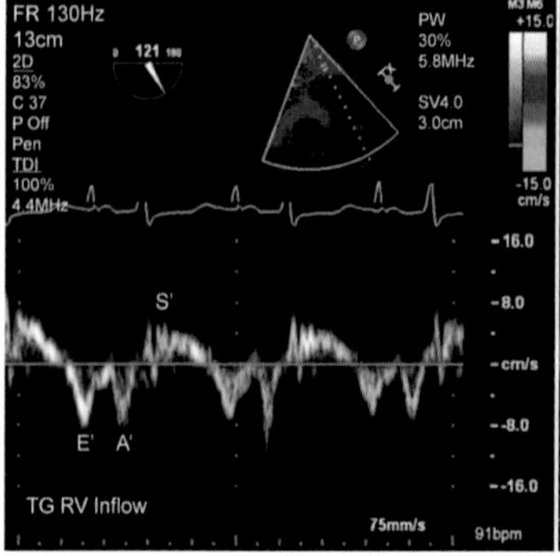

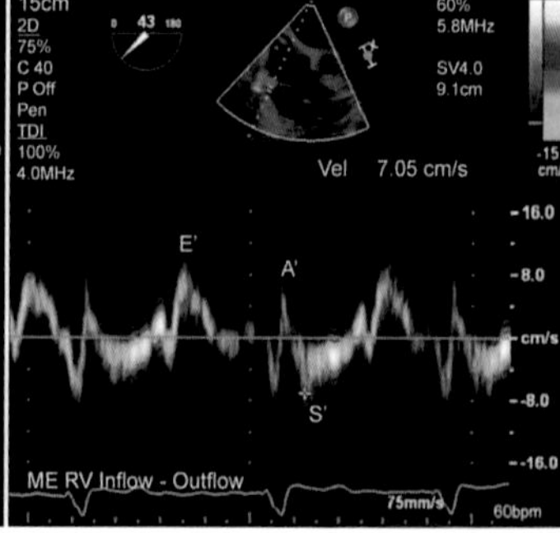

Hepatic Vein Flow (HVF)	Normal
• PW Doppler in TG view use 1–3 mm sample volume in hepatic vein • Sweep speed 50–100 mm/s baseline and scale, so spectral trace fills space • Measure during end-expiration • Reflects RA filling	• Measure S, D, A velocities, A wave duration • Normal HVF: – S/D > 1 – Atrial wave reversal duration (Adur) < half maximum S velocity

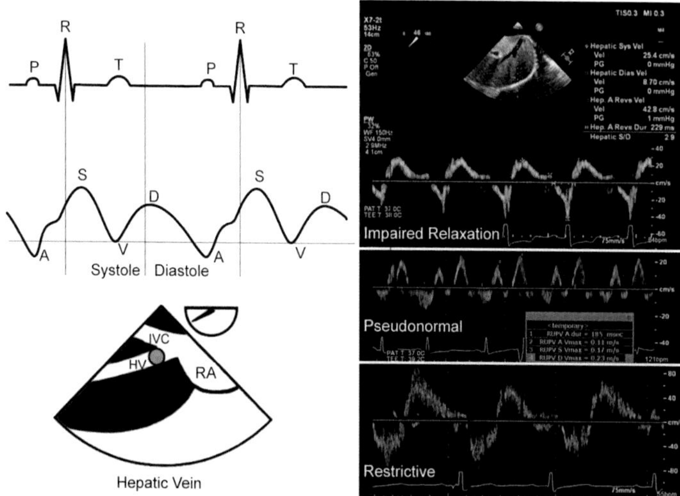

Grading of RV Diastolic Dysfunction			
	Impaired relaxation	Pseudonormal	Restrictive
Tricuspid Valve Inflow	E/A ratio < 0.8[a]	E/A ratio 0.8–2.1[a]	E/A ratio > 2.1[a]
TV Tissue Doppler	e′ < a′[b]	E/e′ ratio > 6[a]	DT < 120 ms[a]
Hepatic Vein Flow	S/D > 1[b] Adur > 50% S Vel[b]	S/D < 1[a]	S reversed[b]

DT, deceleration time
[a]**Rudski LG, et al. J Am Soc Echocardiogr 2010;23:685–713**
[b]**Denault A, et al. Can J Anesth 2006;53:1020–1029**

RV Diastolic Dysfunction (RV DD)

- RV DD is more challenging to assess than LV diastolic function.
- RV DD is present in different pathologies including right heart disease, lung diseases, LV dysfunction, and systemic diseases.
- Grades of RV DD depend on assessing TVI, HVF, and TDI of TV annulus.
- For TTE:
  Mild RV DD is defined by TV E/A < 2, HVF S/D > 1, TV TDI $E_t' < A_t'$, or an atrial reversal (AR) wave more than half of the systolic wave of the HVF.
  Moderate or severe RV DD is present if TV E/A > 1, HVF S wave is reduced or inverted.
- TEE has been used to assess RV DD based on this algorithm. Patients with atrial fibrillation, paced or non-sinus rhythms, severe TR, TV annuloplasty were excluded.

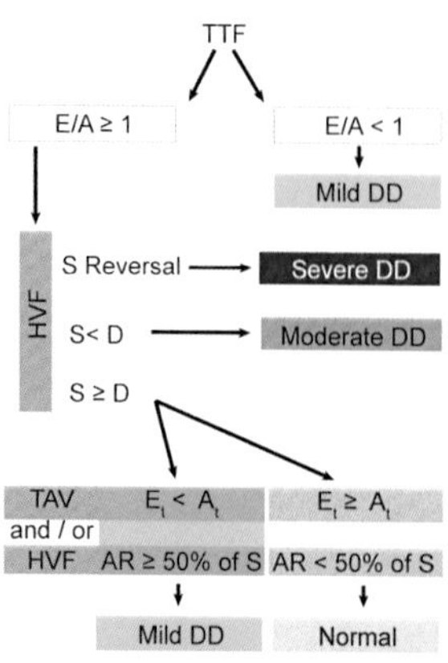

7
Native Valves

A. Vegas, *Perioperative Two-Dimensional Transesophageal Echocardiography*, https://doi.org/10.1007/978-3-319-60902-7_7

Aortic Root Anatomy

- The aortic valve (AV) is part of the aortic root complex which connects the LV and aorta. The cylindrical-shaped aortic root is the dilated proximal portion of the ascending aorta that extends proximally from the basal AV cusp attachments in the LV, to distally at the sino-tubular junction (STJ).
- The centrally positioned aortic root has 3 major components the: (1) AV, (2) sinuses of valsalva, and (3) interleaflet triangles.
- The LVOT comprised of the muscular IVS and fibrous anterior mitral valve leaflet (AMVL) forms the start of the aortic root. The bases of the interleaflet triangles and the AV cusps each share 50% of the base circumference of the LVOT.

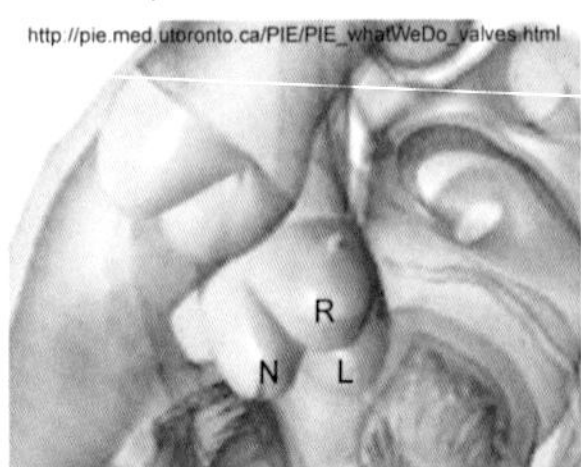

Base of AV Cusps

- Non: AMVL, membranous IVS
- RCC: membranous IVS, anterior LV
- LCC: AMVL, anterior LV

Sinuses of Valsalva

- Non: LA, RA, transverse pericardial
- Right: RA, free pericardium
- Left: LA, free pericardium

Interleaflet Triangles

- Non/R: RA, RV, TV (septal leaflet)
- R/L: potential space aorta and PA
- L/non: LA, AMVL

Source: Ho S. Eur J Echocard 2009;10:i3–10

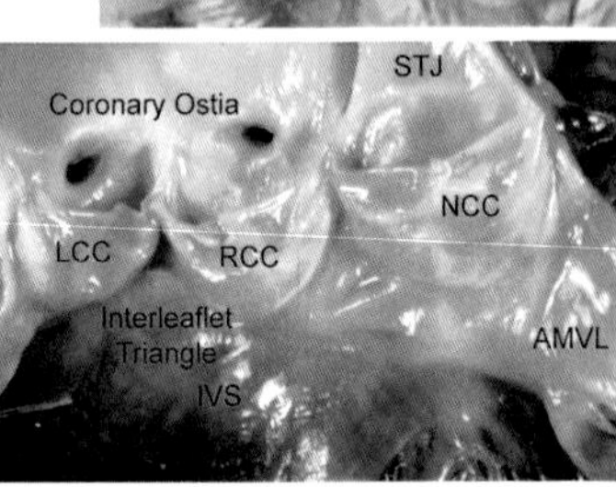

Aortic Valve

- The normal AV consists of three cusps (or leaflets). Each cusp has a similar crescent shape making them indistinguishable from each other.
- Individual cusps have a body, free margin, and base that is attached to the sinus wall at the hinge points. The free margins of each cusp overlap at the lunula and nodule of Arantius during diastole to prevent valvular regurgitation. The commissures are the areas where 2 adjacent cusp margins meet the aorta.
- The cusps are named in relation to the surrounding sinus of Valsalva: left coronary cusp (LCC) near the PA, right coronary cusp (RCC) is the most anterior, and non-coronary cusp (NCC) near the inter-atrial septum.

Interleaflet Triangles

- These are the 3 triangular-shaped spaces in the aortic root between adjacent hinge lines of the AV cusps and the LV.
- Though part of the aortic root, they are considered an extension of the LVOT that reach the STJ at the commissures. In systole, these thin fibrous areas are subjected to LV pressure, making them vulnerable to aneurysmal formation.

Sinuses of Valsalva

- These are an outpouching of the proximal thoracic aorta between the LVOT and STJ that is composed of fibrous tissue. Anatomically, the sinuses are named anterior (right coronary), left posterior (left coronary), and right posterior (non-coronary) and are identifiable by the presence or absence of coronary arteries.
- The sinuses are largest (RCS > NCS > LCS) in diastole to help distribute stress over the closed cusps and a reservoir for blood to perfuse the coronary arteries.

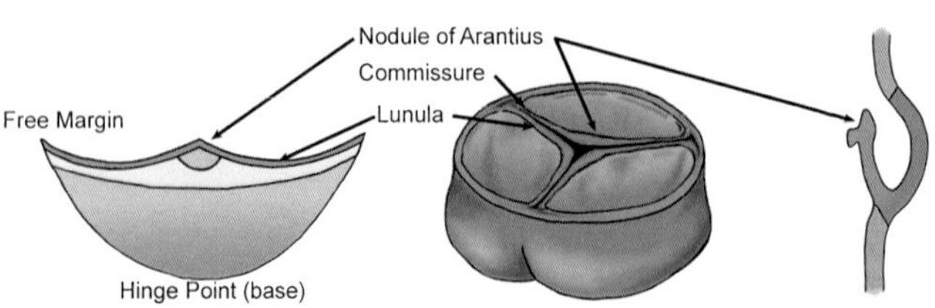

Aortic Root Function

- Normal aortic root function allows unrestrictive unidirectional blood flow from the LV to the ascending aorta during systole. The AV has a passive valve mechanism, opening and closing with minimal pressure differences between the LV and aorta. The aortic root is dynamic, changing shape during the cardiac cycle to assist flow.
- During isovolumic contraction, the MV is closed. LV pressure rises with LV contraction expanding the interleaflet triangles, creating a small central triangular AV orifice but without forward flow.
- The rapid rise of LV pressure during systole further opens the AV to form a larger triangular orifice. Forward flow creates a more circular AV orifice. Expansion at the commissures (aortic root outlet) with LV contraction of muscle at the annulus (aortic root inlet) creates a funnel to assist flow. AV closure begins during systole as LV pressure falls.
- During isovolumic ventricular relaxation, LV pressure is less than aortic pressure and the AV is closed.
- During diastole, the AV remains closed. The AV annulus expands as the LV relaxes with recoil at the commissures to restore the static equilibrium. The STJ diameter is 10–15% smaller than the annulus creating a truncated cone.

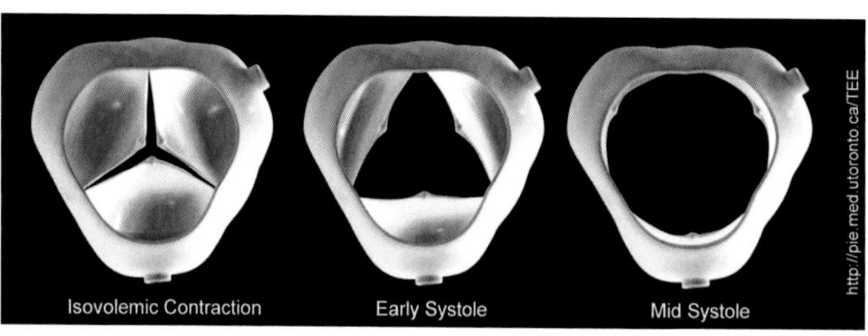

Aortic Root Rings

The aortic root can be described by 4 rings: 3 circular rings and 1 crown-like ring. There is no true AV annulus.

1. **Sino-tubular junction (STJ)**
- This forms the superior border (or outlet) of the aortic root where the sinuses of Valsalva meet the tubular ascending aorta. The STJ is not completely circular in shape, but is scalloped as it follows the bulging sinuses of Valsalva.
- STJ dilatation leads to AV cusp malcoaptation and may cause central AI.

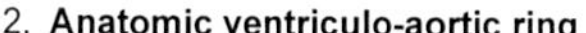

2. **Anatomic ventriculo-aortic ring**
- This ring demarcates the border where the LV myocardium changes to the fibroelastic aortic wall. Note that the hinge points for AV cusp attachment cross this ring. It is a circular-shaped ring located near the base of the sinuses.
3. **Aortic annulus (virtual basal ring)**
- This is a virtual ring formed by joining the base of each of the 3 AV cusp attachments in the LVOT and is often referred to as the "aortic annulus." The elliptical shape changes size during the cardiac cycle and is smallest during systole.
- Annular dilatation reduces commissural height, but does not result in AI.
4. **Physiologic ventriculo-aortic ring**
- This is a crown-shaped ring formed by the hinge attachment of the AV cusps.
- This ring represents the hemodynamic separation or the physiologic ventriculo-arterial junction between the LV structures and the aortic sinuses.
- Parts of the aorta, the interleaflet triangles, are exposed to LV pressures.

- The AV is easily visualized using standard TEE views. The anatomy of the cusps and the aortic root is best examined from the mid-esophageal (ME) views.
- The adequacy of AV function is assessed by using color Doppler in the ME views and by spectral Doppler in the transgastric (TG) views. Pathology may include aortic insufficiency (AI) or aortic stenosis (AS).

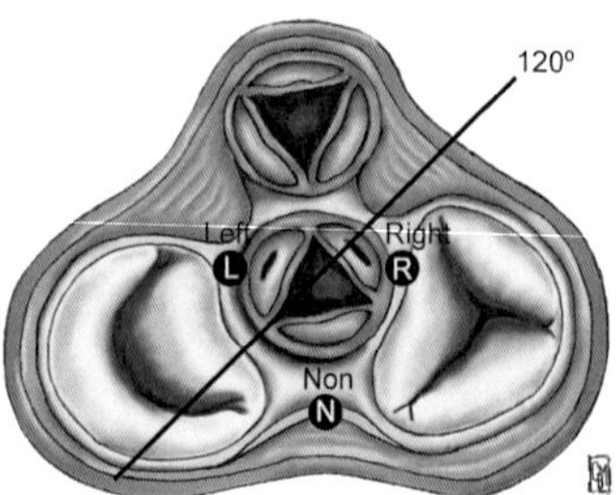

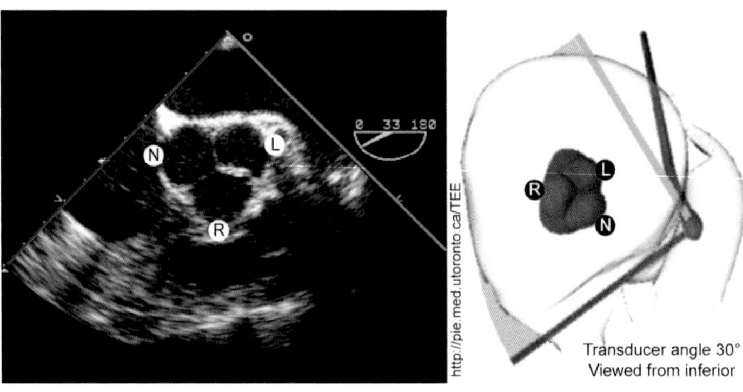

ME AV SAX View (30–60°)

The AV lies at a 30° angle to the sagittal plane of the heart. The transducer angle is varied to ensure the AV is in the center of the screen with all 3 AV cusps appearing symmetric. In diastole as shown here, the cusps, commissures, and coaptation line are identified. Color Doppler in a normal AV shows flow during systole without flow in diastole. In the presence of AI, the jet location is identified as central or commissural. To image the entire aortic root in short axis, the probe is advanced to visualize the LVOT and withdrawn to see the coronary arteries.

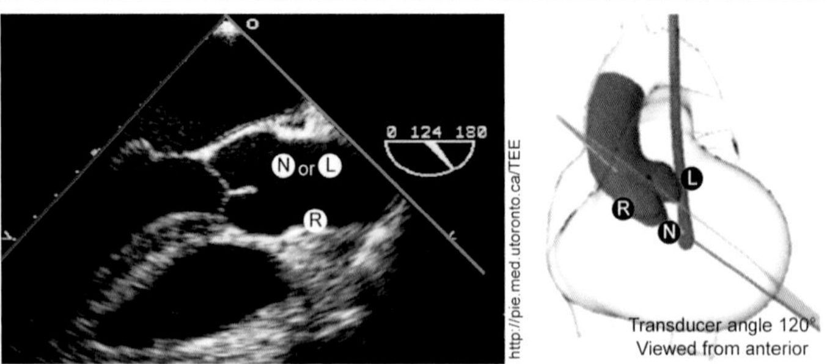

ME AV LAX View (120–150°)

This view is obtained by increasing the transducer angle to 120–150° to show the aortic root in long axis. The RCC is always positioned anterior with the posterior-positioned cusp closest to the probe either the NCC or LCC. Normal cusp coaptation during diastole occurs above the aortic annulus in the sinuses of Valsalva with an adequate length of cusp overlap. Aortic root measurements are obtained (see p. 134). Cusp morphology, prolapse, and root pathology are easily identified. Color Doppler shows normal laminar flow in the LVOT and ascending aorta. Abnormal color Doppler flow in diastole suggests AI with determination of jet direction (central, eccentric). Turbulent antegrade systolic flow suggests obstruction and is identified as subvalvular (LVOT), valvular (aortic stenosis), or supravalvular (membrane).

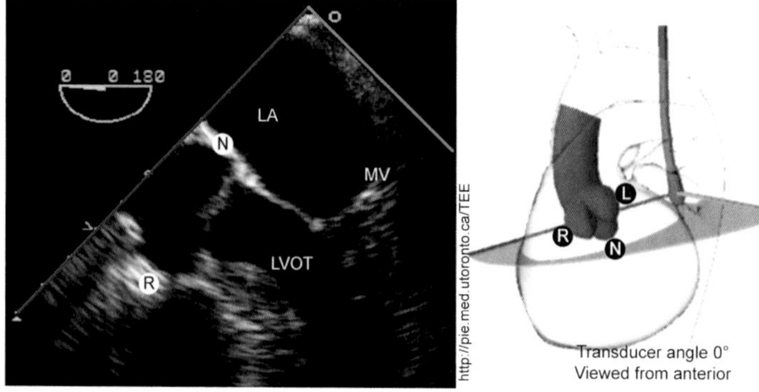

ME 5 Chamber View (0°)
This view is obtained by withdrawing the probe from the ME 4 chamber view to enable visualization of the RCC, NCC, LVOT, and the interventricular septum. Color Doppler shows the presence of AI in diastole. In systole, turbulent flow may be seen in the LVOT (subvalvular obstruction) or at the level of the valve (aortic stenosis).

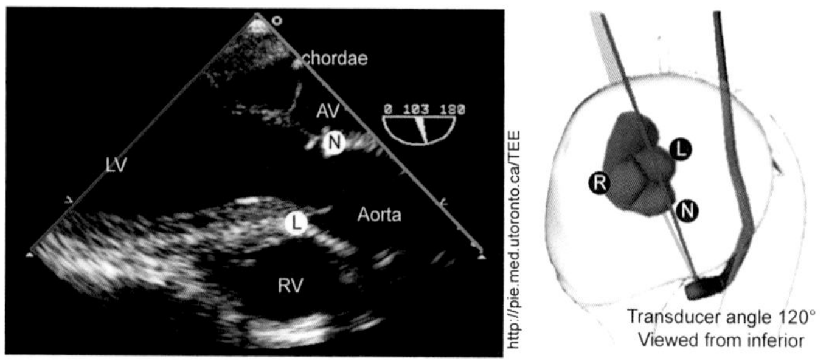

TG LAX View (120°)
This view is obtained by advancing the probe into the stomach and increasing the transducer angle. This TG view is useful to show cusp motion particularly of mechanical prosthetic valves. Color and CW spectral Doppler identifies stenotic and regurgitant valve pathology and can measure any associated pressure gradients.

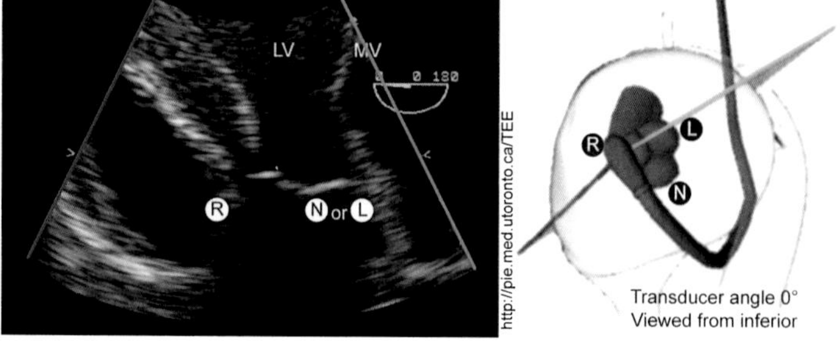

Deep TG View (0°)
This view is obtained by advancing the probe deep in the stomach with anteflexion of the probe tip. Similar information is provided as from the TG LAX view. Color and CW spectral Doppler identifies stenotic and regurgitant valve pathology and any associated pressure gradients. This view is also useful to assess prosthetic valve function and the presence of a paravalvular leak.

Aortic Valve ME SAX (30°) View and Surgeon's Perspective
In 2D or 3D ME AV SAX views, the AV opens as a triangular orifice in systole and, when closed in diastole, forms a Mercedes Benz sign. Rotate 90° for surgeon's view.

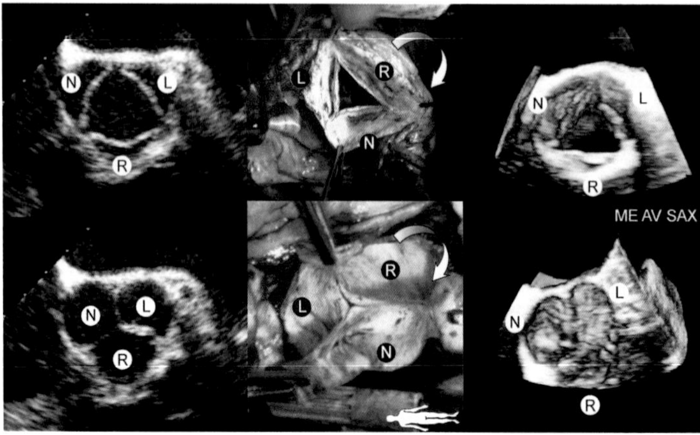

Aortic Root Dimensions

	Male	Female
Systole: inner to inner edges		
Annulus	2.6 ± 0.3	2.3 ± 0.2
Diastole: leading to leading edges		
Sinuses	3.4 ± 0.3	3.0 ± 0.3
STJ	2.9 ± 0.3	2.6 ± 0.3
Ascending aorta	3.0 ± 0.4	2.7 ± 0.4
Source: Lang R, et al. JASE 2015;28:1–39		

- ASE guidelines suggest measurements be made during different points in the cardiac cycle using the ME AV LAX view. Normative values of root size vary with age, sex, BSA, and technique. Measurements are made perpendicular to the long axis to avoid overestimation.
- Root height (normal <22 mm) is the horizontal distance between the STJ and aortic annulus with implications for valve sparing root and TAVI procedures.
- Measurement of the maximum aortic annulus diameter is obtained in the ME AV LAX view preferably by not visualizing the non/left coronary cusps.

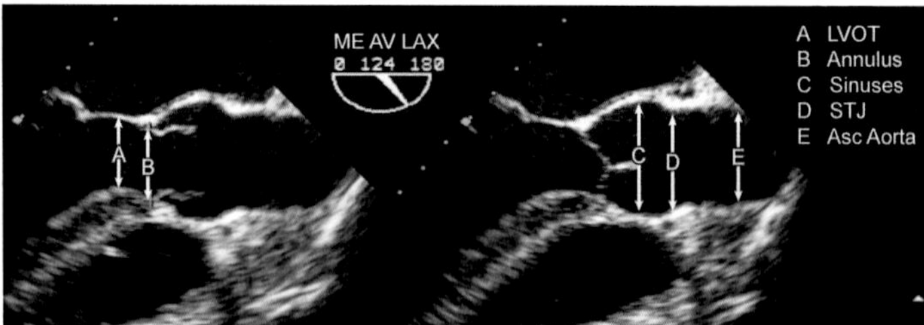

Aortic Cusps Dimensions
Each AV cusp must be of sufficient size, so when combined together cover the AV orifice. The height of each cusp can be measured during systole from the ME AV LAX view as shown above. The length of cusp coaptation can be measured during diastole.

Aortic cusps dimensions
Free margin (FM) length = 28–34 mm
Cusp height = 13–16 mm
Cusp base = 42–59 mm (1.5 × FM length)
Cusp area: non >R >L

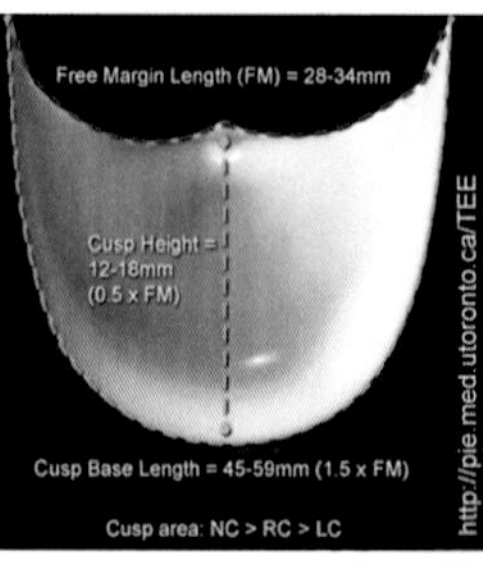

- eSie Valves® by Siemens is on-cart software available for MV and AV analysis of 3D datasets. It is the only software that constructs patient-specific physiologic dynamic 3D AV models. (A) The software is semi-automated as views are automatically extracted, aligned, and tracked producing dynamic models of MV and AV.
- A unique feature is the simultaneous analysis and display of the aortic-mitral complex. (B) The models can be superimposed on the heart and color Doppler added to show flow. In addition, a multitude of morphological quantification and measurements of dynamic variables are displayed.

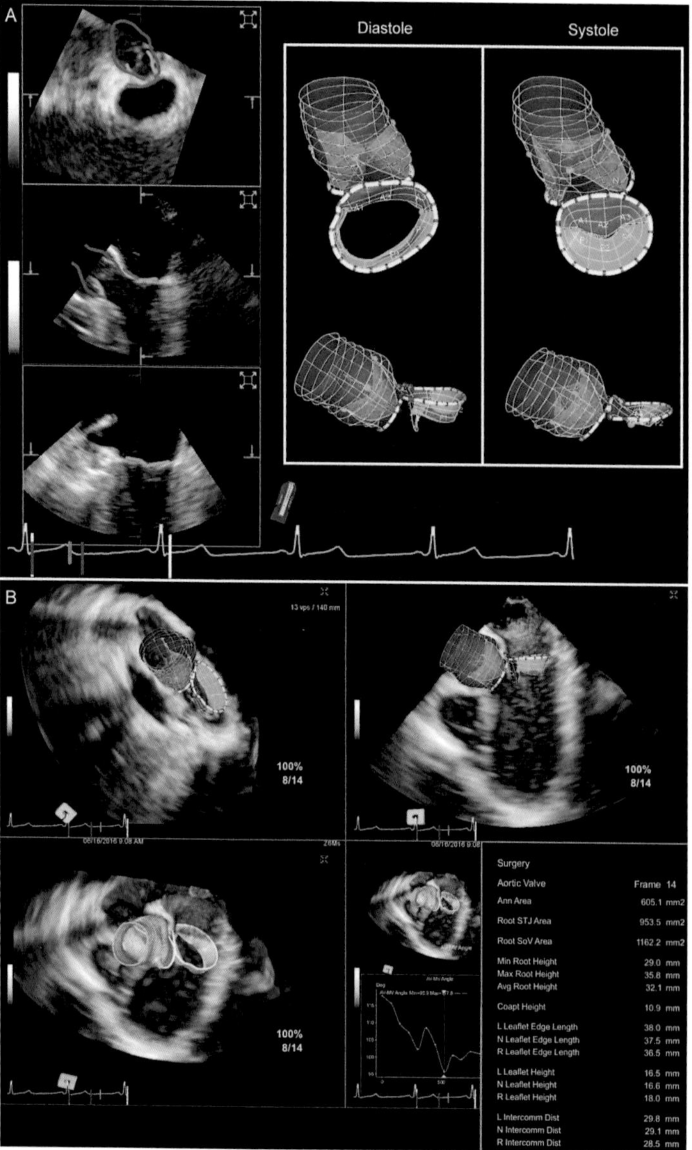

Bicuspid Aortic Valve (BAV)

- There are only 2 aortic valve cusps which make the AV abnormal.
  - Congenital fusion: L + R (86%), R + N (12%), L + N (3%), variable cusp size.
  - Acquired: unequal cusp size from fused commissure.
  - Described by commissure location (4 + 10 o'clock), or ant/post, or right/left.
  - The aortic cusps are thickened.
- Raphe is often present at 90° to the valve orifice.
  - Sievers classification based on # of raphe (0,1,2).
- Usually there are 3 sinuses of Valsalva present.
- Location of coronary ostia (may be 180° apart).
  - Type 1: 2 coronaries on same side of orifice.
  - Type 2: valve orifice separates the coronaries
- Associated pathology:
  - AI, PDA, VSD.
  - Aortopathy: dilatation, aneurysm, dissection.
  - BAV may have coarctation of aorta (<10%), but 50% of aortic coarctations have BAV.

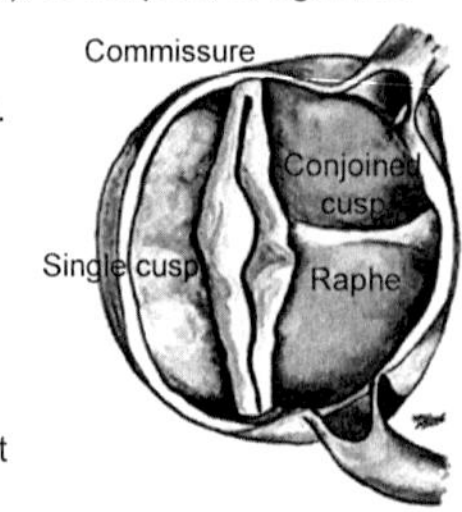

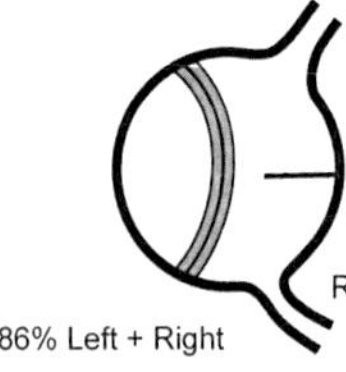

86% Left + Right

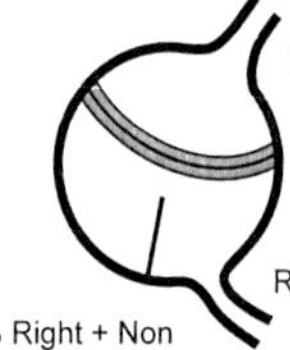

12% Right + Non

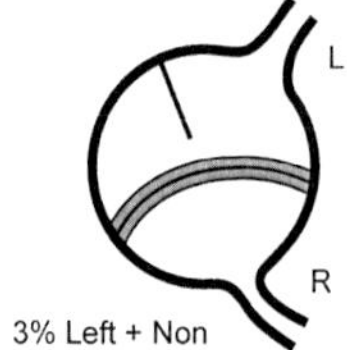

3% Left + Non

TEE Imaging BAV

- The number of AV cusps is determined during systole in the ME AV SAX view. (B) Normal AV with 3 cusps opens with a triangular orifice and 3 commissures. BAV the orifice appears oval or "fish mouth" with 2 commissures (D). During diastole, a BAV raphe (C) may make the "Mercedes Benz" sign like a normal AV (A).
- Normal AV cusps open and close in the center of the sinuses of Valsalva. In the ME AV LAX view, the BAV cusp opening during systole is often eccentric and the cusps appear domed (arrow) from incomplete opening. During diastole, the cusp coaptation line may be eccentric from the different cusp sizes and the body of the cusp may prolapse (diastolic doming).

TEE Bicuspid Aortic Valve
- Systolic elliptical orifice opening (SAX)
- Systolic cusp doming (LAX)
- Diastolic eccentric closure line (LAX)
- Diastolic doming cusp prolapse (LAX)

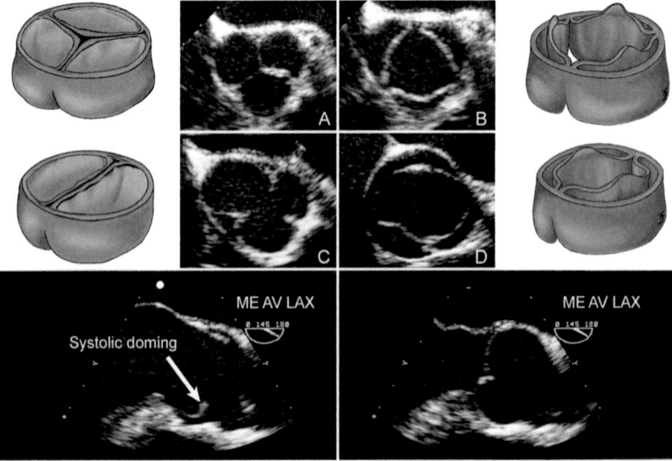

Unicuspid Aortic Valve

- This is a rare (0.02%) congenital abnormality of aortic cusp number. There are two types of unicuspid valves; either acommissural or unicommissural. The acommissural valve has no lateral attachments to the aorta and a central pinhole orifice. The more common unicommissural valve has lateral attachments of the commissure to the aorta (posterior commissure) with an eccentric elliptic-shaped orifice.
- Both types of unicuspid valves are prone to aortic stenosis. Other abnormalities may be present which include aortic aneurysm, aortic dissection, coarctation, and PDA.

ME AV SAX and ME AV LAX views with color compare are shown during systole of a stenotic unicuspid unicommissural AV.

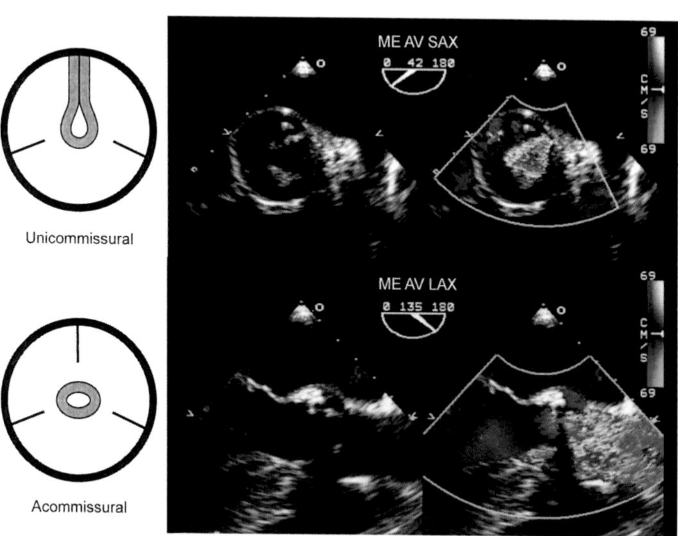

Quadracuspid Aortic Valve

- This is the rarest (0.013%) of cusp number abnormalities. Seven anatomic variants have been described based on the cusp size (as shown below). The commonest are equal cusp size, or 3 large equal cusps with one smaller cusp.
- This anomaly may be an incidental finding, have AI or rarely stenosis.
- Other congenital abnormalities may be present such as VSD, ASD, PDA, subaortic membrane, MV malformation, and coronary abnormalities.

(A, B) ME AV SAX views are shown during diastole and systole of a quadracuspid valve with 3 equal and one small cusps. Note during systole all 4 cusps open widely.

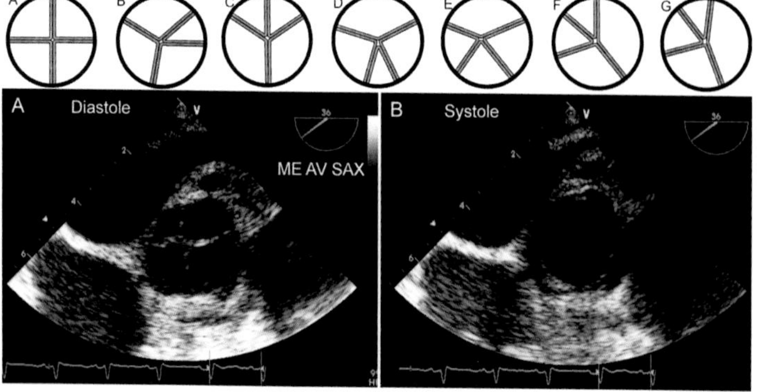

Assessment

1. Etiology: valvular, subvalvular, supravalvular
   - Valvular: degenerative/calcific, rheumatic, congenital bicuspid
   - Subvalvular: membrane, HOCM, SAM
   - Supravalvular: congenital ascending aorta narrowing
   - Aortic sclerosis is thickened AV cusps without hemodynamic significance.
2. 2D findings of AV:
   - Etiology: degenerative vs. rheumatic
   - Valvular calcium location
   - Restricted cusp opening of one or all cusps in SAX and LAX
   - SAX: # of cusps (tri vs. bicuspid), planimetry (difficult if calcified)
   - LAX: systolic doming of cusp (<15 mm opening, angle <90°)
   - Aortic annulus size (in systole), root dimensions in diastole (see p. 134)
   - Location of coronary ostia
3. Doppler:
   - Color: turbulence at level of obstruction
   - PW: locate level of obstruction
   - CW: peak/mean velocity and pressure gradients vary with flow
     - Underestimate: ↓ LV function, MR, poor Doppler alignment, L → R shunt
     - Overestimate: high CO, AI
     - If LVOT V_{peak} >1.5 m/s or AV V_{peak} <3.0 m/s, then use modified Bernoulli: peak gradient = $4\,(\text{AV } V_{peak})^2 - (\text{LVOT } V_{peak})^2$
   - CW: continuity equation VTI (LVOT, AV) for AV area
4. Stenosis severity (see table below)
5. Associated findings:
   - LVH, septal hypertrophy
   - LV RWMA: inferior basal hypokinesis
   - Preserved LV function, if poor LV can underestimate AS severity
   - Post-stenotic aorta dilatation
   - Mitral regurgitation
   - Mitral annular calcification (MAC)

Aortic Stenosis Severity (EACVI, ASE guidelines)

	Aortic Sclerosis	Mild	Moderate	Severe
Peak Velocity (m/s)	≤2.5	2.6–2.9	3.0–4.0	>4.0
Mean Gradient (mmHg)	–	<20	20–40	>40
AVA (cm^2)	–	>1.5	1.0–1.5	<1.0
Indexed AVA (cm^2/m^2)	–	>0.85	0.6–0.85	<0.6
Velocity ratio	–	>0.50	0.25–0.50	<0.25

Adapted from: Baumgartner H, et al. J Am Soc Echocardiogr 2017;30:372–92

What to Tell the Surgeon Aortic Stenosis

PreCPB

- AV etiology: rheumatic, calcific, BAV
- Annulus size (for stentless valve: STJ within 10%)
- AV area (to avoid prosthetic mismatch), pressure gradients
- Aorta: Post-stenotic aorta dilatation, if calcified, may be difficult for minimal access
- Location of coronary ostia
- Calcium bar may extend onto the AMVL restricting leaflet motion, MR
- LVH (concentric) and LV function
- Septal hypertrophy (SAM, LVOT diameter)

PostCPB

- Prosthetic valve stability, leaflet mobility
- Paravalvular, valvular leaks
- Peak/mean pressure gradients
- No LVOT obstruction with SAM or VSD (rare)
- LV and RV function, intra-cavitary gradient (↑ mortality)

Views	2D Findings	Color	Spectral Doppler
ME 5C (0°)	AV, subvalvular	LVOT turbulence	Non-parallel
ME AV SAX (30°)	AV, planimetry	AV	
ME AV LAX (120°)	Sub/supra/AV	LVOT/AV/supra	
TG LAX (120°)	Sub/supra/AV	LVOT/AV/supra	CW (AV)
Deep TG (0°)	Difficult image	LVOT/AV/supra	PW (LVOT)

Calcified Aortic Valve

- Fibrocalcific changes to cusp body
- Thick, stiff cusps, heavily calcified
- Irregular orifice
- Rarely commissural fusion
- Shadowing in 2D ME views
- MAC

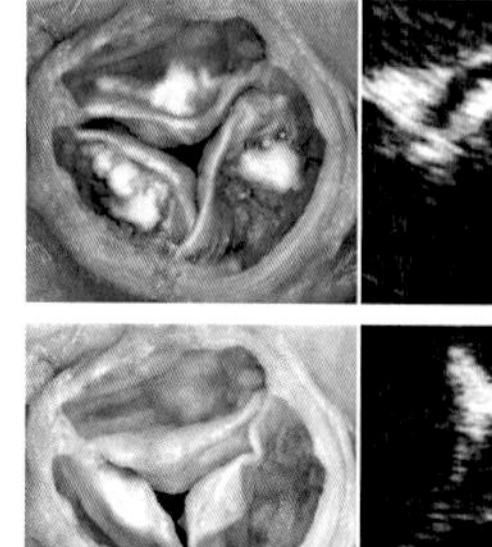

Rheumatic Aortic Valve

- Commissural fusion
- Thick, calcified free edge
- Calcific nodules on both surfaces
- Stellate orifice
- Chordal shortening
- MV always involved

Bicuspid Aortic Valve

- Asymmetric cusp size
- Raphe often present
- Calcified body
- Systolic elliptical orifice (fish mouth)
- Aortopathy

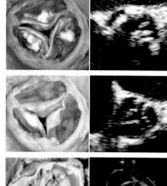

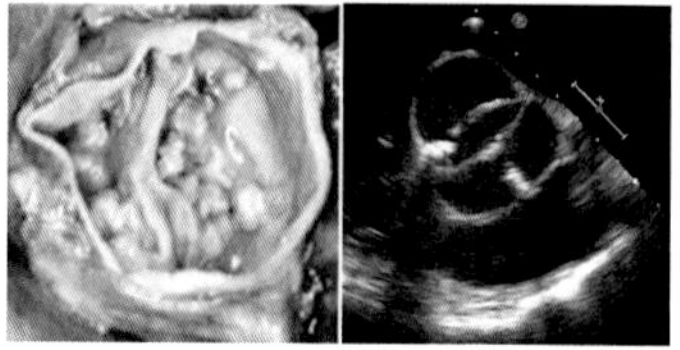

(A) ME AV LAX shows systolic restricted opening and turbulent flow at the AV into ascending aorta with color Doppler. (B) Post-stenotic ascending aorta dilatation may require replacement of the aorta. (C) LV hypertrophy results in a small stroke volume, diastolic dysfunction, and inferior wall hypokinesis. (D) Need to differentiate 2° functional from 1° structural MR, as the latter will need an additional MV repair.

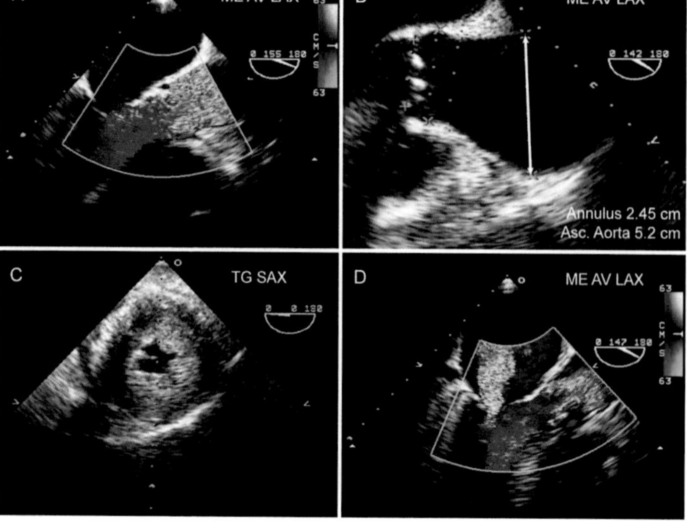

Velocity (V)

CW Doppler in TG views (deep TG, TG LAX)

- Adjust gain to identify peak
- Adjust scale to fill velocity axis
- Incomplete spectral trace if malaligned Doppler cursor

Dense velocity curve with an identifiable peak

- Early peaking in mild AS, mid-systole more severe
- Shape distinguishes obstruction level
  - Smooth mid-systolic: valvular
  - Late peaking dagger-shaped: LVOT (see p. 312)

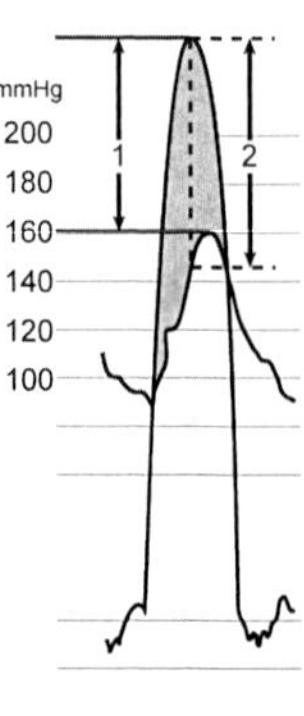

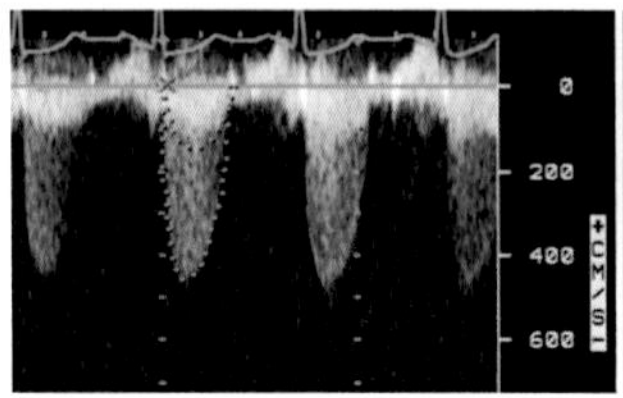

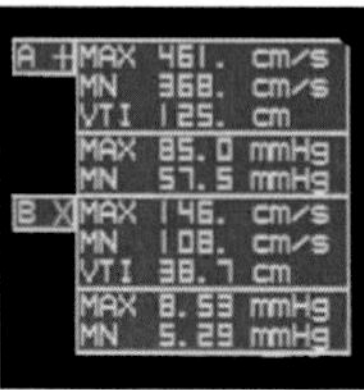

Pressure Gradients (PG)

- Measure the transaortic PG between the LV and aorta in systole
- Trace outer edge for VTI and Pressure gradients (peak and mean)
  - Peak instantaneous PG is estimated by the Bernoullii equation:
  - simplified: ($\Delta P = 4V^2_{max}$) when $V_{proximal}$ <1 m/s
  - modified: ($\Delta P = 4V^2_{max} - V^2_{proximal}$) if $V_{proximal}$ >1.5 m/s or aortic velocity <3.0 m/s
  - The "peak to peak" PG obtained from cardiac catheterization (1) is lower than by Doppler which estimates the peak instantaneous PG (2) as shown above.
  - Mean PG is an average of the instantaneous gradient over the ejection time.
  - The mean Doppler and cath PG are similar.
  - Mean PG is more accurate than peak PG to quantify AS.
- The PG across a stenotic orifice is dynamic and flow-dependent.
  - Less flow underestimates PG: high SVR, low CO, severe MR/MS, shunt.
  - More flow overestimates PG: low SVR (sepsis), severe AI, high CO (anemia, hemodialysis, AV fistula, hyperthyroidism).
  - In these settings, the aortic valve area (AVA) should be estimated.
- Pressure recovery (PR) occurs only if the ascending aorta is small (<30 mm).

Aortic Valve Area

- This is the valve orifice during systole and can be determined as the anatomic (or geometric) area by planimetry or functional (effective) area by Doppler techniques.
- The effective AVA is smaller than the geometric area as it represents flow through the valve (vena contracta). Effective AVA is the primary predictor of outcome.
- Doppler techniques used to estimate the effective AVA include the standard continuity equation, simplified continuity equation, and velocity ratio (dimensionless index). The latter is relatively flow-independent, but has limited supporting data.

Planimetry

- ME AV SAX view
- Trace AV orifice during systole
- Represents the anatomic AVA
- Limited if heavily calcified
- Accurate only if at the smallest orifice

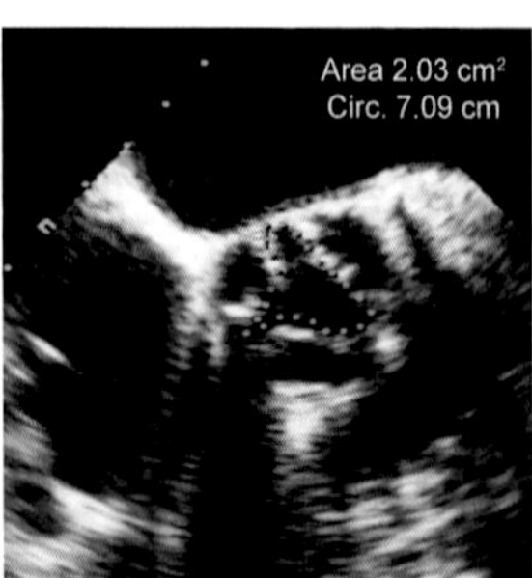

Velocity Ratio (VR)

A **VTI_{LVOT}/VTI_{AV} ratio** <0.25 indicates severe AS. It is a dimensionless number, independent of flow, which represents the size of the effective AVA. It can be used to assess AS severity with poor LV function.

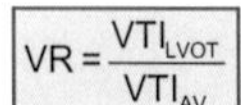

$$VR = \frac{VTI_{LVOT}}{VTI_{AV}}$$

Continuity Equation for physiological (effective) aortic valve area (AVA)

$$AVA = \frac{VTI_{LVOT} \times 0.785\, d^2_{LVOT}}{VTI_{AV}}$$

Simplified Continuity Equation

This uses peak velocities rather than the VTI. It assumes similar-shaped velocity curves in the LVOT and stenotic AV, so the LVOT to aortic jet VTI ratio is nearly identical to the maximum velocity (Vmax) ratio.

LVOT Velocity

PW in TG views

Smooth velocity curve

- Well-defined peak
- Narrow velocity range
- Identify peak velocity
- Trace modal velocity for VTI

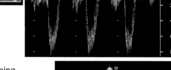

Error: improper position, spectral broadening (filled in) too close to AV (overestimate).

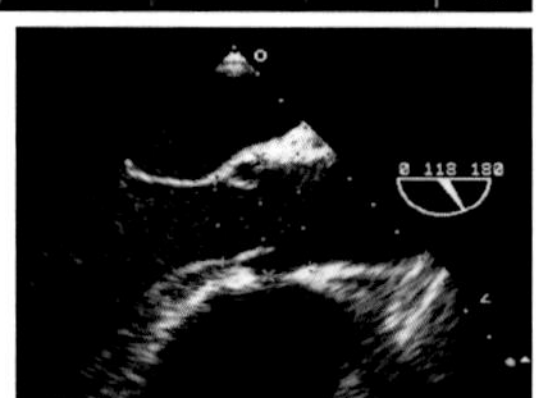

LVOT Diameter

ME AV LAX zoom mode, symmetric aortic root

- Optimal blood tissue boundary
- Inner to inner edge
- Mid-systole
- Parallel to AV plane, within 0.05–1 cm of AV

Assumes a circular CSA

Source of error if inaccurate measurement is made

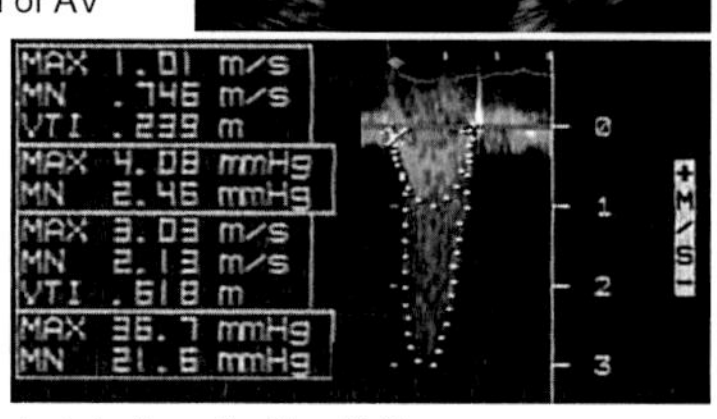

Double Envelope Technique

A single CW Doppler trace is obtained through the AV and LVOT that contains flow from the AV (outer) and LVOT (inner). Both the inner (LVOT) and outer (AV) envelopes are traced for each VTI and inserted in the continuity equation to calculate the effective AVA.

Low Gradient Aortic Stenosis

- Low gradient AS may occur with low EF or normal EF (MR, small stroke volume).
- Low gradient/low EF AS is defined as severe AS (AVA <1.0 cm^2) with a transvalvular mean PG <40 mmHg, LVEF <50%, and SVi <35 cm^3/m^2. There is insufficient forward flow from LV dysfunction or small SV to fully open the stenotic valve, resulting in a low gradient and underestimated AVA.
- Dobutamine stress echocardiogram (DSE) helps differentiate reduced cusp opening in true AS (abnormal valve) from pseudo-AS (normal AV) with reduced flow. Increasing doses of dobutamine (2.5–20.0 μg/kg/min) will change the stroke volume, altering the aortic velocity, mean PG, and AVA. True orifice stenosis will not have an increase in AVA or PG, but pseudo-stenosis will ↑ AVA by ≥0.3 cm^2 or AVA>1 cm^2. DSE is not indicated in a patient with a low EF and a resting AS velocity ≥4.0 m/s or mean PG ≥40 mmHg as this represents a normal LV response to high afterload that will improve after relief of stenosis.
- "Paradoxical" low flow (<4 m/s), low gradient AS (<40 mmHg) with AVA (<1.0 cm^2)-preserved EF may be a result of a small hypertrophied LV with low SVi <35 cm^3/m^2.

Low velocity + Low gradient AS

Effective AVA <1.0 cm^2

LVEF <50%

Mean PG <40 mmHg

SVi <35 cm^3/m^2

Differential Pressure Gradients, Velocity, Valve Area in AS

Abnormally Low Gradient	Abnormally High Gradient	AS Velocity >4 m/s + AVA >1.0 cm^2	AS Velocity ≤4 m/s + AVA ≤1.0 cm^2
LV dysfunction	AI	High CO	Low CO
MR	High CO	Mod-severe AI	Severe MR
LVH (low SVi)		Large BSA	Small BSA

Assessment

1. Etiology of Insufficiency:
   - Related to congenital or acquired pathology of the aortic valve or aorta.
   - Surgical classification of AI is based on functional AV anatomy (cusp motion).

	Aortic Valve	Aorta
Acquired	Rheumatic Calcific ± concomitant aortic stenosis Endocarditis (vegetation, perforation) Traumatic Toxin, radiation	Aneurysm (SOVA, ascending aorta) Aortic dissection Autoimmune: SLE, ankylosing spondylitis Aortitis: Syphilis, Takayasu's arteritis Trauma
Con	Congenital cuspid (bi, quadri, uni) VSD	Annulo-aortic ectasia (annular dilatation) Connective tissue disorders (Marfan's, Ehlers-Danlos)

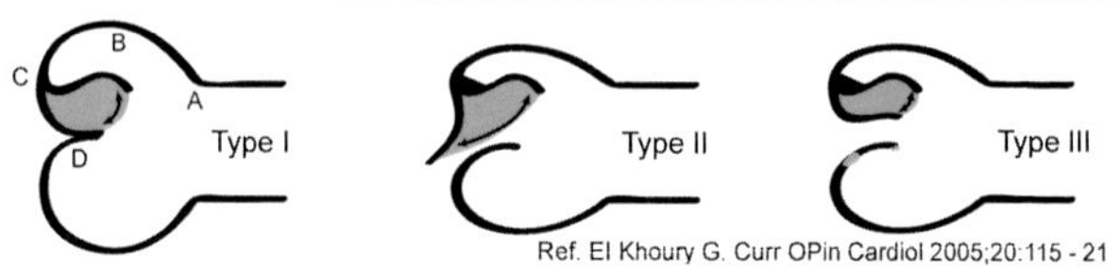

Ref. El Khoury G. Curr OPin Cardiol 2005;20:115 - 21

Type 1	Type 2	Type 3
Normal cusp motion coapts at or above annulus in sinuses of Valsalva	**Excessive cusp motion** cusp body (or belly) falls below the AV annulus	**Restricted cusp motion** results in central malcoaptation of cusps
Subtypes: • Dilatation of (**A**) STJ, (**B**) SOV, (**C**) annulus • Cusp fenestration (**D**)	Prolapse or flail cusps	Calcification Rheumatic

2. 2D findings.
   - AV: # cusps, coaptation (SAX, LAX), diastolic fluttering, lack of cusp closure, prolapse, calcified/fused, bicuspid
   - Root dimensions: LVOT, annulus, sinuses, STJ, aorta (see p. 134)
3. Doppler findings:
   - Color: diastolic turbulence in LVOT, jet direction (LAX): central or eccentric, jet location (SAX): central or commissural
   - Color: measure JH/LVOT (LAX), Jet/LVOT CSA (SAX), vena contracta
   - CW: density, diastolic decay measured as PHT or deceleration slope
   - PW: ↑ LVOT velocity >1.5 m/s
   - PW/CW: diastolic flow reversal in arch/descending/abdominal aorta
   - Calculate ERO area, regurgitant fraction (RegF), regurgitant volume (RegV)
4. LV dilated, function variable
5. Associated findings (indirect effect on MV): premature MV closure, reverse doming AMVL, fluttering AMVL, presystolic (diastolic) MR, jet lesion AMVL
6. Insufficiency severity grade is based on integration of parameters

Aortic Insufficiency Severity (ASE)

	Method	Mild	Moderate	Severe
Qualitative	Jet Width LVOT	Small	Intermediate	Large
	Flow Convergence	None/small	Intermediate	Large
	CW Density	Faint	Dense	Dense
	PHT (ms)	>500	200–500	<200
	Descending Aorta Reversal	Early brief	Intermediate	Holodiastolic
Semiquant	VC Width (mm)	<3	3–6	>6
	Jet/LVOT CSA[a](%)	<5	5–59	≥60
	Jet/LVOT width[a](%)	<25	25–64	≥65
Quant	Regurgitant Volume (cc)	<30	30–59	≥60
	Regurgitant Fraction (%)	20–30	30–49	≥50
	EROA (cm^2)	<0.10	0.1–0.29	≥0.30

All color Doppler at Nyquist limit 50–70 cm/s [a]Central jets
PHT, pressure half time; VC, vena contracta; EROA, effective regurgitant orifice area
Adapted from: Zoghbi W, et al. J am Soc Echocardiogr 2017;30:303–371

Views	2D Findings	Color	Doppler CW
ME 5C (0°)	Root size	Direction AI	Not aligned in ME views
ME AV SAX (30°)	Coaptation # cusps	Location AI Severity AI	
ME AV LAX (120°)	Coaptation Root measure	Direction AI Jet length, width	
TG LAX (120°) Deep TG (0°)	Cusp motion	Paravalvular leak	Doppler aligned CW decay slope

AV Cusp Prolapse
Normal cusps coapt above the annular plane (dotted). Prolapse occurs if a part of the cusp is below the annulus, three types:

1. Flail: cusp tip in LVOT
2. Whole: free edge in LVOT
3. Partial: cusp body in LVOT

In LAX, see cusp below annular plane. In SAX, see double line or gap at cusp coaptation. Color shows AI location.

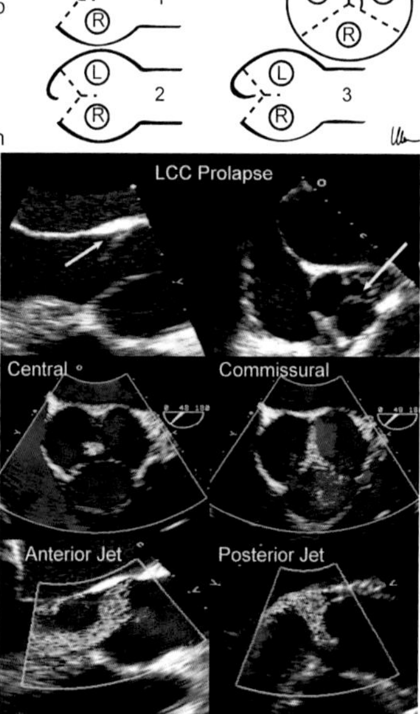

AI Jet Direction/Location
In SAX, AI shows as continuous diastolic flow, locate jet as central or commissural, and which cusp edges (R, L, non) are involved. Note the AI jet direction in LAX of an eccentric jet, consider BAV, prolapsed, or fenestrated cusp. The involved cusp is opposite to AI direction.

Secondary Findings in AI

- AV: Premature opening
- Left Ventricle (LV)
  - Dilatation + sphericity
  - Hyperkinesis, hypokinesis (late)
  - LVOT velocity >1.5 m/s
- Mitral Valve (MV)
  - Premature closure MV
  - Reverse doming, fluttering AMVL
  - Diastolic MR

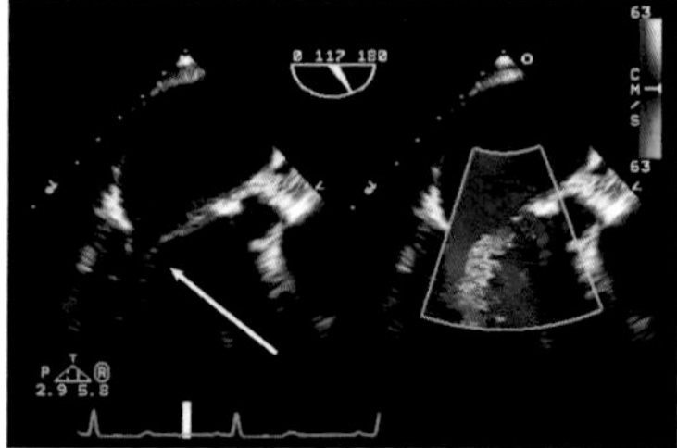

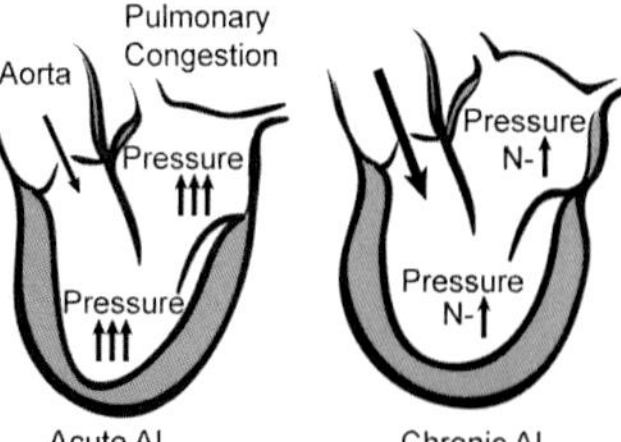

What to Tell the Surgeon Aortic Insufficiency
PreCPB

- Mechanism: Root vs. valve pathology, dimensions of aortic root
- Cusps: Number, morphology, coaptation, prolapse, calcification, fenestration
- Location + direction AI (central, eccentric commissural), AI severity
- Ross procedure: Pulmonic valve annulus size (10–15% of aortic annulus), ±PI

PostCPB

- Valve sparing: Cusp coaptation above annular plane (LAX), AI location + severity
- Prosthetic valve: function, gradient, paravalvular leak
- LV function

Components of Aortic Insufficiency Jet

- Color Doppler in the ME AV LAX view assesses AI jet direction and can help grade AI severity by using the three different components of the AI jet (1) jet area, (2) vena contracta, and (3) flow convergence.
- The appearance of the AI jet varies depending on the ultrasound machine settings (Nyquist limit) and patient hemodynamics.

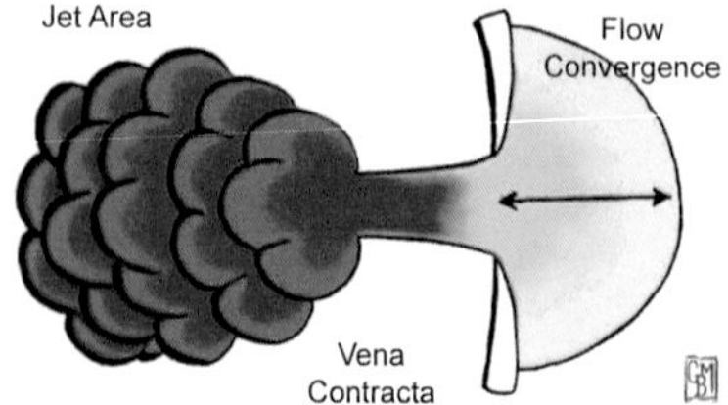

Jet Area or Height (Nyquist Limit 50–60 cm/s)

- Jet length and area into the LV relies on the hemodynamics and ultrasound machine settings, thus it poorly grades AI severity and is no longer used.
- Jet height can more reliably grade a central AI jet as shown below.

(A) The ratio of jet height to LVOT height is the **Perry Index**. Measurements can be made from a color M-mode of the ME AV LAX view, provided the cursor is aligned as parallel as possible to the AV. Color jet height is divided by the LVOT height at the same level (within 1 cm below AV) in the ME AV LAX view.

(B) Jet Area is similar to the Perry index, but instead uses the ME AV SAX view. Cross-sectional area (CSA) of the jet is divided by the area of the LVOT. The measurement is made within 1 cm of the LVOT and not at AV level as shown here.

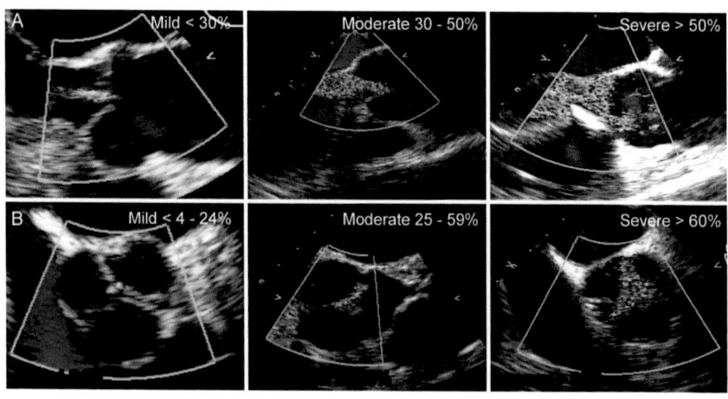

Vena Contracta (VC) (Nyquist Limit 50–60 cm/s)

- This is the narrowest portion of the jet at or just downstream from the orifice, with laminar flow and highest velocity. VC size is independent of flow rate and driving pressure for a fixed orifice, but may change with a dynamic orifice. VC is a sensitive semi-quantitative measure of AI severity and correlates with the EROA.
- VC width should be measured below the region of flow convergence, between the AV cusps. VC may be difficult to accurately measure with TEE in the ME views as the flow convergence region is poorly seen due to color Doppler misalignment with the jet. Eccentric jets are measured perpendicular to the LAX of the jet. VC is not useful for assessing multiple jets. VC size is relatively unaffected by flow rate and is less dependent on loading changes or HR than regurgitant volume/fraction.

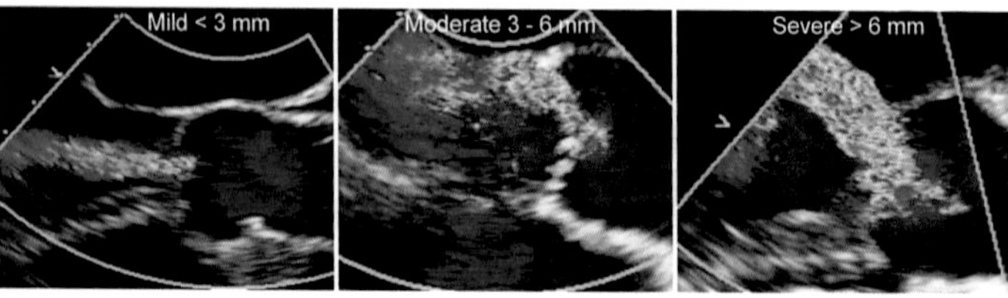

Flow Convergence (Nyquist Variable)

- High velocity flow, termed flow acceleration, proximal to the regurgitant valve orifice results in a series of concentric hemispheres. Adjust the Nyquist limit (Vr) to obtain a rounded flow convergence and measure the aliasing radius (r).
- PISA method can quantify AI severity by calculating the (a) EROA, (b) Regurgitant volume, and (c) Regurgitant fraction.

Effective Regurgitant Orifice Area (EROA) (See p. 59)

- This is the derived area of hemodynamic regurgitation. Corresponds to the vena contracta CSA, the narrowest portion of the jet, which is slightly smaller than the anatomic orifice. EROA is determined using (a) PISA or (b) volumetric methods.
  (a) PISA method
    - Calculate AI flow across the valve: Flow AI (cc/s) = $6.28r^2 \times Vr$ (cm/s)
    - Calculate EROA: ERO_{AI} (cm^2) = Flow $_{AI}$ (cc/s)/Peak V_{AI} (cm/s)

  (b) Volumetric method
    - Calculate Regurgitant Volume: RegV (cc) = $SV_{AV} - SV_{normal}$
    - Calculate ERO_{AI} (cm^2) = RegV (cc)/VTI_{AI} (cm)

Regurgitant Volume (see p. 60)

- Regurgitant volume (RegV) is the volume through the EROA and can be estimated using (a) PISA or (b) volumetric methods.
  (a) RegV (cc) = ERO_{AI} (cm^2) × VTI_{AI} (cm)
  (b) RegV (cc) = $SV_{AV} - SV_{normal}$

Regurgitant Fraction (see p. 60)

- Regurgitant fraction (RegF) is the percentage of regurgitant volume compared with total flow across the regurgitant valve (RegF = RV – SV_{normal}/RV).

Spectral Doppler Tracings

Continuous Wave Doppler (CWD)

- Placed parallel to AI flow (use CFD to help align) in deep TG or TG LAX view to obtain a reliable AI spectral trace (initial peak gradient >40 mmHg (V >3 m/s).
- CW density is a simple qualitative reflection of regurgitant volume; a denser envelope is seen with more severe AI.
- Rate of decline of regurgitant jet can quantify AI by measuring pressure half time (PHT) and slope of deceleration (see p. 57). A larger EROA quickly equalizes pressure between the aorta and LV, creating a steeper slope in regurgitant velocity and shorter PHT. (A) Examples of mild, moderate, and severe PHT are shown.

Pulsed Wave Doppler (PWD)

- Aortic flow reversal is another sensitive qualitative indicator of AI severity.
- The more in the distal descending aorta flow reversal occurs, the worse the AI.
- Absolute velocity of flow reversal does not reflect AI severity as this is affected by PWD angulation. Ratio of flow reversal to forward flow (VTI ratio) better indicates AI severity. (B) Examples of mild, moderate and severe aortic flow reversal.

CWD weak density	**CWD moderate density**	**CWD dense density**
Mild -“flat top”	Moderate - ↑ angle	Severe - steep slope
Decay slope <2 m/s	Decay slope 2–3.5 m/s	Decay slope >3 m/s
PHT >500 ms	PHT 200–500 ms	PHT <200 ms

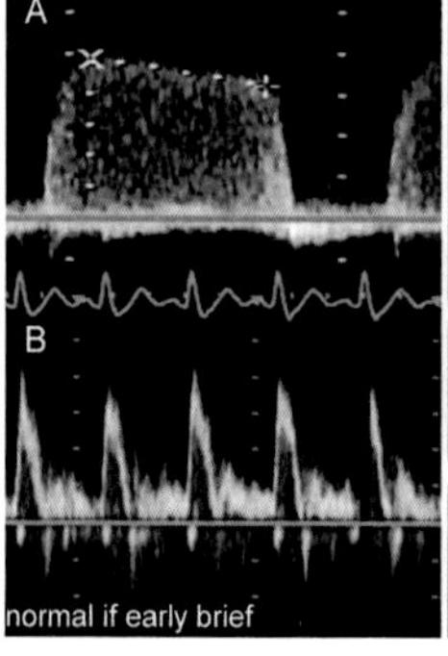

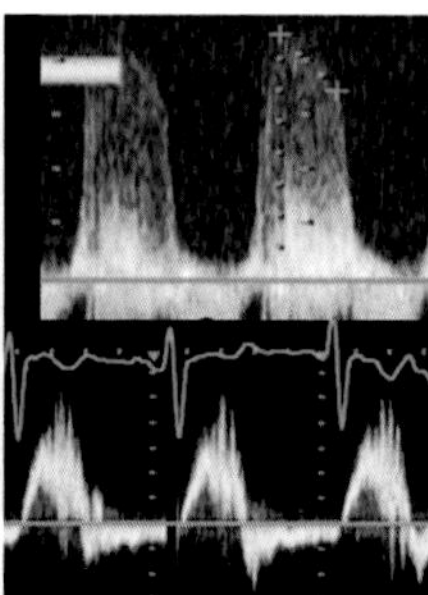

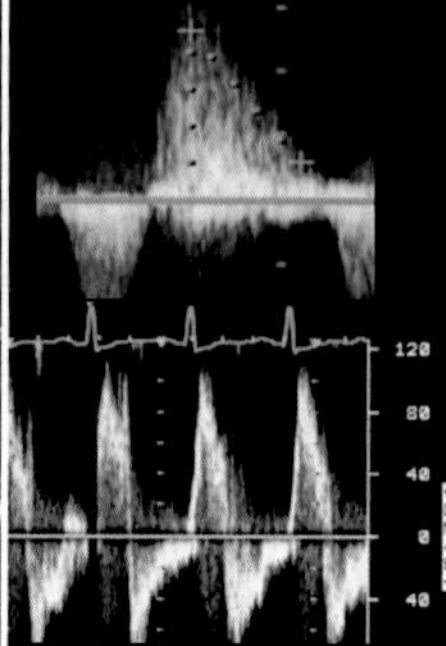

Mitral Apparatus

The MV apparatus is an anatomic term describing cardiac structures associated with MV function. These structures consist of the fibrous skeleton, annulus, leaflets, chordae, and papillary muscle-ventricular wall complex. Normal MV function depends on the integrated function of all the components of the MV apparatus.

Fibrous Skeleton (Three Parts)

This is a dense tissue continuum of rings and trigones that extends around the heart base. The 2 trigones are the right (near NCC) and left (near LCC) and a smaller Tendon of Conus between the RCC and PA. The 4 fibrous rings form the base of the valves, AV and PV annuli are crown-shaped, MV and TV annuli are incomplete ovals. The inter-trigonal region between the right and left trigones has rigid fibrous tissue, the aortic curtain, which is common to both AV and MV.

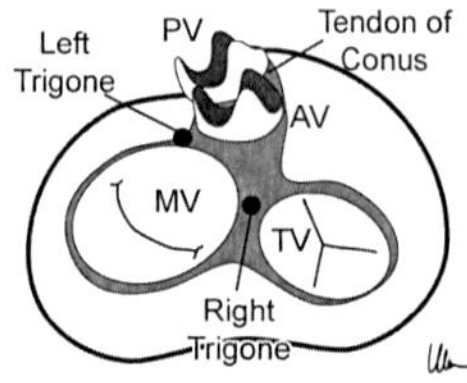

Mitral Annulus

Mitral annuli fibrosi is incomplete becoming thinner as it extends posterior, making it prone to dilatation.

- P2 prolapse commonest
- Saddle-shaped (hyperbolic paraboloid)
  - Highest in ME 120° view
  - Lowest is commissural
- Changes shape during cardiac cycle
  - Circle (diastole): 40% larger
  - "D" shape (systole): smaller
- Measure annulus in diastole in
  - ME AV LAX view (120°)
  - Normal size 29 ± 4 mm

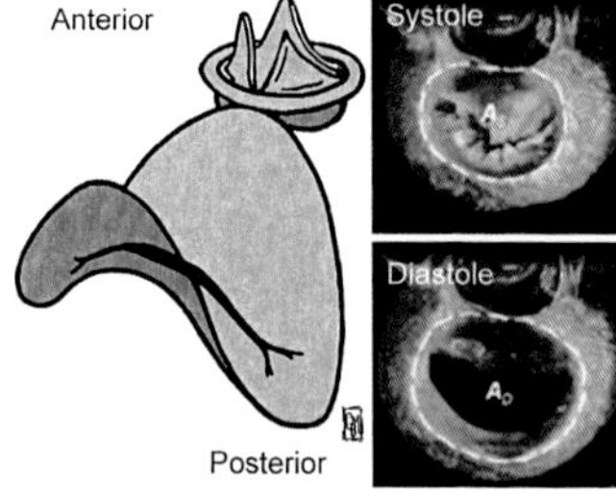

Mitral Valve Leaflets

A curtain of fibroelastic tissue extends from the mitral annulus forming MV leaflets.

- Four anatomic leaflets:
  - Anterior (AMVL): 1/3 MV annulus
  - Posterior (PMVL): 2/3 MV annulus, three scallops
  - Anterior commissure (AC)
  - Posterior commissure (PC)
- Leaflet nomenclature (see p. 147)
- Leaflet thickness ≤4 mm
- Annulus area 4–6 cm^2
- MV leaflet surface area: twice the annulus area
- Large leaflet coaptation area (30%), 1 cm length

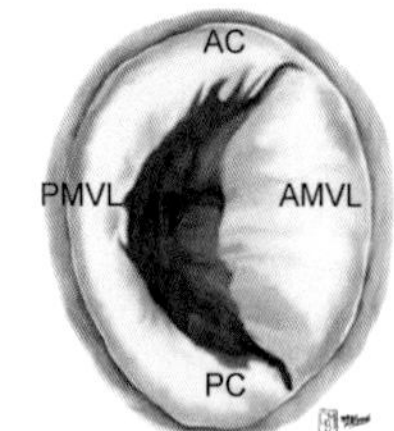
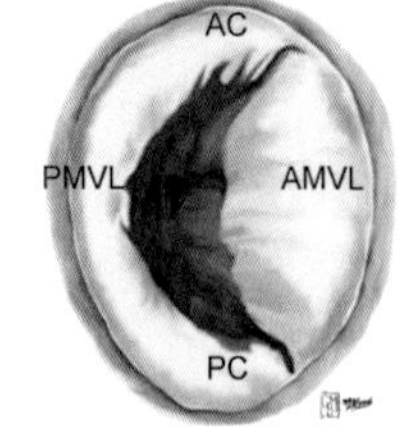

Chordae Tendinea

These fibrous strings radiate from the papillary muscles or the LV free wall (PMVL only) to attach to the mitral leaflets in an organized way. There are three orders:

- Stay chordae are 2° chords that attach to AMVL and are important for MV geometry
- First: leaflet-free margin
- Second: ventricular leaflet aspect
- Third: vent wall to PMVL only

Papillary Muscles (PM)

Papillary muscles are 2 large trabeculae carnae originating from the LV free wall.

- Chordae arising from the anterior PM attach to the anterior half of MV and from posterior PM to posterior half.
  - Anterolateral: A2, A1, Ac, P1, P2
  - Posteromedial: A2, A3, Pc, P3, P2
- Anterior PM has dual blood supply; the posterior PM has single artery supply.

MV Function

- In diastole, the papillary muscles and LV myocardium relax, LA pressure exceeds LV pressure, and the MV passively opens.
- In systole, the papillary muscles contract making the chordae tendinae taut to prevent leaflets from prolapsing into the LA. Leaflet and chordae length is fixed. Excess leaflet area permits a large area of coaptation, analogous to a roman arch.

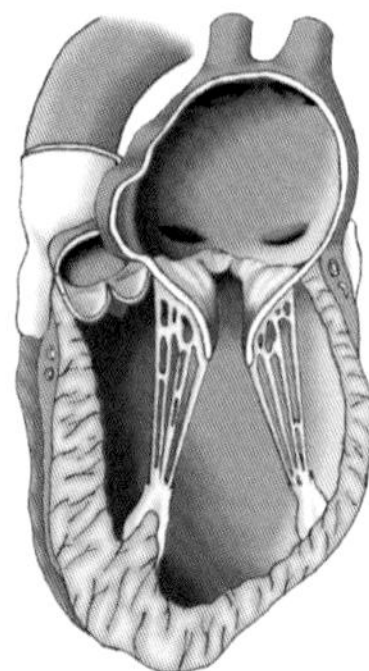

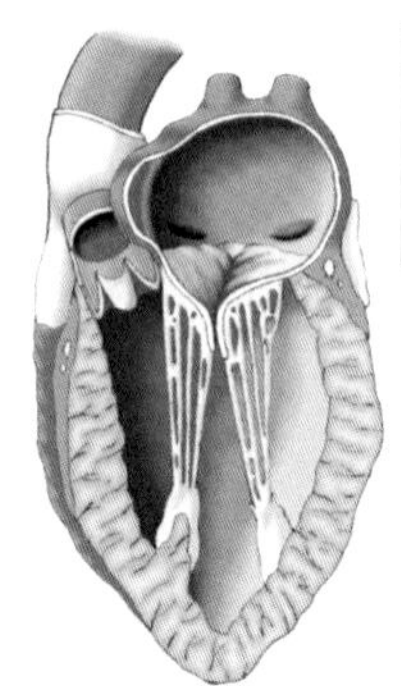

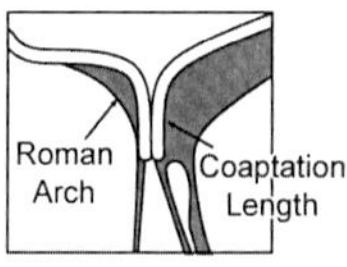

MV Leaflet Nomenclature

Carpentier Classification

- This is used by the ASE and SCA, divides the PMVL using the scallops into P1 (lateral), P2 (middle), and P3 (medial) and the AMVL into corresponding A1 (lateral), A2 (middle), and A3 (medial) portions.

Duran Classification

- This is based on which papillary muscle supply chordae to the segments.
- PMVL: P1 (lateral), PM (middle), and P2 (medial) with PM further subdivided into PM1 (anterior PM) and PM2 (posterior PM).
- AMVL: A1 (anterolateral PM) and A2 (posteromedial PM) portions. Other valve parts include the anterolateral commissure (Cl), posteromedial commissure (C2), PM1 (anterolateral PM), PM2 (posteromedial PM), inter-trigonal distance (T1-T2).

Leaflet Nomenclature		
Anatomic	Duran	Carpentier
Posterior leaflet (scallops)		
Lateral	P1	P1
Middle	PM (1/2)	P2
Medial	P2	P3
Commissural leaflets		
Anterolateral	C1	Ac com
Posteromedial	C2	Pc com
Anterior leaflet (segments)		
	A1, A2	A1, A2, A3

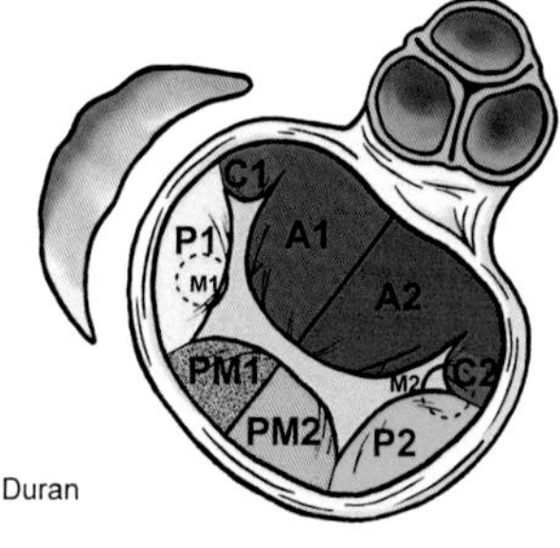

Duran

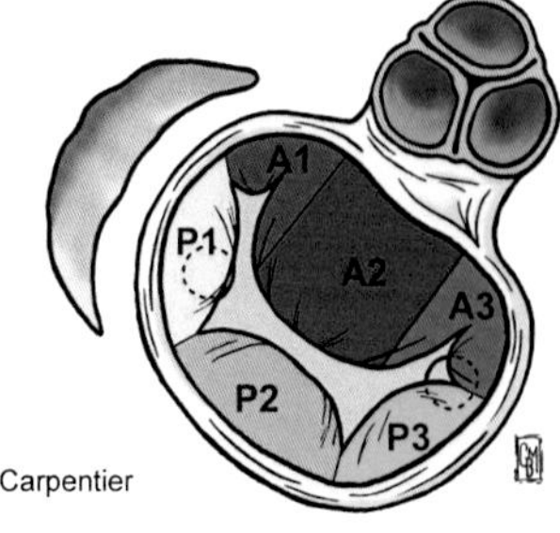

Carpentier

- MV is examined from 6 standard TEE views (ME 4C, ME commissural, ME 2C, ME AV LAX, TG basal SAX, and TG 2C). Beyond 90°, the image transitions to show the AMVL on the display right and PMVL on left. In the MC view (60°), turning the probe right images the AMVL and left the PMVL.
- Individual segments/scallops are identified using systemic evaluation of ME views.
- Imaging of MV segments should not be based on the TEE transducer angles, but on the reliable identification of the structures in each view. The most reliable views are the ME 4C (A2, P2), ME commissural (P3, A2, P1), and ME AV LAX (P2, A2).
- Withdrawing the probe in the ME 4C view images a more anterior portion (A1,P1) of the MV, while advancing the probe images the more posterior part (A3, P3).
- In the TG SAX view, the MV is imaged from posterior, so the PMVL is closest to the probe in the near field and the AMVL is in the far-field.

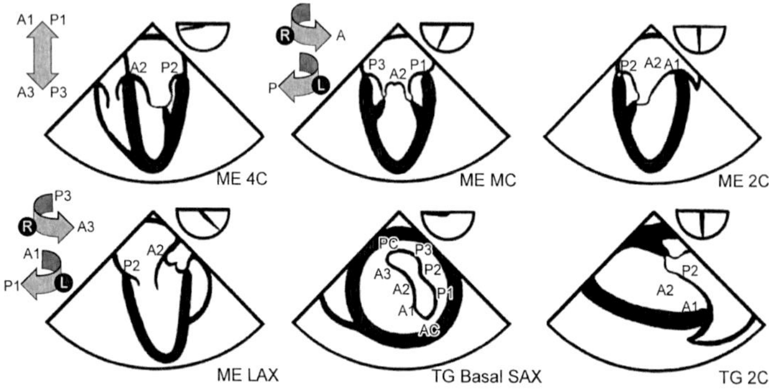

Surgeon's View and 3D TEE

The MV as viewed by the surgeon through a left atriotomy is displaced 90° counterclockwise from the 2D ME TEE views. The AMVL is superior and the PMVL is inferior, shown here with MV annuloplasty ring. The MV as imaged using real-time 3D TEE can be orientated to display it in the surgeon's perspective as seen from the LA. In this image, the scallops of the PMVL are apparent. Note the aortic valve (AV) is displayed at the top of the image and the left atrial appendage (LAA) to the left.

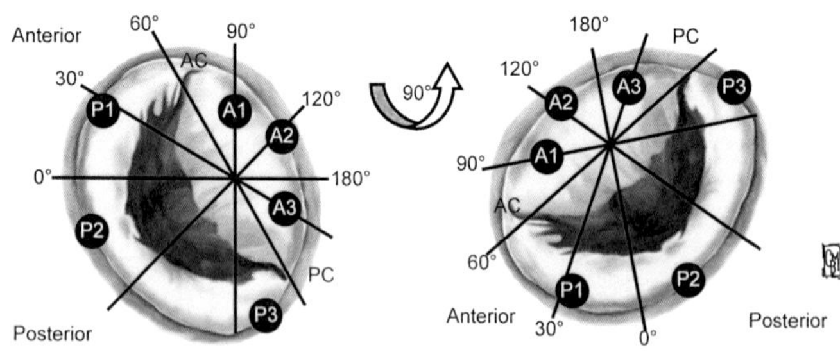

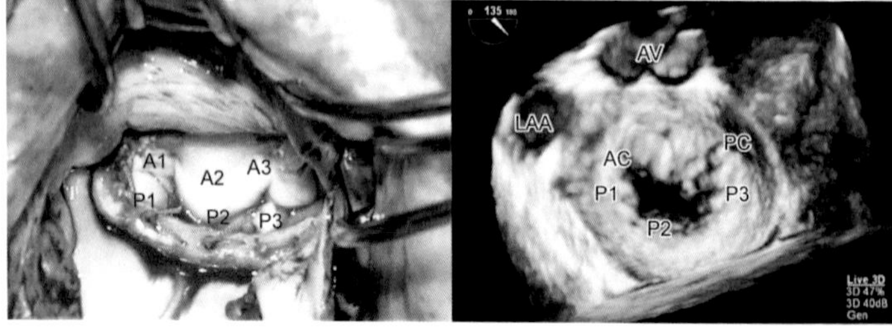

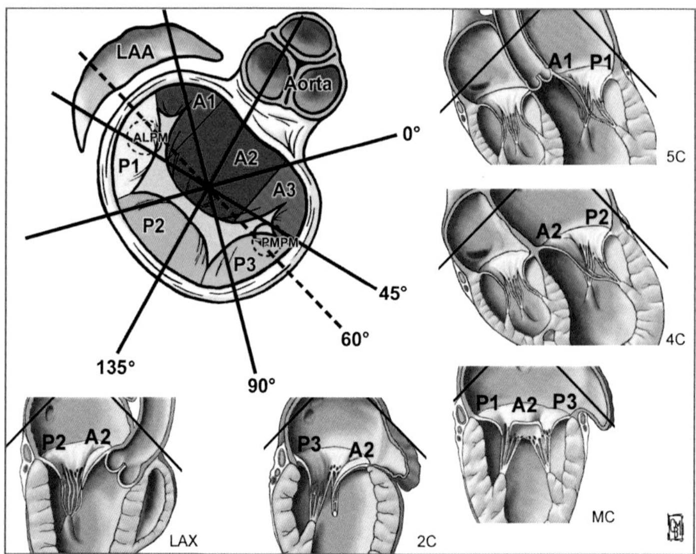

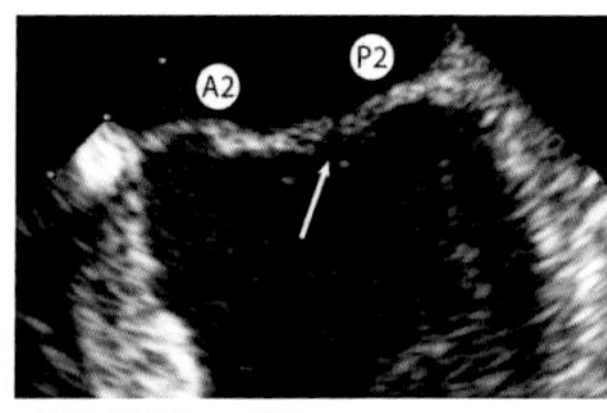

ME 4C View (0°)
Anteflex (5C) view: A1/A2 + P2/P1
Retroflex (4C) view: A3/A2 + P2/P3

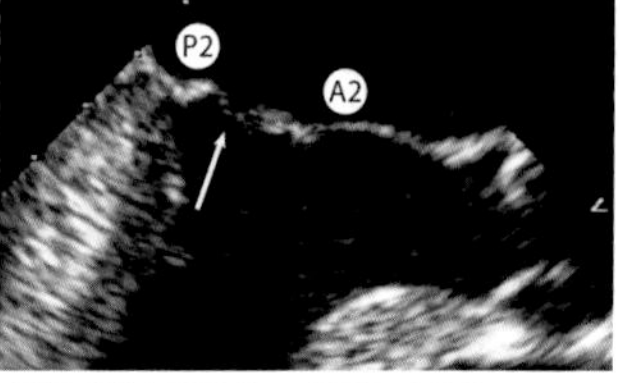

ME AV LAX View (120–135°)
Reliably image A2, P2
Annulus high point to detect prolapse

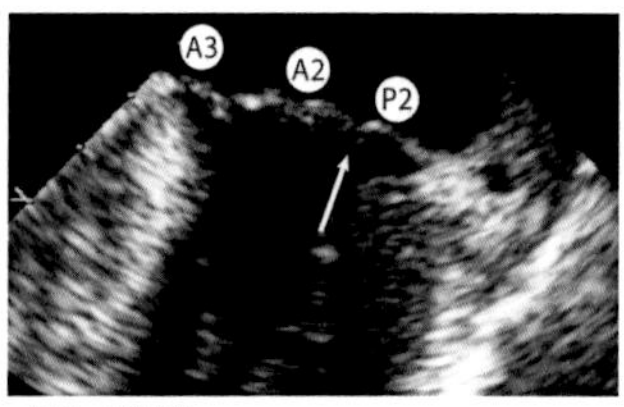

ME 45° View
AMVL is on the display left
AMVL (A3, A2) is long and coapts (arrow) with short P2

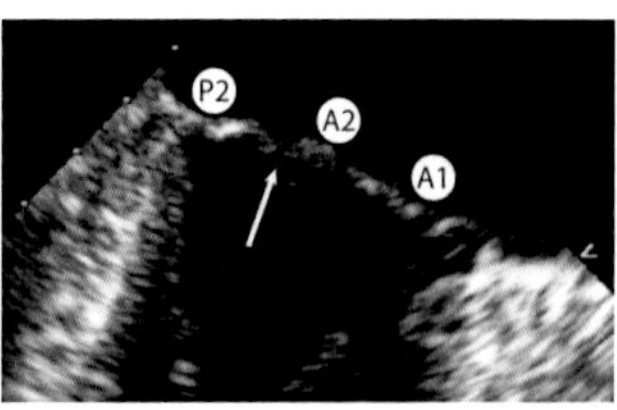

ME 2C View (90–105°)
AMVL is on the display right
AMVL (A1, A2) is long and coapts (arrow) with short P2

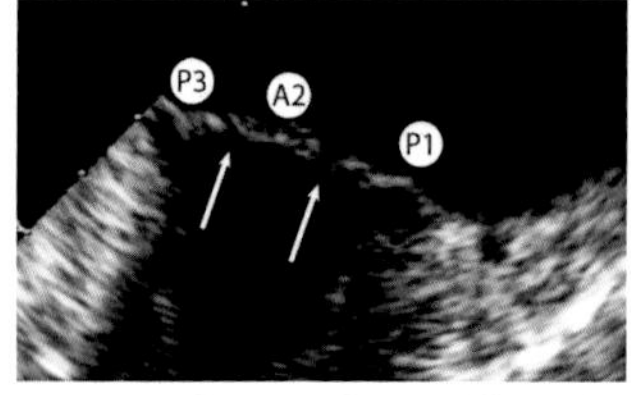

ME Mitral Commissural View (60–75°)
Image 3 distinct segments (P3, A2, P1)
See 2 coaptation points (arrows)
Mobile center A2 disappears in diastole
LAA is seen

Source: Omran AS, et al. J Am Soc Echocardiogr 2002; 15:950–7

Assessment

1. Etiology of Regurgitation:
    - Normal finding in 40% of patients (trace MR)
    - Primary MR (structural): failure of any component of the MV apparatus
        - Leaflet: degenerative, myxomatous, rheumatic, endocarditis, congenital
        - Annulus: mitral annular calcification (MAC)
        - Chordae: rupture, elongation, shortening
        - Papillary muscle: rupture
    - Secondary MR (functional): structurally normal MV leaflets (see p. 153)
        - Annular dilatation
        - LV dysfunction
        - Aortic stenosis, SAM
    - Diastolic MR: LV pressure exceeds LAP during diastole
2. 2D findings:
    - Leaflets: thick (>5 mm), calcified, malcoapt, prolapsed, flail, vegetation
    - Annulus: MAC, size (mid-diastole 29 ± 4 mm)
3. Doppler findings:
    - Color: turbulent systolic flow from LV to LA, flow acceleration below MV
        - 3 components: area mapping (trace mosaic area), vena contracta (narrowest width), proximal flow convergence (PISA)
        - Jet direction: central, posterior, anterior
    - CW: systolic flow above baseline, velocity 5–6 m/s, density α MR, contour parabolic or early peaking, triangular shape in severe MR
    - PW: mitral inflow velocity >1.5 m/s with moderate-severe MR (no MS), A-wave predominance excludes severe MR
    - PW: pulmonary vein systolic flow reversal-specific, but not sensitive, absent if large LA. Eccentric jet look in contra-lateral pulmonary vein
4. LA enlarged (>55 mm AP diameter), LA:RA ratio >1
5. LV size + systolic functions are important prognostic factors and surgical indicators
    - LV size: ESD >55 mm, dilated from volume overload
    - Systolic function: initially good, but worsens over time
6. Regurgitation Severity (2017 ASE) (See Next Page)
    - Classify onto 3 Grades (overlap in moderate/severe)
    - Consider the mechanism (1° or 2°)
    - Determine LA/LV size to establish chronicity of MR
    - Consider the duration and timing of MR in diastole
    - Assess MR at a clinically relevant systolic BP (SBP >120), note HR + rhythm
    - All parameters have limitations and are imprecise, use an integrative approach
    - If more than mild MR, use quantitative indicators when possible
        - Regurgitant volume for an estimate of volume overload
        - Effective regurgitant orifice area (EROA) for lesion severity
    - Specific criteria have high positive predictive value for MR severity.
        - Structural defect in MV
        - Vena contracta width ≥7 mm
        - Pulmonary vein flow S-wave reversal in >1 vein

What to Tell the Surgeon Mitral Regurgitation

PreCPB

- Mechanism MR (Carpentier classification Type I, II, IIIa, IIIb)
- Leaflet pathology: myxomatous, calcified, prolapsed/flail segments
- Annular size, MAC
- Direction and severity of MR jets, pulmonary vein flow (blunted/reversed)
- LA, LV size, and function

PostCPB

- Post-repair mitral leaflet morphology, Prosthetic valve function
- Residual MR, impaired mitral inflow (?stenotic)
- Complications repair: SAM, posterior wall (circumflex art), atrioventricular groove separation, AV non-coronary cusp trauma
- LV/RV function, severity TR

Mitral Regurgitation Severity Doppler Assessment (AHA/ASE)				
	Method	Mild	Moderate	Severe
Qualit	Color Flow Jet Area[a]	Small	Variable	Large
	Flow Convergence (cm)[b]	<0.3	Intermediate	≥1.0
	CW Doppler Signal Strength	Faint	Dense, partial	Holodiastolic
Semiquant	Vena Contracta Width (cm)	<0.3	Intermediate	≥0.7
	Pulmonary Venous Doppler (S-wave)	Normal	Normal/blunt	Reverse
	Mitral Inflow	A-wave	Variable	E-wave
Quant	Effective Regurgitant Orifice Area (cm^2)	<0.20	0.20–0.39	≥0.4
	Regurgitant Volume (cm^3)	<30	30–59	≥60
	Regurgitant Fraction (%)	<30	30–49	≥50

Assess regurgitation severity under physiologic conditions (SBP, afterload, and LV function)
Use appropriate Nyquist velocity, [a]50–70 cm/s and color gain, [b]40 cm/s
Adapted from: Zoghbi W, et al. J Am Soc Echocardiogr 2017;30:303–371

Jet Area Mapping
- Trace mosaic jet area
- Nyquist 50–60 cm/s
- Physiology-dependent, so less reliable
- Underestimates if eccentric jets, acute MR
- Useful if multiple jets

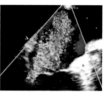

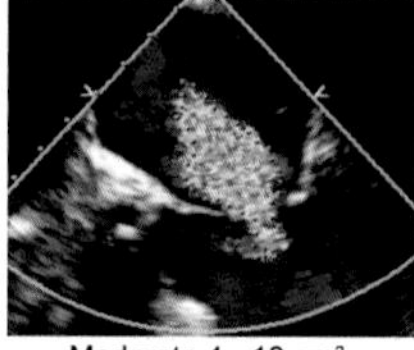
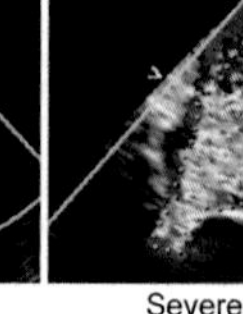
Moderate 4 - 10 cm^2 Severe > 10 cm^2

CW Doppler
- Density, compare with forward flow
- Contour (complete)
- High velocity (>5 m/s)
- ↑ MV E velocity >1.5 m/s

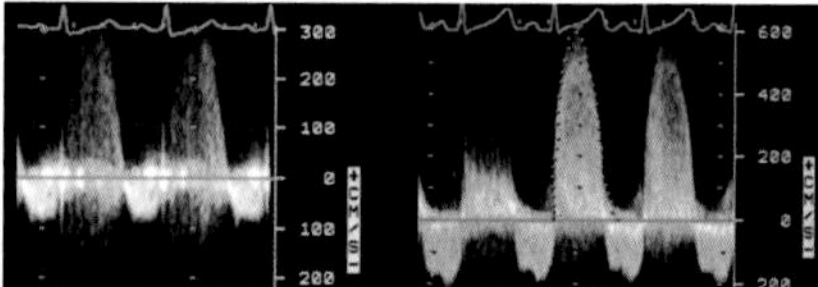

Vena Contracta
- Narrowest diameter, measure above flow acceleration
- Nyquist 50–60 cm/s
- Useful if eccentric jets
- Not used if multiple jets
- Best measured in ME AV LAX or 4C views
- Correlates with EROA, RegV

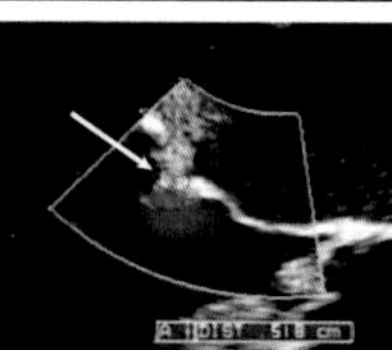
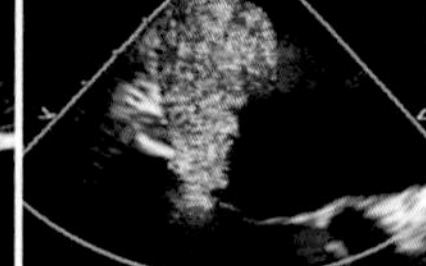
Moderate 4 - 6 mm Severe > 7 mm

Pulmonary Vein Doppler
- Normal pattern mild MR
- Blunted nonspecific
- Reversed specific for severe MR
- Multiple veins
- Eccentric MR sample contra-lateral vein

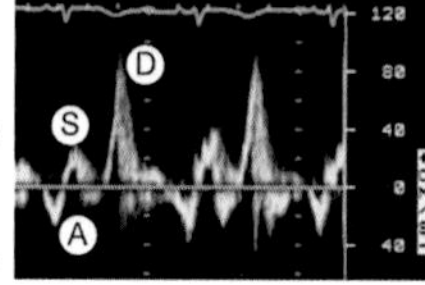

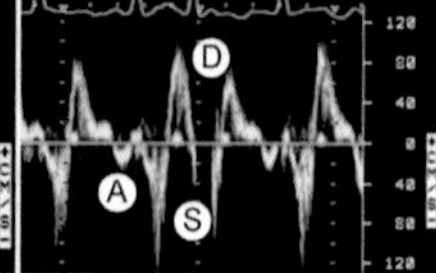

PISA (EROA)
- Radius of proximal flow convergence
- Nyquist 40 cm/s
- Less useful if eccentric
- Not used if multiple jets
- Calculate EROA (p. 59)

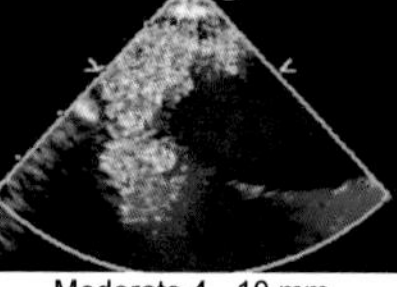
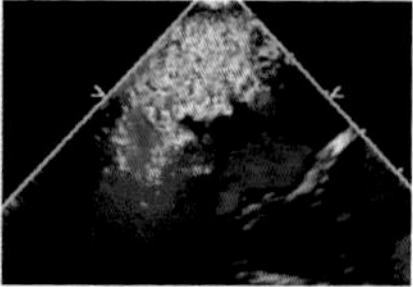
Moderate 4 - 10 mm Severe > 10 mm

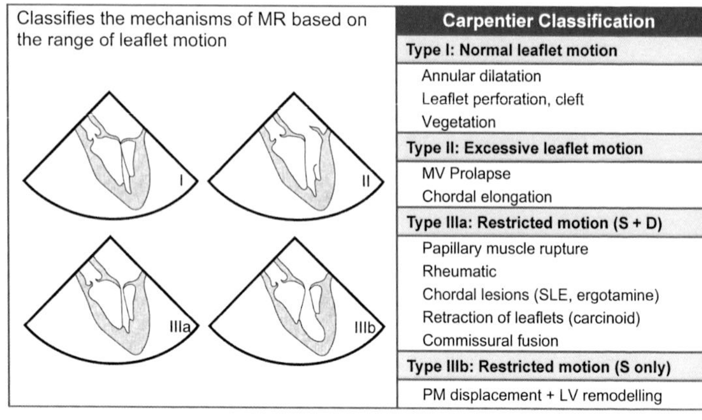

Classifies the mechanisms of MR based on the range of leaflet motion

Carpentier Classification
Type I: Normal leaflet motion
Annular dilatation Leaflet perforation, cleft Vegetation
Type II: Excessive leaflet motion
MV Prolapse Chordal elongation
Type IIIa: Restricted motion (S + D)
Papillary muscle rupture Rheumatic Chordal lesions (SLE, ergotamine) Retraction of leaflets (carcinoid) Commissural fusion
Type IIIb: Restricted motion (S only)
PM displacement + LV remodelling

Excessive Mitral Leaflet Motion

- MV annulus is saddle-shaped with the highest points at 0 and 120°.
- Normal leaflet tip coaptation is below the annular plane in the LV.
- Excessive leaflet motion occurs if any portion of the MV leaflet is above the annular plane and is described using different terms.

Billowing Leaflet

Part of the leaflet body is above the annulus during systole, but the coaptation point (arrow) is below the annulus

Prolapsed Leaflet

Body and leaflet tip (arrow) is above the annulus during systole, thus preventing leaflet coaptation. Leaflet tips point to the LV

Flail Leaflet

Leaflet tip is above the annular plane and points towards the LA. Often has mobile torn chordae that are attached (arrow)

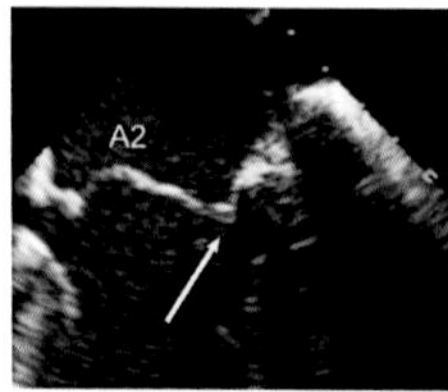

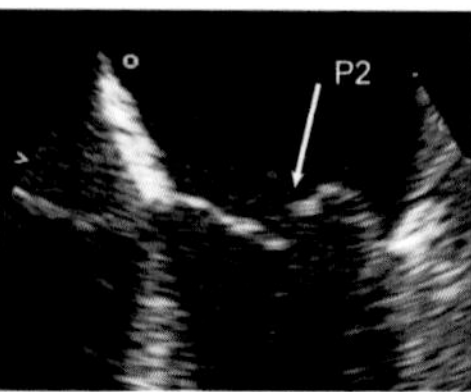

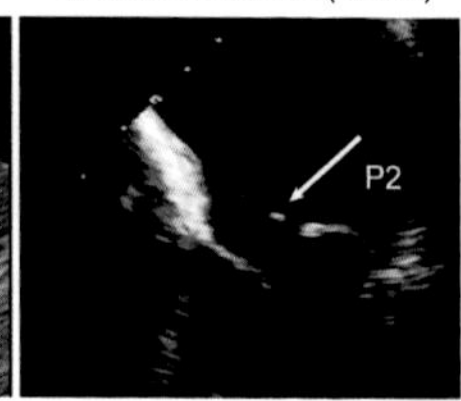

Jet Direction and MR Mechanism

The direction of the MR jet can help establish the mechanism of MR:

- Anterior jet
  - Typically from prolapsed posterior leaflet, rarely restricted anterior leaflet or perforation. Jet hugs the AMVL, wraps around the LA towards right pulmonary veins.
- Posterior jet
  - Typically from prolapsed anterior leaflet, rarely restricted posterior leaflet or perforation. Jet hugs the PMVL, wraps around the LA towards left pulmonary veins.
- Central jet
  - Typically bileaflet prolapse, annular dilatation, or LV dysfunction which restrict the motion of both leaflets. Any or all 4 pulmonary veins may be affected.

The **Coanda Effect** may underestimate the severity of an eccentric MR jet as there is a loss of energy when the jet adheres and flows around the LA wall.

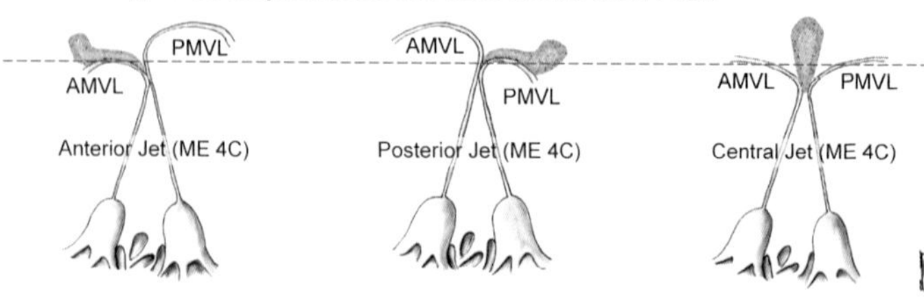

Functional MR

Parameter	1° MR	2° MR
EROA (cm^2)	≥0.4	≥0.2
VC width (cm)	≥0.7	≥0.7
RegFr (%)	≥50	≥50
RegVol (cm^3)	≥60	≥30

Source: AHA/ACC Guidelines. JACC 2014; 63 (22): e57–188

- Recent AHA guidelines endorse lower cut-off values for functional (2°) MR (see p. 109) compared with primary (1°) organic MR. The 2017 ASE guidelines do not distinguish MR severity based on the mechanism.
- Vena Contracta width (VCW) is the diameter of the MR jet measured perpendicular to the line of leaflet coaptation above the flow acceleration region at any Nyquist in the ME AV LAX or 4C views. Measurement in other views is not used to avoid overestimating severity. This is a linear measure that is representative of the regurgitant orifice area.
- EROA has a circular shape in 1° MR and is elongated in 2° MR. The cut-off value for severe chronic ischemic MR is lower at 0.2 cm^2 compared with 1° MR 0.4 cm^2. Tracing the vena contracta area (VCA), which is a surrogate measure of EROA using 3D echocardiography, may provide more accurate measurements. The PISA radius can be used to calculate EROA, but varies in size in 2° MR with early and late peaks, so care must be taken if using the PISA radius in this setting.
- There is a difference in prognostic values for regurgitant volume based on the presence of 1° organic (>60 cc) versus 2° functional (>30 cc) disease. Smaller volumes indicate greater severity of 2° MR.

(A–C) Shown here is a 3D TEE dataset of a functional (2°) MR jet in a multiplanar reconstruction (MPR) format. The (A) ME 4C view in the green plane and (B) ME 2C view in the red plane display orthogonal views of the MR jet. (C) The blue plane is positioned at the vena contracta in both ME 4C and 2C views and displayed. Tracing the elongated-shaped vena contracta area (VCA) yields a value of 1.22 cm^2 which represents severe MR.

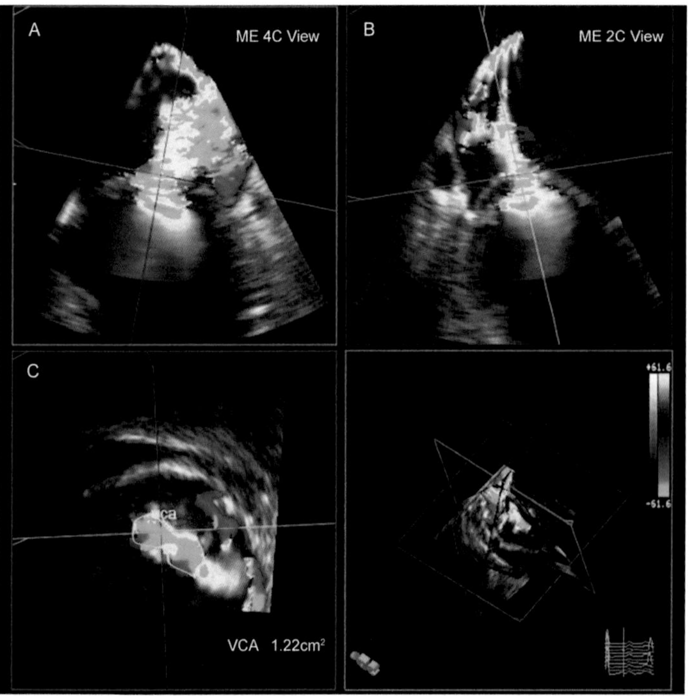

Posterior Mitral Regurgitation Jet

An eccentric posterior-directed MR jet is shown. (A, B) Anterior mitral valve leaflet prolapse/flail (in red) results in a posterior-directed MR jet (in green). This is shown in multiple ME views with and without color Doppler imaging (Nyquist 55 cm/s). The appearance of the MR jet varies depending on the view. The MR jet is posterior-directed and wraps around the LA seen best at 0° (4C) and 137° (ME AV LAX). Quantification of MR severity relies on examination under adequate physiological conditions with measurement of the vena contracta (VC) width and calculation of EROA. Tracing of the jet area is not recommended and will underestimate severity due to the Coanda effect. Abnormal left pulmonary vein flow is expected.

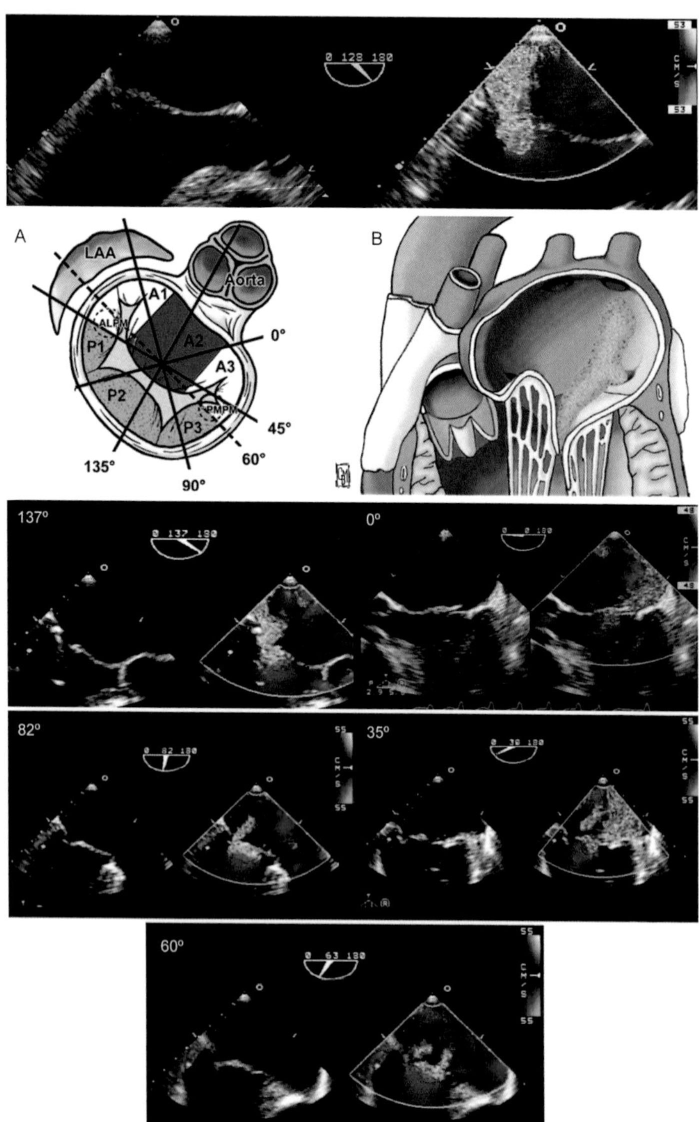

Anterior Mitral Regurgitation Jet

An eccentric anterior-directed MR jet is shown. (A, B) Posterior mitral valve leaflet prolapse/flail (in red) results in an anterior-directed MR jet (in green). This is shown with and without color Doppler imaging (Nyquist 55 cm/s). The MR jet is anterior-directed and wraps around the LA seen best at 0° (ME 4C) and 129° (ME AV LAX). Quantification of MR severity relies on measurement of the vena contracta (VC) width and regurgitant volume. The EROA may be hard to calculate using the PISA method as it will be difficult to measure a complete spectral Doppler trace. Abnormal right pulmonary vein flow is expected.

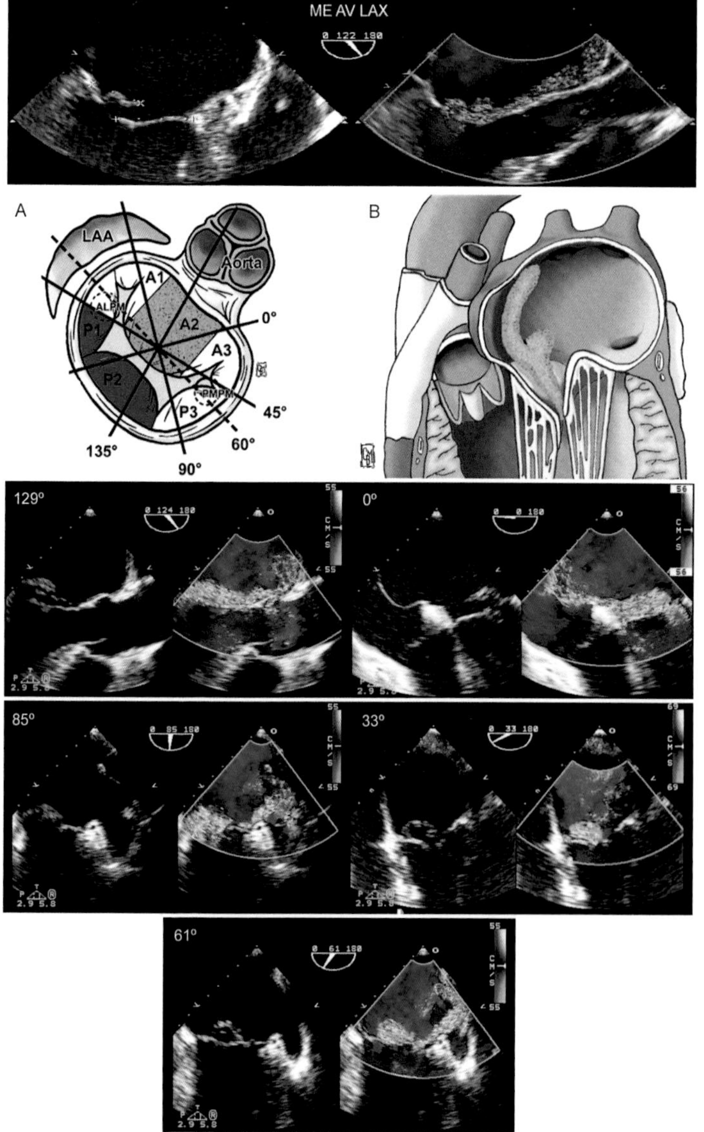

Barlow's Disease

This is a degenerative disease of the MV from mucopolysaccharide deposits resulting in excessive leaflet tissue. An example is shown from the LA side (A) using 3D TEE, (B) at surgery and in the (C) 2D TEE ME Mitral Commissural view with bileaflet prolapse and severe central MR. (D) The MV annulus is often displaced into the LA (arrow) complicating the repair. (E) A static MV 3D model reconstruction shows bileaflet prolapse. There may be concurrent other valve prolapse: tricuspid (30%), pulmonic (10%), aortic (2%).

Source: Eriksson M, et al. J Am Soc Echocardiogr 2005; 18:1014–22

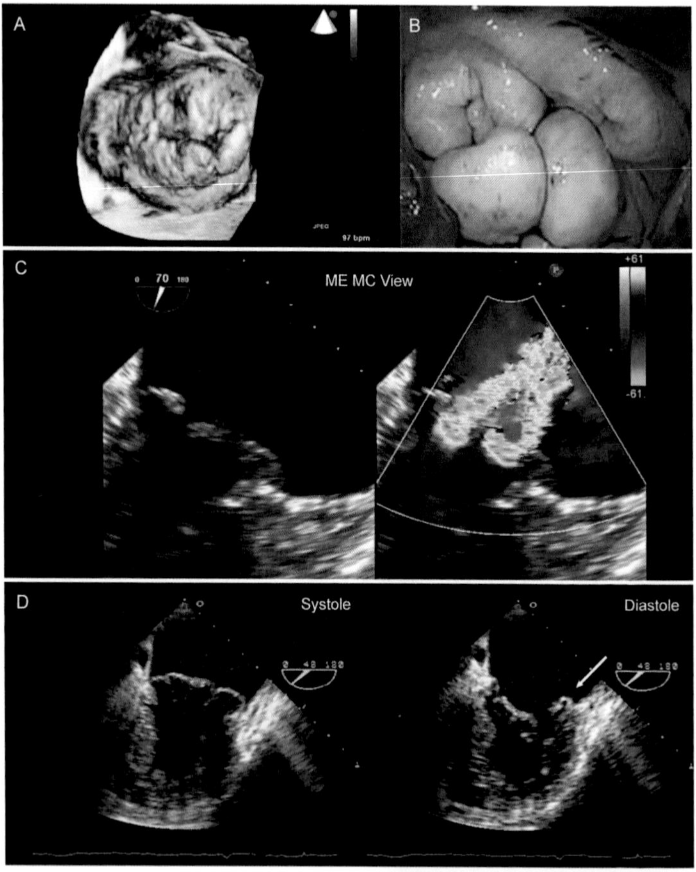

TEE Barlow's Disease

- Thick leaflets (>4 mm)
- Prolapse both leaflets
- Central or eccentric MR
- Annular dilatation (ESD >36 mm)
- Annulus displacement into LA
- Chordal elongation and thickened
- Chordal rupture uncommon
- Associated secundum ASD
- Complex repair

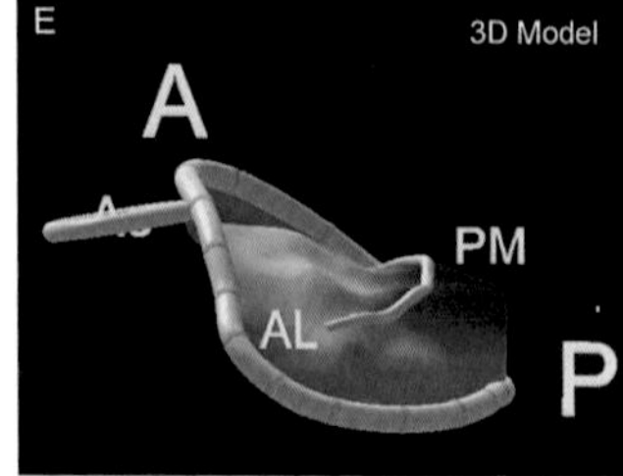

Fibroelastic Degeneration

This is a degenerative disease of the MV characterized by deficiency of fibroelastic tissue, resulting in thin MV leaflets and chordae. The weakened chordae frequently rupture leading to a flail segment as shown in these examples of two patients with an isolated P2 prolapse with flail tip (P2) and torn chordae (arrow). (A, B) Examples are shown from the LA side in the surgeon's orientation using real-time 3D TEE. (C) Compare 2D ME 4C view of the MV with color Doppler showing severe anterior-directed MR. (D) Reconstructed static MV 3D model shows the prolapsed segment.

Source: Anyanwu A and Adams D. Semin Thorac Cardiovasc Surg 2007;19: 90–96

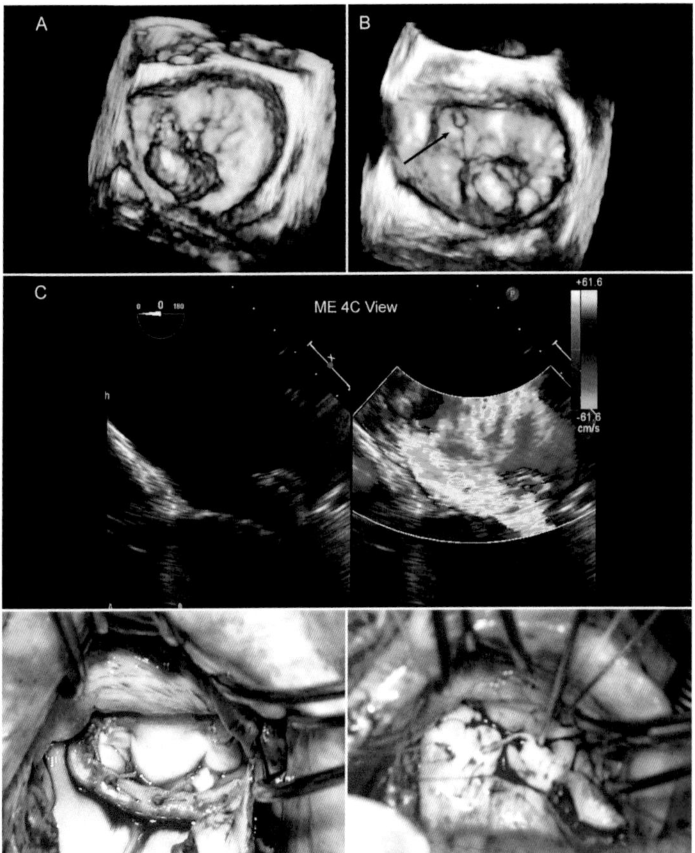

TEE Fibroelastic Disease

- Normal leaflet thickness of MV
- Isolated segment prolapse/flail
- Prolapsed segment may be thickened
- Eccentric MR
- ± Annular dilatation
- No annulus displacement
- Chordal rupture common
- Simple repair

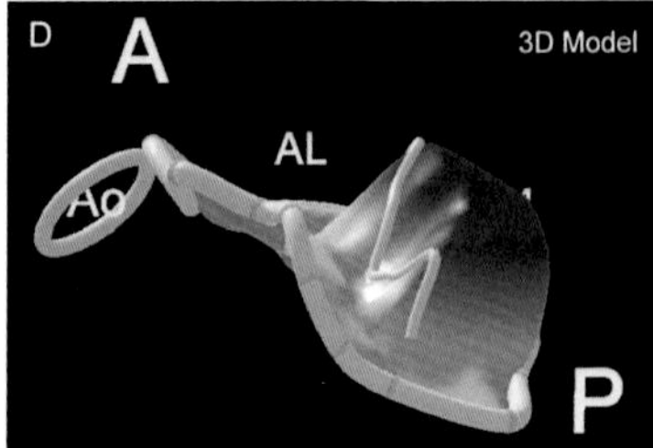

Assessment

1. Etiology of stenosis:
    - Valvular: rheumatic (75%), calcific (25%), carcinoid, SLE, congenital, drugs
    - Subvalvular: mass, myxoma
2. 2D findings:
    - Annulus: Ca^{2+}, size (end-diastole)
    - Leaflets: Ca^{2+}, thickness (>4 mm), mobility, diastolic doming "hockey stick"
    - Chordae: Ca^{2+}, thickened, extent of subvalvular involvement
    - Planimeter MV area (MVA) TG basal SAX view (often underestimates MVA)
3. Doppler findings:
    - Color: turbulent diastolic flow, proximal flow acceleration
    - PW/CW: peak velocity >3 m/s, peak/mean pressure gradient (PG)
        - MV flow is determined by diastolic transvalvular gradient, influenced by LA compliance, LV diastolic dysfunction, HR, and cardiac output
        - Note an elevated transmitral inflow also occurs with high cardiac output, MR, and restrictive diastolic filling
        - Coexisting MR have high peak PG (>20 mmHg), low mean PG <10 mmHg
    - Pressure half-time (PHT) for native MVA (see p. 58)
4. Stenosis severity (severe).
    - Peak velocity >3 m/s
    - Mean pressure gradient >10 mmHg
    - MVA <1.0 cm^2 (2D planimetry, PHT)
5. LA enlargement (LAX view: A-P diameter >45 mm), smoke, thrombus in LAA
6. LV function: small underfilled, RWMA (postero-basal segment)
7. Right heart changes due to pulmonary hypertension
    - PASP (estimate from TR jet)
    - RV function: dilated, hypertrophy, IVS paradoxical motion
    - Coexisting TR severity, may require surgical intervention

Severity Assessment (EAE/ASE Guidelines)				
	Valve Area (cm^2)	Mean Gradient (mmHg)	PHT (ms)	Peak Pulmonary Artery P (mmHg)
Normal	4–6		40–70	20–30
Mild	>1.5	<5	70–150	<30
Moderate	1.0–1.5	510	150–200	30–50
Severe	<1.0	>10	>220	>50
Adapted from: Baumgartner H, et al. J Am Soc Echocardiogr 2009;22:1–23				

The assessment of MS severity should not rely on a single measure, but rather a multimodal approach that establishes the pressure gradient, MVA, and peak PAP. MVA should be used to determine MS severity if Doppler gradients are unreliable, as with concurrent MR. MVA can be estimated by several methods, each has limitations, so choosing the best method is based on image quality and other pathology.

- Planimetry: difficult in heavily calcified valves
- Pressure half-time (PHT): avoid in $\uparrow$ LVEDP (AI, LV dysfunction), $\uparrow$ LA (ASD)
- Continuity: avoid in LVOT obstruction, MR, atrial fibrillation
- Proximal isovelocity surface area (PISA): use in AI, MR, prosthetic valve, a fib

What to Tell the Surgeon Mitral Stenosis

PreCPB

- Calcific vs. rheumatic valve
- Chordal involvement.
- Annulus size (diastole)
- Mitral annular calcification (MAC)
- LA size (severe >50 mm), LAA thrombus
- RV function, TR severity, TV annulus size

PostCPB

- Peak/mean Pressure gradients
- Residual MR
- Prosthetic valve function

Mitral Stenosis	2D Echo	Color/Spectral Doppler
ME 4C (0°)	Annulus: Ca^{2+}, size	Turbulent diastolic flow
ME commissural (60°)	Leaflets: Ca^{2+}, thick, mobile	PISA
ME 2C (90°)		MV inflow: peak/mean
ME AV LAX (120°)	Chordae: Ca^{2+}, thick	Pressure half time (PHT)
TG SAX (0°)	Ca^{2+}, planimetry	Commissural MR origin color
TG 2C (90°)	Subvalvular apparatus	

Grading of MV Characteristics in Mitral Stenosis				
Grade	Mobility	Leaflet Thickened	Subvalvular	Calcification
1	Tips restricted	4–5 mm	Minimal	Minimal
2	Base-mid normal	5–8 mm	1/3 chordae	Leaflet margins
3	Base normal	5–8 mm	2/3 chordae	Mid leaflet
4	No movement	>8–10 mm	Total	Majority leaflet

The echo score quantifies the severity of the rheumatic MV morphologic derangement to establish a predictor of outcome after percutaneous balloon valvuloplasty. Valve score <8 has a good outcome. Increased score associated with suboptimal outcome, mortality, restenosis, heart failure, need for cardiac surgery
Source: Wilkins G. Br Heart J 1988; 60:300

(A) Fusion of the rheumatic leaflet edges with elevated LAP pushes the more mobile body of the AMVL toward the LV producing diastolic doming of the AMVL, thus giving it a hockey stick appearance. (B) The subvalvular chordae, best seen in the TG 2C view, are short and thickened resulting in restricted leaflet motion. (C) Color Doppler shows proximal flow acceleration and turbulent antegrade flow through the stenotic MV. (D) Spectral Doppler (PW/CW) can be traced to measure the peak and mean pressure gradients and analyzed for the pressure half-time (PT1/2) to estimate the MV area (see p. 58). (E) ME 4C view shows left atrial enlargement with smoke and (F) thrombus in the left atrial appendage in this ME commissural view.

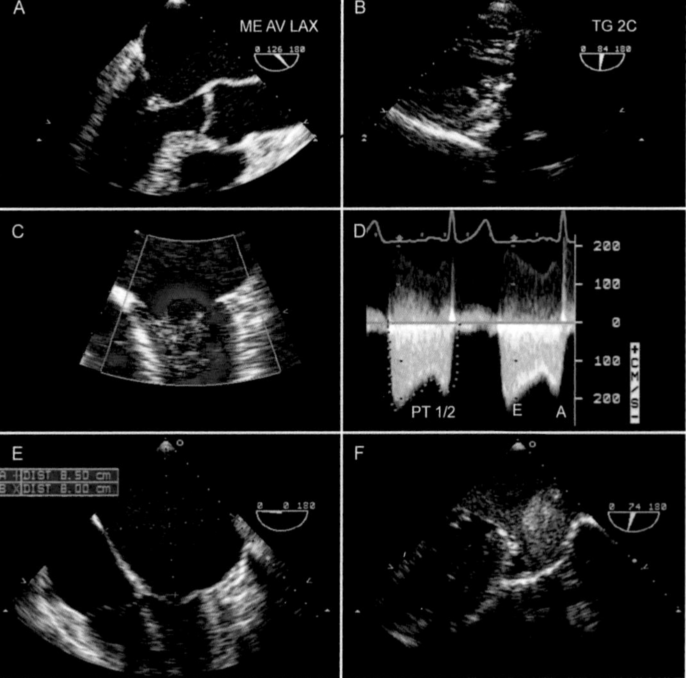

The TV apparatus is similar in structure to the other atrioventricular valve, the mitral valve, comprising an annulus, valve leaflets, chordae, papillary muscles, and RV.

Tricuspid Annulus

- This is an incomplete fibrous ring to which the leaflets attach.
- Septal leaflet hinge point is apically displaced below the MV annulus. This feature distinguishes the more apically displaced TV from the MV in the ME 4C view.
- The annulus has a non-uniform 3D shape with high points anterior and posterior, and the low points that are medial-lateral (see below).
- It has a distensible size:
  - Tricuspid Annulus Diameter (TAD): end-systole 28 mm ± 5, end-diastole 31 mm ± 4
  - Annulus measurements are underestimated using 2D vs. 3D TTE.
  - In TEE, the TG RV Inflow measurement is better correlated than the ME views.
- TV annulus area 10 ± 2.9 cm^2, TV orifice area 4.8 ± 1.6 cm^2, circumference 12–14 cm
- Tricuspid annulus fractional shortening (TAFS), normal >25%
  - TAFS = end-diastolic TAD – end-systolic TAD/end-diastolic TAD

Leaflets

- TV has 3 valve leaflets of variable sizes:
  - Anterior > septal > posterior
  - 3 incomplete commissures do not meet at the annulus to separate the leaflets
- Normal leaflet thickness is 3 mm.

Chordae

- Chordae support the leaflets during systole, preventing leaflet prolapse.
- Attach from papillary muscles to the leaflets
  - Anterior PM to anterior + posterior leaflets
  - Posterior PM to posterior + septal leaflets
  - Septal PM to septal + anterior leaflets
- Also have attachments from the septal leaflet directly to the septal wall (unlike MV)

Papillary Muscles

- The RV has 3 or more papillary muscles:
  - Anterior (largest), posterior, ± septal
  - Anterior and posterior PM connected by the moderator band

Right Ventricle

- RV dilatation from RV pressure or volume overload from any cause can lead to tricuspid annular dilatation.
- Left heart failure or pulmonary hypertension may also cause tricuspid annular dilatation.

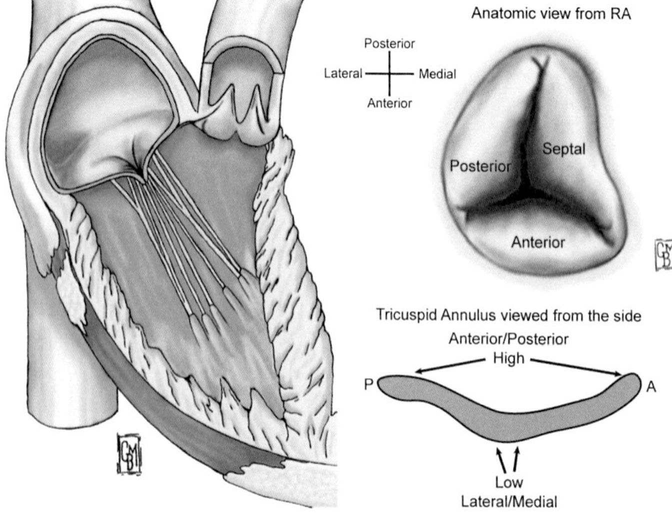

TV Function

Normal TV inflow is diastolic laminar flow (blue) with color Doppler and has the lowest velocity (<70 cm/s) of all valves as measured with PW spectral Doppler.

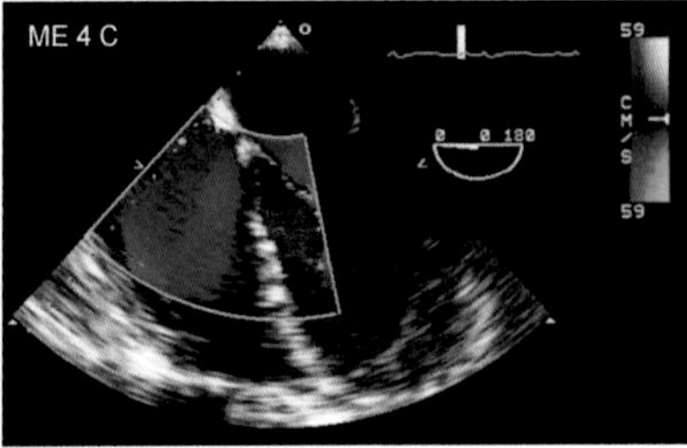

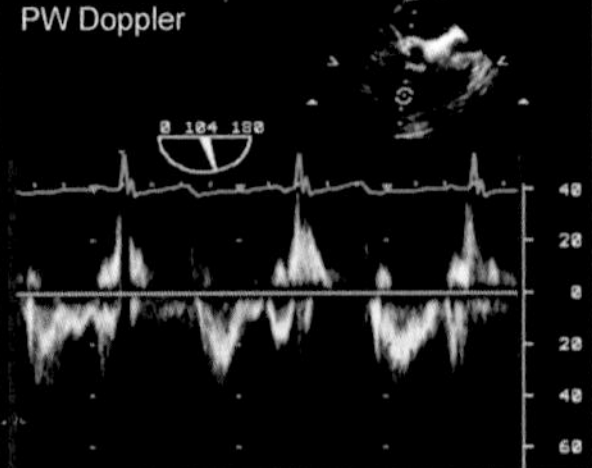

Tricuspid Annular Function and Size

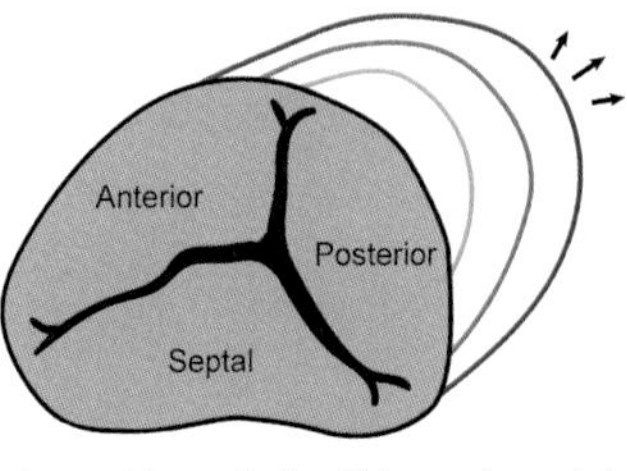

- The TV annulus has a more complex 3D shape than the MV, with peaks in the antero-posterior position and nadirs in the medio-lateral position. The annulus size decreases by 20% during systole. The septal leaflet is anchored by the fibrous trigones making it less mobile. Tricuspid annular descent takes place along the margins of the anterior and posterior leaflets, which move to meet the septal leaflet during diastole. The lateral tricuspid annulus descent towards the RV apex in systole is measured as the Tricuspid Annulus Plane Septal Excursion (TAPSE), an indicator of RV systolic function (see p. 94).
- Tricuspid annular dilation occurs primarily along the antero-lateral annulus at the attachments of the anterior and posterior leaflets to the RV-free wall. The annulus initially maintains a triangular shape, but may become circular from annular dilatation. The annular plane also becomes flatter with functional TR. There is often little correlation with TV annulus size, leaflet malcoaptation, and the amount of TR.

TV Repair Surgery

- TV surgery is indicted in isolation or as part of left-sided valve surgery for primary and secondary TV pathologies. Severe TR requires surgical intervention. Mild to moderate functional TR reduces patient survival.
- TV repair should be considered in patients with mild or moderate functional (2°) TR undergoing left-sided valve surgery if the annulus is dilated (systolic TAD $\geq$40 mm or $\geq$21 mm/m^2), TAFS <25%, right heart failure, or pulmonary hypertension.
- TV repair consists of reducing the TV annulus size (<24 mm) and eliminating TR. This may require insertion of a full or partial annuloplasty band through a right atriotomy. The partial band shown here is placed around the dilated anterior and posterior portion of the annulus. Note the surgical orientation of the TV. Alternatively, a DeVega repair consisting of a suture plication with or without pledgets around the TV annulus is performed.

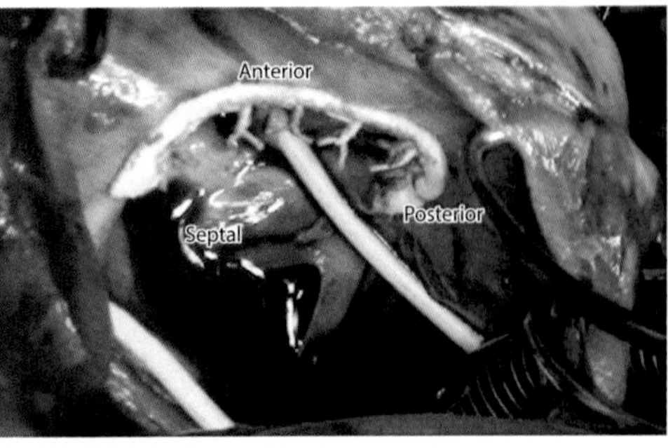

- TV is examined from standard TEE ME 4C, ME RV Inflow-Outflow, ME Bicaval, coronary sinus, TG SAX RV, and TG RV Inflow views.
- Normal TV leaflets are thin and in the far-field, making them difficult to image in most patients. Systematic examination will identify the different leaflets in each view.
- Spectral Doppler alignment is often best in ME RV Inflow-Outflow view (see p. 16) or ME modified Bicaval TV views (see p. 17, 37).

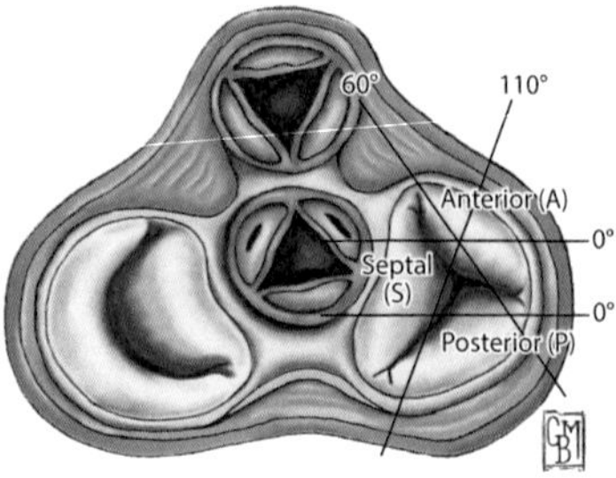

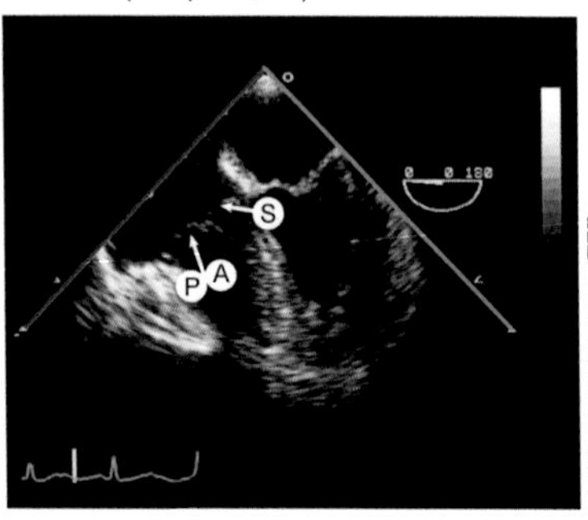

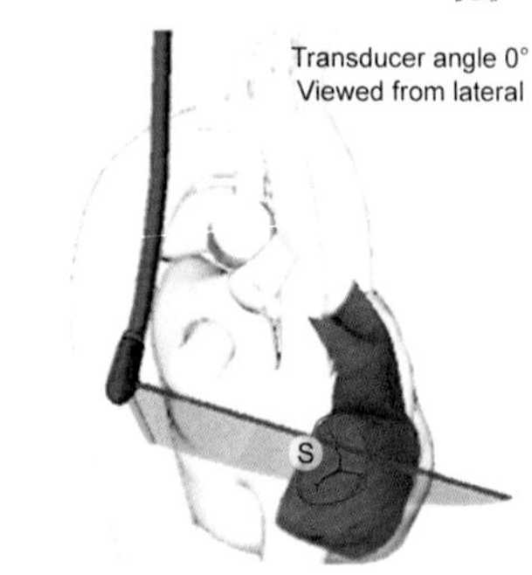

ME 4C View (0°)

This standard view is obtained by positioning the probe to maximize the TV diameter and measure annular dimensions (normal ESD 28 ± 5 mm, EDD 31 ± 5 mm). The TV leaflets seen are the septal (near the IVS) and either the anterior or posterior leaflet depending on the amount of probe tip ante/retroflexion. Color Doppler will demonstrate the presence and direction of TR.

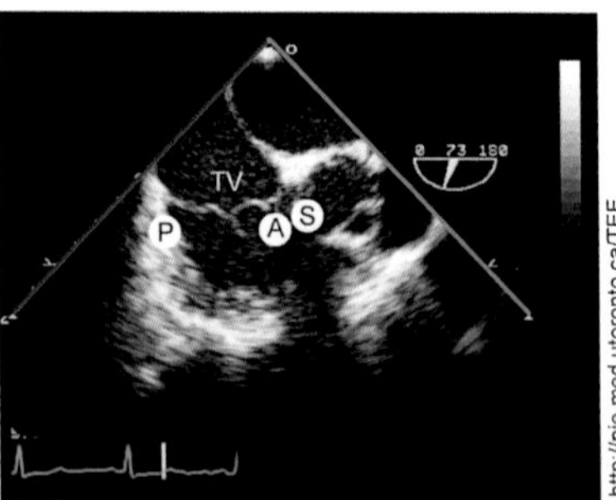

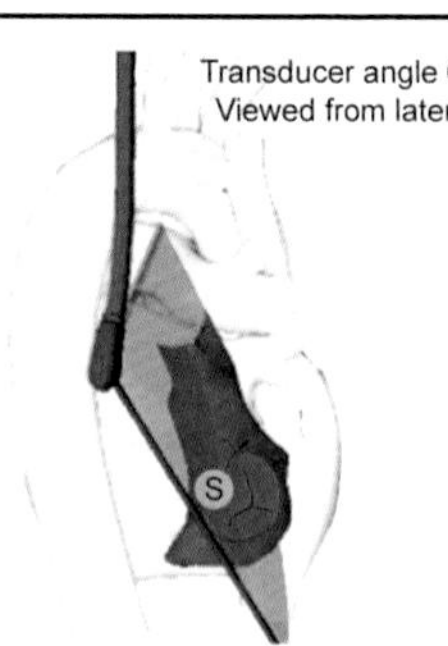

ME RV Inflow-Outflow View (60–75°)

From the ME 4C view, the transducer angle is rotated around the TV to image different leaflets. The posterior leaflet is in the far-field and either the septal or anterior leaflet is near the AV. Color Doppler shows TR, often directed towards the IAS. There is better Doppler alignment for both TV inflow as well as the TR jet.

TEE View	Display Left	Display Right
ME 4C (0°)	A (anteflex), P (retroflex)	Septal
ME RVOT (60°)	Posterior	Septal, Anterior (right turn)
ME bicaval (120°)	Posterior, Septal (anteflex)	Anterior
ME coronary sinus (0°)	Posterior	Septal
TG RV Inflow (90–120°)	Anterior	Posterior

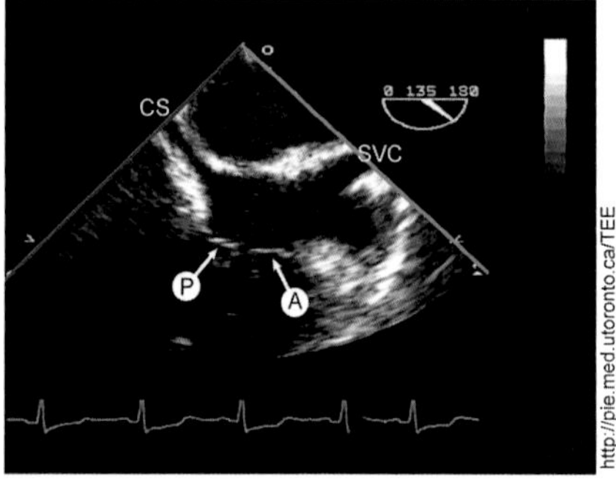

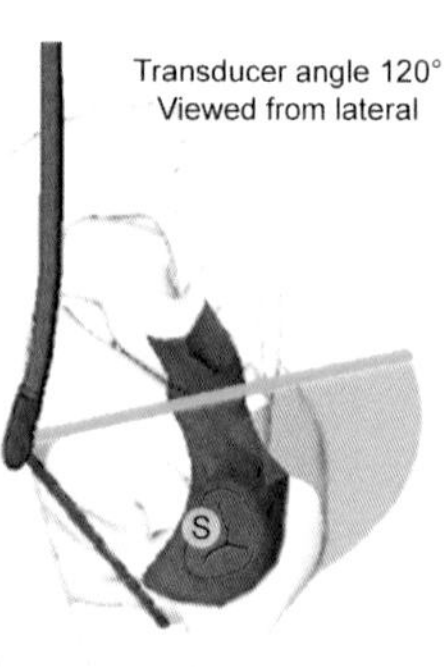

Modified Bicaval View (110–140°)

This view is obtained by increasing the transducer angle to 110–140° from the ME Bicaval view (90°). The TV is centered on the display. The anterior leaflet appears adjacent to the right atrial appendage (RAA) and the other is the posterior leaflet. There is good spectral Doppler alignment for both TV inflow and TR.

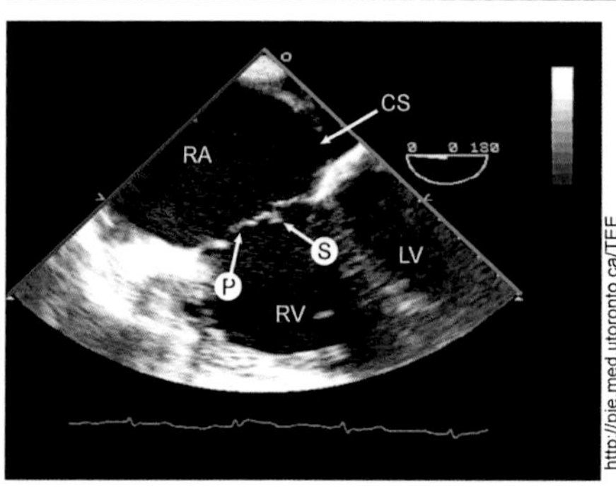

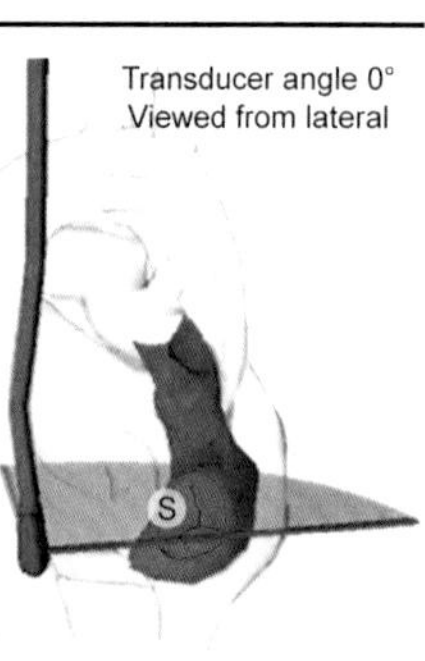

Coronary Sinus (CS) View (0°)

This view is obtained by advancing the probe from the ME 4C view to the GE junction to see inflow from CS into the RA and the TV. The septal leaflet is adjacent to the IVS and the posterior leaflet is seen.

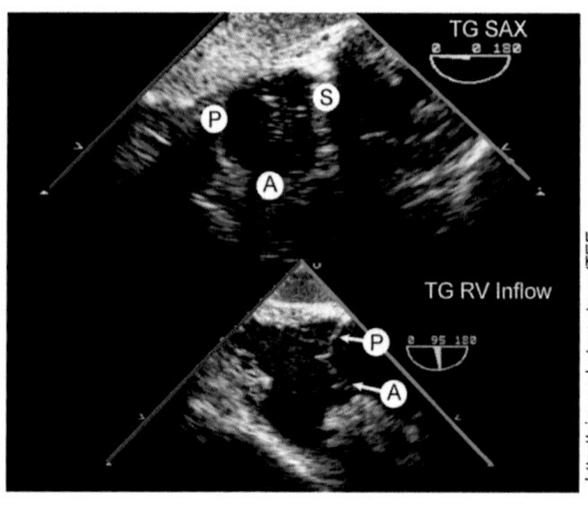

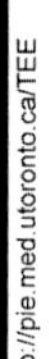

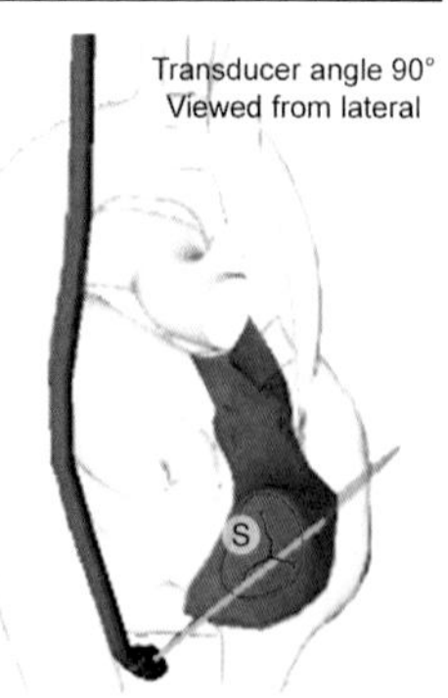

TG SAX View (0–40°)

All three leaflets imaged simultaneously
Poor spectral Doppler alignment

TG RV Inflow View (90–120°)

Subvalvular apparatus, chordae
Poor spectral Doppler alignment

Assessment

1. Etiology of TR is mostly acquired and rarely congenital.
   - Physiological TR is the commonest valve lesion in adults (>90%).
   - Functional TR (2°) may occur from a dilated annulus related to RV dysfunction, left heart disease (MS, MR), high PAP (Eisenmenger's, cor pulmonale).
   - Primary (1°) TR has a structural abnormality of the TV leaflets:
     - Degenerative, myxomatous (25% of patients with myxomatous MV)
     - Rheumatic: thickened leaflets, TR > TS
     - Carcinoid: thickened, shortened immobile leaflets
     - Endocarditis
   - Catheter, pacer
   - Trauma
   - Congenital: Ebstein's anomaly (see p. 250), TV dysplasia
2. 2D findings
   - Leaflets: thickened, calcified, prolapse, malcoaptation, flail
   - Annulus: dilated >34 mm end-systole (normal ESD ≤28 mm, EDD 31 ± 5 mm)
3. Doppler findings
   - Color: turbulent (mosaic) retrograde flow, jet direction is usually toward IAS
     - Laminar (red) retrograde flow if severe RV failure
     - Identify 3 components: area, vena contracta, PISA radius
   - CW: systolic flow towards transducer, peak velocity unrelated to TR severity
   - PW: hepatic vein flow systolic reversal is 80% sensitive
   - PW: TV inflow ↑ E-wave velocity >1 m/s.
4. Associated findings
   - RA, RV, IVC hepatic vein dilated
   - Paradoxical IVS motion (volume overload), IAS bulges to left "D" shape
5. Regurgitation Severity
   - Color map area: for central jet, not sole parameter, invalid with eccentric jets
   - Vena contracta >0.7 cm, EROA ≥0.4 cm^2, Reg Vol ≥45 cc is severe
   - Hepatic vein systolic flow reversal
     - May be absent in chronic TR if RA dilated
     - Unreliable if atrial arrhythmias, v pacing, A-V dissociation
   - IVC > 2 cm, no respiratory variation, normal IVC size if acute TR

Tricuspid Regurgitation Severity (ASE)

		Mild	Moderate	Severe
Qualitative	Jet area (cm^2)[a,b]	<5	5–10	>10
	Flow convergence	Small	Moderate	Large
	CW jet density	Soft, parabolic	Dense, variable shape	Dense, triangular
Semi-quantitative	Jet Area (cm^2)	Not defined	Not defined	>7
	VC width (cm)[a]	<0.3	0.3–0.69	≥0.7
	PISA (cm)[c]	≤0.5	0.6–0.9	>0.9
	Hepatic vein flow	S dominance	S blunting	S reversal
	Tricuspid inflow	A-wave	Variable	E-wave
Quant	EROA (cm^2)	<0.20	0.20–0.39	0.4
	Reg Vol (cc)	<30	30–44	≥45

Nyquist limit: [a](50–70 cm/s), [b]not valid with eccentric jets, [c](28 cm/s); S = systolic
Adapted from: Zoghbi W, et al. J am Soc Echocardiogr 2017;30:303–371

What to Tell the Surgeon Tricuspid Regurgitation

- Leaflet morphology: myxomatous, prolapse, endocarditis
- Annulus size: normal ESD 28 ± 5 mm, EDD 31 ± 5 mm
- TR jets number + direction, severity (color map area/RA area)

PostCPB

- Annulus size
- TR severity
- TV inflow (rule out stenosis)

Grading TR Severity

- (A) Color flow mapping (Nyquist 61 cm/s) of a moderate TR jet appears mosaic in the presence of adequate RV function. Color map area should not be used as the sole criteria to grade TR severity. (B) Color Doppler of severe TR (Nyquist 59 cm/s) may appear laminar with severe RV dysfunction.
- In the hepatic vein view, systolic reversal of hepatic vein flow (HVF) with severe TR is seen (C) as mosaic color using color Doppler (Nyquist 48 cm/s) and (D) PW Doppler S-wave (arrow). Note that HVF reversal can also be seen with atrial arrhythmias and ventricular pacing. In chronic severe TR with a dilated RA, HVF reversal may not be seen.
- The density of the TR spectral trace is an indicator of TR severity (see below). Severe TR is triangular, early peaking, with a density equal to TV inflow.

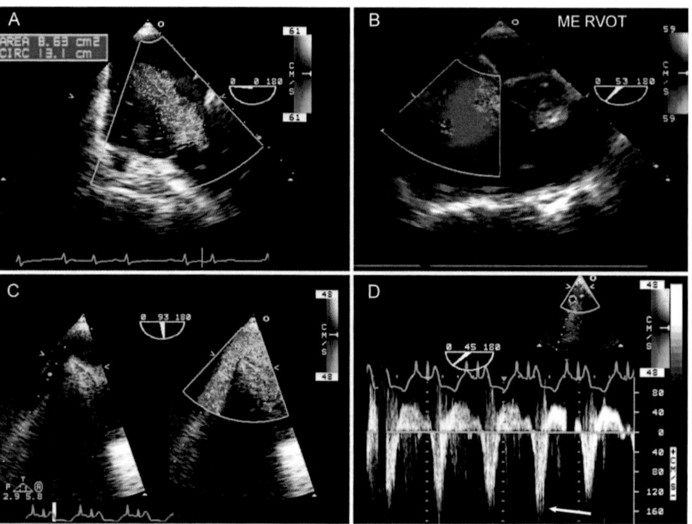

Right Ventricular Systolic Pressure (RVSP)

- Peak TR jet velocity does not reflect TR severity, but rather the peak instantaneous pressure gradient between the RA and RV across a closed TV. This pressure difference when added to right atrial pressure (RAP) estimates RVSP and represents PA systolic pressure (see p. 56).
- Laminar TR jet may underestimate RVSP as RA and RV act as a single chamber.

(A, B) shown here have similarly dense TR spectral Doppler traces, but with different peak velocities. (A) The higher velocity indicates pulmonary hypertension (52 mmHg) compared with (B) normal PASP (23 mmHg).

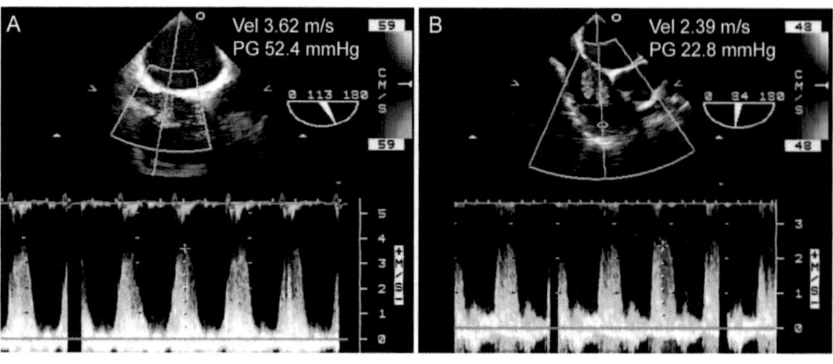

Assessment

1. Etiology of stenosis:
    - Valvular: rheumatic (+mitral), carcinoid (+pulmonic)
    - Obstruction: tumor, vegetation, thrombus, extra-cardiac compression
2. 2D findings:
    - Leaflets: thickened
    - Decreased leaflet mobility, tethered leaflet tips (diastolic doming)
3. Doppler findings:
    - Color: turbulent diastolic flow, may also have TR (systolic flow)
    - CW: HR between 70–80, TV inflow peak E velocity >1.0 m/s
      Mean Pressure gradient
        - Mild <2 mmHg
        - Moderate 2–5 mmHg
        - Severe >5 mmHg
      CW for PHT of TV area (TVA)
5. Associated findings: RA enlarged, IVC dilated (>2.3 cm)
6. Stenosis severity (severe), ASE guidelines*.
    - TV area <1.0 cm^2
    - Peak velocity >1.5 m/s, mean pressure >5 mmHg, VTI >60 cm
    - PHT valve area is not validated (use TVA = 190/PHT), continuity, PISA

***Source: Baumgartner H, et al. J Am Soc Echocardiogr 2009;22:1–23**

(A, B) Turbulent diastolic color flow through the TV with proximal flow acceleration (Nyquist 55 cm/s) and a CW Doppler mean gradient >5 mmHg suggests severe tricuspid stenosis. This occurred in a patient after TV repair.

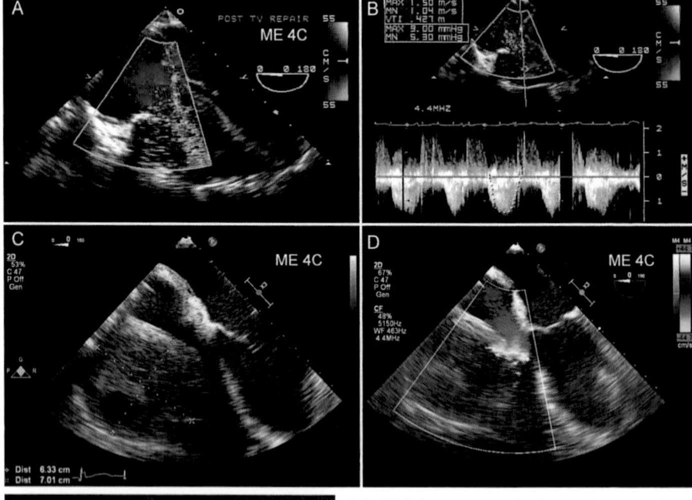

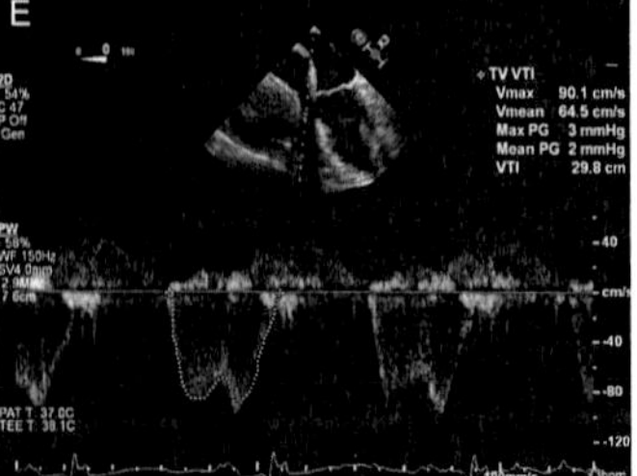

(C, D) These ME 4C views show extrinsic compression of the TV annulus by a large extra-cardiac hematoma, This results in turbulent diastolic color flow through the TV with proximal flow acceleration as shown by color Doppler (Nyquist 44 cm/s).
(E) CW Doppler shows a mean pressure gradient of 2 mmHg, which suggests moderate tricuspid stenosis (TS). Removing the hematoma resolved the functional TS.

Carcinoid heart disease results from serotonin produced by a carcinoid tumor in the intestinal tract or pancreas. Serotonin deposits may form on the right heart endocardium causing valvular dysfunction and RV failure.

TEE Carcinoid
- TV leaflets
  - thickened
  - immobile fixed
- TR >> TS
- Increased mean PG, mild TS
  - E <1.0 m/s
  - Mean gradient 1.0–2.0 mmHg
- PV involvement finding similar to TV
- Endocardial plaques

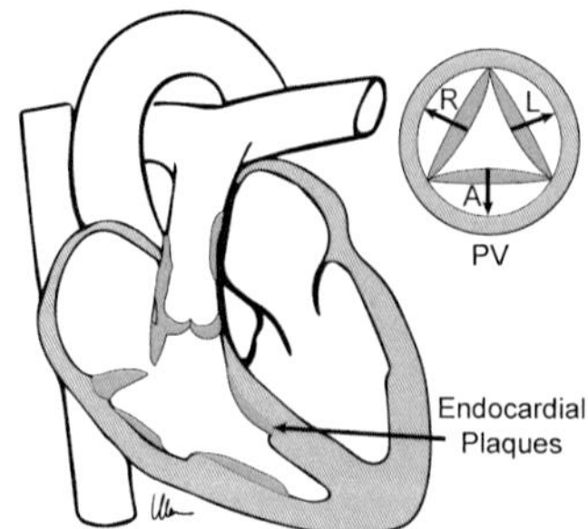

(A) Modified ME 4C view rotated to the right to show the TV during systole. The leaflets appear thickened and immobile with poor central coaptation. Color Doppler (Nyquist 61 cm/s) demonstrates severe TR. (B) The pulmonic valve (PV) is also thickened and dysfunctional. (C) Spectral Doppler shows to and fro flow through the PV suggesting severe pulmonic insufficiency. (D, E) Color Doppler (Nyquist 60 cm/s) shows turbulent flow during systole and diastole in the UE Aortic Arch SAX view.

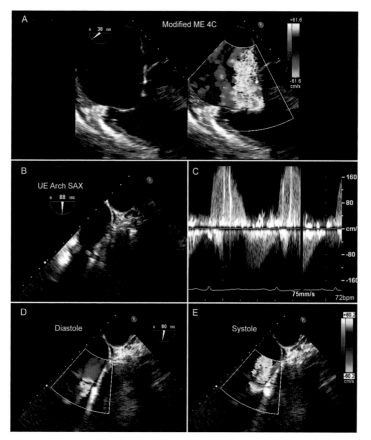

Pulmonary Root Complex

- Similar to the aortic root complex, the pulmonic valve (PV) is part of the pulmonary root complex that connects the right ventricular outflow tract (RVOT) to the pulmonary artery (PA).
- In the normal heart, it lies superior, anterior, and to the left of the AV with an orthogonal (90°) orientation. The cylinder-shaped pulmonary root has 3 major components: (1) pulmonic valve, (2) RVOT infundibulum, (3) pulmonary artery.

Pulmonic Valve

- The normal PV is a semilunar valve with 3 crescent-shaped cusps of equal size.
- The cusps are named in relation to the:
  - Aortic valve: Right (R), Left (L), Anterior (A)
  - Commissure between AV and PV: right facing, left facing, non-facing
- The size of the PV is slightly larger than the AV with a similar design, but thinner cusp body, coapting free edge, and central nodule.

Right Ventricular Outflow Tract

- The PV is enclosed in the cylindrical muscular RV infundibulum that is independent of the IVS and tricuspid valve. There is no fibrous support for the PV.
- The ventricular muscle is in direct continuity with the fibrous sinuses of the PA at the anatomic ventriculo-arterial junction. Individual cusps attach across the anatomic ventriculo-arterial junction to reach the sino-tubular junction (STJ) of the PA and form a coronet-shaped hemodynamic ventriculo-arterial zone.
- Interleaflet triangles are the 3 triangular-shaped areas of the arterial wall proximal to the hinge lines of the PV cusps that are incorporated within the RVOT.
- There is no well-defined PV annulus, though measurement is made at the level of cusp insertion (ESD normal 21 ± 3 mm).

Pulmonary Artery

- The PA dilates slightly forming sinuses of Valsalva defined proximally by the cusp hinge points and distally by the STJ in the PA.
- The STJ is the distal point of insertion of the PV cusps and the zone of apposition between the cusps and the PA wall at the commissures.
- PA dilatation can contribute to PV malcoaptation and pulmonic insufficiency (PI).

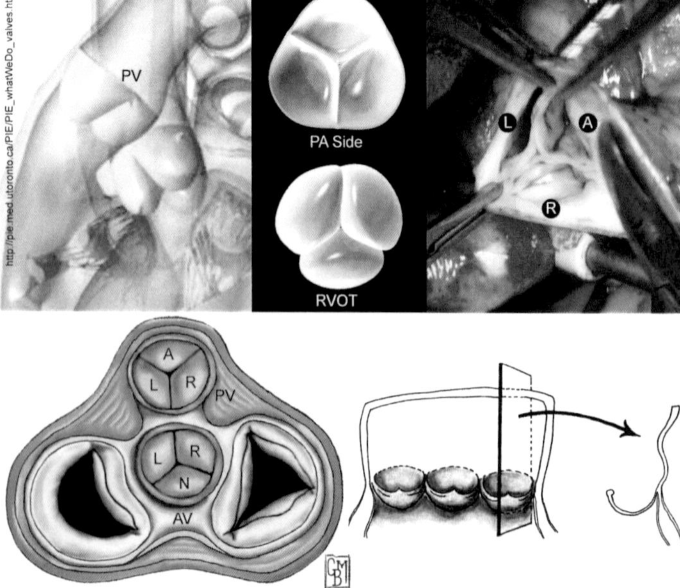

- Morphology and function of the PV are assessed using standard TEE views: ME RV Inflow-Outflow, UE Arch SAX, and modified TG RV Inflow views.
- A normal PV is often difficult to image by TEE and is better imaged using TTE.
- Best spectral Doppler alignment is in the UE Arch and modified TG PV views.
- AV and PV normally lie at 90° planes to each other. ME RVOT view images AV SAX (PV LAX) and ME AV LAX view, (PV SAX) but difficult to see as it is anterior.

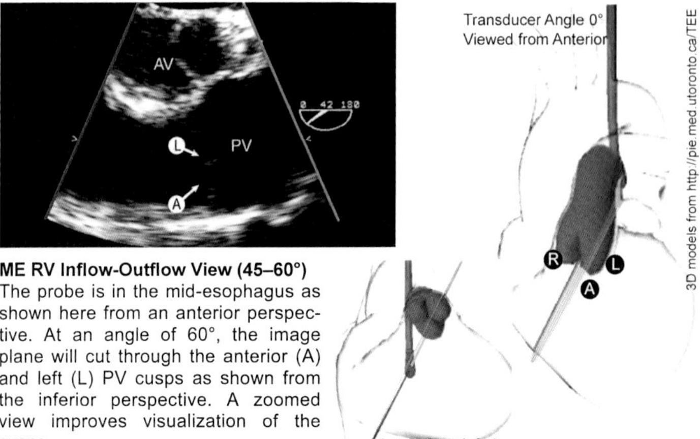

ME RV Inflow-Outflow View (45–60°)
The probe is in the mid-esophagus as shown here from an anterior perspective. At an angle of 60°, the image plane will cut through the anterior (A) and left (L) PV cusps as shown from the inferior perspective. A zoomed view improves visualization of the cusps.

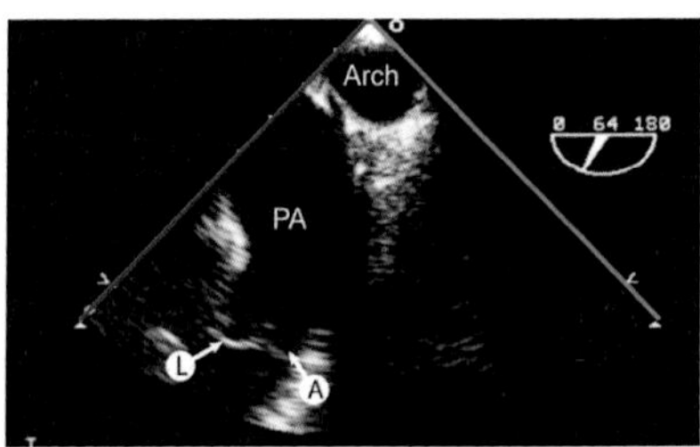

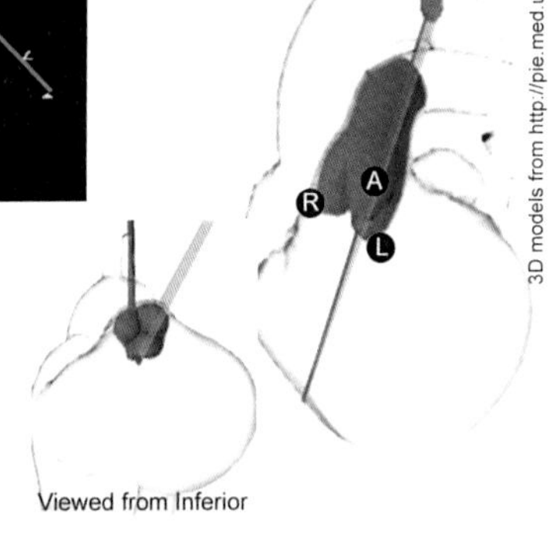

UE Aortic Arch SAX View (60–90°)
The probe is in the upper esophagus as shown here from an anterior perspective. At an angle of 60°, the image plane will cut through the anterior (A) and left (L) PV cusps as shown from the inferior perspective. The cusps are closer to the probe and often better seen.

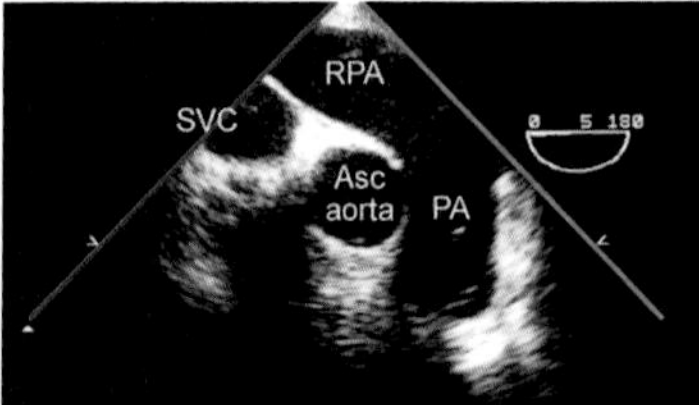

ME Ascending Aortic SAX View (0°)
Useful for Doppler alignment of PA flow
Normal diameter main PA: 20 ± 5 mm

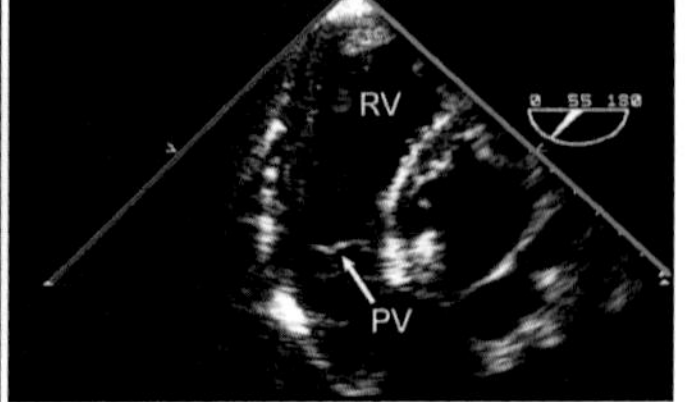

TG RV Modified View (30–60°)
Useful for Doppler alignment
Normal PV peak velocity 0.5–1.0 m/s

Assessment

1. Etiology of insufficiency:
   - Physiologic PI occurs in 80% of patients
   - 1° Valvular: congenital, rheumatic, carcinoid, trauma, endocarditis, prosthetic
   - 2° Dilated PA or RVOT, ↑ PA pressures
2. 2D findings of PV:
   - Difficult to image cusps well using TEE as the PV is an anterior structure
   - Immobile or calcified cusps, dysplastic or absent cusps
   - PV annulus or PA dilated
3. Doppler findings:
   - Color: blue or turbulent diastolic flow in RVOT, may be brief in duration
   - PW/CW: diastolic flow away from baseline
     - Spectral Doppler alignment best in UE or TG views
     - Assess density and deceleration slope
   - PW PV flow: ↑ peak systolic velocity, compare with systemic (AV) flow
4. Associated findings
   - RV dilated and round in shape, leftward displacement of IVS
   - TV annulus dilated, TR
5. Severity of insufficiency is difficult to quantify
   - Mild PI is common, Swan-Ganz only causes mild PI
   - Severe PI: PI jet width/PA annulus 0.7, deceleration time PI trace <260 ms, PHT PI jet <100 ms, prominent flow reversal in main PA by PW

PI Severity (ASE)

	Mild	Moderate	Severe
Morphology	Normal	Normal, abnormal	Abnormal
RV size	Normal	Normal or dilated	Dilated
Jet size[a]	Thin, <10 mm length	Intermediate	Large, wide origin
CW density	Soft	Dense	Dense
PI Index		<0.77	<0.77
PA: Systemic flow	Slight increase	Intermediate	Greatly increased
Reg F (%)[b]	<20	20–40	>40

[a]Nyquist limit (50–60 cm/s)
[b]MRI based, poor with Echo, PI index = duration PI/duration of diastole
Adapted from: Zoghbi W, et al. J Am Soc Echocardiogr 2017;30:303–371

Severe PI has holodiastolic flow reversal in main PA by color Doppler (blue) with equally dense forward and reverse CW Doppler flow in the UE Aortic Arch SAX view.

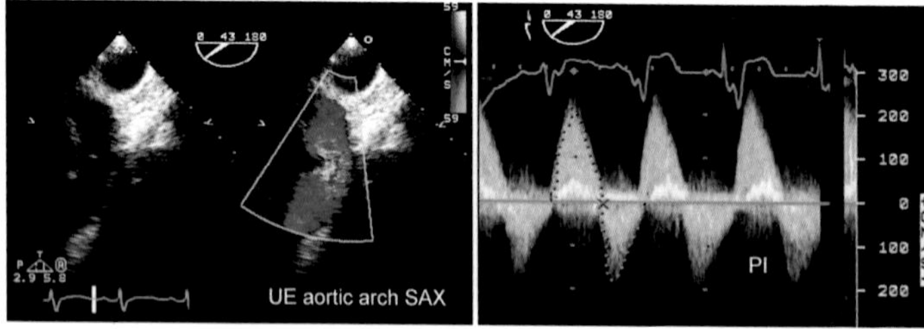

What to Tell the Surgeon Pulmonic Insufficiency

PreCPB

- Valve morphology: calcified, prolapse, endocarditis, prosthetic failure
- PA dilated: >20 mm
- Difficulty to quantify severity, color, and spectral Doppler
- RV size and function
- TV annulus size and TR

PostCPB

- Prosthetic valve function: peak, mean gradients, paravalvular leaks
- Left main coronary artery flow

Assessment

1. Etiology of stenosis:
   - Normal pulmonic valve area 2 cm^2/m^2
   - Valvular: rheumatic, carcinoid, prosthetic
   - Congenital
   - Dynamic: Infundibular (RV hypertrophy)
2. 2D findings:
   - Valve: thickened, calcified, immobile, systolic doming
   - RVOT narrowed in infundibular PS
   - RVH >5 mm thick (pressure overload), RV dilated
   - Post-stenotic PA dilatation (>20 mm)
   - Other congenital lesions
3. Doppler findings:
   - Color: turbulent systolic flow at the level of obstruction, also may have PI
   - PW to locate level of obstruction (valvular, subvalvular)
     - Valvular has early/mid-peak
     - Subvalvular has late peak, dagger shape
   - CW velocity and peak pressure gradients
     - Overestimate gradients if PI
     - Best alignment in UE Aortic SAX or TG views
     - Color Doppler to help align sample cursor
   - PASP does not equal RVSP in the presence of PS
     - PASP = RVSP (from TR + RAP) – PV pressure gradient
4. Stenosis severity (severe by ASE guidelines)
   - Peak velocity >4 m/s
   - Peak gradient >64 mmHg
   - Continuity equation for valve area (<0.5 cm^2)

PS Severity (ASE[a])

	Mild	Moderate	Severe
Velocity (m/s)	<3	3–4	>4
Peak Pressure Gradient (mmHg)	<36	36–64	>64
Valve Area (cm^2)			<0.5

[a]Adapted from: Baumgartner H, et al. J Am Soc Echocardiogr 2009;22:1–23

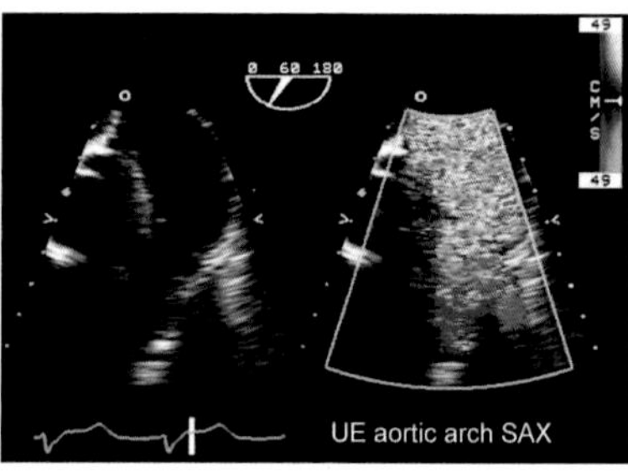

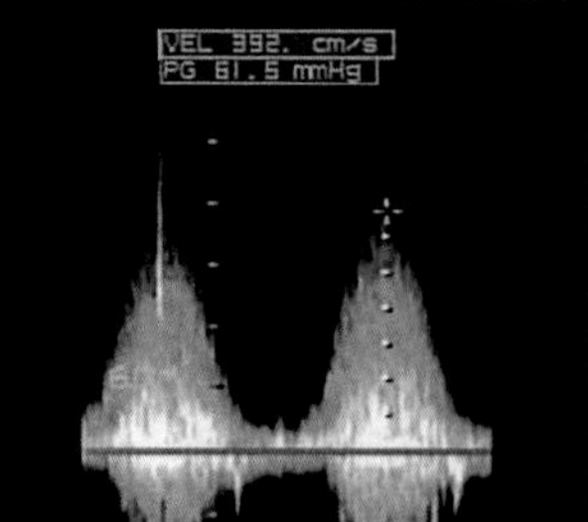

What to Tell the Surgeon Pulmonic Stenosis

PreCPB

- Valve morphology: prosthetic failure, calcified
- Annulus size 21 ± 3 mm (systole)
- Stenosis severity: peak, mean pressure gradients
- Post-stenotic PA dilatation >20 mm
- RV size and function
- Calculate RVSP (see above)

PostCPB

- Prosthetic valve function: peak, mean gradients, paravalvular leaks
- Left main coronary artery flow

8
Prosthetic Valves, Transcatheter Valves and Valve Repairs

A. Vegas, *Perioperative Two-Dimensional Transesophageal Echocardiography*, https://doi.org/10.1007/978-3-319-60902-7_8

- Prosthetic valves can be grouped into 2 broad categories: mechanical (bileaflet, tilting disc, caged ball) or bioprosthetic/tissue (stented, unstented, homografts).
- Percutaneous valves are inserted using a transcatheter system. These valves have a metal frame onto which bovine or porcine pericardium is attached creating 3 leaflets. The valves can be deployed into native valves and prosthetic valves as valve in valve procedures.
- The choice of prosthesis balances the (1) need for anticoagulation, (2) durability, and (3) valve function.
- Despite improving patient survival and quality of life, prosthetic valve implantation is palliative, not curative, as all prosthetic valves have inherent problems. Prosthetic valvular dysfunction may result from structural failure, endocarditis, thrombosis, pannus formation, or technical issues during implantation.
- Surgical implantation involves selecting the correct (1) prosthesis size and height, (2) valve orientation, and (3) insertion level (valvular or supravalvular). Interrupted sutures are used to secure the valve sewing ring to surrounding tissue.
- Intraoperative TEE during prosthetic valve surgery, a SCA/AHA class I indication, determines baseline prosthetic valve function, detects any issues which require immediate reintervention, and monitors cardiac function.

Prosthetic Heart Valves			
Tissue		**Mechanical**	
Stented		**Tilting Disc**	**Bileaflet**
Porcine	**Bovine**	Medtronic Hall	Edwards MIRA
CE S.A.V.	CE PERIMOUNT	Sorin Allcarbon	On-X
Medtronic Hancock	CE Magna	Bjork-Shiley*	Sorin Bicarbon
Medtronic Mosaic	SJM Trifecta		SJM Regent
SJM Epic	Sorin Mitroflow		Sorin Carbomedics
Stentless		**Caged Ball: Starr-Edwards***	
Edwards Prima Plus (porcine) Medtronic Freestyle (porcine) SJM Quattro SJM T-SPV*		*These valves are no longer implanted Valves named after company and product: CE, Carpentier-Edwards; Medtronic; On-X; SJM, St Jude Medical; Sorin	
Homograft: aortic, mitral			

Prosthetic Valve Pressure Gradients (PG)						
Type	Mitral			Aortic[a]		
	Vmax (m/s)	Pmax (mmHg)	Pmean (mmHg)	Vmax (m/s)	Pmax (mmHg)	Pmean (mmHg)
Starr-Edwards	1.9 ± 0.4	14 ± 5	5 ± 2	3.2 ± 0.6	38 ± 11	23 ± 8
St. Jude[a]	1.6 ± 0.3	10 ± 3	4 ± 1	2.4 ± 0.3	25 ± 5	12 ± 6
Bjork-Shiley	1.6 ± 0.3	10 ± 2	3 ± 2	2.5 ± 0.6	23 ± 8	14 ± 5
CE	1.8 ± 0.2	12 ± 3	6 ± 2	2.5 ± 0.5	23 ± 8	14 ± 5
Hancock	1.5 ± 0.3	9 ± 3	4 ± 2	2.4 ± 0.4	23 ± 7	11 ± 2
Stentless	none	none	None	2.2	19	3 ± 1

- [a]PG varies with valve size (aortic position): 19 mm (20 mmHg), 23 mm (12 mmHg)
- Pressure recovery overestimates St Jude AVR gradient
- Valve sizes describe the outer valve diameter, not the internal orifice diameter
- Prosthesis patient mismatch: normal function with high transvalvular gradient (see p. 179)

What to Tell the Surgeon PostCPB Prosthetic Valve

- Valve well-seated
- Leaflets mobile (2D and color Doppler)
- Valvular functional leaks (washing jets, physiologic)
- Paravalvular leaks (color Doppler)
- Peak and mean valve pressure gradients
- Effective orifice area (aortic valve)
- Obstruction LVOT (MV strut), SAM of AMVL (if AV prosthesis is too small)

Mechanical Valves		
Valve Type	Flow Through Valve	Echocardiographic Findings
Starr-Edwards (discontinued 2007) 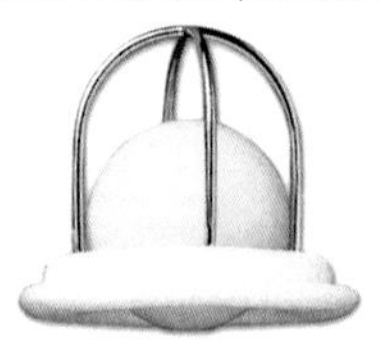	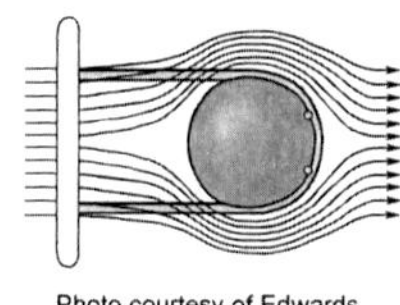 Photo courtesy of Edwards Lifesciences LLC, Irvine, California	**Ball Cage** • Ball larger than orifice • Turbulent antegrade flow through valve periphery • High profile • Small orifice, high pressure • ↑ Thromboembolism risk • Trivial valve regurgitation • No washing jets • Image in LAX to avoid acoustic shadowing
Medtronic-Hall (below), Bjork-Shiley (discontinued) 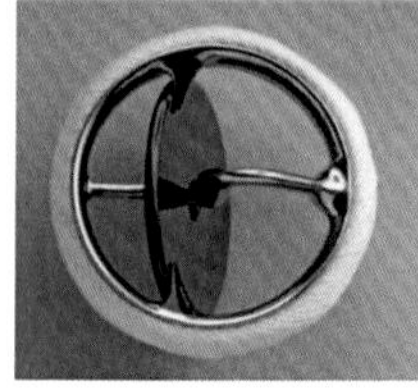	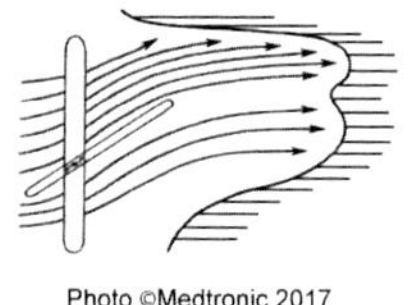 Photo ©Medtronic 2017	**Tilting Disc** • Single disc + eccentric strut/ hinge • Opening angle 60–70° • Back pressure on larger disc portion closes disc • 2 antegrade flow orifices across valve (major, minor) • 3 washing jets large central jet + smaller jets around occluding disc + sewing ring • Acoustic shadowing
St. Jude (below), Carbomedics, On-X 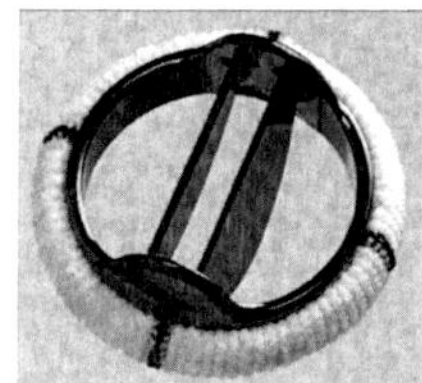	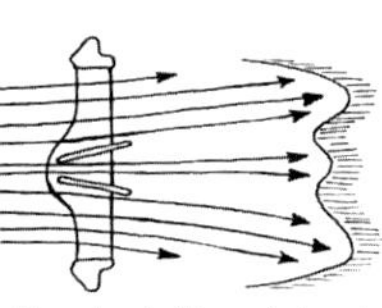 Reproduced with permission of St. Jude Medical, ©2017	**Bileaflet** • 2 symmetrical leaflets + 2 hinges, low profile • Bileaflet pivot motion, opens to 80° • Antegrade flow through 3 orifices • Less obstructive, lowest P • 4 regurgitant washing jets: 2 central + 2 peripheral • Most regurgitant fraction (10%)
St. Jude (below), Medtronic-Hall 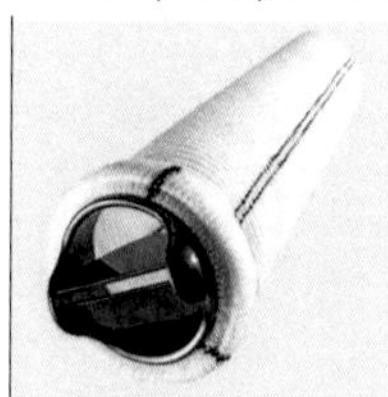	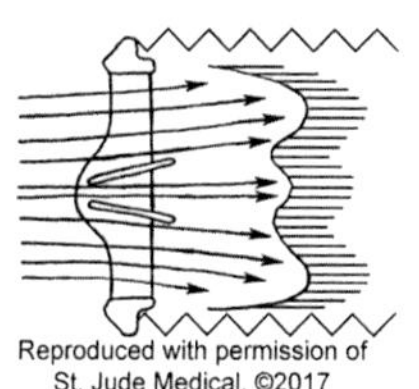 Reproduced with permission of St. Jude Medical, ©2017	**Valved Conduit** • Typically, mechanical valve attached to Dacron conduit • Sewn in as a single unit • Cannot have paravalvular leak, as all leaks would appear outside the heart • Washing jets depend on the valve type

- Mechanical valves have a sewing ring, occluder, and retaining mechanism to maintain occluder position.
- Antegrade flow is across the open valve.
- Retrograde flow across the closing valve has 2 components:
  - Closing volume that pushes the occluder closed
  - Backflow (washing jets) is continuous flow that prevents thrombus formation
- Each mechanical valve type has specific flow patterns

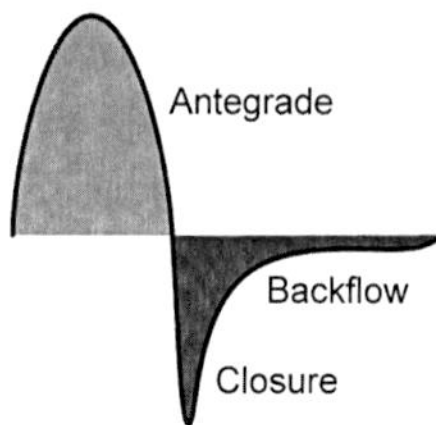

Mechanical Bileaflet

- The valve comprises two symmetric leaflets and two hinges which pivot open.
- Pressure opens both leaflets (80° arc), backpressure closes the leaflets.
- Antegrade flow is through 3 orifices, small central, and outer 2 large orifices.
- Washing jets prevent blood stasis: 3 washing jets: 1 central + 2 peripheral
- Largest closing regurgitant fraction (10%)

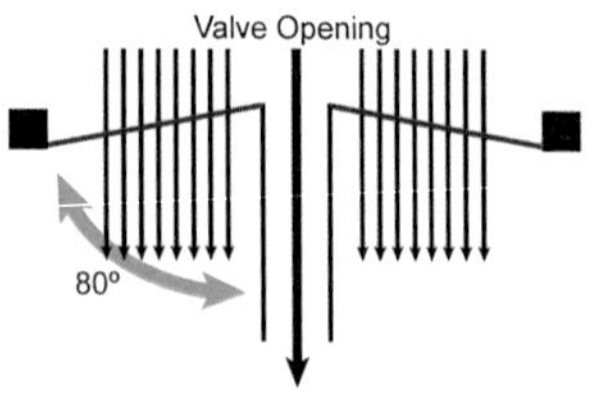

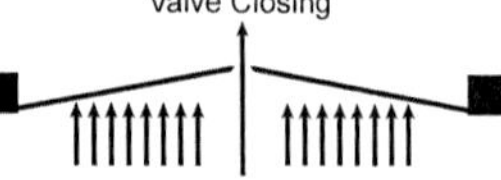

Valve Orientation

- Correct valve orientation of the mechanical valve is important for optimal function and to prevent complications.
- **Mitral Position**: orientate valve to minimize disc entrapment by submitral chordae
  - Anti-anatomic: This is the typical implantation for single disc valves and bileaflet valves with pivot points at 90° to the native MV commissures. The open leaflets are best seen in ME 120° view.
  - Anatomic: Unusual to orientate the pivot points with the native MV commissures. Leaflet opening is best seen in 0° view.
- **Aortic Position**: orientate valve with one pivot between the LCC and RCC to allow for smooth opening of valve discs without obstructing the coronary arteries. Leaflet opening is best seen in the TG views.
- Mechanical valves are seldom implanted in the tricuspid or pulmonic position, as there is insufficient pressure to open and close the valve.

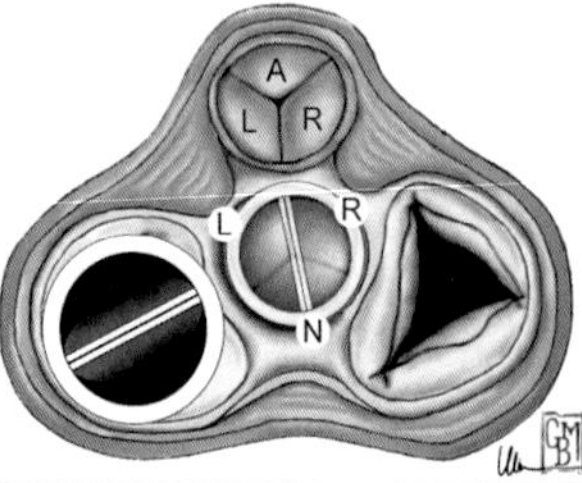

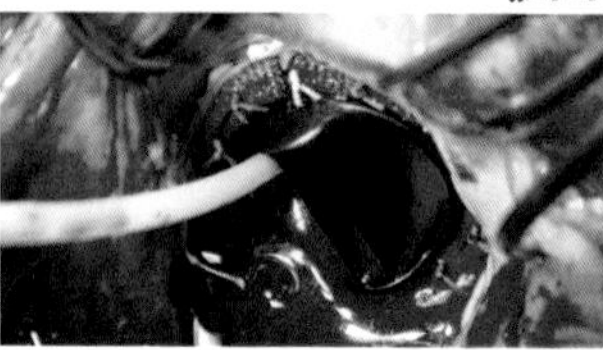
Anti-anatomic

Mitral Position

Mechanical bileaflet valve shown (A) open during diastole with laminar flow and (B) closed (valve inset) during systole with washing jets. The valve is imaged with 3D Live mode (C) open, (D) closed, and with (E) 3D full volume color Doppler, showing washing jets at the hinge points.

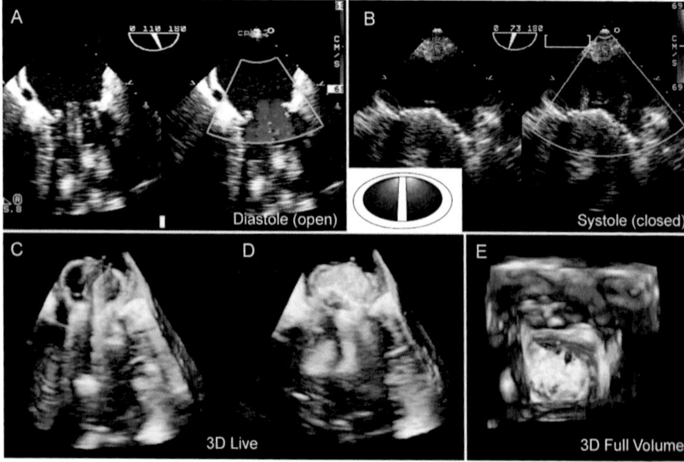

TEE Assessment

- Assessment of the bileaflet mechanical valve immediately after implantation ensures adequate function.
- 2D Imaging
  - Ensure both leaflets open and close fully
  - MVR is easy to assess from any ME view
  - AVR use TG views as shadowing prevents adequate assessment in the ME views
  - Assess valve stability
- Color Doppler
  - Laminar flow through all valve orifices
  - Washing jets inside sewing ring
  - Paravalvular leaks outside the sewing ring (see p. 185)
- Spectral Doppler
  - Use PW or CW to assess valve pressure gradients
  - Measure from the larger orifices to avoid error
  - Calculate EROA or dimensionless valve index (DVI) for AVR

TEE Assessment
Bileaflet Mechanical Valve

- Symmetric leaflet mobility
- 2–3 washing jets
- Laminar flow through valve
- Peak/mean pressure gradients
- EROA, DVI

Aortic Position

Mechanical bileaflet valve shown (A) open during systole with laminar flow (Nyquist 57 cm/s) in the deep TG view. Probe manipulation and angle adjustment may be required to adequately visualize the full movement of both leaflets. (B) Shadowing in the ME views may prevent adequate assessment of leaflet motion.

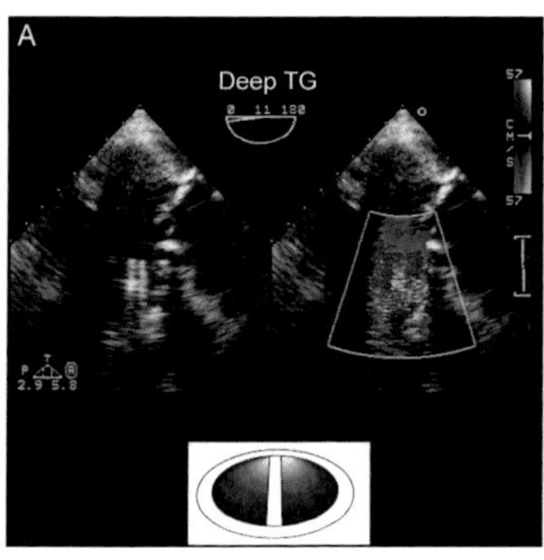

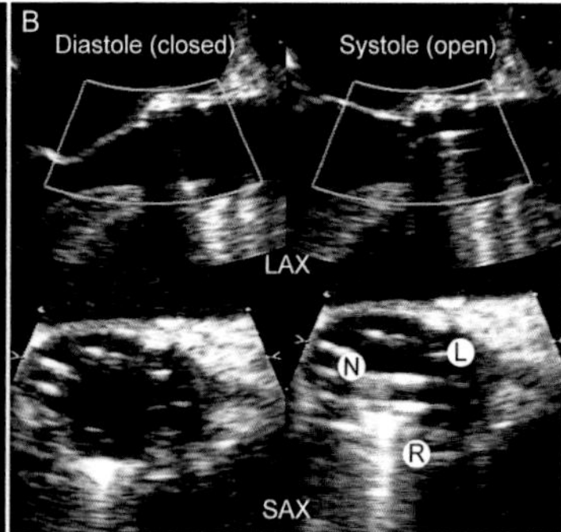

Mechanical Tilting Disc

- Single disc + eccentric strut/hinge
- Opening angle 60–70°
- 2 antegrade orifices (major, minor)
- 2–3 washing jets
  - Medtronic-Hall (diagram below): large central + small peripheral jets
  - Bjork-Shiley (TEE shown): small peripheral jets

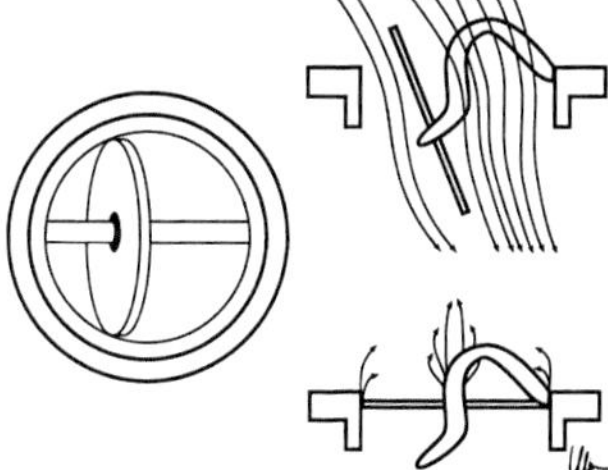

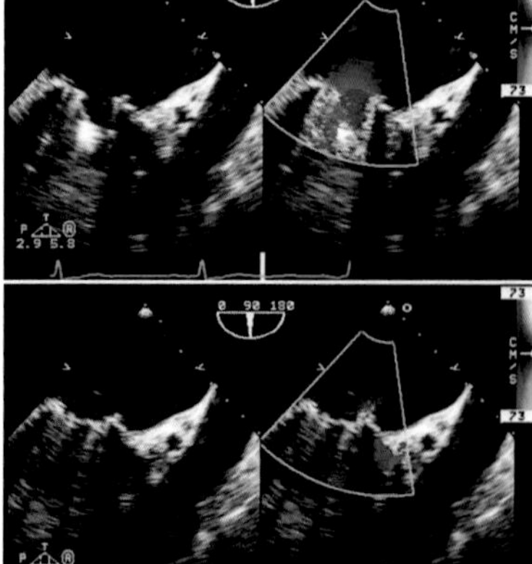

Stented Valve

- 3 stents or struts
- Constructed of bovine pericardium (CE) or porcine heterograft (Hancock)
- 3 leaflets
- Smaller orifice than stentless valve
- Sized to aortic annulus
- Central gap in pericardial valve

Carpentier-Edwards (CE) MagnaEase

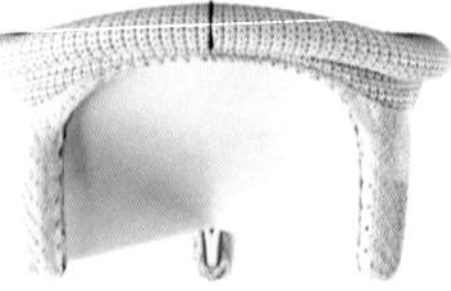

Photo courtesy of Edwards Lifesciences LLC, Irvine, California

Hancock

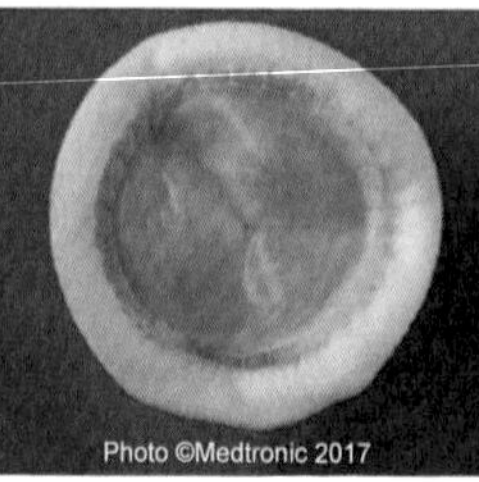

Photo ©Medtronic 2017

The struts of a bioprosthetic valve are positioned to avoid obstruction of structures:

- Mitral: LVOT
- Aortic: coronary ostia

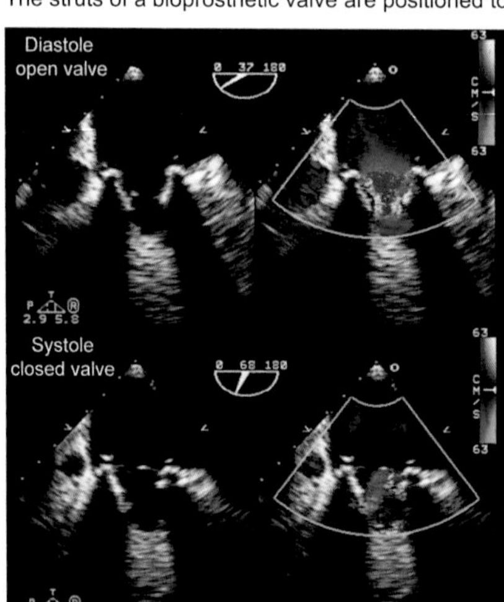

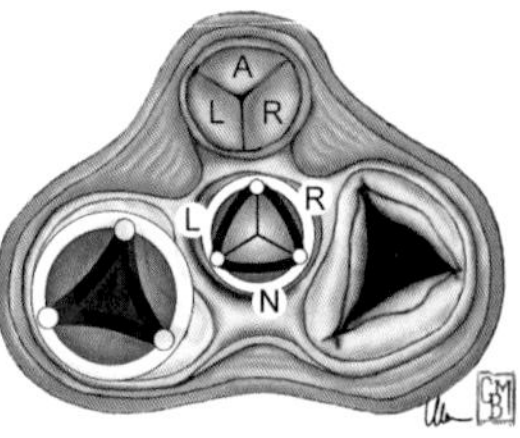

Mitral Position

- Easily image in ME views
- Assess leaflet mobility
- Trace valvular MR
- Peak/mean pressure gradients
- LVOT obstruction by stent
- Paravalvular leaks outside the sewing ring in 2 views

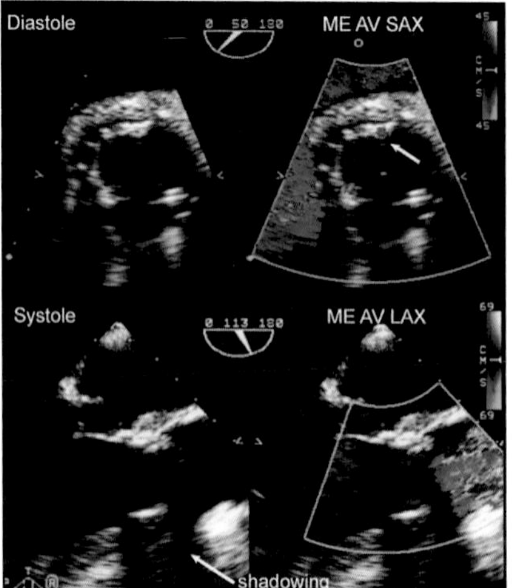

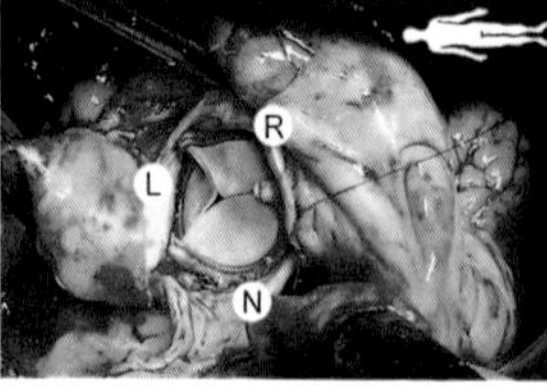

Aortic Position

- Shadow from struts seen in LAX view
- Leaflet mobility, struts (SAX)
- Trace valvular AI central or commissural (SAX arrow)
- Peak/mean pressure gradients CW Doppler in TG views
- Paravalvular leaks outside sewing ring below valve in the LVOT (SAX, LAX)

Stentless Valve
(FreeStyle™)

- No stent
- Porcine aortic heterograft
- 3 leaflets
- Larger orifice than stented valve
- Only implanted in aortic position
- Sized to sinotubular junction

TEE Findings

- Little acoustic shadowing
- 3 leaflets similar to native AV
- Implantation involves valve (SPV) or valve + root (FreeStyle)
- Thickened aortic root
- Trace valvular AI
- Small pressure gradient
- Paravalvular leaks are not possible

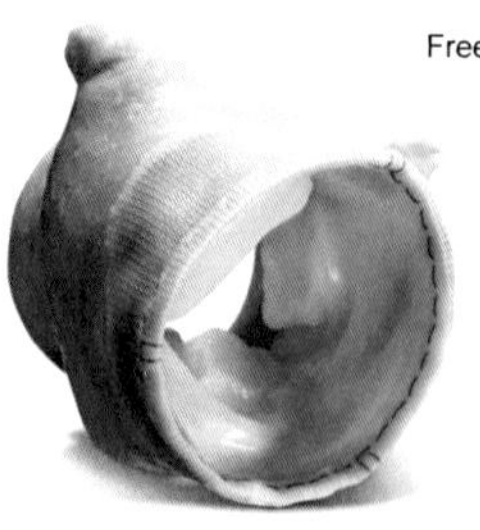
FreeStyle™

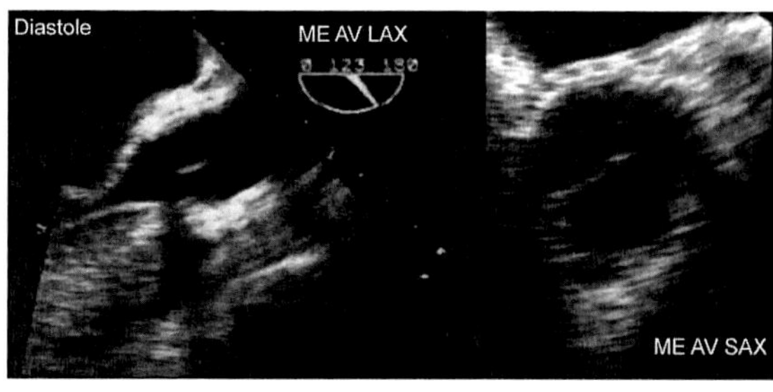

Patient Prosthetic Mismatch (PPM)

- PPM occurs if the prosthesis-effective orifice area (EOA) is too small for the patient's size, resulting in abnormally high transvalvular pressure gradients.
- PPM may be less relevant in obese patients.
- Well studied with AVR (see below) and can occur with MVR:
    - PPM MVR if $\leq$1.2–1.3 cm^2/m^2 occurs in 39-71% of patients
    - suspect if persisting pulmonary hypertension
- When PPM is present after AVR patients have reduced short- and long-term survival, particularly if there is LV dysfunction.
- Avoidance of PPM may necessitate AVR implantation that is:
    - after patch root enlargement
    - in the supra-annular position
    - tilted from the standard intra-valvular position

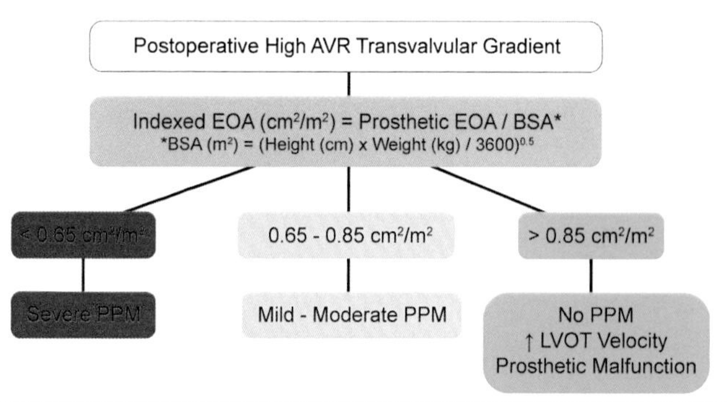

Aortic Valve Prosthesis

1. 2D assess: valve opening and closing, calcification
2. Doppler:
   - Color: laminar (normal), turbulent, regurgitation (valvular, paravalvular)
   - CW Spectral (see below): flow-dependent, avoid being too close to prosthesis
     Normal: triangular, early peaking, short acceleration time (AT) < 80 ms
     Obstructed: rounded, mid-peaking, AT > 100 ms, AT/ET > 0.4
     Differential of high gradient in a normal valve: small size, PPM, increased stroke volume, obstruction
     Can have low gradient despite stenotic valve, if there is poor LV function
   - Flow-independent parameters: EOA and DVI (Dimensionless Valve Index)

$$EOA = \frac{CSA_{LVOT} \quad VTI_{LVOT}}{VTI_{PrAV}} \qquad DVI = \frac{PW\,Peak\,Velocity_{LVOT}}{CW\,Peak\,Velocity_{PrAV}}$$

3. Associated: LV size and function, coronary blood flow

Mechanical and Bioprosthetic AVR Stenosis			
Method	**Normal**	**Possible Stenosis**	**Significant Stenosis**
Peak velocity (m/s)	<3	3–4	>4
Mean gradient (mmHg)	<20	20–35	>35
DVI	≥0.30	0.29–0.25	<0.25
EOA (cm^2)	<1.2	1.2–0.8	<0.8
CW Doppler through valve	Triangular early peak	Triangular to intermediate	Rounded symmetric
Acceleration time (ms)	<80	80–100	>100

Adapted from: Zoghbi WA, et al. J Am Soc Echocardiogr 2009; 22: 975–1014

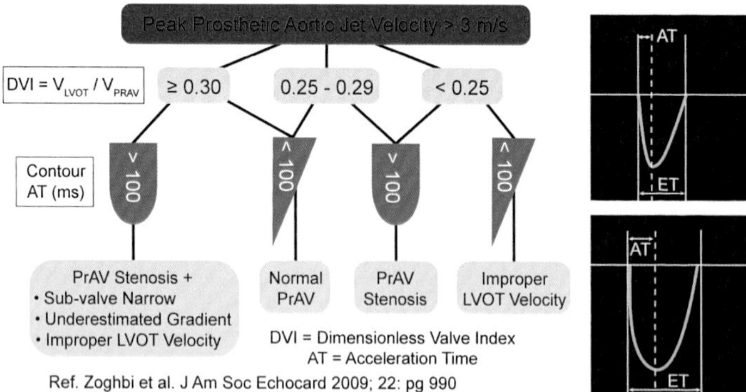

Ref. Zoghbi et al. J Am Soc Echocard 2009; 22: pg 990

Prosthetic Aortic Valve Regurgitation			
Method	**Mild**	**Moderate**	**Severe**
Jet height/ LVOT d[a] (%)	<25	25–64	>65
CW density	Weak "flat top"	↑ Angle on CW	Dense, Steep slope
PHT (ms)	>500	200–500	<200
PW LV Q:pulmonary Q	Slight ↑	Intermediate	Greatly ↑
Desc. aorta reversal	Early mild	Intermediate	Holodiastolic abd
Regurgitant volume (cc)	<30	30–60	>60
Regurgitant fraction (%)	20–30	30–50	>50

[a]Nyquist limit 50–60 cm/s. Q, flow; PHT, pressure half time; PW, pulse wave; CW, continuous wave
Adapted from: Zoghbi WA, et al. J Am Soc Echocardiogr 2009; 22: 975–1014

Mitral Valve Prosthesis

- Peak velocity and mean pressure gradient are flow-dependent, increasing with: hyperdynamic state, tachycardia, small valve size, valve stenosis, or regurgitation
- VTI is less dependent on HR
- Effective orifice area (EOA):
  - Assess by continuity and not pressure half time (PHT)
  - Bioprosthetic and tilting disc valves

$$EOA_{PrMv} = \frac{\text{Stroke Volume}}{VTI_{PrMV}} = \frac{CSA_{LVOT} \times VTI_{LVOT}}{VTI_{PrMV}}$$

- Pressure half time (PHT):
  - Dependent on loading conditions and AI
  - Not valid with tachycardia, first degree AV block
  - Not valid immediately post-implantation

Mechanical and Bioprosthetic MVR Stenosis			
Method	Normal	Possible Stenosis	Significant Stenosis
Peak velocity (m/s)	<1.9	1.9–2.5	>2.5
Mean gradient (mmHg)	≤5	6–10	>10
VTI_{MV}/VTI_{LVOT}	<2.2	2.2–2.5	>2.5
EOA (cm^2)	>2.0	1.0–2.0	<1.0
PHT (ms)	<130	130–200	>200

- MR results in hyperdynamic LV with reduced LV systemic output
- CW regurgitation jet with early maximum velocity
- Paravalvular leak is outside the sewing ring, identify origin, eccentric direction

Mechanical MVR TTE Findings of Prosthetic MR with Normal PHT			
Method	Normal	Sensitivity	Specificity
Peak E velocity (m/s)	≥1.9	90%	89%
VTI PrMV/VTI LVOT	≥2.5	89%	91%
Mean gradient (mmHg)	>5.0	90%	70%
TR jet velocity (>3 m/s)	>3.0	80%	71%
LV stroke volume	>30%	Moderate	Specific
Flow convergence	Present	Low	Specific

Tricuspid Valve Prosthesis

1. 2D assess: valve opening and closing
2. Doppler: inspiratory variation so average over 5 cycles, (* increased with TR)
   - Peak velocity*: >1.7 m/s
   - Mean gradient*:≥6 mmHg
   - PHT ≥ 230 ms
   - EOA and V_{PrAV}/V_{LVOT} not validated
3. Associated findings: RV size and function, RA size, IVC size with respiratory variation, hepatic vein flow

Pulmonic Valve Prosthesis

1. 2D assess: cusp thickening and mobility
2. Doppler findings of stenosis:
   - Color: turbulent antegrade flow
   - Peak velocity/mean gradient
     Homograft: >2.5 m/s, >15 mmHg
     Bioprosthetic: >3.2 m/s, >20 mmHg
   - Elevated RVSP
3. Pulmonic Insufficiency (PI) assessment similar to native valve (see p. 170)
   - Color: broad base retrograde jet
   - CW: dense, mid to late peaking, to and fro = sine wave

- Immediate intraoperative TEE assessment after implantation of a prosthetic valve includes the evaluation of valve function, ventricular function, and excluding any associated complications.
- This involves the use of multiple TEE views (ME and TG), color, and spectral Doppler.
- Epicardial echocardiography may be required to assess coronary blood flow.
- Late prosthetic valve dysfunction may occur years after implantation and is often a result of wear and tear on the valve.

Prosthetic Valve TEE
Prosthetic Valve
Stability
Flow color Doppler
Regurgitation: valve, paravalve
Pressure gradients
Other Findings
Injury coronary arteries/sinus
New WMA/LV + RV function
Aortic root hematoma
AV groove separation

Prosthetic Valve Dysfunction			
	Early	**Late**	**Findings**
Stenosis	Stuck leaflet PPM Pressure recovery High cardiac output LVOT obstruction	Pannus Calcification Thrombus PPM	Turbulent color ↑ Pressure gradient Calculate EOA Valve motion Calcification
Regurgitation	Suture Stuck leaflet Paravalvular	Degeneration Paravalvular Hemolysis	Color Doppler ↑ Pressure gradient Valvular or paravalve
Mass	Suture	Thrombus Vegetation	Mobile mass
Valve bed	Hematoma Sutures	Dehiscence Abscess Fistula Pseudoaneurysm	Thick bed Abnormal color flow

Valve Regurgitation

(A) ME view shows late mechanical MVR dehiscence (arrow) with severe paravalvular MR. The valve has an abnormal rocking motion independent of the surrounding tissue. (B) ME AV LAX view shows a newly implanted MV bioprosthesis with moderate valvular MR from leaflet suture. (C) ME AV LAX view of an infected bioprosthetic MV with leaflet vegetation (arrow) and severe valvular MR.

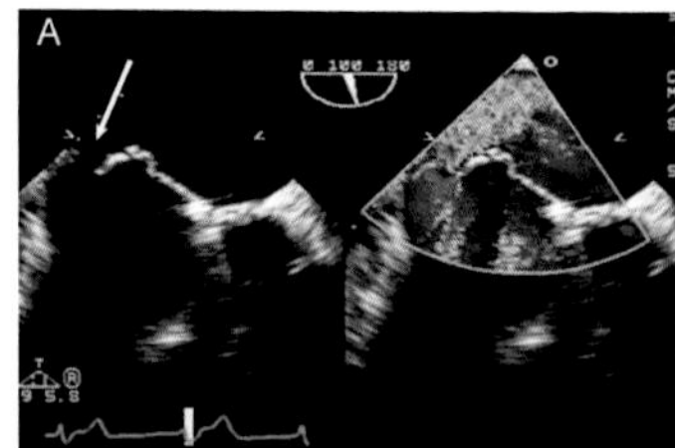

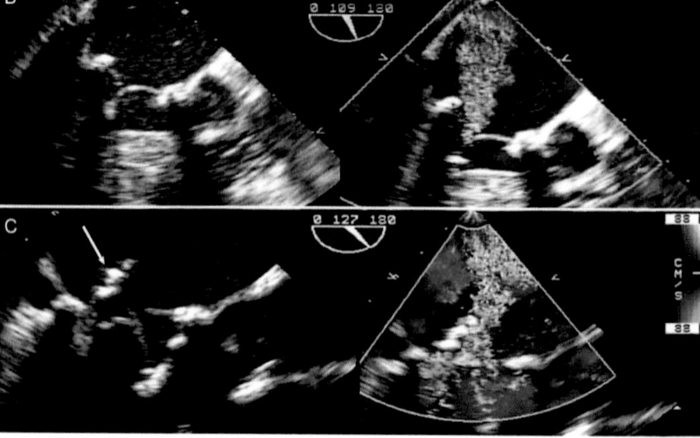

Stuck Leaflet

- Bileaflet or tilting disc valves
- Caused by: subvalvular apparatus, sutures
- Identified by:
  - Immobile leaflet: stuck open, closed, or in between,
  - Check in multiple views
  - Turbulent or no flow through valve
  - Partially open has regurgitation
- Treatment:
  - Remove debris, suture
  - Rotate valve

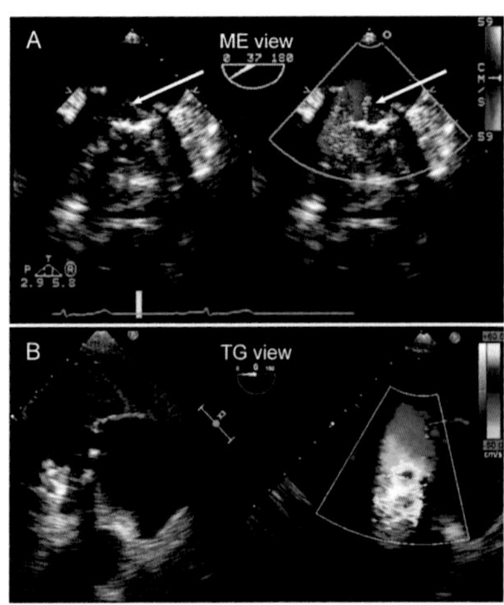

(A) ME view showing mechanical MVR (St Jude) with partially stuck leaflet (arrow) without diastolic color flow. (B) TG view of a mechanical AVR (St Jude) showing stuck leaflet with systolic flow acceleration through the valve orifice by color Doppler.

Hematoma

- Blood or edema (arrow) may collect around the suture line during valve insertion.
- This typically resolves in days. This early finding is important to document; should the patient become febrile, it should not be confused with an abscess.

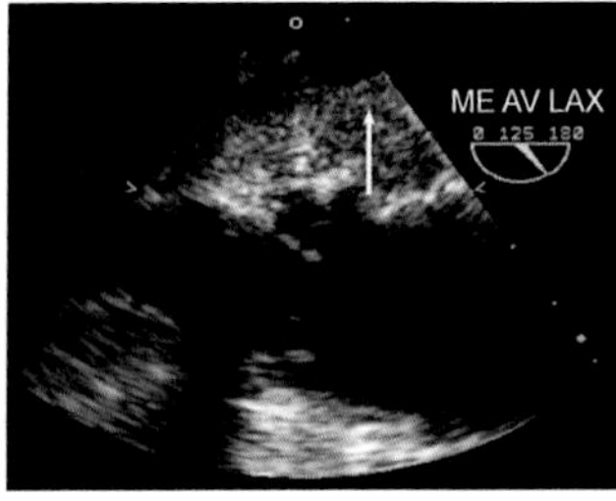

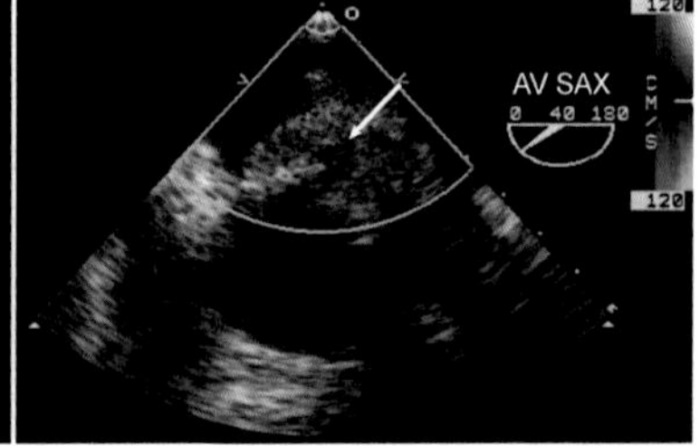

Atrioventricular Groove Separation

- This involves disruption of the mitral annulus from the LV results in flow outside the heart. This is evident by profuse bleeding in the surgical field.
- The ME 4C view shows systolic flow (green) outside of the heart as seen during mechanical MVR implantation.
- Treatment includes removing the prosthesis and patch repair to restore continuity.

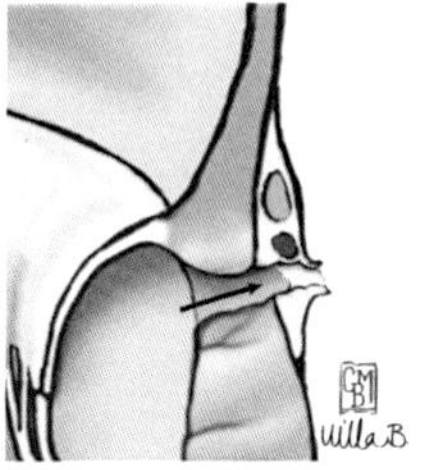

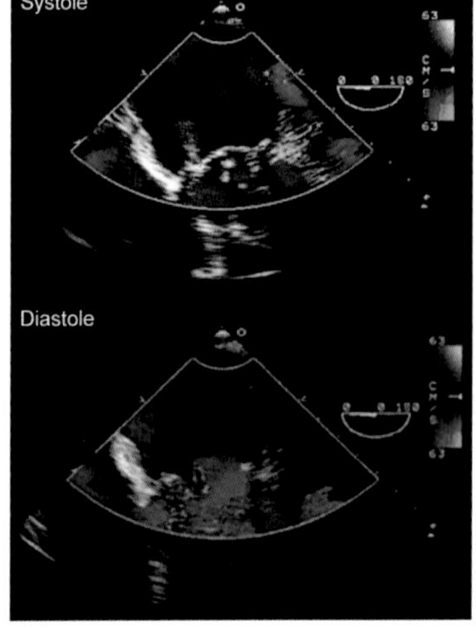

Mechanical Bileaflet

- Washing jets are normal regurgitant jets that originate from the hinge points or between the leaflets and valve stent. A mechanical bileaflet valve has 4 washing jets which appear within the sewing ring.
- When the imaging plane shows both leaflets opening and closing, 4 diverging jets are seen and when it is parallel to the closed disc, 2 converging jets are seen.

(A) MVR in ME LAX view shows one of the discs and converging jets. (B) MVR in a commissural view shows 4 washing jets. (C) AVR in ME AV LAX view shows converging washing jets and (D) in SAX, 2 of 4 washing jets are seen.

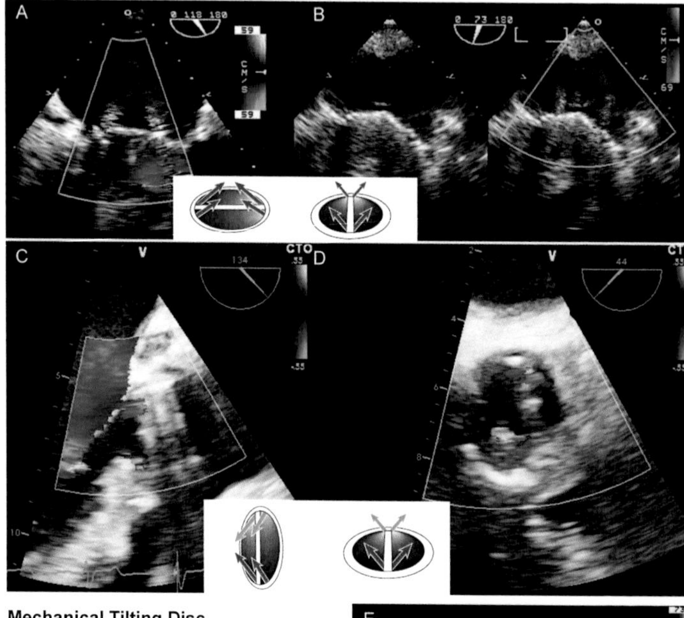

Mechanical Tilting Disc

- 2–3 washing jets
- Medtronic-Hall (diagram below): large central + small peripheral jets
- Bjork-Shiley (TEE shown in E): small peripheral jets

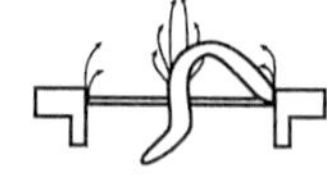

E

Paravalvular Leak

- Incomplete seal between sewing ring / annulus
- Incidence: AVR (1–17%), MVR (up to 30%)
- Risk factors: annular calcium
- Difficult to quantify regurgitation, as an eccentric jet
- Trivial leaks common, resolve after protamine
- If uncorrected, may cause hemolysis, dehiscence

TEE Findings Paravalve
Differentiate washing jets
Outside sewing ring
Eccentric
Difficult to quantify
Multiple views

Washing (Regurgitant) Jets	Paravalvular Leaks
• Inside sewing ring • Short duration • Pattern depends on prosthesis	• Outside sewing rings • Longer duration • Eccentric • Flow acceleration

Paravalvular Leak Location

The location of the paravalvular leak can be identified using TEE.

Mitral Valve

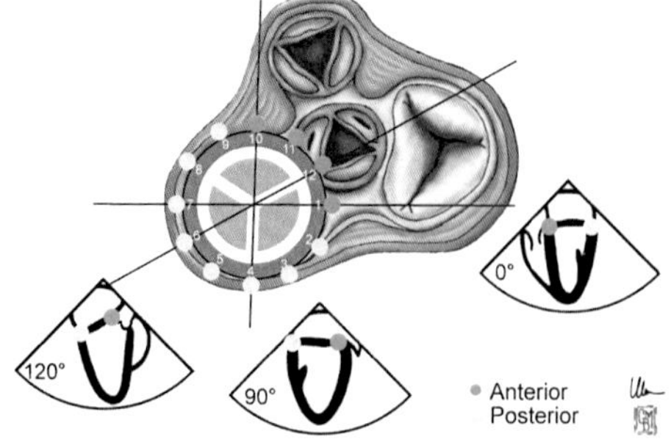

- MV paravalvular leak is easily identified by scanning the prosthetic valve using color Doppler (Nyquist 50–60 cm/s) through 180° in multiple ME views from ME 4C to ME LAX.
- Based on the findings in different views, the leak size and location are identified.
- These leaks can be described to the surgeon in relation to a clock face in the MV en-face orientation with 12 o'clock in the middle of A2.

Aortic Valve

- AV paravalvular leaks are more difficult to identify from the ME views (LAX, SAX) alone and often require the use of TG views.
- The leak can also be related to a clock face (as described below), the sinuses (Non, Right, or Left), the stents, or the coronary arteries.

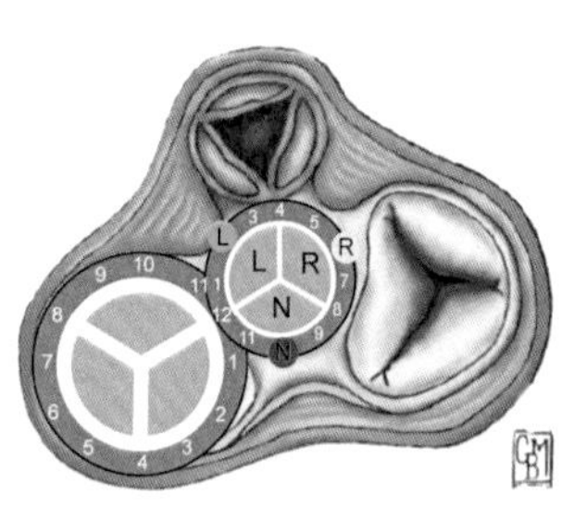

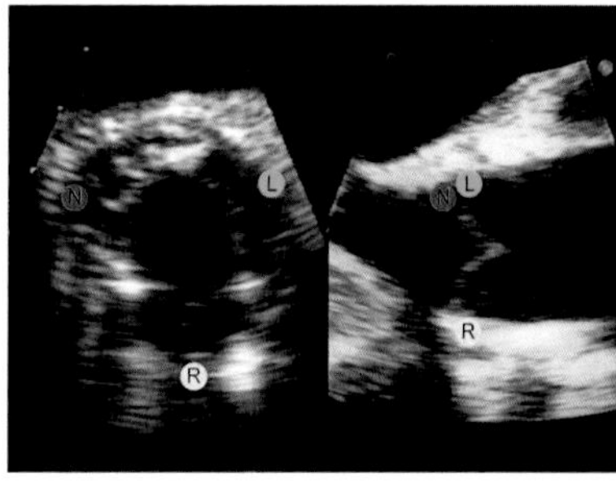

(A, B) Mechanical bileaflet AVR in the ME AV LAX and SAX views showing (A) a posterior paravalvular leak (11 o'clock) and (B) an anterior (8 o'clock) paravalvular leak. (C) Mechanical MVR with paravalvular leak at 145° (near the P2 region, 8 o'clock). (D) Tissue MVR with small anterior paravalvular leak (at 6 o'clock).

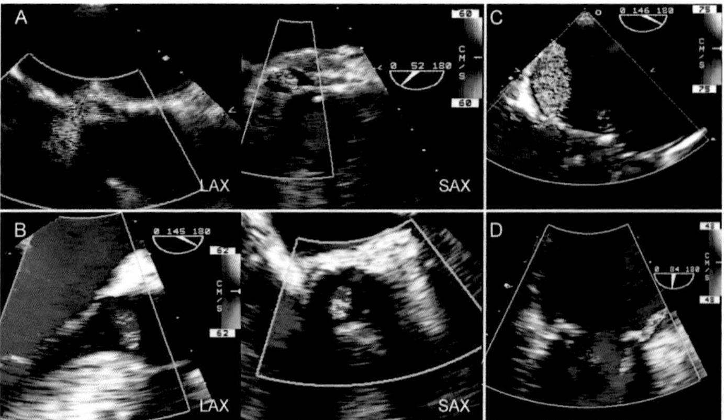

- There are 2 commercial systems used for transcatheter aortic valve implantation (TAVI). (A) Edwards SAPIEN XT™ or SAPIEN 3™ Transcatheter Heart Valve (THV) made from bovine pericardium is externally mounted and deployed during inflation of a balloon catheter. (B) Medtronic CoreValve® made from porcine pericardium is internally contained and self-deploys during catheter withdrawal.
- The TAVI procedure involves placement of a catheter-mounted valve delivered either retrograde through a trans-femoral approach or antegrade through a transapical or trans-aortic approach (only for the THV). The valve is carefully positioned across the native AV, using fluoroscopy and/or TEE guidance.

A

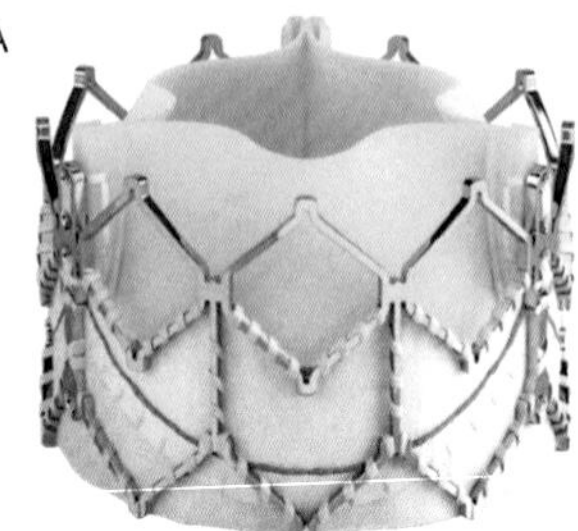

Photo courtesy of Edwards Lifesciences LLC, Irvine, California

B

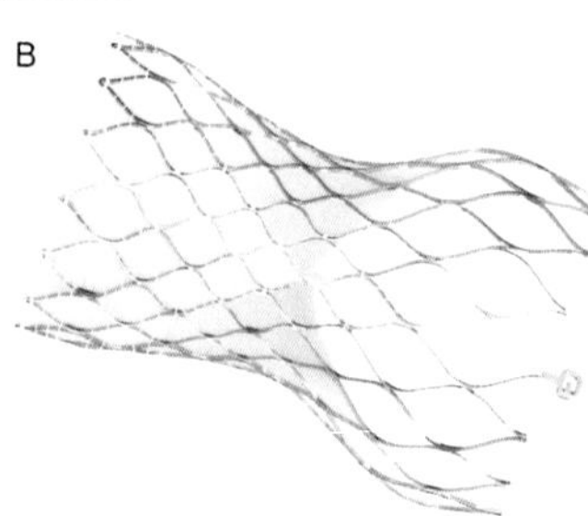

Photo ©Medtronic 2017

Valve Size	20	23	26	29	31
(all measurements in mm)	SAPIEN SXT™				
Annulus Bicuspid AV	16–18	18–21 23	22–24 23–25	25–27 25	–
Valve height	13.5	14.3	17.2	19.1	–
Distance coronaries		10	10	11	–
	CoreValve®				
Annulus Bicuspid AV	–	17–19 20	19–22 20–23	22–26 23–26	25–28 26
Valve height	–	45	55	53	52
Sinus width	–	25	27	29	29
Ascending aorta	–	≤34	≤40	≤43	≤43
Source: Hahn R, et al. J Am Coll Cardiol Imag 2015;8:261–87					

TEE for TAVI

- TEE is used during TAVI procedures when the patient has a general anesthetic. For patients receiving only sedation, TTE is performed before and after the procedure, with fluoroscopy used to position the valve.
- TEE has an important role pre-, during, and post-deployment of the valve.
- Currently, the valve size is often chosen based on annulus dimensions obtained by CT. 2D TEE is less reliable than 3D TEE to measure AV and root dimensions.
- Complications may be life threatening and can be promptly identified using TEE.

TEE TAVI		
Pre-deployment	**Deployment**	**Post-deployment**

Assess AV morphology
  Calcium (2D + 3D)
  Mobility (LAX, SAX)
  Annulus size
RV/LV function
Mitral valve (MR)
LVOT/Root morphology
Coronary ostia
Atheromatous disease
	Position wires
	Post-balloon AI
	Valve position
		Valve function
		  Stability
		  Color Doppler
		  Pressure gradient
		  DVI
		Paravalvular leak
		LV function
		MR
		Complications

AI, aortic insufficiency; MR, mitral regurgitation; DVI, dimensionless valve index **Source: Klein A, et al. Anesth Analg 2014;119:784–98**		

(A) 3D TEE is more accurate for measuring the aortic annulus diameter using multiplanar reconstruction by aligning the short and long axes of the AV. The distance of the coronary ostia from the aortic annulus can also be measured. The average 3D annulus diameter of the LAX and coronal planes in this example is 22 mm. (B) Compare this with the measurement of 19 mm obtained by 2D imaging in the ME AV LAX view. Ideally, the non/left coronary cusp should not be seen in this view as the maximum diameter is in the commissure. (C) The stenotic native AV is first dilated by balloon valvuloplasty as shown in ME AV 3D Live views. This may lead to significant aortic insufficiency. (D) The catheter with the undeployed Edwards SAPIEN THV is positioned with one-half to two thirds of the prosthetic valve in the LVOT. During deployment, the THV moves forward slightly, so the final prosthetic valve position is at the mid-point of the native aortic valve annulus. (E) The balloon is inflated during a period of rapid ventricular pacing to prevent valve embolization with deployment.

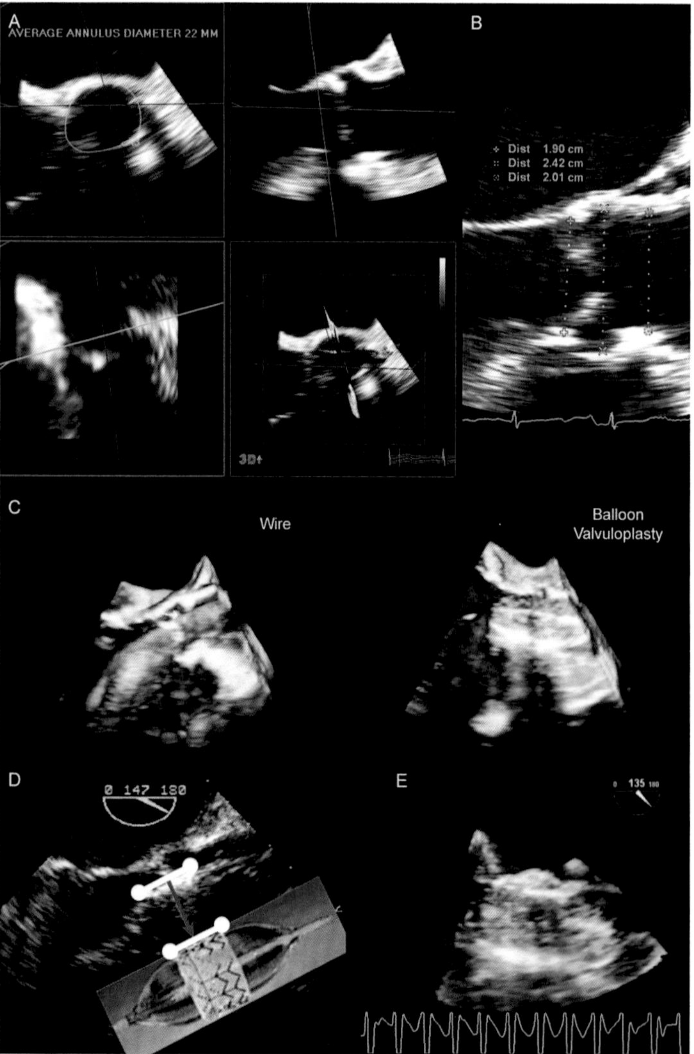

Post-valve deployment TEE assessment includes:

- Confirmation of adequate valve position and stability.
  - High valve position may obstruct the coronaries.
  - Low valve position may impair MV function.
- Leaflet motion and flow through the valve are assessed using color Doppler from ME views and spectral Doppler from TG views.
- The presence of a paravalvular leak is common.

TEE Post TAVI
Location
Stability
Leaflet motion
Flow color Doppler
Pressure gradient
Calculate DVI
Paravalvular leak

(A, B) Systemic valve embolization to the mid-aortic arch occurred during valve deployment seen with (A) fluoroscopy and (B) UE Aortic Arch LAX view. (C, D) Paravalvular leak of an Edwards SAPIEN™ THV in (C) ME AV SAX and (D) LAX views. (E, F) CoreValve® in (E) TG and (F) posterior paravalvular leak in ME AV LAX views.

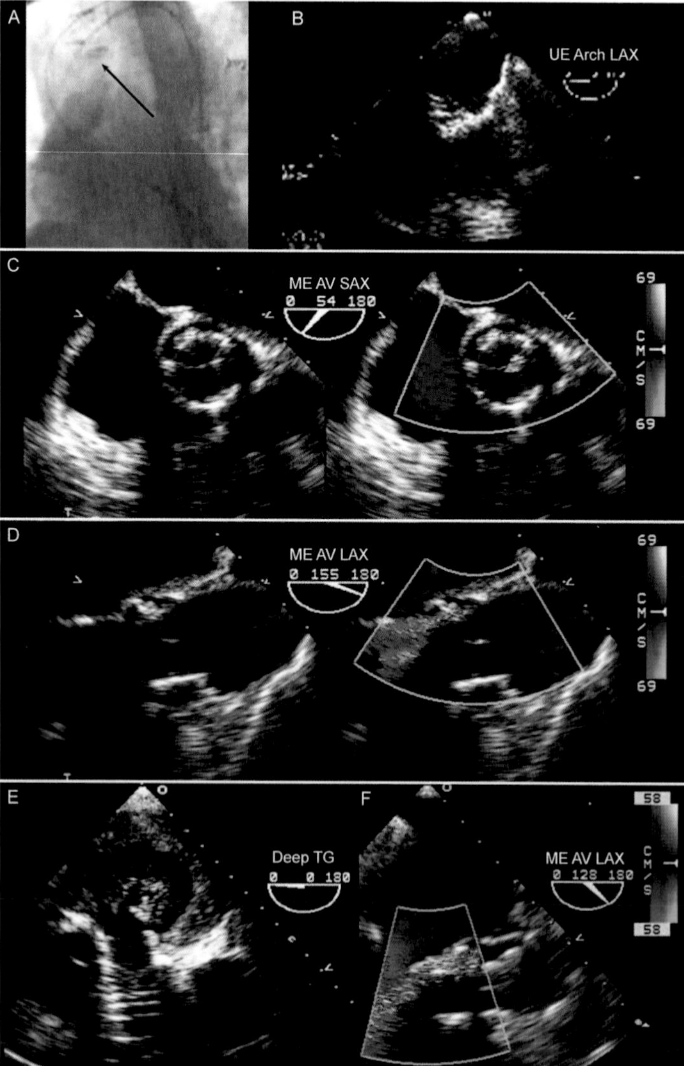

- In addition to valve-related problems, other early and late complications may occur after TAVI as listed here. Some may be life threatening requiring prompt diagnosis.
- LV dysfunction may occur from hypotension during pacing for valve deployment, assess for global, and RWMA.

(A) MR may worsen if the valve is mal-deployed too low and interferes with normal leaflet motion as seen in this ME AV LAX view.

(B) Pericardial effusion (arrow) in the TG mid-SAX view may arise from ventricular perforation during catheter positioning or annular disruption and result in tamponade.

(C) Iatrogenic aortic dissection during wire manipulation occurred in this patient. UE Aortic arch LAX and SAX views show the wire (arrow) in the smaller lumen. The patient required an open repair with CPB to fix this problem.

(D) Acute left main (LM) coronary occlusion from displaced calcium following balloon valvuloplasty diagnosed with angiography. This can cause regional or global LV dysfunction. Urgent coronary stent placement may be required.

(E) Early postoperative LV apical pseudoaneurysm following a transapical approach in the (E) ME 4C and (F) ME 4C color Doppler views.

Complications TAVI
Ventricular dysfunction
New RWMA
MR severity
Pericardial effusion
Cardiac tamponade
Aortic dissection
Aortic rupture
Coronary occlusion
LV pseudoaneurysm

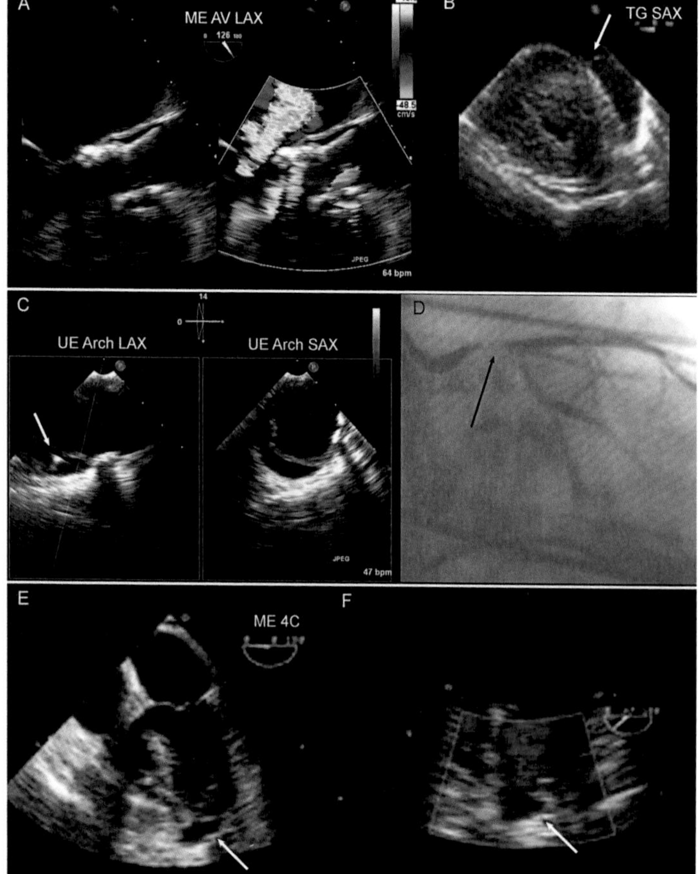

- Patients at prohibitive surgical risk for redo valve surgery are now being offered Valve in Valve (ViV) procedures as an alternative. This procedure positions a transcatheter valve inside a previously surgically implanted valve.
- The technique has been reported for any valve position, the most common are the aortic and pulmonic with increasingly the mitral and less so the tricuspid positions.
- TEE can provide procedural guidance to (1) assess the existing lesion, (2) position guide wires, (3) position the transcatheter valve, (4) assess the deployed valve position, and (5) assess prosthetic valve function.

(A) Aortic Valve in Valve: A 72 year old patient with a previous 27 Freestyle AVR 13 years ago now has severe AI (inset), MR, and refractory CHF. Because of the large annulus size, a 29 CoreValve® was successfully positioned across the old prosthetic AVR retrograde via the femoral artery with mild residual paravalvular AI. (B) Mitral Valve in Valve: A 46 year old patient presented 12 years after MVR (Hancock) with prosthesis failure (MR and MS), poor LV function, cardiogenic shock, and renal failure. Using a trans-septal approach, after balloon dilatation of the valve, a 29 Edwards SAPIEN™ THV was successfully placed under RV pacing.

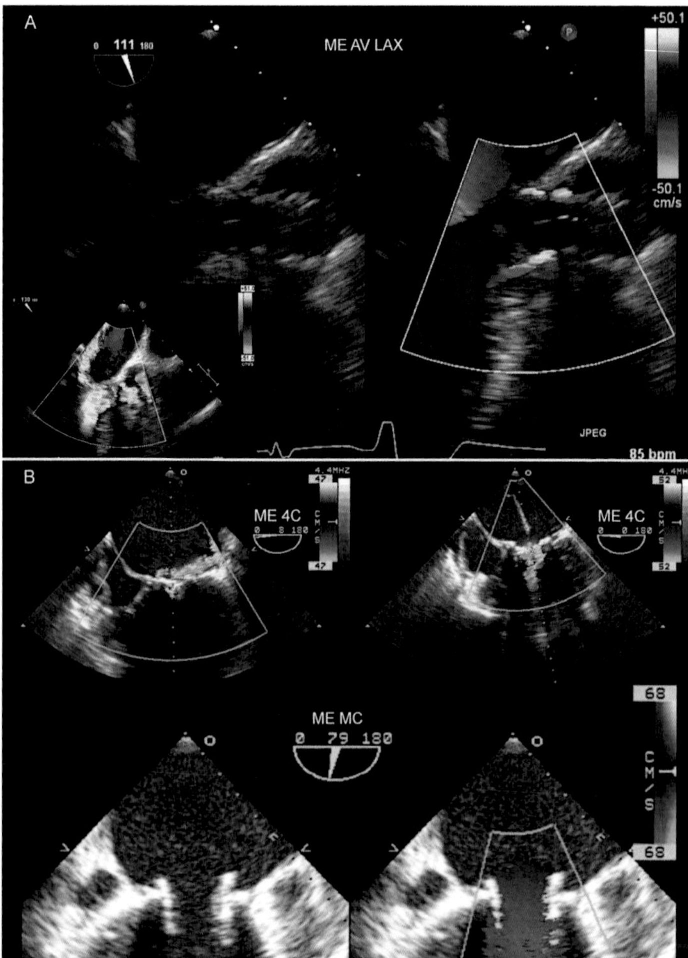

Mitraclip®

- MitraClip® (Abbott Laboratories, Abbott Park, IL, USA) is an edge to edge MV leaflet clip that alters MV morphology and reduces MR in 1° or 2° MV disease.
- The clip is delivered using a percutaneous transcatheter method and trans-septal approach to connect the middle scallops of the anterior and posterior leaflets.
- TEE is useful to (1) assess existing MV morphology, (2) guide delivery, and (3) assess post-procedure MV function.

(A) ME view showing the clip attached to the MV during systole. (B) ME MC view shows the double orifice opening of the MV with laminar flow post-deployment.

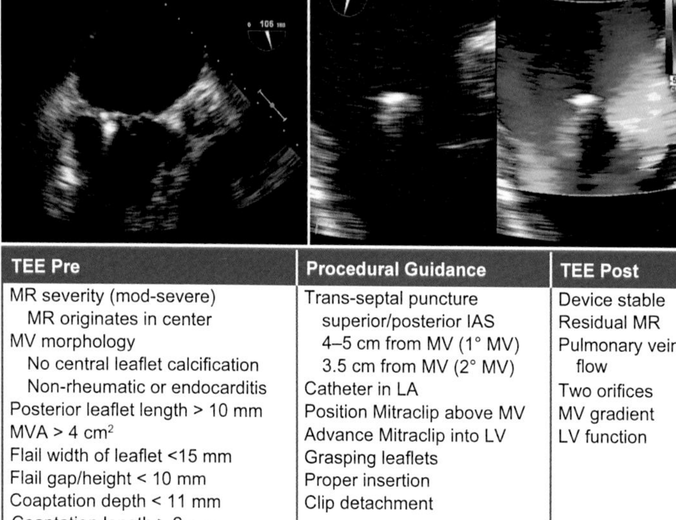

TEE Pre	Procedural Guidance	TEE Post
MR severity (mod-severe)	Trans-septal puncture	Device stable
MR originates in center	superior/posterior IAS	Residual MR
MV morphology	4–5 cm from MV (1° MV)	Pulmonary vein flow
No central leaflet calcification	3.5 cm from MV (2° MV)	Two orifices
Non-rheumatic or endocarditis	Catheter in LA	MV gradient
Posterior leaflet length > 10 mm	Position Mitraclip above MV	LV function
MVA > 4 cm²	Advance Mitraclip into LV	
Flail width of leaflet <15 mm	Grasping leaflets	
Flail gap/height < 10 mm	Proper insertion	
Coaptation depth < 11 mm	Clip detachment	
Coaptation length > 2 mm		
Source: Wunderlich NC, Siegel RJ. Eur Heart J Cardiovasc Imaging 2013;14 (10):935–949		

FORMA® Device

- Transcatheter-based treatment option for severe tricuspid regurgitation (TR)
- FORMA® device (Edwards Lifesciences, Irvine CA, USA) uses a foam-filled polymer balloon spacer to reduce TR by occupying the regurgitant orifice area and providing a surface for coaptation of native valve leaflets.
- Implantation is performed via the left axillary vein in much the same way as a pacemaker. The device is anchored to the RV apex.
- Intraoperative TEE helps to guide the device anchor to the apex of the RV.
- Overall, TR severity is reduced but not eliminated.

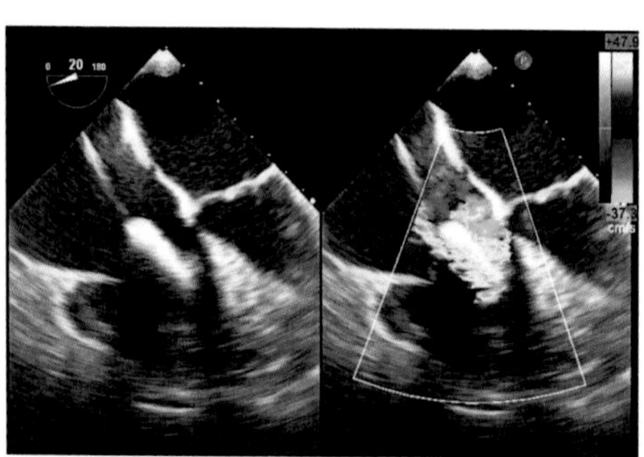

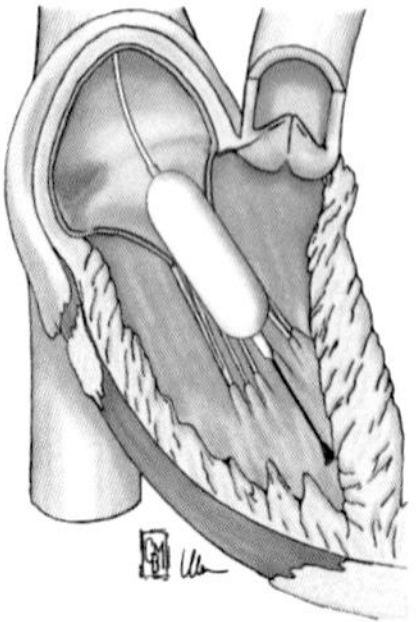

Indications for MV Surgery (Class 1B)*

- Symptomatic chronic severe 1° MR, LVEF >30%
- Asymptomatic chronic severe 1° MR, LVEF 30–60%, and/or LVESD ≥40 mm
- Chronic severe 1° MR undergoing other cardiac surgery

***Source: AHA/ACC Guidelines. JACC 2014; 63 (22): e57–188**

Difficult Predictors Mitral Repair

- Central MR
- Annular calcification
- Severe annular dilatation
- Bileaflet or multiple segment (>3)

Risk of SAM post-MV Repair

1. PMVL length > 19 mm
2. AMVL/PMVL lengths < 1.3
3. Septal leaflet contact length < 25 mm
4. Mitro-aortic angle ≤ 130°

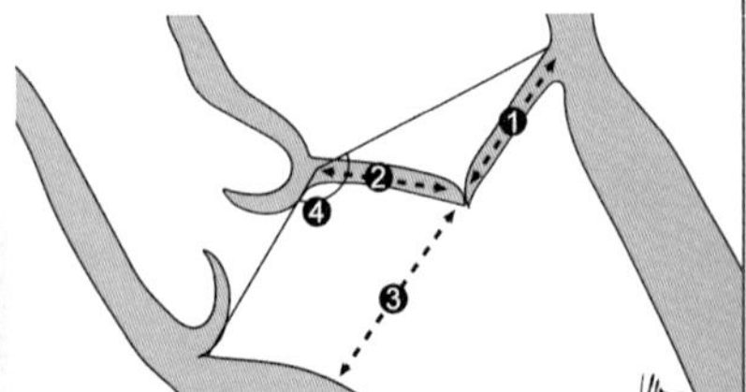

Annuloplasty

This repair is used for a dilated posterior annulus causing poor central leaflet coaptation. Sutures are placed in the annular tissue and passed through an annuloplasty ring. The sutures are placed closer together in the area of the commissures and the posterior leaflet, which results in a "gathering up" of the posterior annulus. A complete or incomplete, flexible or rigid ring can be used. Image the annular ring near the MV annulus in ME 4C, commissural, 2C, and AV LAX views. The incomplete ring is absent anteriorly in the ME 4C view, but present in 60–120° views.

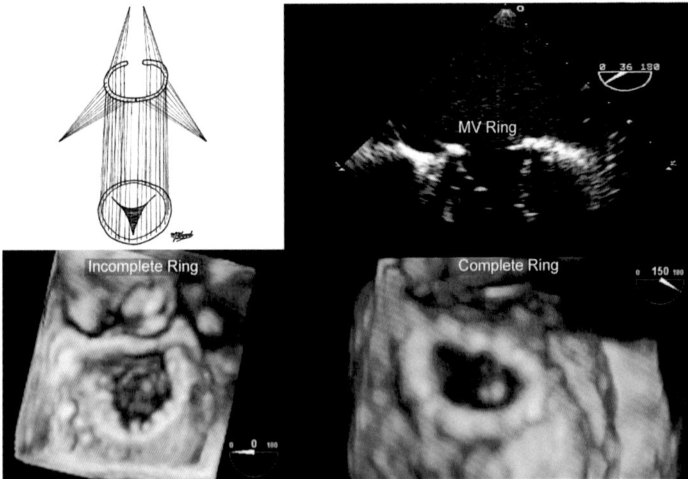

Artificial Chordae

Repair of chordae, using Gortex, to create artificial chordae. The suture is attached to papillary muscle tips, through the mitral leaflet edge, and tied at an approximate length.

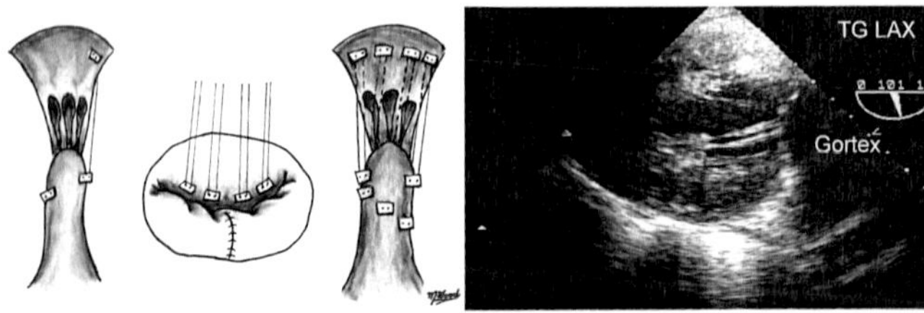

Quadrangular Resection (+ Sliding Plasty)

- This repairs ruptured chordae to the posterior leaflet. It consists of resecting the ruptured chordae and a leaflet portion, reapproximating the leaflet, and reconstructing the annulus. To support the repair and adapt the annulus to the amount of tissue remaining, a ring annuloplasty (partial or complete) is often performed.
- Note the short fixed P2 segment of the posterior leaflet (ME 4C, AV LAX views). The large anterior leaflet moves to coapt with the fixed (P2) segment.

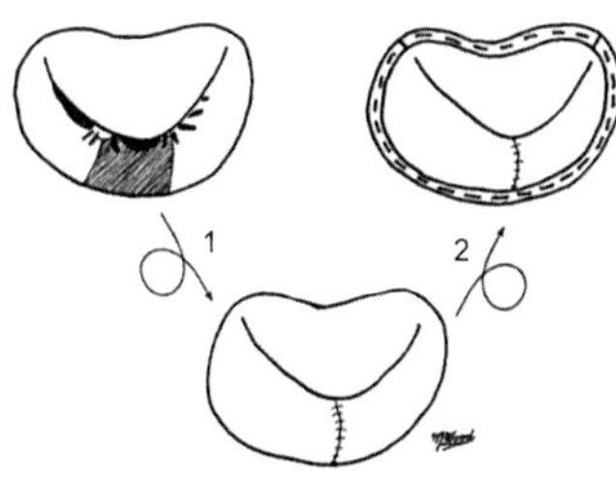

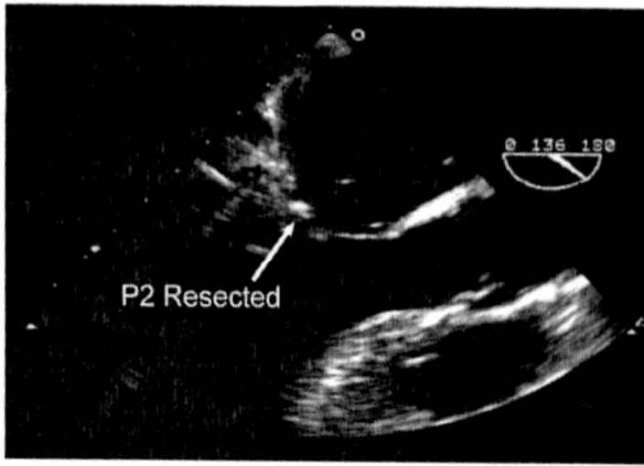

Alfieri Repair

- Repair technique for AMVL/bileaflet prolapse, commissural lesions, and PMVL prolapse with severe MAC. Anchors' free edge of the prolapsing leaflet to the corresponding free edge of the opposing leaflet (Edge-to-Edge), creating a valve with two openings; prolapse close to a commissure has a smaller valve opening.
- In this example, P2 and A2 segments are sutured together. In the ME 60° view, this is seen as a fixed leaflet, shown here with color Doppler. In the TG basal SAX view, the leaflets form a figure of 8. Planimetry of each orifice will give the MV area.

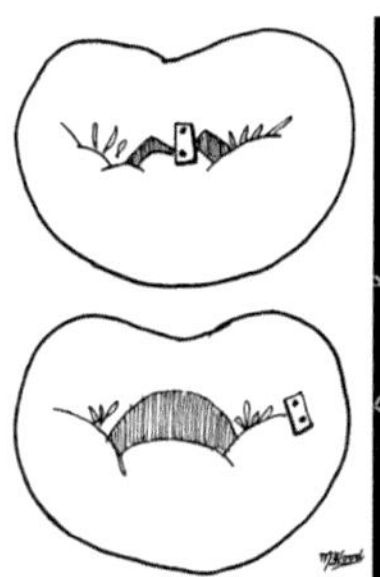

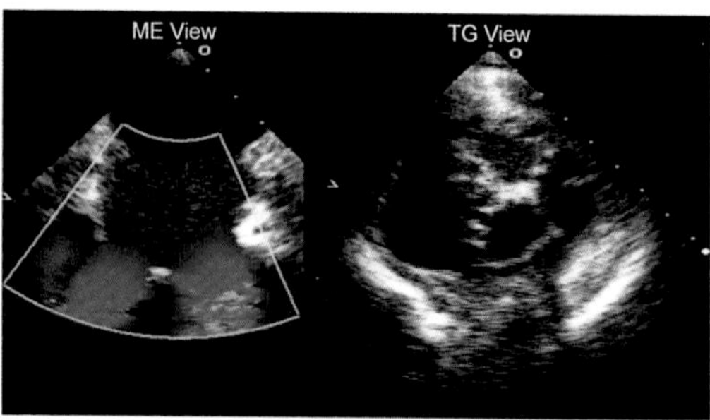

Anterior Leaflet Repair

- Repair technique for a ruptured chordae of the AMVL. A triangular section with the ruptured chordae is resected and the leaflet reapproximated. This may be combined with artificial chordae, if needed, to support the valve mechanism.
- The patient underwent resection of A2 with a complete ring annuloplasty, seen here in the ME AV LAX view.

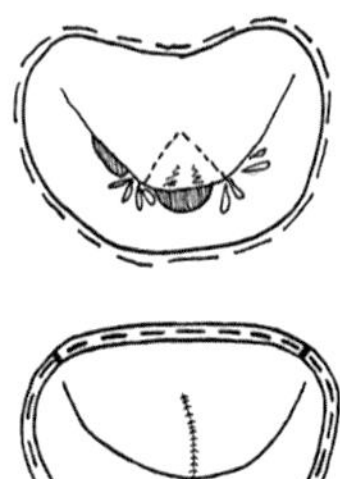

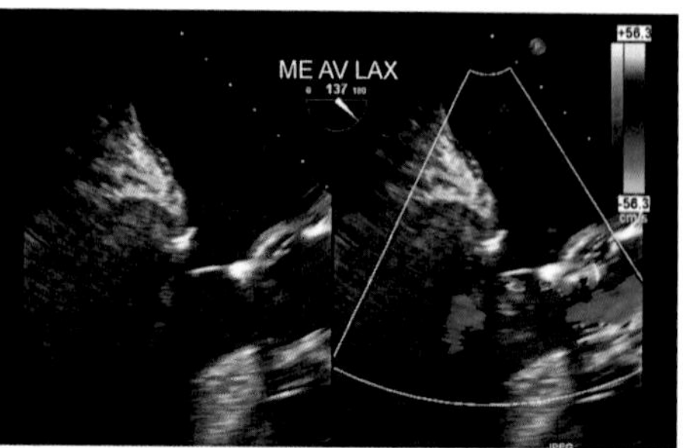

Aortic Valve Repairs

The surgical classification of AI (by El Khoury) is related to the functional AV anatomy. It is based on aortic cusp mobility much like mitral regurgitation is related to MV leaflet mobility (Carpentier classification, see p. 152). Surgical repair depends on the mechanism of AI, which can be identified through careful TEE examination.

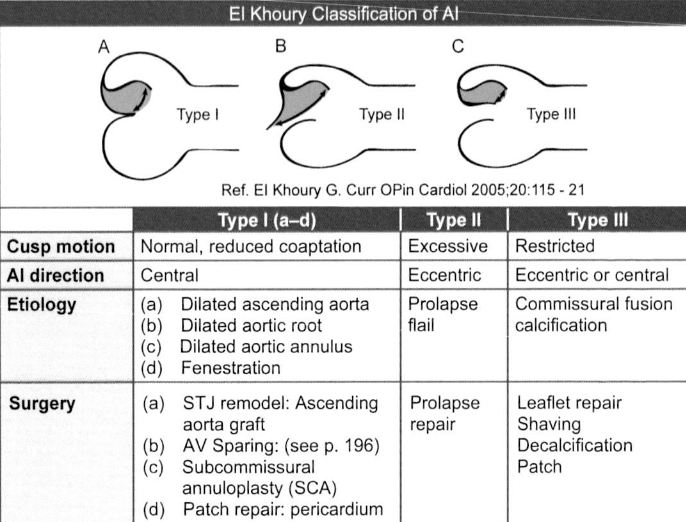

	Type I (a–d)	Type II	Type III
Cusp motion	Normal, reduced coaptation	Excessive	Restricted
AI direction	Central	Eccentric	Eccentric or central
Etiology	(a) Dilated ascending aorta (b) Dilated aortic root (c) Dilated aortic annulus (d) Fenestration	Prolapse flail	Commissural fusion calcification
Surgery	(a) STJ remodel: Ascending aorta graft (b) AV Sparing: (see p. 196) (c) Subcommissural annuloplasty (SCA) (d) Patch repair: pericardium	Prolapse repair	Leaflet repair Shaving Decalcification Patch

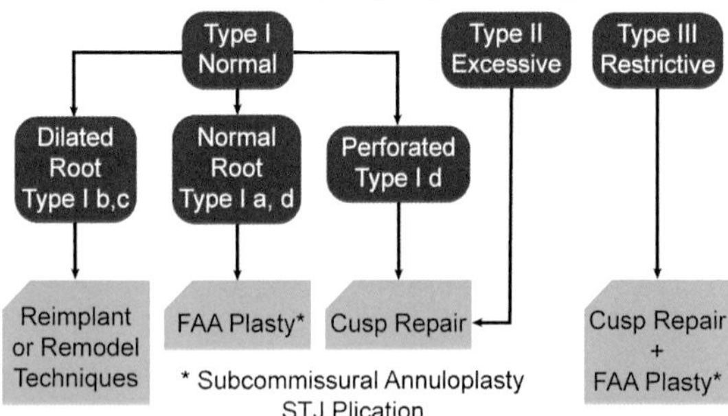

Aortic Insufficiency PreCPB
- Etiology (cusp vs. aortic root)
- AI direction and severity
- Measure aortic root
- LV size, function, RWMA

Aortic Insufficiency PostCPB
- Adequacy of repair (<mild AI)
- Root morphology restored
- LV function global/RWMA

PERF (perforation), SCL (sclerosis), ANN (annulus), RH (rheumatic heart), PLP (prolapse), BAV (bicuspid)

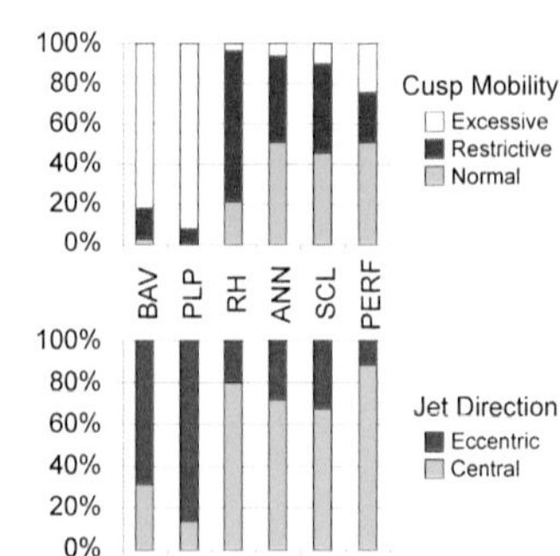

Source: Cohen GI, et al. J Am Soc Echocardiogr 1996;9:508-15

Annular Dilatation and Plication/Annuloplasty

STJ widens with downward stretching of the commissures. Repair sutures are placed around the commissures (not cusps) reducing the commissural area. This plicates the aortic wall displacing the commissures medially, preserving cusp function. The lower down the suture is placed, the greater the plication and leaflet coaptation area.

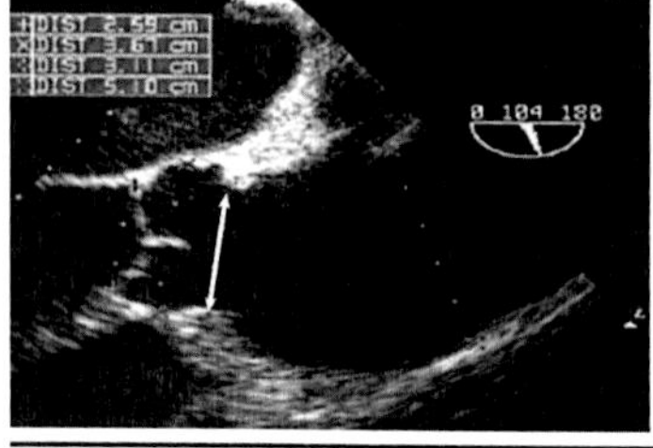

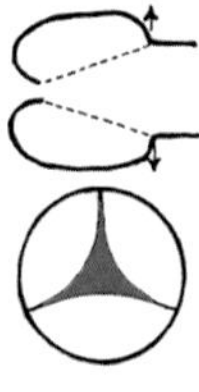
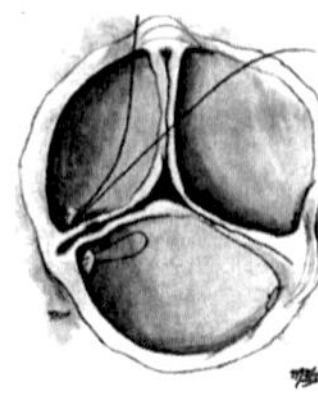

Cusp Perforation and Patch Closure

Cusp perforations cause AI jets that originate at the cusp level. Autologous pericardium repairs the hole in the cusp. Primary closure may cause cusp malcoaptation.

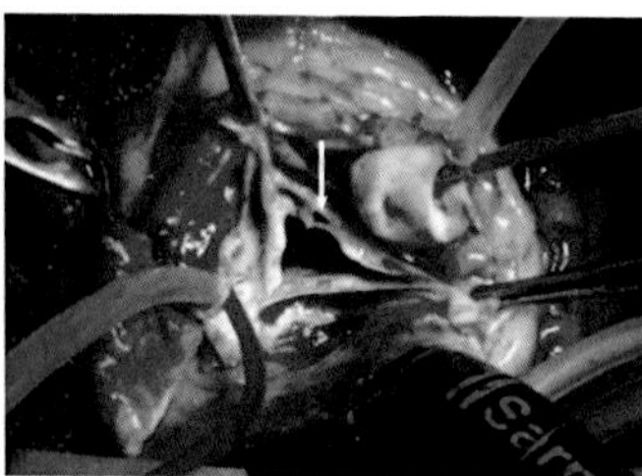
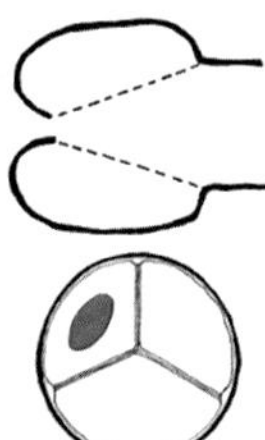
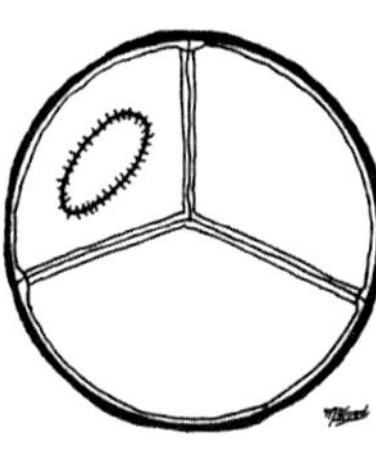

Cusp Prolapse and Cusp Resuspension

Cusp prolapse results from lack of commissural support or an elongated cusp. Repair shortens the elongated cusp edge by suturing the cusp-free edge to the aortic wall.

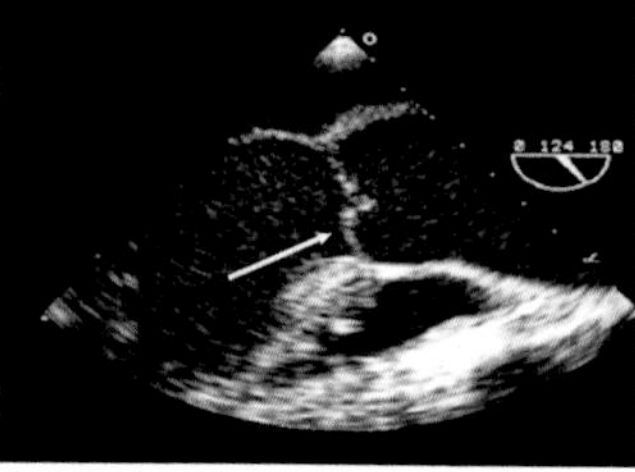

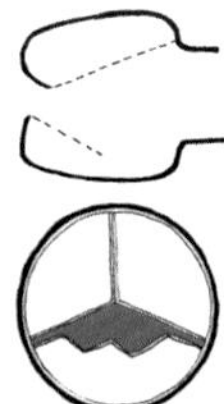
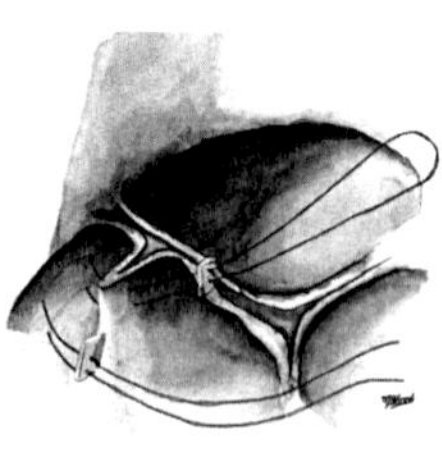

Commissural Prolapse and Resuspension

Aortic dissection that extends into the root disrupts the commissure, leading to cusp prolapse. Repair involves commissural resuspension.

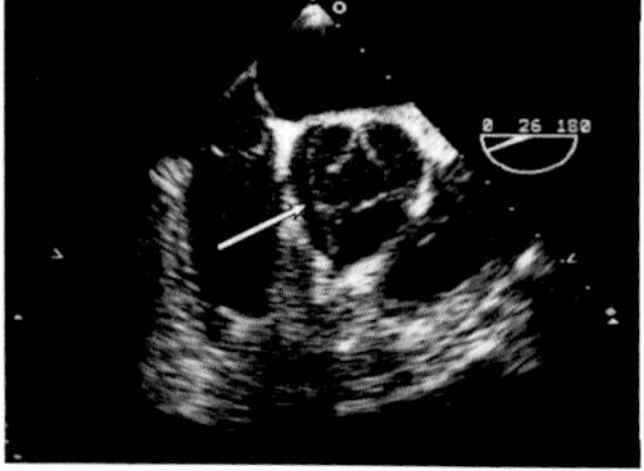

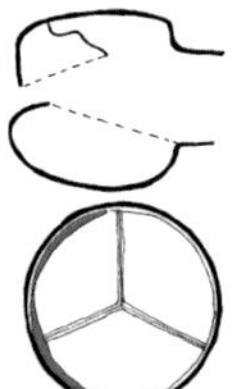
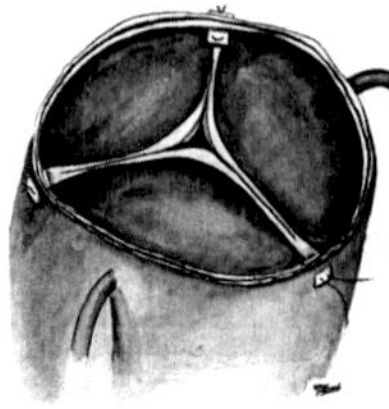

Aortic Valve Sparing Procedures

Surgery for aortic root pathology can involve sparing the native AV and repairing the aortic root. This is possible if the AV cusps are non-calcified, not excessively thinned, and are sufficiently mobile. Aortic root dimensions are less important. There are 2 types of AV sparing root procedures: (a) Reimplantation and (b) Remodelling.

	Reimplantation David/Feindel Procedure	Remodelling Yacoub/David II Procedure
Technique	The native AV is suspended within a straight Dacron graft at the native commissural pillars.	The native AV is sutured to a sculpted Dacron graft at the native commissural pillars
Advantages	Hemostatic Annulus stable Reproducible procedure	2 suture lines Neo-sinuses
Disadvantages	3 suture lines Lack of sinuses	No annulus support Difficult to reproduce

The technique for both procedures involves similar steps:

1. The aorta is transected above the STJ.
2. Sculpted aortic root is dissected, retaining the commissural pillars
3. Dacron graft is sutured to the heart using reimplantation or remodeling technique
4. Coronaries are reimplanted
5. Ascending aorta is re-anastomosed

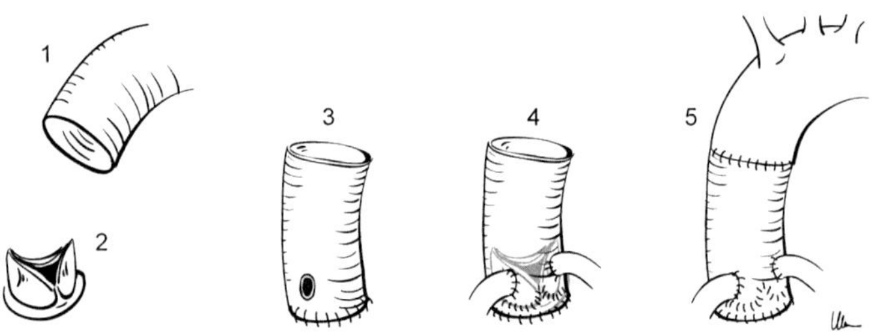

Intraoperative photos of the (A) reimplantation AV sparing procedure in which the native AV is suspended in a straight Dacron graft. (B) A sculpted Dacron graft is used in the remodeling AV sparing procedure.

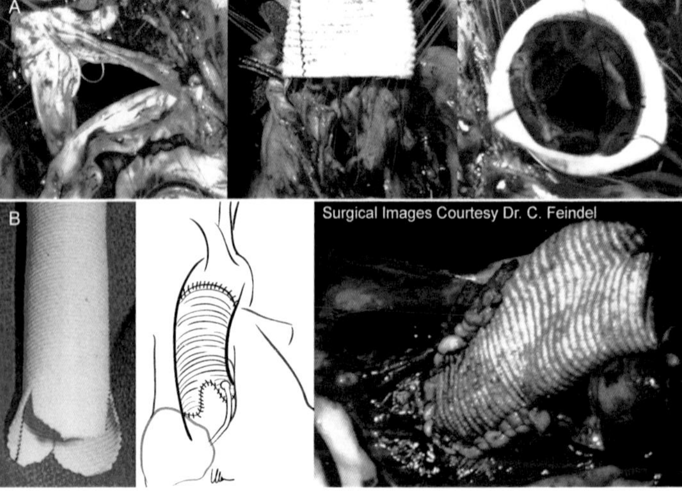

TEE Assessment During Aortic Valve Sparing Procedures

The decision to preserve the AV during aortic root surgery is aided by perioperative TEE. The single most important criterion in selecting patients for valve sparing root procedures is the morphological appearance of the aortic valve cusps. This assessment is best done through visual inspection by the surgeon.

TEE PreCPB
Root measurements
Cusps: morphology
AI: direction severity
Aorta: calcium
TEE PostCPB
Cusps above annular plane
Coaptation length
Coaptation height
AI: direction severity
LV function

PreCPB TEE

- Aortic cusp abnormalities are identified.
  - Uni/bi/tri or quadracuspid (ME AV SAX)
  - Thinned, fenestrated, curled edges
  - Calcified
  - Prolapse
  - Coaptation point in the aortic root

  Absence of calcification and significant cusp prolapse improves the chance of valve sparing. Cusps may become thinned, with curled edges and fenestrations making them unsuitable for repair.
- Severity and direction of AI jet is assessed.
  - No AI is seen if there is enough cusp coaptation.
  - Central AI jet results from symmetric dilatation of the aortic root.
  - Eccentric AI jets imply an additional cusp pathology (prolapse, fenestration) that may further complicate valve sparing procedures.
- Root dimensions are measured in diastole.
  - Root height (>20 mm) or root height/annulus ratio of >1 precludes valve sparing
  - Dilated aortic annulus (>28 mm) may need an additional aortic annuloplasty.
  - The STJ may be severely dilated making it difficult to identify and accurately measure.
- LV size and function

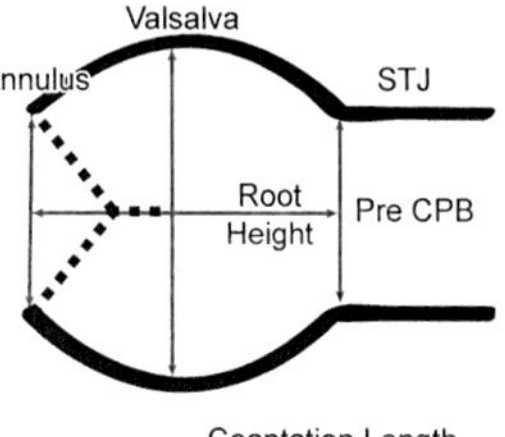

PostCPB TEE

- Evaluation of cusp morphology and coaptation
  - Entire cusp is above the annular plane
  - Cusp coaptation length > 5 mm
  - Coaptation height > 8–9 mm distance from the aortic annulus to the end of cusp coaptation
- Residual AI (severity, jet direction)
  - Trace to mild AI is acceptable
  - Moderate or eccentric AI is more likely to require early surgical intervention
- Root dimensions
- Aortic root hematoma
- LV function

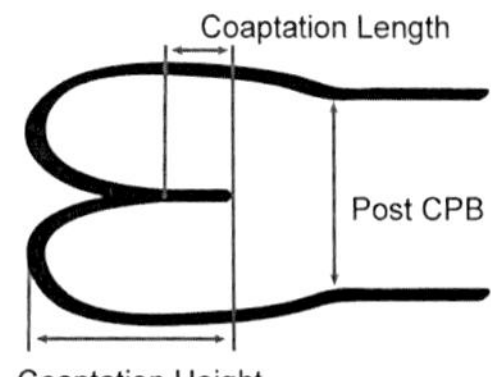

Aortic Root Aneurysm

Pre: normal annulus size, dilated sinuses of Valsalva and STJ (no waist), reduced cusp coaptation with AI

Post-valve sparing: Zoom of the aortic root shows coaptation above annular plane, thin root without patch annuloplasty, measured coaptation length ≥ 7 mm (arrow).

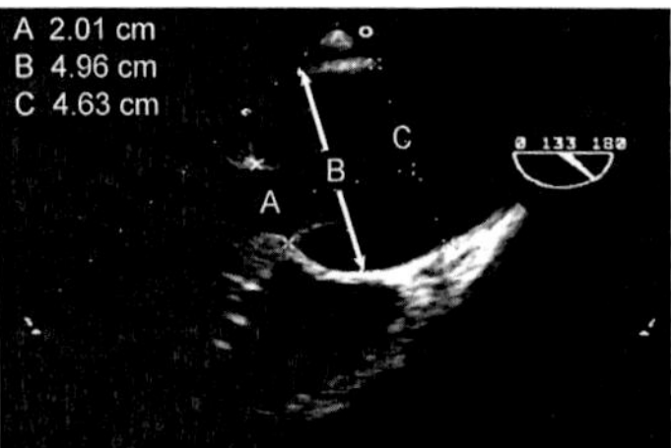

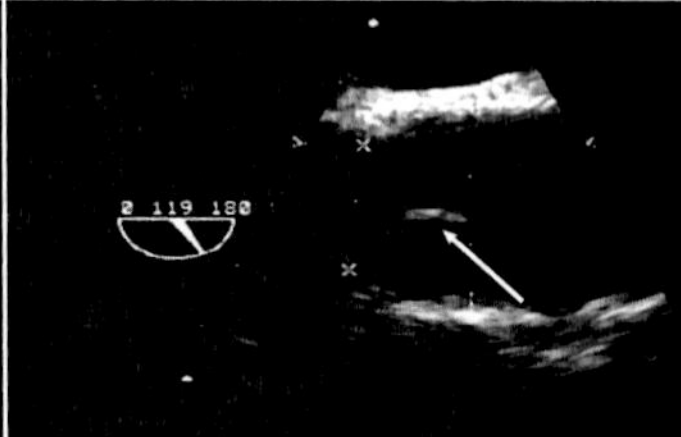

9
Aorta

A. Vegas, *Perioperative Two-Dimensional Transesophageal Echocardiography*, https://doi.org/10.1007/978-3-319-60902-7_9

Aorta Anatomy

- The thoracic aorta is a tubular structure that is divided into 5 segments (level 1–5):
    1. Aortic root: from the aortic valve (AV) to the sinotubular junction (STJ)
    2. Ascending aorta: STJ to innominate artery
    3. Aortic arch: innominate artery to left subclavian artery (LSCA)
    4. Descending thoracic aorta: LSCA to diaphragm
    5. Abdominal aorta: below diaphragm
- The ascending aorta has an average length of 7–11 cm, arch 2.2–3.6 cm, and the descending aorta 20–30 cm.
- Normal aortic diameter varies with the measurement method (US, CT, MRI), age, sex, BSA, and the location, but typically it is up to 35 mm (±2 mm).
- The aortic wall is 1–2 mm thick and comprises 3 layers: thin adventitia, elastic media, and a smooth intima (see p. 205).

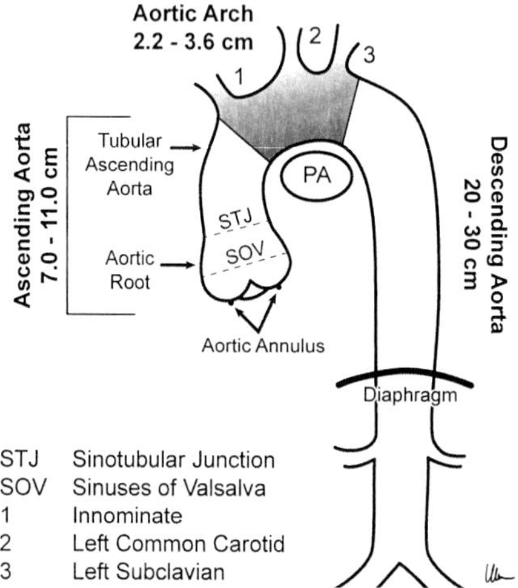

Source: Evangelista A, et al. Eur J Echocardiogr 2010;11(8):645-58

Aorta Function

- The aorta is the main artery from the heart that carries oxygenated blood with high pressure and pulsatile flow during systole. TEE imaging of the aorta can assess both structure (see pp. 202–203) and flow within the aortic lumen.
- Color Doppler imaging of the aorta (Nyquist 50–70 cm/s) shows intermittent laminar antegrade systolic flow. Aortic flow is unidirectional, but in relation to the probe, may appear red (towards), blue (away), or black (perpendicular to flow) depending on the aortic segment being imaged. Low Nyquist scale (30 cm/s) shows intercostal artery flow.
- Spectral Doppler assessment of flow is easily performed using PW Doppler in the ascending aorta (deep TG views), arch (UE Arch LAX), and descending aorta (Desc Aorta SAX or LAX). The direction of flow varies with position of the sampling volume. Normal systolic flow has low velocity <1 m/s.

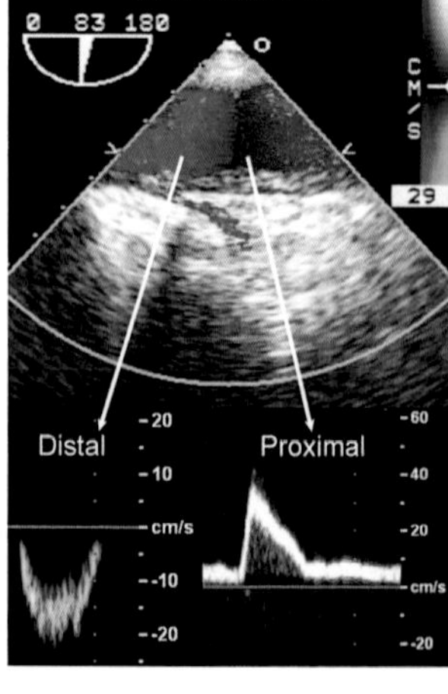

Right-Sided Aortic Arch

- Aberrant development of the symmetric embryonic pharyngeal arch system results in aortic arch (AA) anomalies. Regression of portions of the distal right 4th and 6th arches creates the typical left-sided AA. Regression of the same left-sided portions results in persistence of an abnormally positioned right-sided arch with variable configurations of branch vessel anatomy (Types I–III).
- Type I is a mirror image of the normal left-sided arch; Type II with an aberrant LSCA is the commonest variant. Type III is the rarest form with the LSCA disconnected from the arch. The three variants are indistinguishable by TEE.
- A right-sided arch is associated with other congenital heart anomalies, most often Tetralogy of Fallot.

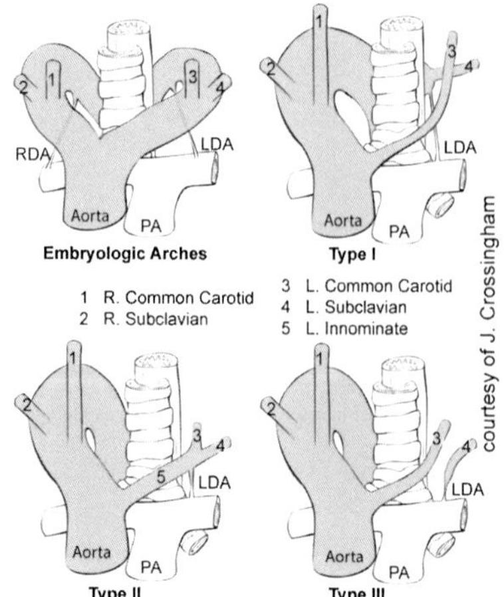

(A) A right-sided arch is shown in an UE Arch LAX view (0°) as it courses upwards from right (proximal) to left (distal) in the display. (B) Compare this with a normal left side aortic arch which is shown in an UE Arch LAX view (0°) as it courses upwards from left (proximal) to right (distal) in the display. The arrows in both (A, B) indicate a prominent innominate vein beneath the arch.

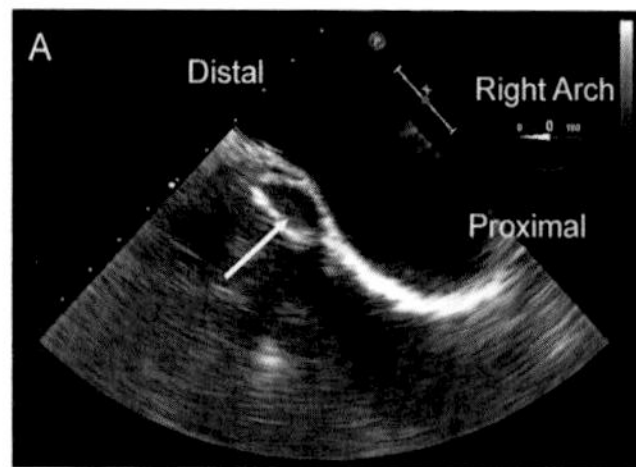

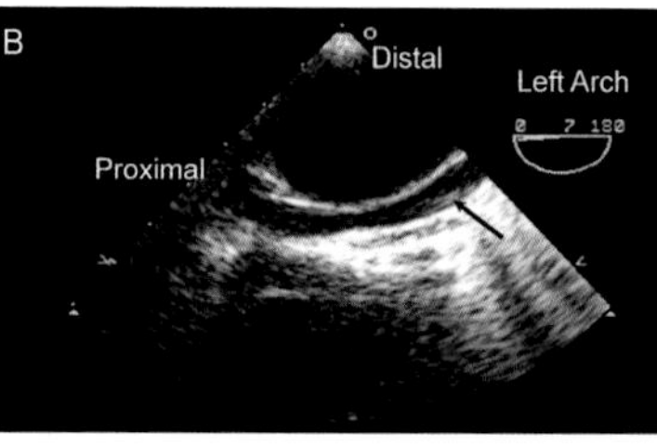

Aorta Pathology

- The thin aortic wall is exposed to high pressure pulsatile flow and may develop acute or chronic pathologies.
- Acute aortic syndromes (AAS) are aortic pathologies in which layers of aortic wall are disrupted causing aortic pain with a risk of rupture and death. These pathologies include aortic dissection, intramural hematoma (IMH), penetrating aortic ulcer (PAU), and aortic aneurysm. Non-invasive imaging such as Computed Tomography Angiography (CTA), TTE, TEE, and MRI are used to diagnose these conditions.
- Atheromatous disease is common in most patients. Complex plaque may rupture or form thrombus and become a source of embolus to the brain causing stroke or ischemia of any peripheral artery.

Acute Aortic Syndromes
Aneurysm (>50 mm)
Dissection (intimal flap)
Intramural hematoma
Penetrating aortic ulcer

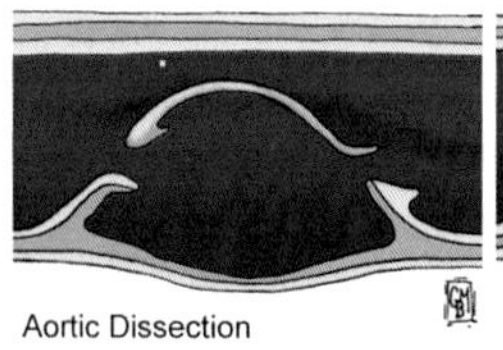
Aortic Dissection

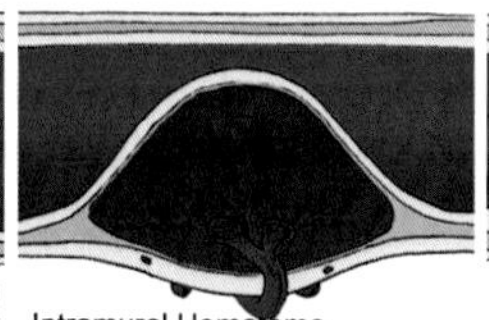
Intramural Hematoma

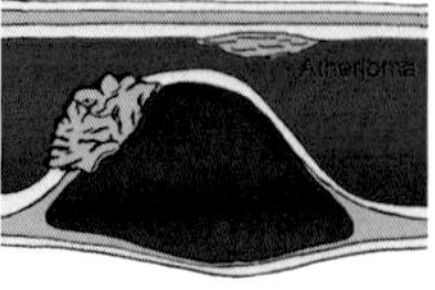

Penetrating Aortic Ulcer

TEE Assessment of Aorta

- Different levels of the thoracic aorta are examined sequentially in SAX and LAX using six basic TEE views: Desc Aorta SAX, Desc Aorta LAX, UE Aortic Arch LAX, UE Aortic Arch SAX, ME Asc Aorta SAX, and ME Asc Aorta LAX.
- The esophagus has a tortuous relationship with the aorta, so the aortic walls are hard to determine with precision. Near-field clutter may obscure the aortic wall closest to the probe and may be reduced by decreasing gain using the near-field TGC sliders.

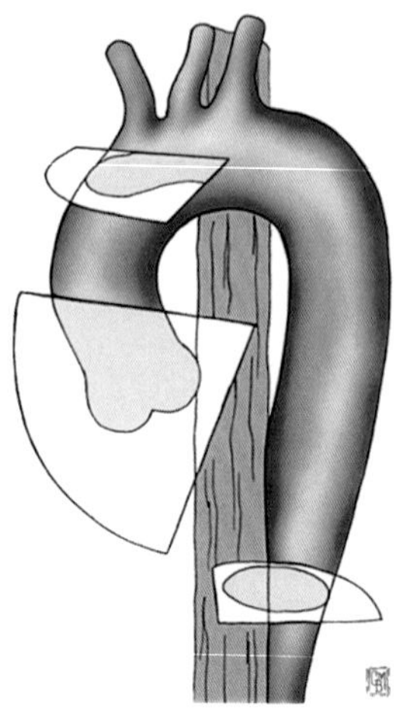

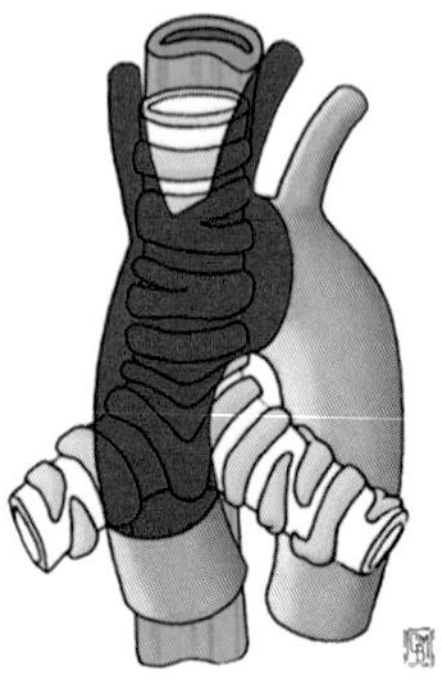

- Only the most proximal 5 cm of the aorta is imaged well by TEE. The distal ascending aorta and proximal arch is obscured by the air-filled trachea creating a blind spot for TEE imaging. Visualization of this region of the aorta can be better obtained by using epiaortic scanning (see p. 206).

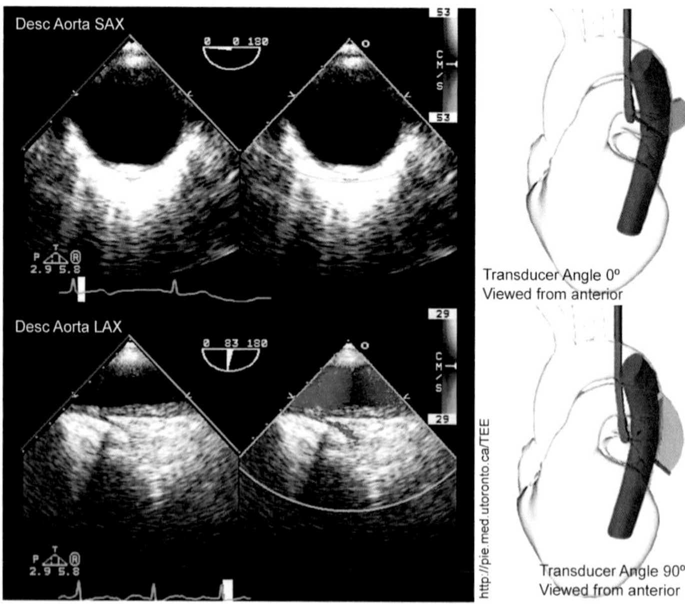

Descending Aorta

The descending aorta is easily imaged in SAX (0°) as a circular shape and in LAX (90°) from the stomach through to the mid-esophagus by withdrawing or advancing the probe with slight manipulation to keep the aorta in the center of the display. The distal portion is on the display left in the LAX view. The near-field image of the circular aorta represents the right anterior aortic wall with the rightward structures on the screen's left and leftward structures on the right.

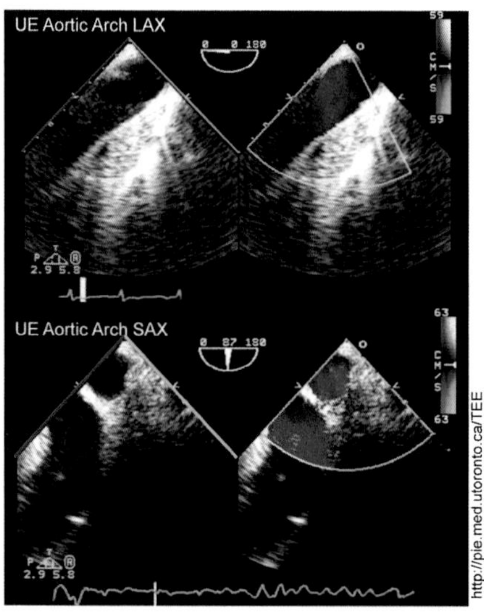

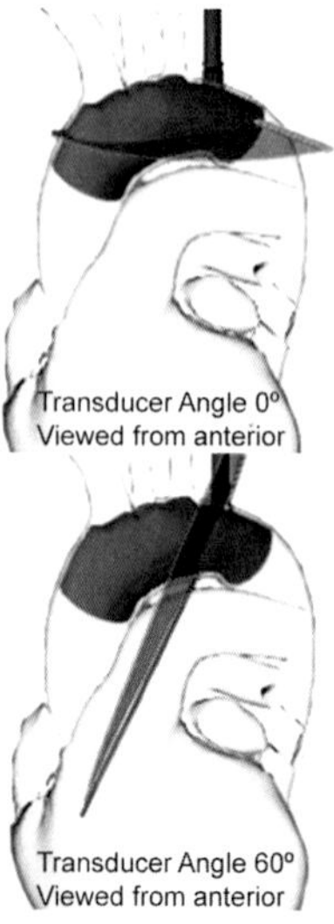

Aortic Arch

Further withdrawing the probe as it passes the left subclavian artery changes the aorta into the oblong aortic arch in LAX (0°). The distal portion is closest to the probe. Rotation of the transducer angle between 60 and 90° images the aortic arch in SAX with the pulmonary artery (PA) in LAX. The diameter of the aortic arch is more easily measured from the circular aorta in the UE SAX view (superior-inferior walls) as compared with the UE LAX view (anterior-posterior walls).

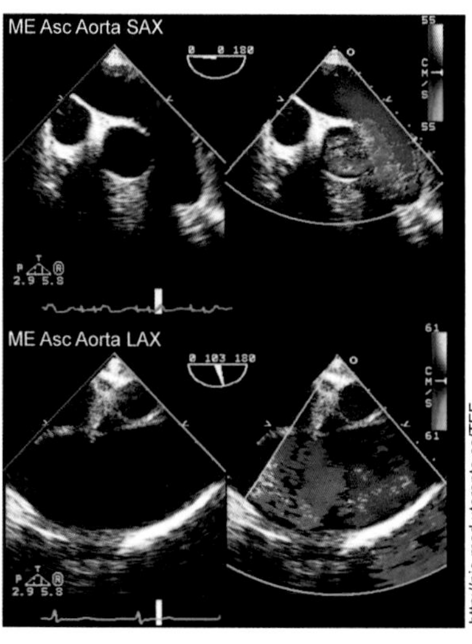

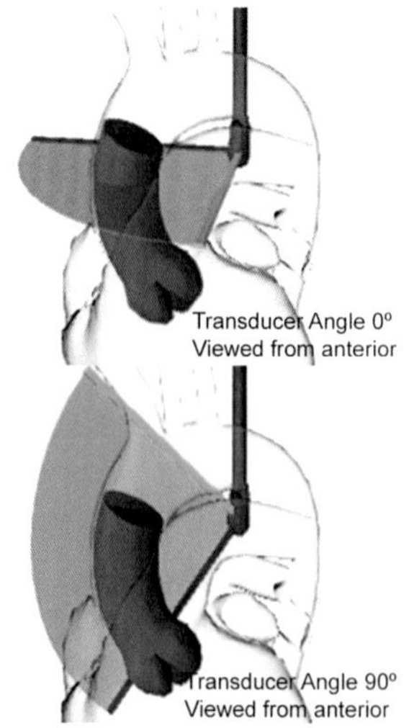

Ascending Aorta

Ascending aorta in LAX (100–120°) is seen by withdrawing the probe from the ME AV LAX view and reducing the transducer angle. The ascending aorta is seen in SAX (0–30°) just above the aortic valve by withdrawing the probe from ME AV SAX view. Alternatively, either view can be obtained by increasing or decreasing the transducer angle by 90° to show the LAX or SAX view from the previously described views.

Aortic Arch Arteries

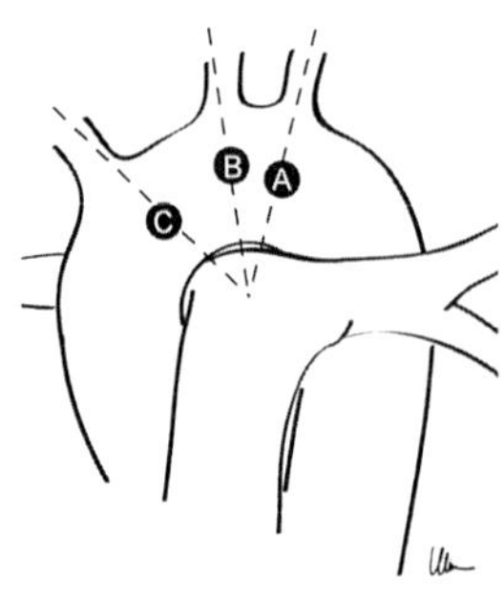

- Upper esophageal views of the transverse aorta and proximal arch vessels are shown with anatomic correlation.
- Views of the arch vessels are obtained with a left to right rotation of the TEE probe from an UE Aortic Arch SAX view at 90°.

(A) The discrete appearing distal left subclavian artery (LSCA) is the first vessel imaged. (B) Further rightward probe rotation images the main pulmonary artery (MPA) in LAX and the broader-based origin of the left common carotid artery (LCCA). (C) The most proximal is the innominate (or brachiocephalic) artery (BCA) that gives rise to the right carotid and subclavian arteries. The aortic arch is seen off-axis with the innominate artery in LAX.

Source: Orihashi K, et al. J Thor Card Surg 2000;120:460–72

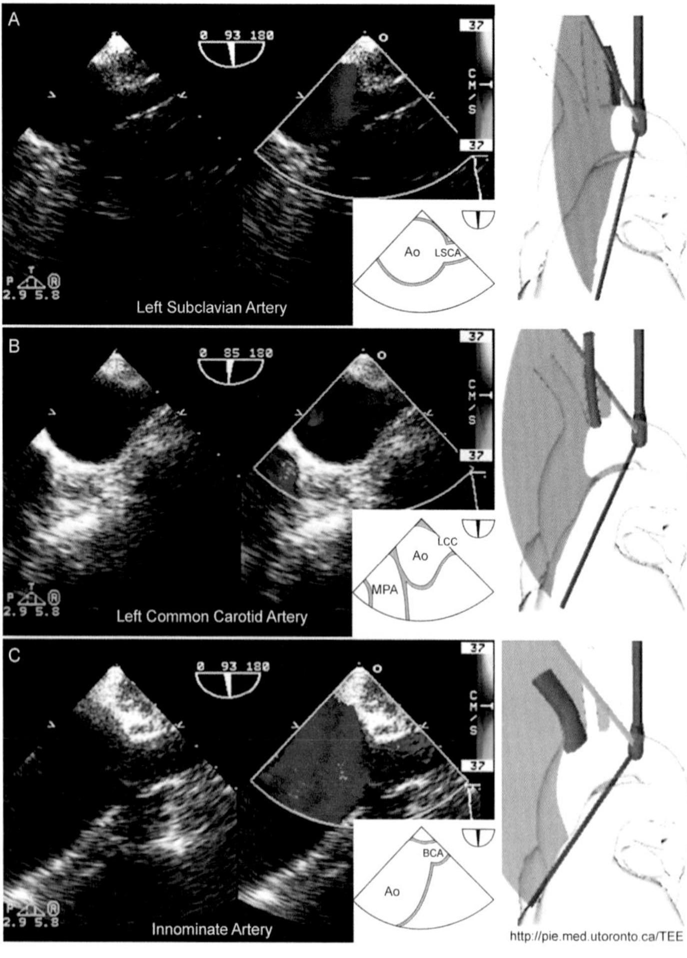

A

Ao LSCA

Left Subclavian Artery

B

Ao LCC MPA

Left Common Carotid Artery

C

BCA Ao

Innominate Artery

http://pie.med.utoronto.ca/TEE

- Atherosclerotic plaques are defined as complex in the presence of protruding atheroma of 0.4 mm in thickness, mobile debris, or plaque ulceration. Simple aortic atheroma have irregular intimal thickening of at least 2 mm.
- Atheroma are least common in the ascending aorta (7.6–9.4%), more common in the arch, and most prevalent in the descending thoracic aorta. The likelihood of a neurologic event (6.4–10.5%) correlates with more severe disease.
- TEE has greater sensitivity in detecting aortic arch atheroma than angiography and CT scanning.
- TEE characterizes plaque by assessing thickness, ulceration, calcification, and superimposed mobile thrombi.
- Different atheroma grading systems exist based on the echocardiographic appearance of atheromatous plaques; none has proven superior to another.
- Optimal strategies for the treatment of atheroma have not been evaluated.

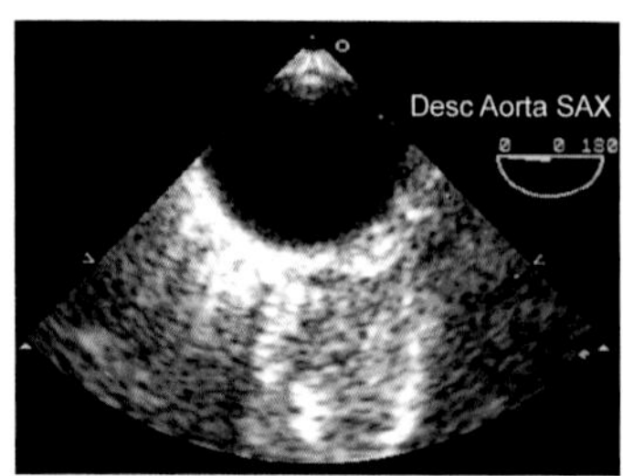

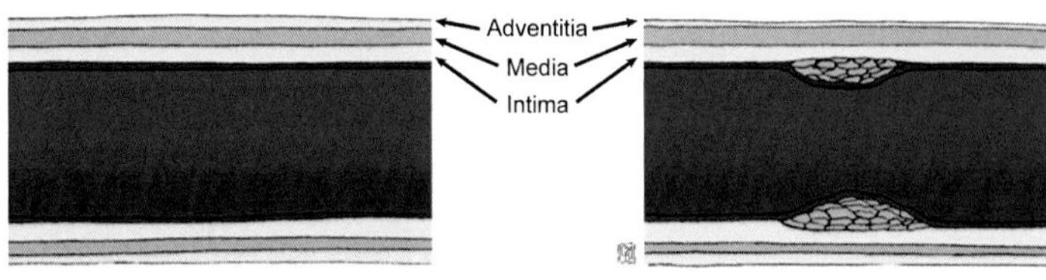

Atheroma Grade **(Source: Katz ES, et al. J Am Coll Card 1992; 20:70–77.)**

1. Normal aorta, no intimal thickening
2. Extensive intimal thickening <3 mm, smooth
3. Protrudes <5 mm into aortic lumen, irregular, sessile
4. Protrudes <5 mm into aortic lumen, irregular, sessile (↑ stroke risk)
5. Mobile atheroma of any size (↑ stroke risk)

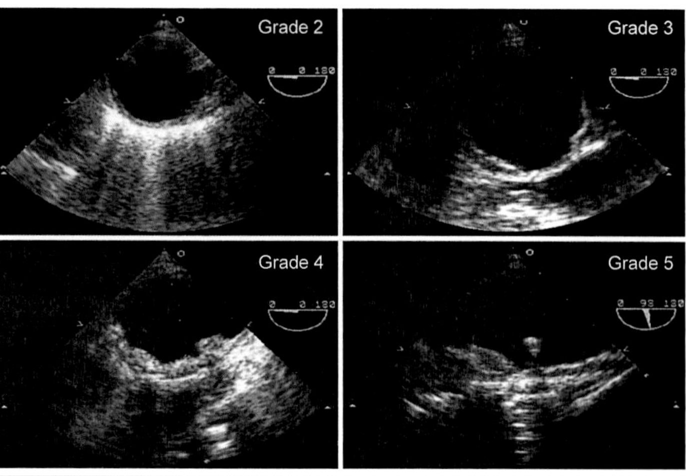

What to Tell the Surgeon Aortic Atheroma

1. Size: Measure thickness and atheroma height from intima to adventitia
2. Location of maximal plaque
3. Identify presence of mobile components
4. Atheroma burden: ratio of plaque area/aortic area

- Epiaortic scanning uses a high frequency (>7 MHz) ultrasound probe in a sterile sheath placed directly on the aorta by the surgeon.
- A linear probe gives a rectangular image. A standard transthoracic probe gives a fan-shaped sector, so a stand-off with saline or a saline-filled glove may be preferred to optimize imaging of the anterior wall of the aorta.
- Consider epiaortic scan if calcified descending, arch, or proximal ascending aorta.

Source: Glas K, et al. J Am Soc Echocardiogr 2007;11:1227–35

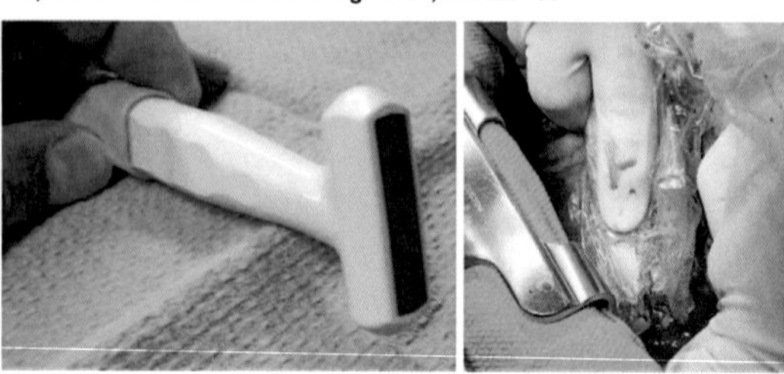

Epiaortic images of a normal ascending aorta in (A) SAX and (B) LAX are obtained using a linear array probe. The image width is the width of the probe; the anterior aortic wall is closest to the probe. (C–E) Aortic atheromatous plaques (arrows) are imaged by an epiaortic scan in the ascending aorta and proximal arch. The location, size, and complexity of atheroma can be better identified using this technique. (F, G) Large mobile thrombus on an atheroma is shown by an epiaortic scan and during surgery.

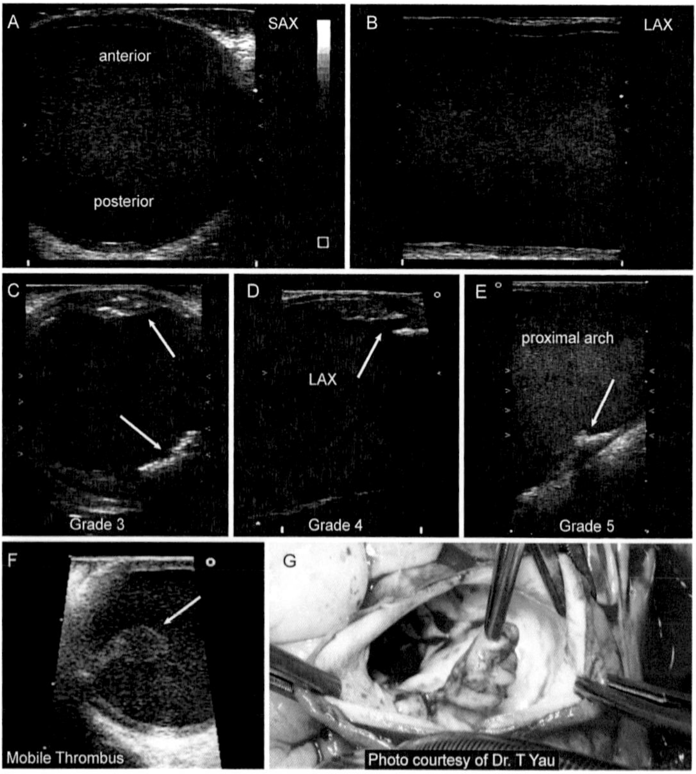

Aortic Intramural Hematoma (AIH)

- By definition, aortic intramural hematoma (AIH) is a localized separation of the aortic wall layers by partially or totally clotted blood without an intimal tear.
- The natural history of AIH is variable. The hematoma may entirely resolve, convert to a classic aortic dissection (Type A or B), or enlarge and rupture.
- Imaging criteria of AIH are based on the appearance of fresh thrombus in the aortic wall, including ≥7 mm circular thickening extending 1–20 cm longitudinally along the aortic wall, without intimal flap, intimal tear, or flow into a false lumen.

Penetrating Atherosclerotic Ulcer (PAU)

- This is an atherosclerotic lesion with ulceration that penetrates the internal elastic lamina with formation of intramural hematoma, aneurysm, dissection, or rupture.
- Common in descending aorta (90%), an ascending aorta lesion is more malignant.
- PAU with an initial depth >10 mm or maximal diameter >20 mm has a high risk for disease progression. It is seen on echo as a crater-like defect with jagged edges located within a complex atherosclerotic plaque.

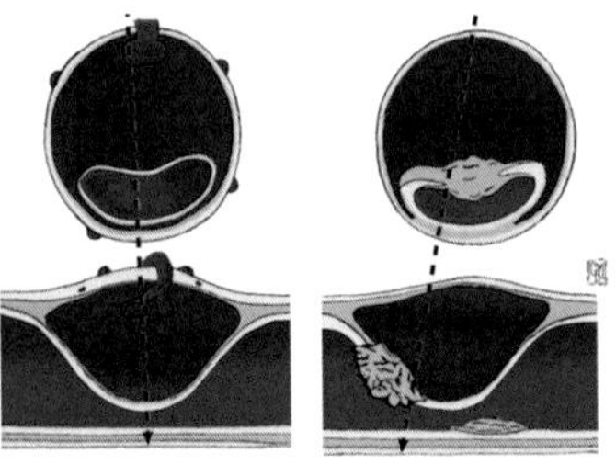

Aortic Intramural Hematoma
Aorta thickening >7 mm
Inner intima to outer adventitia
Longitudinal extent 1–20 cm
Layered appearance
Absence of intimal tear
No flow into hematoma
Penetrating Atherosclerotic Ulcer
Ulcerated atheroma
Central displaced intimal calcification
>10 mm deep

Aortic hematoma in the aortic root localized near the right sinus of Valsalva in (A) ME AV SAX and (B) ME AV LAX views. (C, D) More extensive hematoma of the ascending aorta in ME Ascending Aortic LAX views without and with color Doppler. (E, F) Contained rupture of the descending aorta shows a PAU, surrounding hematoma, and false aneurysm. In Desc Aortic SAX, it looks like a left pleural effusion and, in LAX, the contained space appears adjacent to the aorta without flow by color Doppler.

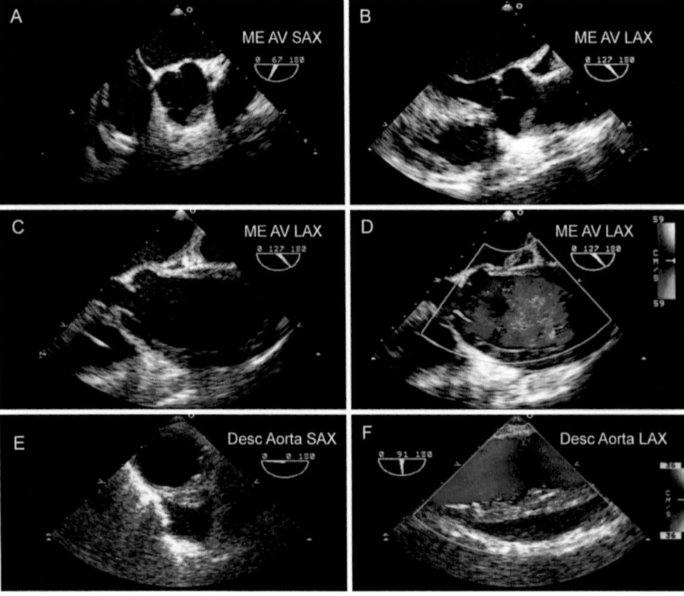

- Aortic aneurysms are a permanent, localized dilatation of all aortic wall layers with a diameter at least 1.5 times the expected normal diameter of a given segment. Ectasia is 1–1.5 dilatation of the aorta. Thoracic aneurysms are further classified by their shape (fusiform >> saccular) and location; ascending (50%), arch (10%), and descending (40%) thoracic aorta. Up to 25% of patients with thoracic aortic aneurysms have additional aneurysms involving other parts (brain) of the body.
- Etiology, natural history, and treatment for each aneurysm differ depending on the location. Patients may be asymptomatic (40%), with the diagnosis made as an incidental finding on imaging studies. The most worrisome consequences are from rupture or dissection of the aneurysm.
- TEE diagnosis is based on demonstrating aortic enlargement relative to the expected aortic diameter. There may be low blood flow represented by swirling smoke and mural thrombus in the aneurysm.

Aortic Aneurysm
Dilatation of aorta involves all wall layers
Location: ascending/root, arch, descending
Size: >1.5 × normal diameter
Associated findings: AI, thrombus, atheroma
Etiology: atherosclerosis, HBP, AS, Marfan's

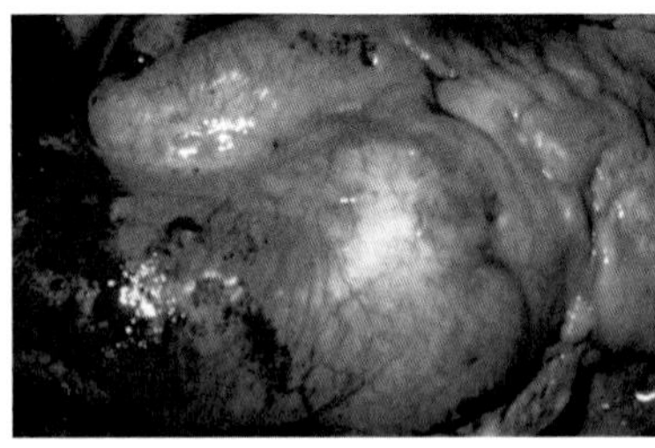

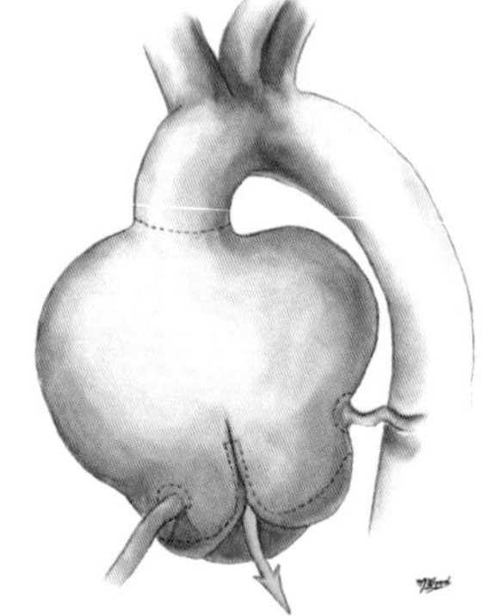

Ascending aortic aneurysm may also have dilatation of aortic annulus, sinuses, STJ, or arch. (A) Measure each site of the aortic root for the extent of pathology (see p. 134). (B) Nomograms for aorta size are indexed to BSA as shown here for the sinuses of Valsalva. (C, D) Poor central AV cusp coaptation causes central AI shown with color Doppler (Nyquist 59 cm/s) in the ME AV LAX and SAX views.

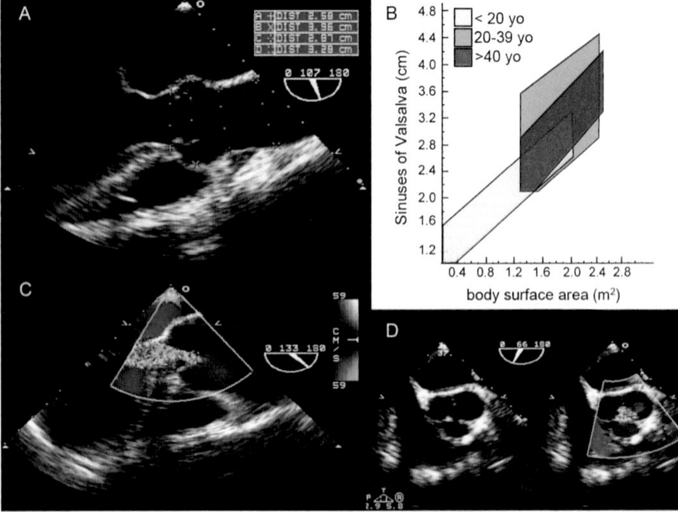

- Aortic aneurysm surgery indications vary with the level and aortopathy.
- At each level, the aorta diameter is measured in a plane perpendicular to the long axis of the aorta.

Aortic Aneurysm Surgery Indications
Sinuses >40 mm
Ascending aorta >50 mm with aortopathy
Ascending aorta >55–60 mm no aortopathy

Annuloaortic Ectasia involves dilatation of annulus, sinuses, STJ (no waist), and ascending aorta. The AV cusps are thinned with reduced coaptation and AI. Following a valve sparing root procedure (see p. 196), there is a thickened aortic root from patch annuloplasty of the aortic annulus (arrow), lack of sinuses, and a tapered STJ.

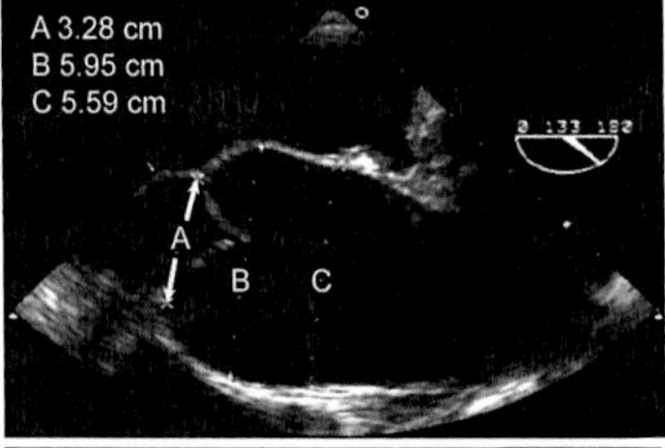

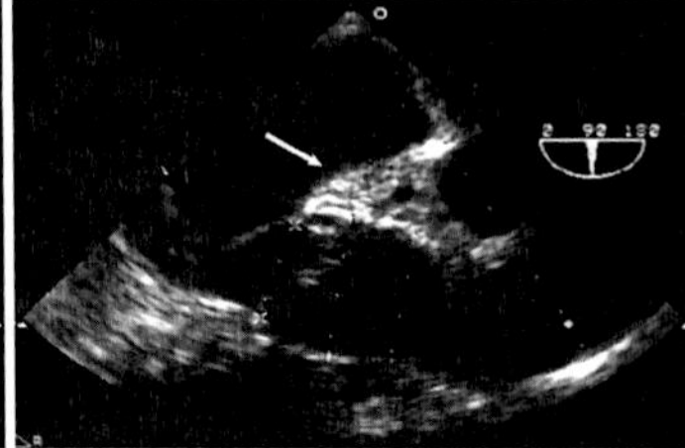

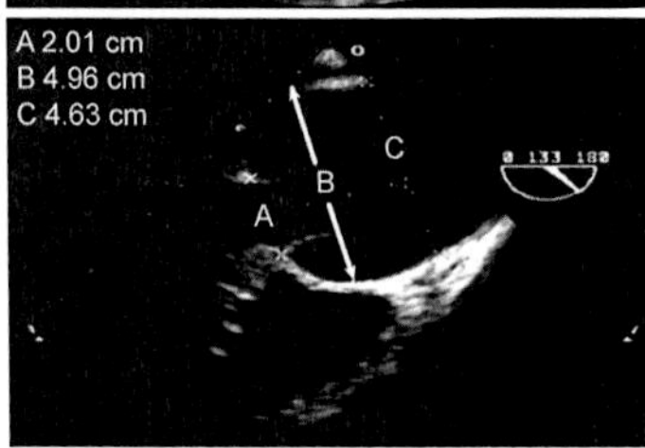

Aortic Root Aneurysm may have symmetric or asymmetric (most often non-coronary sinus) dilatation of the sinuses. There is a normal annulus size, dilated sinuses of Valsalva and STJ (no waist), and reduced cusp coaptation during systole often with central AI.

Ascending Aortic Aneurysm often occurs as a result of hypertension or aortic stenosis. There is normal size annulus and sinuses of Valsalva. Dilatation occurs after the STJ in the ascending aorta, which allows for good AV cusp coaptation without AI. These aneurysms are the easiest to perform aortic valve sparing root surgery with a Dacron graft sutured at the STJ (arrow). The "ball shape" of the native aortic root at the sinuses of Valsalva is retained.

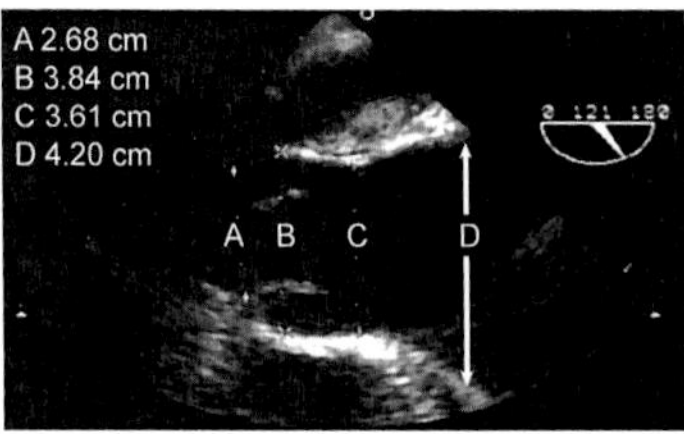

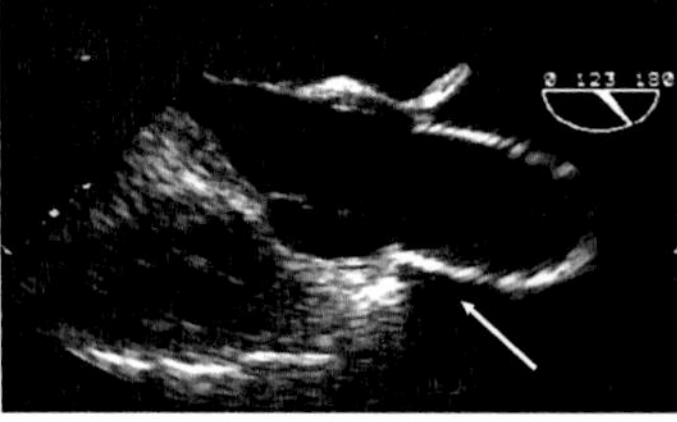

Aortic Arch Aneurysm is often present with an ascending aortic aneurysm. Measurement of the aortic arch is best performed in the UE Arch SAX view at 90° with a circular-shaped aorta. Compare the measurements in UE arch LAX and SAX views.

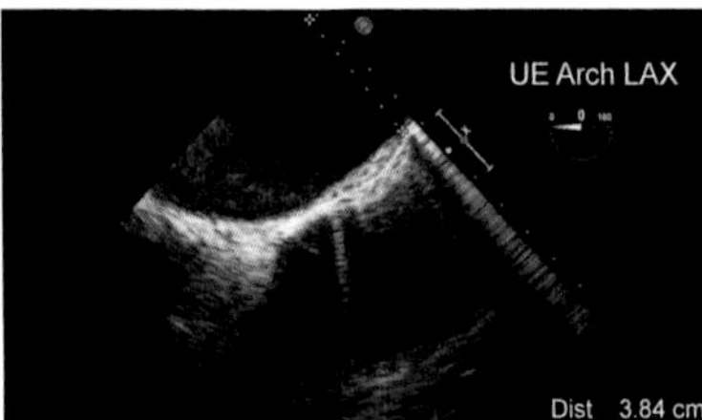

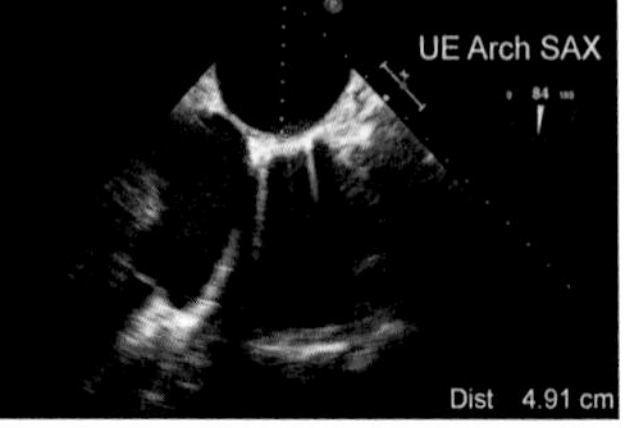

Sinus of Valsalva Aneurysm (SOVA)

- This is a pathology of aortic wall weakness with a true aneurysm or a focal "windsock" deformity.
- Etiology:
  - Congenital: single sinus
  - Acquired: diffuse 2° to Marfan's, syphilis, trauma
  - male (4) >female (1)
- Location: right (65–85%), non (10–30%), left (<5%)
- Associated findings: VSD, bicuspid AV, AI, pulmonic stenosis, coarctation, ASD
- Complications: rupture (RA > RV > LV > PA/IVS), endocarditis, thrombus, MI
- 2D imaging:
  - Sinus dilatation: single (congenital) or multiple (acquired)
  - Location + size of defect
  - Cardiac chamber penetrated
  - Windsock deformity of the sinus
  - Thrombus in sinus
  - Rupture: RV/LV volume overload/dilatation, systolic function
- Doppler findings:
- Color: flow into aneurysm
  - Location of rupture, fistula
  - Shunt direction
- Spectral: peak/mean pressure gradients across an intracardiac fistulae
  - Aortic-intracardiac fistula continuous (S + D) high velocity unidirectional flow
  - VSD demonstrate high velocity systolic flow + low velocity diastolic flow

---

Right SOVA

- There is a bulge of the right sinus which can be seen in the ME AV SAX and LAX views.
- Thrombus in the sinus may cause RCA ischemia.
- Rupture of right SOVA results in communication between the aorta and RV (in the RVOT) or RA.

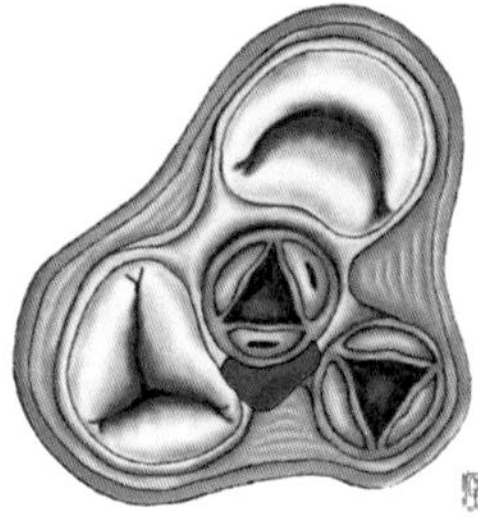

Right SOVA (arrow) is seen in (A) 2D ME AV LAX and SAX views with the windsock orifice in (B) 3D AV LAX view from the aorta. Color Doppler does not show AI in the (C) AV LAX view, but flow from the aorta into the RV is shown in the (D) RVOT view. (E) CW Doppler shows a peak gradient of 51 mmHg.

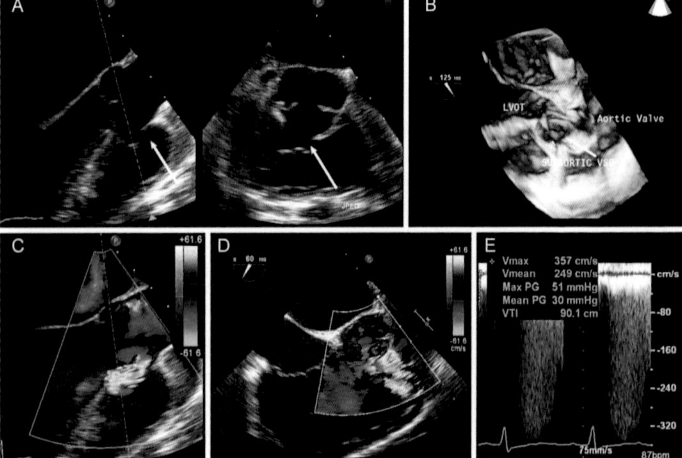

Left SOVA

- Bulge of the left sinus which can be seen in the ME AV SAX and 4C views.
- Thrombus in the sinus may cause LCA ischemia.
- Rupture results in communication between the aorta and LV (in the LVOT) or LA.

(A) Ruptured large left SOVA is seen contained by pericardium in the ME AV SAX views with thrombus and minimal flow by color Doppler (Nyquist 26 cm/s). (B) ME 4C view the thrombus is seen extending to the lateral MV annulus. (C) Diagram of ruptured SOVA thrombus as seen in relation to the base of the heart.

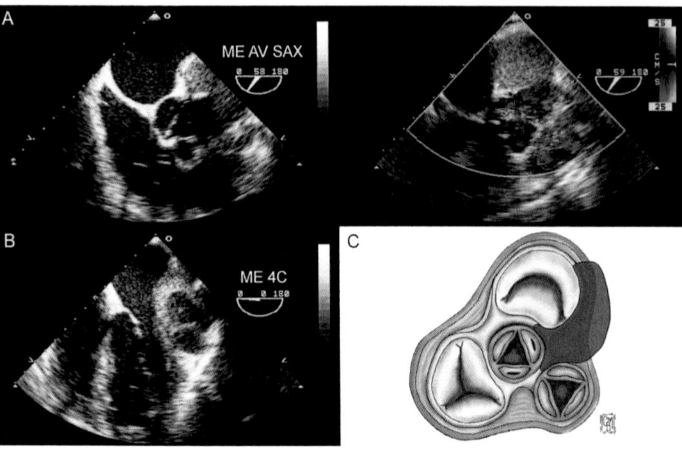

Non-Coronary SOVA

- There is a bulge of the non-coronary sinus which can be seen in the ME AV SAX view.
- Rupture of the non-SOVA results in communication between the aorta and RV (in the RVOT) or RA.

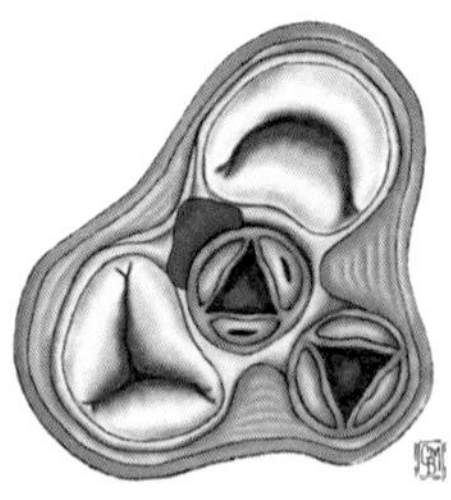

Despite AI, the pathology is not obvious in the (A) ME AV LAX, but is seen in the (C) ME RVOT view. Compare the (B) 3D full volume of the SOVA showing the classic windsock deformity (arrow) with the (D) intraoperative findings.

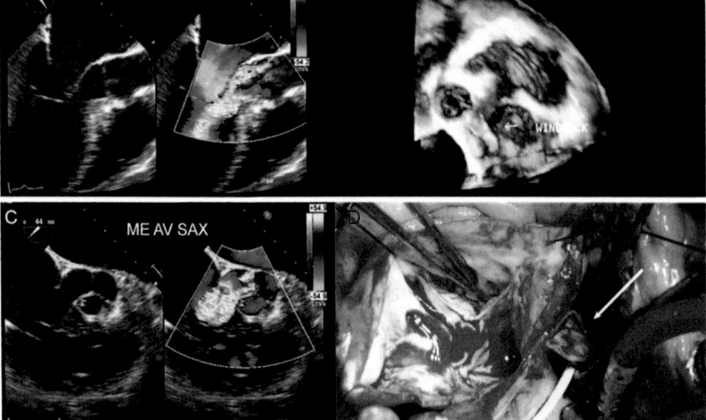

- Aortic dissection begins with an intimal tear causing bleeding within the medial layer and along the aortic wall. There are 5 classes of intimal tears:
  1. Classic: intimal flap between true and false lumen with re-entry
  2. Intramural hematoma: medial disruption, no intimal tear is imaged, but one is found at surgery (see p. 207).
  3. Limited dissection: intimal tear without hematoma, eccentric bulge at tear site, may lead to rupture.
  4. Penetrating atherosclerotic ulcer (PAU) rupture leading to surrounding hematoma to the adventitia (see p. 207), may progress to Class 1.
  5. Iatrogenic (catheter) and traumatic (deceleration) injury.
- Dissections have been defined by two classification schemes, **DeBakey** and modified **Stanford** criteria, which have important clinical and prognostic implications.
- Tears occur in decreasing frequency at an increasing distance from the aortic annulus. Over 50% of primary tears are located within the first 2 cm of the ascending aorta (AA) near the aortic valve (Type A dissection) followed by the aortic isthmus at the ligamentum arteriosum (Type B dissection), where the flexible portion connects to the fixed distal segment.

DeBakey		
Site of Tear Origin		
Type	Intimal tear	Dissection
I	AA	AA, arch, DA
II	AA	AA
II	Distal LSCA	DA
Stanford		
Segment of aorta involved, regardless of origin of intimal tear Type A: with involvement of AA Type B: without involvement of AA		

- Surgery is often required for thoracic aortic aneurysms to prevent rupture or dissection and improve life expectancy; though the timing remains challenging. Thoracic endovascular aortic repair (TEVAR) is a minimally invasive approach that may treat Type B dissection.
- Aortic dissection is acute within 2 weeks; subacute from 2 to 6 weeks; and chronic beyond 6 weeks.

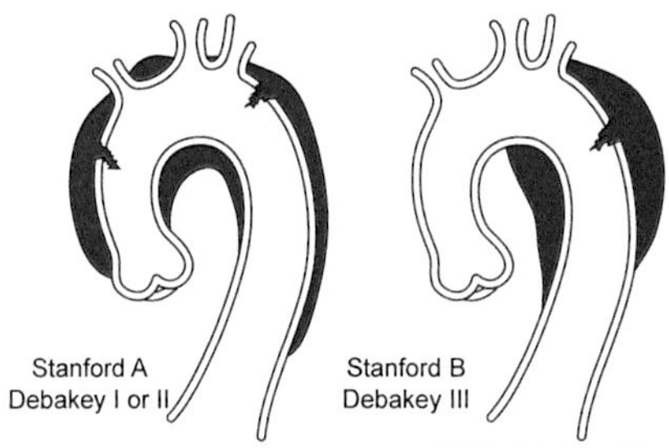

Diagnosis

- In aortic dissection, the ideal initial diagnostic test is one that can be performed most accurately and expeditiously. MRI and angiography are slightly more accurate (specific), but TEE is superior for expediency, safety, and economics.
- Diagnoses of intramural hematoma and penetrating aortic ulcers are also best made by cross-sectional imaging modalities such as MRI, 64 slice CT, and TEE.
- **Angiography** had been the gold standard (95% accuracy) for diagnosing aortic dissection, determining the site of intimal tear, extent of dissection, side branch involvement including coronary arteries, and AI severity. Angiography is invasive, fallible, and requires contrast.
- **CT scanning** with contrast is rapid and easily available with high diagnostic accuracy in identifying the dissection and false lumen. It does not reliably show the site of intimal tear, coronary involvement, or AI.
- **TEE** is a convenient bedside diagnostic modality, but poor imaging in the blind spot may miss a dissection in the distal descending aorta or proximal arch.
- **MRI** has superior diagnostic accuracy and can detect associated complications, but requires time and has limited availability.

Test Modality	Sensitivity (%)	Specificity (%)
TTE	85	60–96
TEE	97–100	100
CT	67–100	98–100
MRI	98–100	94–100

What to Tell the Surgeon Aortic Dissection

- Intimal flap location
- Intimal tear location (multiple)
- Location of entry and exit sites (color Doppler)
- Extent of dissection (distal to proximal)
- Identify true vs. false lumens
- Complications:
  - LV function: global, regional wall motion abnormality (RWMA)
  - Aortic insufficiency (50–70%)
  - Coronary dissection (10–20%)
  - Pericardial effusion, pleural effusion

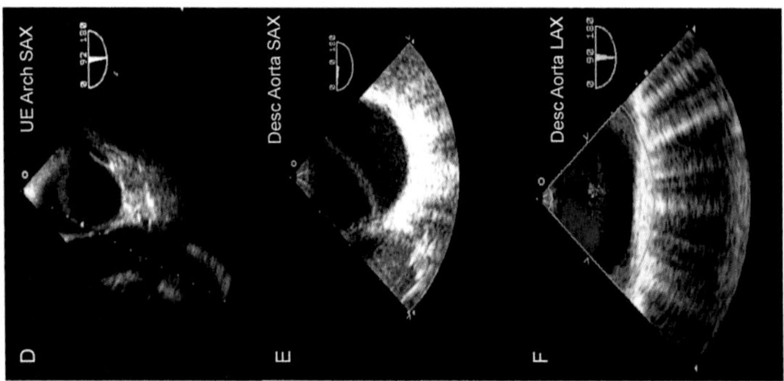

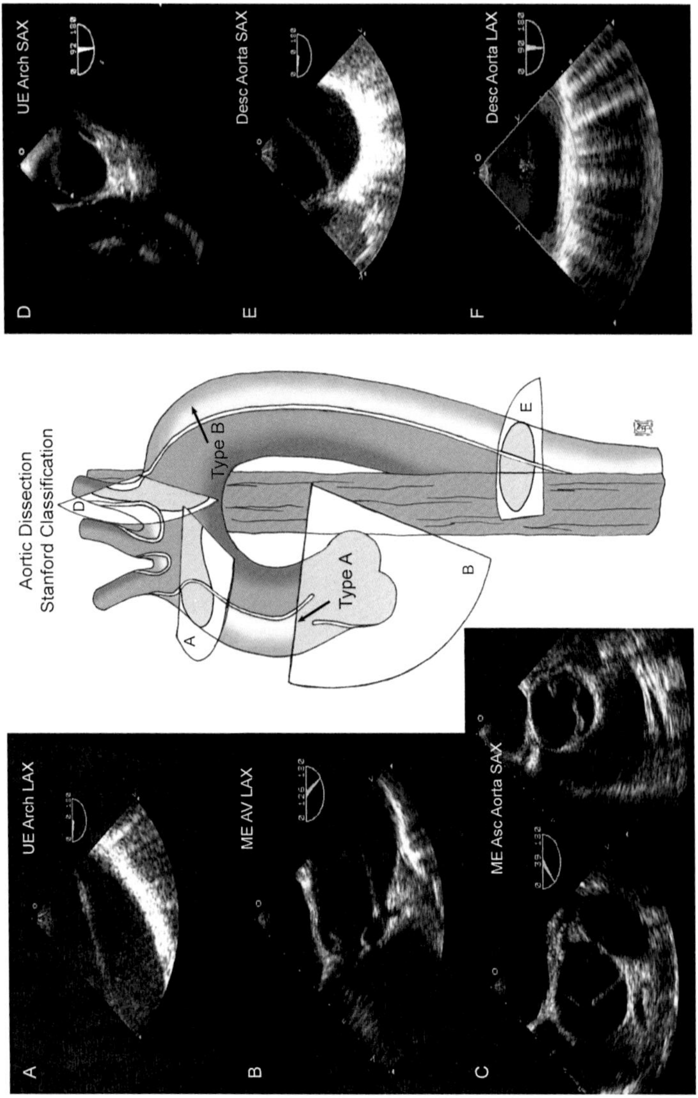

TEE Diagnosis

Blood flow between the intimal and medial/adventitial layers creates a false lumen. As blood separates these layers, the intima is compressed creating a smaller true lumen. TEE diagnosis and evaluation of aortic dissection relies on identifying the presence of an intimal flap and 2 lumens, origin of the intimal tear, dissection extent, perfusion in the lumens, LV function, and the presence of complications.

Intimal Flap

- Multiple TEE views are required to identify the intimal flap separating true (TL) and false (FL) lumens. A real flap is seen in different views, is independently mobile, does not cross anatomic boundaries (outside aortic wall), and has oppositely directed color Doppler flow on both sides.
- The flap must be distinguished from mobile linear artifacts such as mirror or reverberation in the aortic root (anterior LA wall) and ascending aorta (posterior RPA wall). M-mode can differentiate location and movement of intra-luminal structures; as artifacts are twice as far from the transducer with movement parallel to posterior aortic wall.

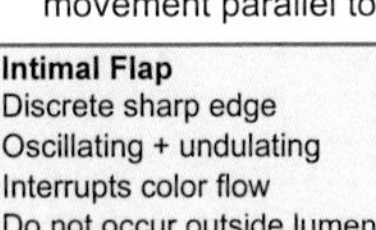

Intimal Flap	Linear Artifact
Discrete sharp edge	Longitudinal, fuzzy
Oscillating + undulating	Moves with heart
Interrupts color flow	May interrupt color flow
Do not occur outside lumen	Occur outside aorta

Intimal Tear

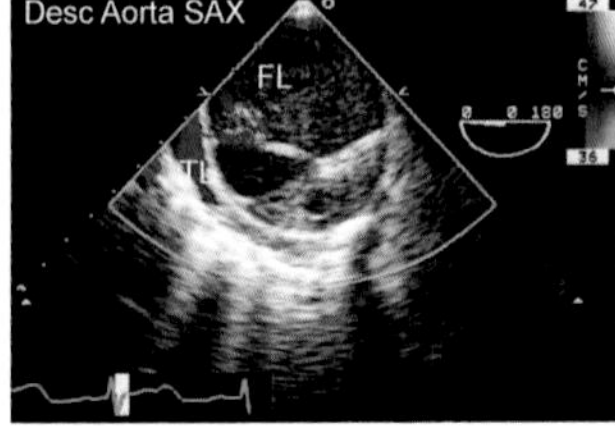

- The tear is seen as a gap in the flap with a diameter >5 mm. Between 5 and 10% of dissections, don't have an obvious intimal tear.
- Color Doppler shows flow through the gap from true to false lumen.
- Commonest site of intimal tear is ascending aorta, with 90% within 1 cm of the AV. The second commonest site is just distal to the left subclavian artery.

True and False Lumens

- Smaller true lumen expands in systole, with higher velocity brighter color Doppler flow and no spontaneous echo contrast (SEC) or clot.
- The false lumen exhibits diastolic expansion, evidence of SEC, complete or partial thrombosis, and reversed, delayed, or absent blood flow.

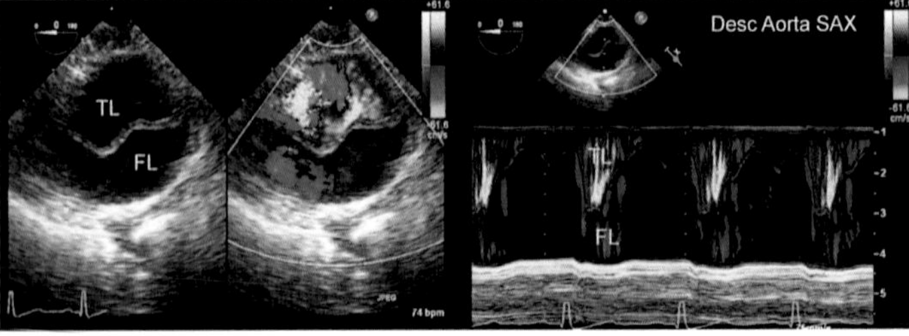

True Lumen (TL)	False Lumen (FL)
Smaller lumen	Larger lumen
Expands in systole (M-mode)	Expands in diastole
Color brighter (higher velocity)	Color less prominent
No smoke	Clot/smoke present

Dissection Complications
Aortic dilatation
Aortic insufficiency (p. 216)
Pericardial effusion
Pleural effusion
Coronary artery

Aortic Dissection

- Local complications associated with aortic dissection are as listed. In addition, end-organ hypo-perfusion may lead to renal, gastrointestinal, cerebral, and limb ischemia.

Aortic Dilatation

- Aortic dilatation is an enlarged diameter of the aorta that involves all 3 walls. An aneurysm is present if the diameter is >1.5 the normal size or the term ectasia is used for diameters 1.1–1.5.
- Patients with an aortic aneurysm have thinned aortic walls that are prone to dissect, often as a result of high blood pressure. Not all dissections involve patients with aortic dilatation.

Shown here is a biplane view of a patient with a dilated aortic root and a Type A dissection. The prominent intimal flap is seen prolapsing through the aortic valve during diastole in both the ME AV SAX and LAX views. This limited the amount of AI that occurred.

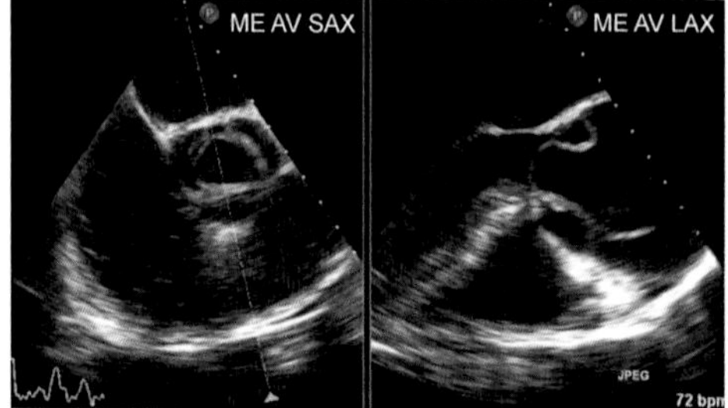

Pleural, Pericardial Effusion
(A) ME AV LAX view shows a pericardial effusion (arrows) that often forms from inflammation of the aortic wall or less often from aortic perforation of the false lumen. Rarely, cardiac tamponade may be present. (B) The presence of a left hemothorax may compromise ventilation, as shown in this Descending Aortic SAX view.

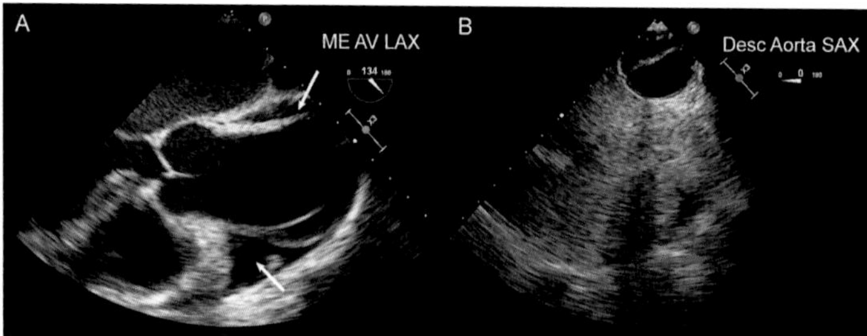

Coronary Malperfusion
(A) Flap invagination into the RCA (10–15%) or, less often, the left main coronary artery (arrow) may be seen in the ME AV SAX view. (B) Use color Doppler in the ME AV SAX view to assess flow in both arteries. Shown here is flow in the left main coronary artery (arrow) during systole in a type A dissection (double arrow). RCA involvement causes RV dysfunction and LV inferior RWMA. Global and regional LV systolic function should be assessed.

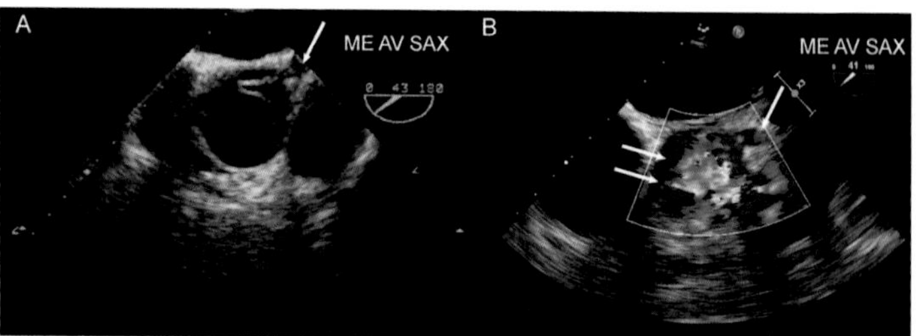

Mechanisms of Aortic Insufficiency (AI)

- AI occurs in 40–60% of type A dissections. Identification of the mechanism of AI has important implications as to whether the AV can be spared or needs to be replaced at the time of surgery.

A. The intimal tear dilates the aortic root and AV annulus causing failure of adequate cusp coaptation (arrow) with central AI.
B. An asymmetric intimal tear depresses one cusp below the coaptation line resulting in cusp prolapse (arrow) and eccentric AI.
C. Annular support is disrupted by the tear, resulting in a flail cusp and eccentric AI.
D. Prolapse of the intimal flap through the AV in diastole prevents cusp coaptation resulting in a variable amount of AI.

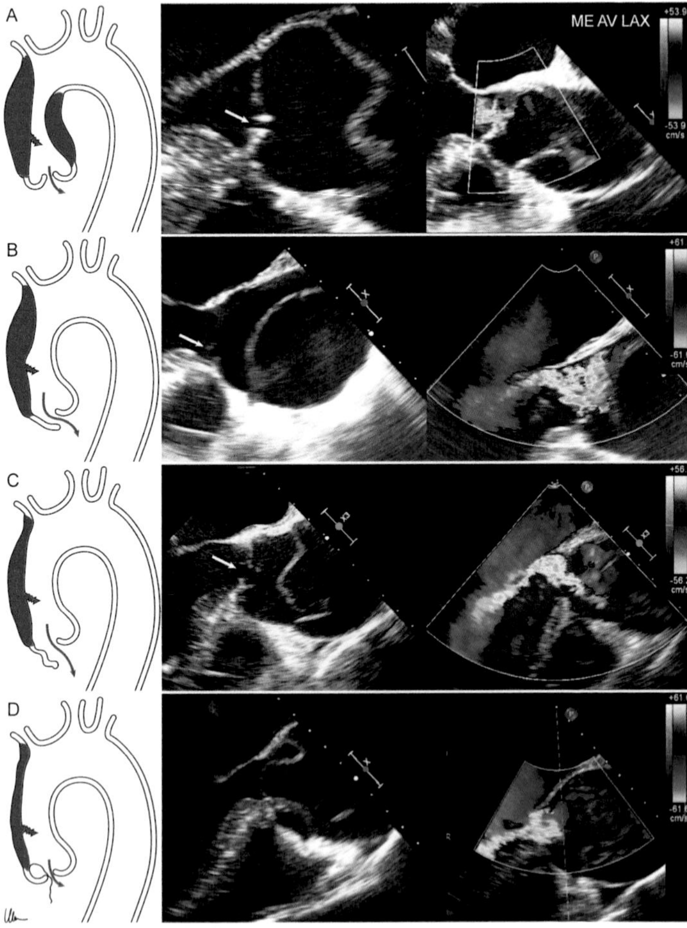

TEE Post-Dissection Repair

- The role of TEE in post-aortic dissection repair is mostly to assess aortic valve function (native or prosthetic) and flow in the true lumen.
- The proximal intimal tear is eliminated.
- The false lumen may thrombose or have persistent flow through multiple entry and exit points.

TEE Post-Dissection
Aortic valve function
AI severity
Paravalvular leak
LV function
Flow in aorta
Entry/re-entry

Cannulation

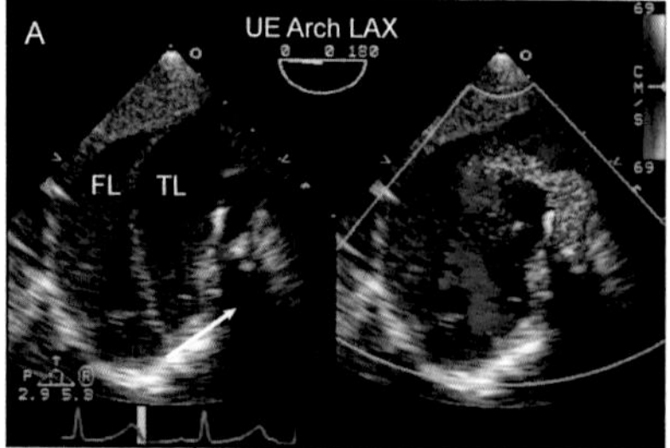

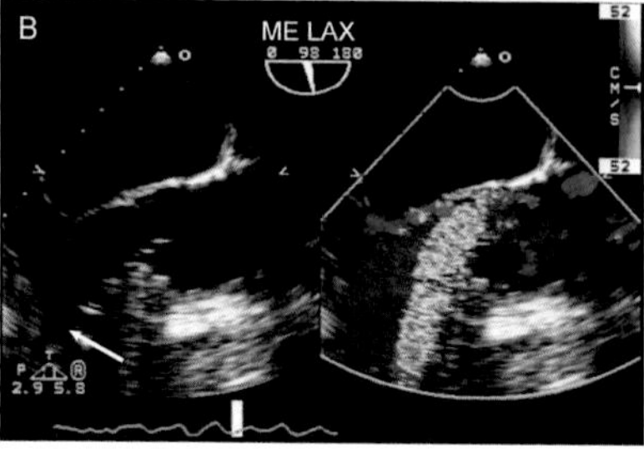

- Typically, a sternotomy is safely performed followed by venous cannulation of the right atrium. Rarely, femoral-femoral CPB may be required prior to sternotomy if there is an associated large aneurysm.
- Arterial cannulation is crucial for cerebral protection and may involve the use of peripheral or central arteries.
- Femoral artery cannulation of the true lumen permits retrograde flow into the descending aorta and antegrade flow through arch vessels.
- Subclavian/axillary/common carotid artery cannulation allows antegrade arch perfusion with improved neurological outcome. (A) UE Arch LAX view shows the correct position of an axillary artery cannula in the true lumen.
- Ascending aorta by direct cannulation of true lumen with ultrasound guidance is followed by circulatory arrest.
- LV apex cannulation allows antegrade perfusion followed by circulatory arrest. This location is chosen if the peripheral vessels are small. (B) ME LAX view shows an apical LV cannula with continuous flow by color Doppler.

Surgical Repair

- Surgical repair of a Type A aortic dissection depends on the location of the tear and whether there is aortic arch and/or AV involvement. Repair involves using a Dacron graft to replace the aorta from the location of the initial intimal tear.
- Identification of arch involvement is important as a tear in this region can lead to early aneurysm formation or rupture. The risk is higher if the intimal flap is circumferential, or the tear enters one or more branch vessels.
- Moderate to severe AI needs to be addressed during surgery. Most often, the AV can be spared, but if not it is replaced. The mechanisms of AI were previously described. Right/non-commissural cusp prolapse is the most common location.

Shown below are surgical photos of (A) aortic dissection with thrombus in lumen, (B) simple repair using a Dacron graft, and (C) complex hemiarch repair.

	Simple Repair	Intermediate	Complex Repair
Arch	Not involved	Involved	Involved
AV	Not involved	Not involved	Involved
Repair	Tube graft from STJ to ascending aorta	Tube graft from STJ to hemiarch	Valve sparing root procedure or Bentall + hemiarch

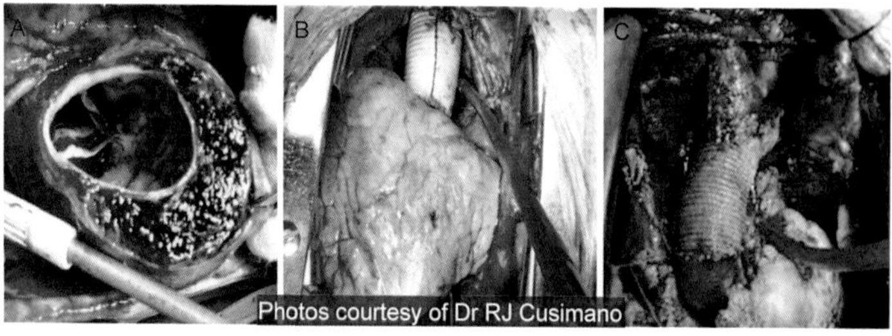

Photos courtesy of Dr RJ Cusimano

10
Congenital Heart Disease

Page

A. Vegas, *Perioperative Two-Dimensional Transesophageal Echocardiography*, https://doi.org/10.1007/978-3-319-60902-7_10

- Congenital heart disease (CHD) is a problem in the structure of the heart that is present at birth.
- Congenital heart lesions may have normal or abnormal relationships of chambers, valves, and vessels that may alter blood flow in the heart.
- Different classification systems exist for CHD.

Classification CHD
Cyanotic (blue) or acyanotic
Simple or complex lesions
Physiologic
Anatomic
Embryologic

Acyanotic	**Cyanotic**
VSD	D-TGA
ASD	TAPVD
PDA	Truncus Arteriosus
Pulmonic Stenosis	TOF
Coarctation	Tricuspid Atresia
Ebstein's Anomaly	Univentricle

Physiologic Congenital Heart Disease Classification

1. Septal defects
    - Atrial septal defects (ASD)
    - Ventricular septal defects (VSD)
    - Atrioventricular septal defects (A-V canal defects)
2. Disorders of mitral valve inflow
    - Anomalous pulmonary venous drainage (total-TAPVD, partial-PAPVD)
    - Cor-Triatriatum
    - Mitral stenosis: supravalvular, parachute
    - Mitral atresia
3. Diseases of left ventricular outflow tract (LVOT)
    - Subaortic, supravalvular stenosis
    - Valvular stenosis
    - Sinus of Valsalva aneurysm
4. Diseases of aorta
    - Patent ductus arteriosus (PDA)
    - Coarctation of the aorta, aortic atresia
    - Truncus arteriosus
    - Vascular anomalies
5. Diseases of tricuspid valve
    - Ebstein's anomaly
    - Tricuspid atresia
6. Diseases of right ventricular outflow tract (RVOT)
    - Subvalvular: tetralogy of fallot (TOF)
    - Valvular: stenosis, pulmonic atresia
7. Chambers and valves are in *abnormal* sequence
    - Atrioventricular discordance (corrected transposition)
    - Ventriculo-great arterial discordance (transposition of great vessels)
    - Double-inlet ventricle (with univentricular heart)
    - Double-outlet right and left ventricles

Normal Connections	Abnormal Connections
Shunt predominates	Atria and ventricles
Atrial septal defects	Double-inlet right ventricle
Ventricular septal defects	– Univentricular heart
Patent ductus arteriosus	Atrioventricular discordance
Stenosis or obstruction predominates	– Corrected transposition
Absent atrioventricular connections	Ventricles and great vessels
– Tricuspid + mitral atresia	Tetralogy of Fallot
Absent ventriculo-great arterial connections	Truncus arteriosus
– Pulmonic + aortic atresia	Double-outlet right/left ventricles
Obstructed great arteries	Ventriculo-great arterial discordance
– Coarctation of aorta	– Transposition of great vessels
Obstructed venous inflow	
– Total anomalous pulmonary venous return	
Anomalous valve position	
Ebstein's anomaly	

Surgery in CHD

- Refined surgical techniques have improved survival for even the most complex of congenital lesions; with 85% of infants with CHD surviving to adulthood. As a result, there is a growing population of adult congenital heart disease (ACHD) or grown-up congenital heart (GUCH) patients.
- Repair of CHD offers three options: correction, partial correction, or palliation.
- Corrective surgery establishes an anatomically normal sequence of blood flow.
- Surgery is considered corrective only if ventricular function and life expectancy are normal, without the need for any further interventions. This applies to the minority of congenital lesions (ASD, VSD, PDA) that are corrected in childhood.
- Palliative surgery does not correct the lesion, but rather minimizes the problems for a given pathology. Most ACHD patients have been palliated, not corrected, and are still at risk of morbidity and mortality from their CHD.

TEE Imaging in Adult CHD

- Several approaches are used for performing a comprehensive TEE examination to acquire anatomic, functional, and hemodynamic information in a patient with CHD.
- These approaches use standard TEE views as well as additional off-axis views.

View-Based Approach

- This is based on obtaining in any sequence the specific 28 predefined views as defined by the ASE.
- Each view is examined for the presence of pathology and the findings of all the views are integrated into an overall assessment.

Structure-Based Approach

- This focuses on TEE imaging of cardiovascular structures of interest using complementary views to permit a detailed examination.
- This type of exam may be useful if only a limited amount of time is available.

Sequential-Segmental Approach

- This methodically interrogates the three major cardiac segments (atria, ventricles, and great arteries) and their relationships to each other (connections or alignments between the segments), to define a patient's anatomy.
- In this setting, one follows the course of blood as it flows through the heart. The exam begins with identifying inflow into the subpulmonic structures.

Indications for TEE in Pediatric CHD
Diagnostic Indications • Suspected CHD, nondiagnostic TTE • PFO + shunt direction (agitated saline contrast) – Etiology for stroke – Right-to-left shunt, before transvenous pacemaker • Evaluate baffles after Fontan, Senning, or Mustard procedure • Aortic dissection • Evaluate for vegetation or suspected abscess • Evaluate intracardiac thrombus before cardioversion • Evaluate pericardial effusion or cardiac function evaluation in postoperative patient with open sternum or poor acoustic windows • Evaluate prosthetic valve **Perioperative Indications** • Immediate preoperative definition of cardiac anatomy + function • Postoperative surgical results + function **TEE-guided Interventions** • Guide placement of ASD or VSD occlusion device • Guide blade or balloon atrial septostomy • Catheter tip placement for valve perforation and dilation • Guide radiofrequency ablation procedure • Results of minimally invasive or video-assisted cardiac procedure
ASD atrial septal defect, *CHD* congenital heart disease, *PFO* patent foramen ovale, *TTE* transthoracic echocardiography, *VSD* ventricular septal defect **Source: Ayres N, et al. J Am Soc Echocardiogr 2005;18:91–8**

Segmental Approach Overview

- Echocardiography in ACHD is challenging as it requires integration and understanding of (1) altered anatomy, (2) compensatory changes, (3) associated lesions, and (4) surgical correction(s) during scanning.
- The sequential-segmental approach is a standardized systematic four-step process, which does not rely on embryology and identifies the descriptive terminology used in ACHD. Familiarity with CHD terminology is required to effectively communicate findings.

Segmental Approach 4 Step Process

1. **Determine Cardiac Sidedness (Situs)**

This relates to the position of the morphologic RA relative to other structures.

- Situs (arrangement): solitus (usual, R of LA), inversus (mirror image, L of LA), ambiguous (R or L)
- Abdominal situs: solitus (usual), inversus (mirror), heterotaxia (different)

2. **Determine Cardiac Position**

- Based on the cardiac position in the thorax: dextro/meso/levo-position
- Based on the cardiac apex orientation: dextro/meso/levo-cardia

3. **Identify 3 Segments**

Each cardiac chamber has intrinsic morphologic features that help define it as right or left, irrespective of whether it supports the systemic or pulmonic circulation.

- Atrial segments are differentiated by the atrial appendage appearance
- Ventricular segments are differentiated as described below
- Arterial segments: PA bifurcates into LPA/RPA
  Aorta originate the coronaries and head vessels.

Right Atrium Morphology		**Left Atrium Morphology**
Appendage wide neck, triangular Extensive pectinate muscles in RAA Terminal crest (crista terminalis) Valves of IVC and coronary sinus		Appendage narrow neck hook-like Smooth walled except for appendage No terminal crest
	Right Ventricle	**Left Ventricle**
Atrioventricular valve	Trileaflet	Bileaflet (unless cleft leaflet)
Chordal attachment	To the septum	Not to the septum
Annulus location	More apical	More basal
Apex	Prominent	Less prominent trabeculations
Moderator band	Present	Absent
Infundibulum	Present	Absent
Ventricular size, shape and wall thickness does not distinguish the RV and LV. Morphologically indeterminate ventricle: coarse trabeculations + no IVS (univentricular heart) Tricuspid valve always attaches to the RV, Mitral valve always to the LV		

4. **Define the Connections**

A connection is the anatomic (physical) link between two structures, whereas drainage is the hemodynamic blood flow direction.

Atrioventricular Connection

- Concordant: RA to RV, LA to LV
- Discordant: RA to LV, LA to RV
- Ambiguous: isomeric
- Double inlet (univentricular) has A-V valves from one ventricle, with three possible connections: absent R (mostly LV), absent L (mostly RV), indeterminate
- Atrioventricular valve (A-V) morphology: straddling, overriding, stenotic, regurgitant, dysplastic, imperforate

Ventriculo-Arterial Connection

Two arterial trunks:

- Concordant: RV to PA, LV to Aorta
- Discordant: RV to Aorta, LV to PA
  Valve morphology: AV always attaches to aorta, PV always attaches to PA
- Double outlet: both great vessels originate from one ventricle: one arterial trunk + ½ more than half of the other trunk is connected to the same ventricle

One arterial trunk:

- Single outlet: truncus arteriosus (Types I–IV)
- Outflow tract: muscular (RVOT), fibrous (LVOT)

Segmental Approach Congenital Heart Disease

1. Determine Cardiac Sidedness (Situs)

Based on position of morphological RA

Situs Solitus
RA lies to right of LA

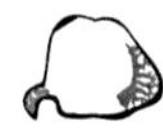

Situs Inversus
RA lies to left of LA

Situs Ambiguous
Indeterminant/Isomersim
Paired mirror image sets of normally single non identical organs

Right	Left
R Bronchi (x2)	L Bronchi (x2)
R Atria (x2)	L Atria (x2)
No spleen	Polyspleen

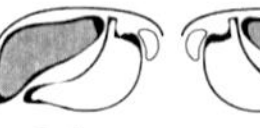

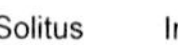

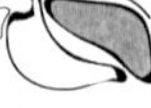

Abdominal Situs
Position of major unpaired organs

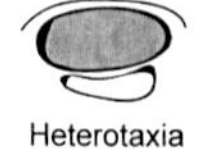

2. Determine Cardiac Position

Cardiac Position
Based on position in thorax

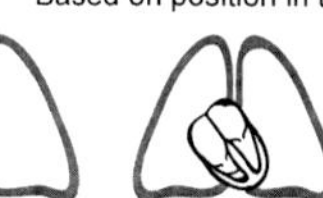

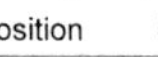

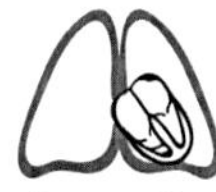

Cardiac Orientation
Base to apex axis

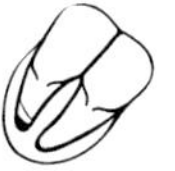

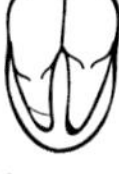

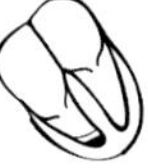

3. Identify 3 Segments

Atrial Segment

Right
- Triangular RAA
- Broad based RAA
- Terminal crest
- Pectinate muscles
- (SVC/IVC)

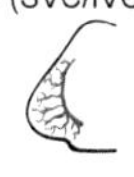

Left
- Narrow LAA
- Hook shaped
- No terminal crest

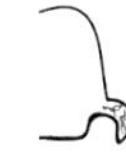

Ventricular Segment

TV/RV
- Apical SLTV*
- SLTV* chords IVS
- Coarse trabecula
- Moderator band
- Supraventricular crest

*Septal Leaflet Tricuspid Valve

MV/LV
- Fibrous continuity
- No chords to IVS

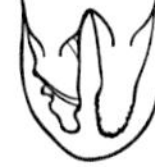

Arterial Segment

Pulmonary Trunk
- Bifurcation to RPA and LPA

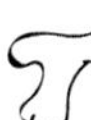

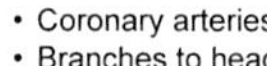

Aorta
- Coronary arteries
- Branches to head

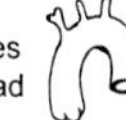

4. Define the Connections

Veno-Atrial
- IVC/SVC
- Pulmonary veins

Atrio-Ventricular

Concordant
- RA → RV
- LA → LV

Discordant
- RA → LV
- LA → RV

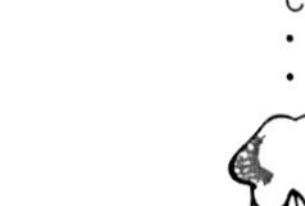

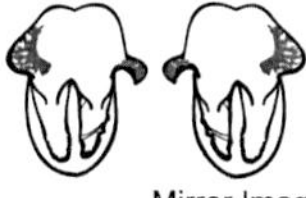

Ventriculo-Arterial

Discordant
- RV → Aorta
- LV → PA

Concordant
- RV → PA
- LV → Aorta

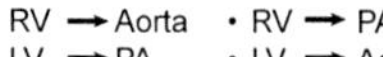

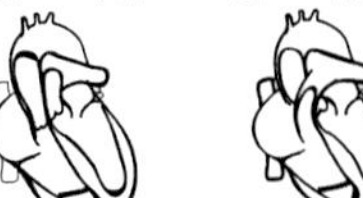

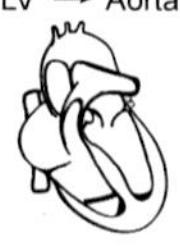

Double Inlet Ventricle
Connection of both AV valves to predominantly one ventricle

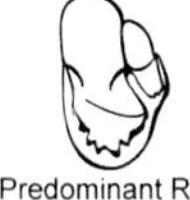

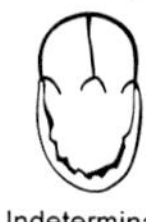

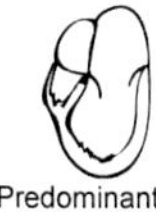

Double Outlet Ventricle
Both great arteries arise from predominantly one ventricle

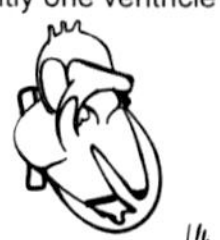

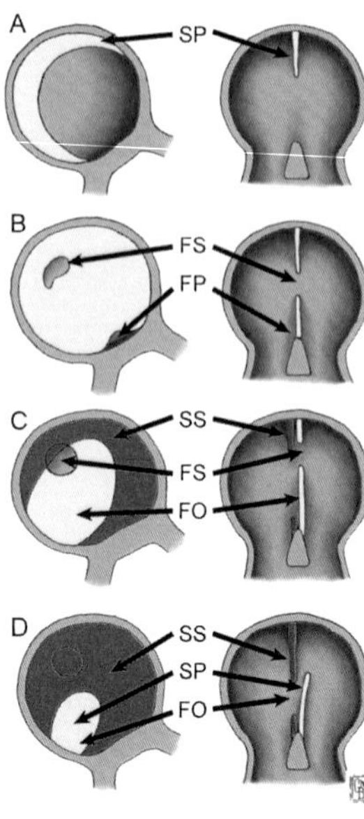

Embryology of the Inter-Atrial Septum (IAS)

A. Formation begins with the septum primum (SP) growing down from the dorsocranial wall of the atria towards the endocardial cushions. Above the endocardial cushions, a space, the foramen primum (FP) remains.

B. Perforations appear in the upper SP and form the foramen secundum (FS); this allows for partial reabsorption of the SP.

C. The septum secundum (SS) grows from the ventrocranial wall and covers the FS and FP. But leaves an opening, the foramen ovale (FO), which is covered by the septum primum (SP).

D. The upper septum disappears and the lower portion becomes the valve of the foramen ovale.

Normal Variants of the IAS

(**A**) Lipomatous hypertrophy is a benign fatty infiltration of the surrounding tissue of the IAS with sparing of the thin membranous fossa ovalis.

(**B**) IAS aneurysm (arrow) is defined by a mobile IAS with excursions of >10 mm from the plane of the IAS or a total excursion of >15 mm as shown with mMode in the ME Bicaval view. The hypermobile IAS may be associated with a PFO and an increased risk of stroke. A prominent Eustachian valve is also seen in this patient.

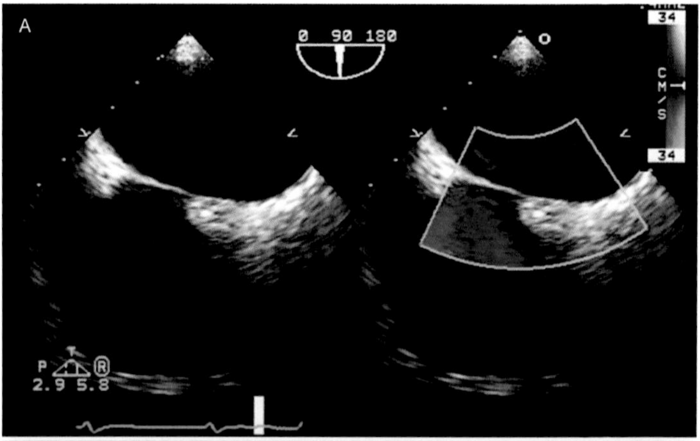

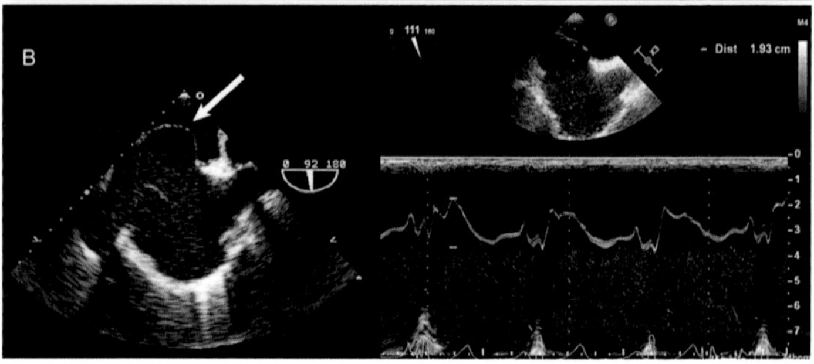

Standard TEE views of the IAS include the (**A–C**) ME 4C, (**D**) ME RVOT, (**E**) bicaval, and (**F**) right upper pulmonary vein (RUPV) (see p. 19). In the ME 4C view, the parallel alignment of the imaging plane to the IAS makes the tissue appear thin and absent from dropout. Advancing and withdrawing the probe helps image most of the IAS as (**A**) high near the aortic valve, (**B**) mid near the mitral valve, and (**C**) low near the tricuspid valve. (**D**) ME RVOT view shows the IAS at 60° with the AV in the center. (**E**) The optimal view for imaging the IAS is the bicaval view as the image plane is perpendicular to the IAS tissue with the fossa ovalis in the display center. There is good spectral Doppler alignment to assess flow through the IAS. (**F**) Modifying the view by increasing the angle and rotating the probe right can better image the SVC and IVC regions and drainage of the RUPV into the LA.

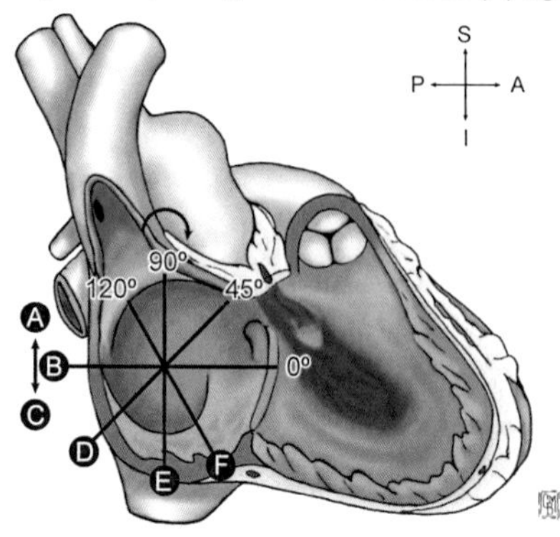

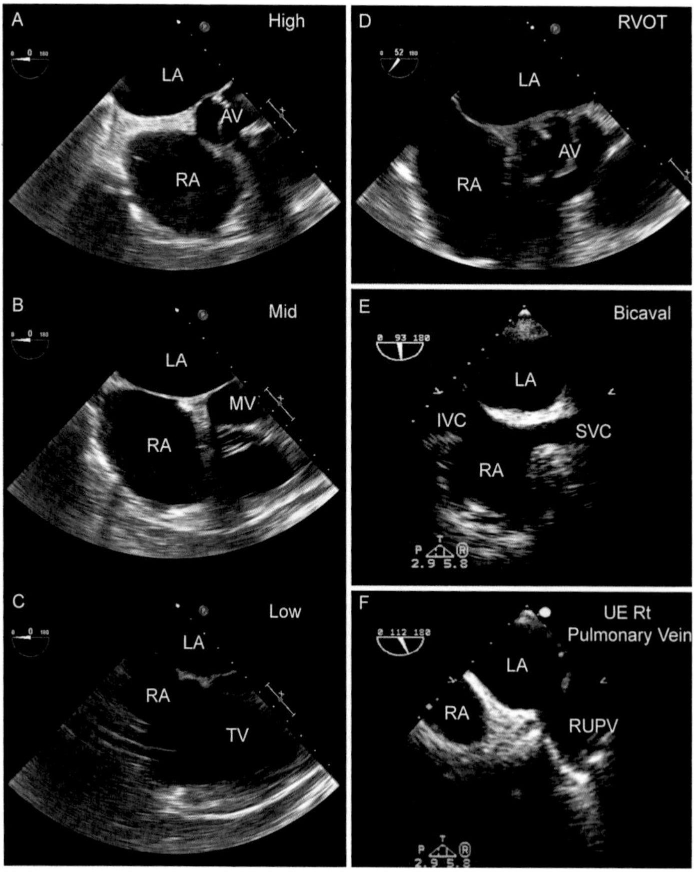

Atrial Septal Defects

- A true ASD by definition should have an absence of IAS tissue. Not all inter-atrial shunts involve a deficiency of IAS tissue, thus these should not be classified as an ASD.
- True ASDs involve defects in different portions of the IAS.
- There may be associated findings.

Atrial Shunts	
Deficiency IAS tissue	(%)
Secundum ASD	70
Primum ASD	20
No deficiency IAS tissue	
Sinus venosus defect	5
Coronary sinus defect	Rare
Patent foramen ovale (PFO)	20–25

2D Imaging

- 2D views (ME 4C, RVOT, bicaval, RUPV)
- Type, location, size of defect
- Volume overload is proportional to the defect size, results in a dilated right side:
  - RA, PA dilate from the increased flow
  - RV is dilated with paradoxical motion and flattening of the IVS, RVH if ↑ PAP
- Associated lesions: Primum (cleft MV), Secundum (MV prolapse), Sinus Venosus (PAPVD)
- Agitated saline contrast (bubble) study is sensitive in diagnosing shunt.
- Atrial septal aneurysms may have a shunt.
- PFO occur in 25% of patients, some only shunt R to L post-Valsalva maneuver.
- Device closure is used for PFO, secundum (≤38 mm) defect with rim of tissue.

Doppler

- Color: laminar vs. turbulent flow, ± reduce Nyquist limit <30 cm/s
  - Direction of shunt (usually L→R, R→L, bidirectional)
- PW of IAS defect shows continuous phasic flow (see p. 228)
- TR is often present from TV annulus dilatation
  - Estimate RVSP (for the presence of pulmonary hypertension)
- PI if dilated PA, may have turbulent flow in the PA from ↑ flow
- MR if cleft mitral valve leaflet
- Identify drainage of all four pulmonary veins into LA
- Qp/Qs shunt ratio by measuring the stroke volume at different sites (see p. 61).
  - ASD: Qp is PA/Qs is aortic or mitral valve
  - Hemodynamically significant shunt is >1.5:1.

Patent Foramen Ovale (PFO)

- This is a small flap-like opening in the IAS between the septum primum and the septum secundum; as there is no tissue deficiency, this is not a true ASD.
- In the ME bicaval or AV SAX views, look for small gap (flap) in the IAS
- Confirm flow with color Doppler (see image below)
  - R→L flow termed "PFO", without deficiency in IAS tissue
  - L→R flow termed "stretched PFO", atrial pressure creates a gap in IAS tissue
- Saline contrast (SC)/Bubble study (see p. 228)
- Incidence PFO:
  25% autopsy
  +5–10% TEE color
  +5% SC at rest
  +25% SC cough, Valsalva
- PFO identification is important in patients with:
  - Stroke to determine source of embolism
  - Refractory hypoxemia
  - VADs (avoid hypoxemia)
- Management of the finding of an incidental PFO is controversial particularly for closed cardiac procedures.
- PFO can be closed using a percutaneous device.

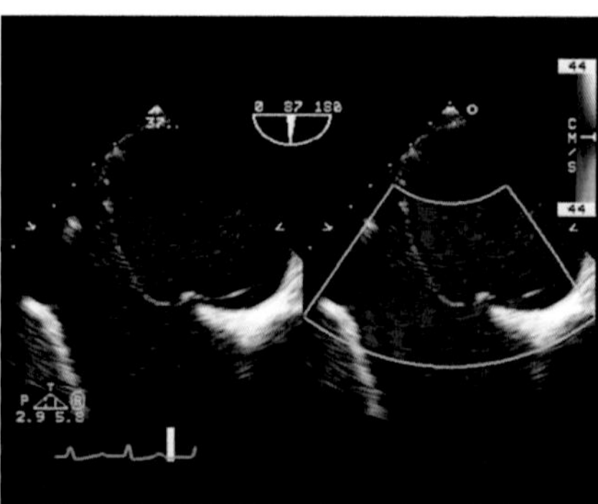

What to Tell the Surgeon ASD	
PreCPB • Defect type • Single or multiple defects • Location, size of defect • Identify all four pulmonary veins • RV size and function • RA, PA size • RVSP from TR jet • Shunt fraction (Qp:Qs) • Agitated saline contrast (bubble) study • Associated lesions – MV prolapse – Cleft A-V valve (regurgitation) – PAPVD	**PostCPB** • Persistent shunt post-repair • RV function • RVSP from TR jet Primum repair • Atrioventricular valve regurgitation Sinus Venosus Repair • SVC patency • RUPV drains into LA • Persistent shunt post-repair
Source: Silvestry FE, et al. J Am Soc Echocardiogr 2015;28:910–58	

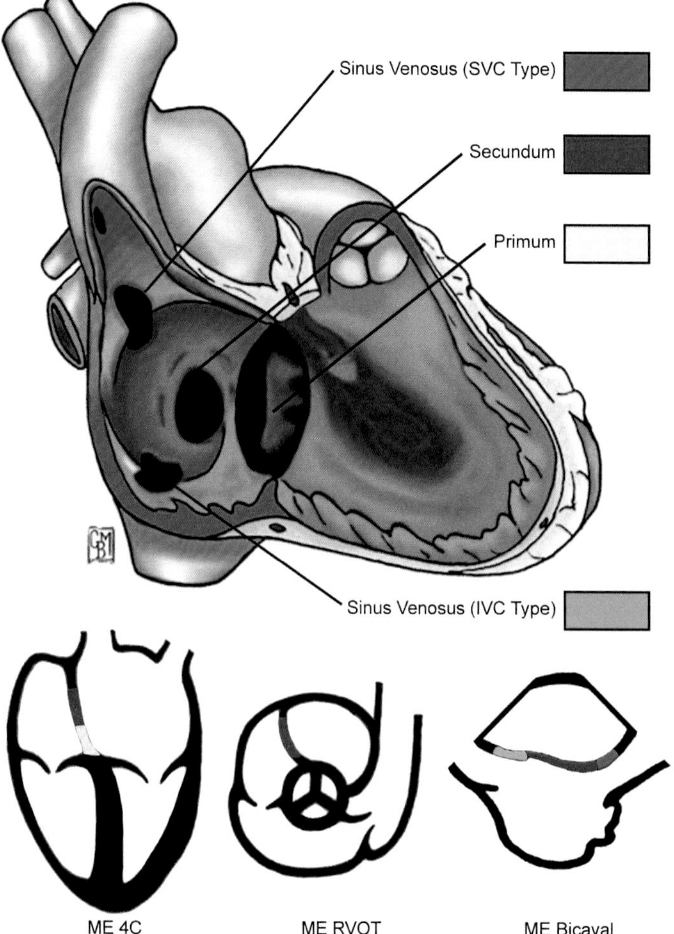

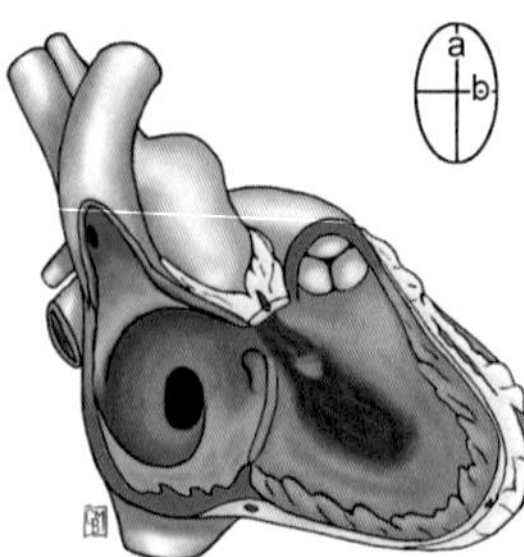

ASD Secundum

- Commonest type of ASD (80%)
- Located in center of IAS within the fossa ovalis
- Bound on all sides by tissue, results from deficiency of septum primum tissue
- Round or elliptical in shape
  a. Major axis (bicaval view)
  b. Minor axis (RVOT view)
- May be isolated or part of complex congenital heart lesions
- Associated with mitral valve prolapse (30%), PAPVD right pulmonary veins (rare)

- ME 4C, AV SAX, RVOT, Bicaval view
- IAS gap (measure size, oval shape)
- Color Doppler (Nyquist 50–70 cm/s)
  - Laminar flow (large non-restrictive)
  - Turbulent flow (small restrictive)
- PW Doppler
  - Low velocity <1.5 m/s
  - Peak velocity inverse relation to size
  - Direction of flow, biphasic
    - ◊ L→R in midsystole + diastole
    - ◊ Flow reversal early systole (arrow) may worsen R→L shunt with IPPV

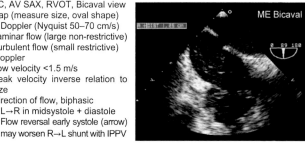

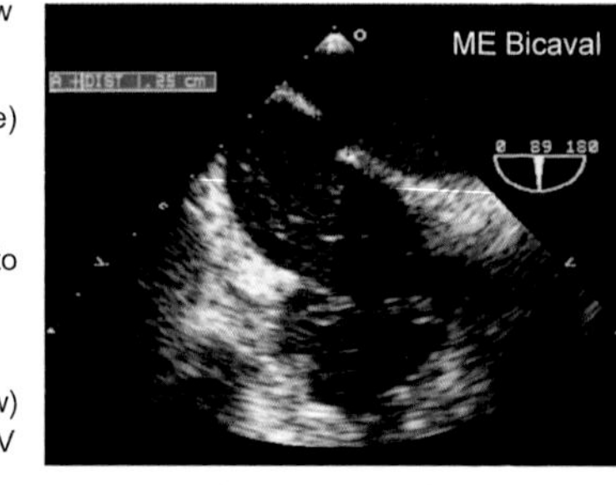

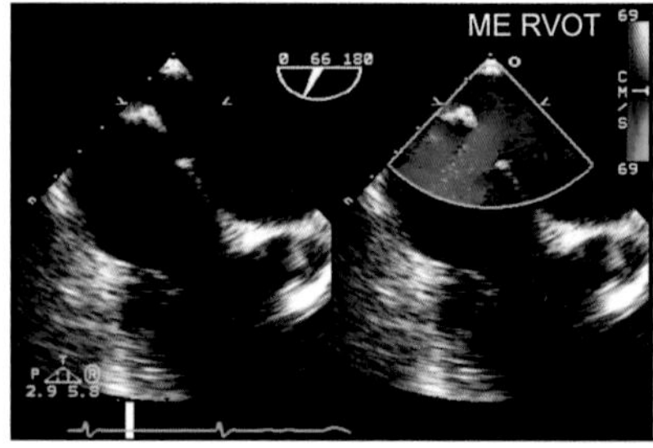

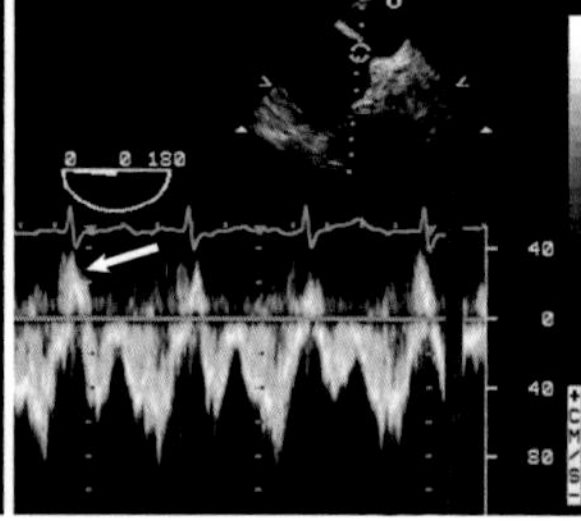

Saline Contrast/Bubble Study

Saline contrast may help to detect an intra-cardiac shunt. Typically, 1 cc of air is agitated with 5–9 cc of saline, propofol, or blood through a three-way stopcock using two syringes and injected rapidly through a peripheral vein. At rest, the RAP is usually less than the LAP, so bubbles will only opacify the RA.

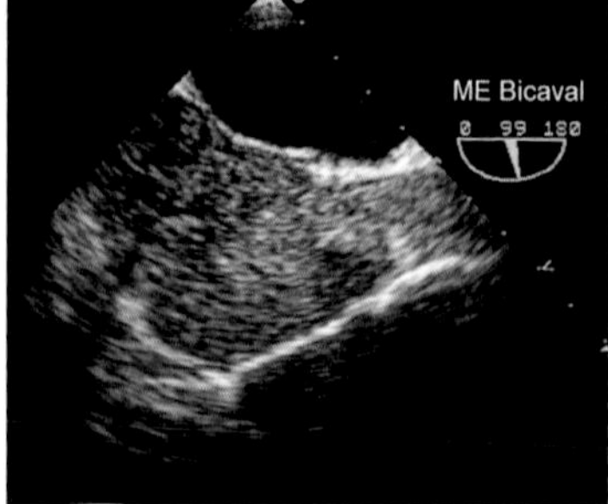

To demonstrate a shunt, the RAP is elevated by either a cough in a spontaneously breathing patient or a Valsalva maneuver in a ventilated patient.

- A positive contrast study occurs with the presence of microbubbles in the LA within five heartbeats. This indicates right to left shunting. A false positive study may occur in the presence of a pulmonary arterial-venous malformation.
- A negative contrast study represents no flow of bubbles across the IAS.
- However, if there is left to right shunting, non-contrasted blood will appear in the contrast-filled RA to identify a shunt.

Device Closure

A transvenous percutaneous-delivered umbrella device placed across the IAS is now the preferred method to close an ASD secundum or large PFO. Suitability for device closure is a defect size <40 mm with a sufficient rim (>5 mm) of IAS tissue to ensure stable device deployment and avoid complications. Specific TEE views can define the tissue rim. TEE may guide device insertion, but this requires a general anesthetic. Multiple septal defects may require the use of additional devices. Post-deployment, the device is assessed for stability and for residual shunt flow. A small shunt may be present which resolves after endothelialization of the device.

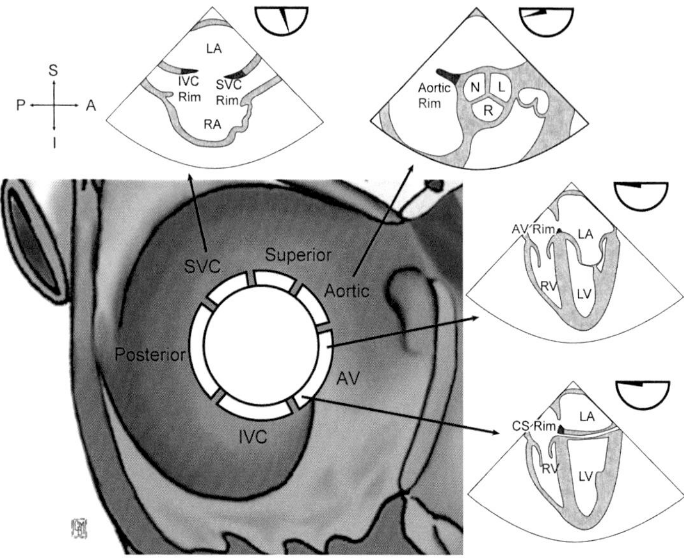

View	Structure	IAS Rim
ME 4C (0°)	TV, MV	Anterior-inferior
ME 4C (0°) low	Coronary sinus	Inferior
ME RVOT (45°)	Aorta, AV	Anterior-superior
ME Bicaval (90°)	SVC, IVC	Posterior-superior/inferior

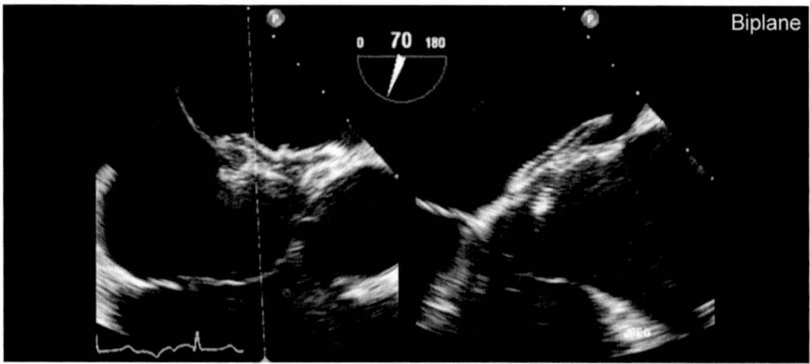

Suitable ASD Anatomy	Device Complications
Defect size ≤40 mm	Clot, thrombus
Tissue rim ≥5 mm	Device instability
PA pressure ≤2/3 systemic	Erosion (Aorta → LA fistula)
PVR is reversible, or ≤2/3 systemic	Residual shunt

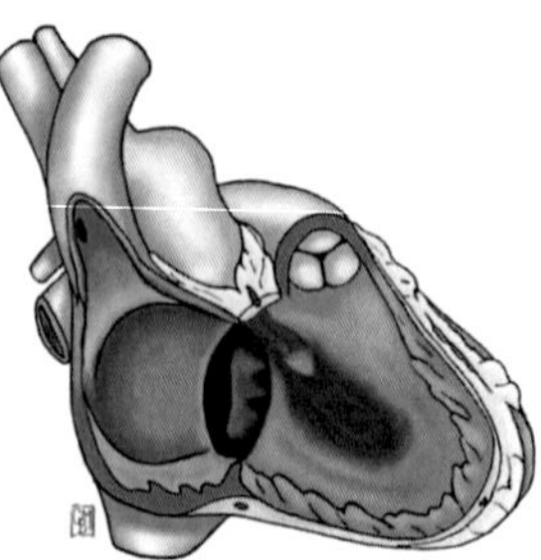

Primum ASD

- Second commonest type of ASD (20%)
- Located in the inferior portion of the IAS, involves the atrioventricular septum
- Atrioventricular valves in the same plane
- Form of endocardial cushion defect, also called A-V canal defect (see p. 231)
- Associated defects:
  - Atrioventricular valve abnormal (cleft MV)
  - Subaortic stenosis
  - Double orifice MV
  - Coarctation of aorta
  - PDA, TOF

2-D Image (ME 4C View)

- Absence of IAS above the atrioventricular valves
- Both atrioventricular valves (MV, TV) are in the same plane
- Measure largest gap with and without color
- RA, RV, PA dilated

Color Doppler

- Color turbulent (restricted) or laminar (unrestricted) flow
  - Usually L→R, through defect, may be R→L or bidirectional
- Atrioventricular valve regurgitation: systemic (MV → MR), venous (TV → TR)

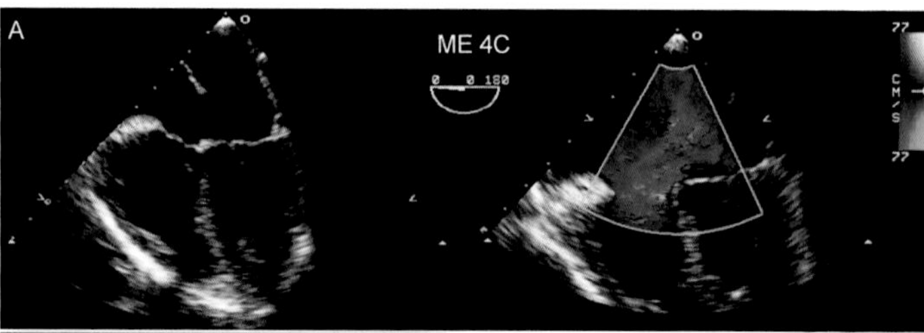

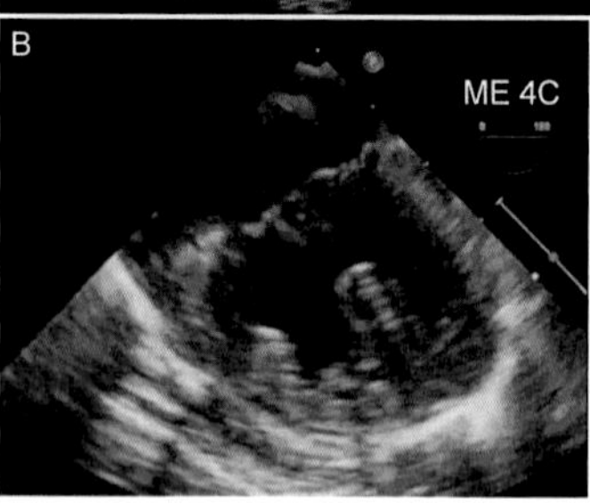

(**A**) ME 4C view with color Doppler shows a defect in the IAS above the atrioventricular valves, which both insert into the IVS at the same level. The laminar blue flow, despite the high Nyquist, (77 cm/s) suggests a large unrestricted primum ASD. No VSD is present.
(**B**) ME 4C view shows a complete atrioventricular (A-V) canal defect including a primum ASD and a VSD. A common bridging atrioventricular valve is present (see pg 231)

What to Tell the Surgeon Primum ASD	
PreCPB	**PostCPB**
• Defect type ASD, (±VSD) • Single or multiple: location, size • Doppler: direction of flow • RV size and function • RA, PA size • RVSP from TR jet • Atrioventricular valve: type, function • Septal chordae: LVOT obstruction • Mitral regurgitation • Associated lesions	• Persistent shunt post-repair • RV function • RVSP • Residual A-V valve regurgitation, stenosis • LVOT obstruction

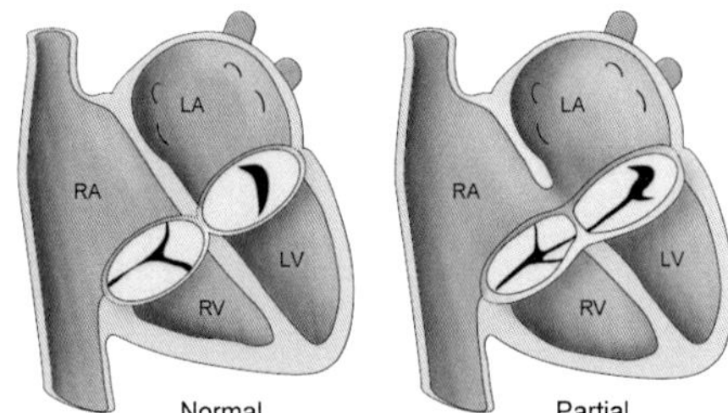

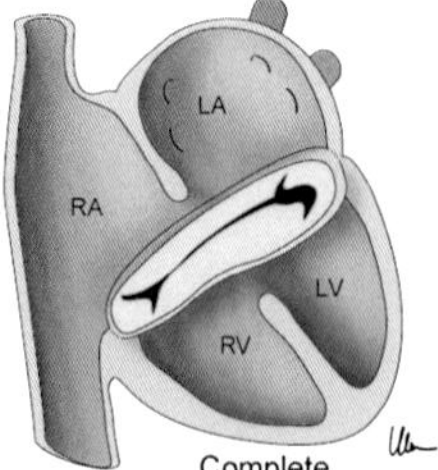

Atrioventricular Septal Defect (AVSD)

- AVSD is also referred to as "common A-V canal" or endocardial cushion defects
- This pathology encompasses a spectrum of defects of the IAS and IVS and lesions of the atrioventricular (A-V) valve:
  - Complete: single annulus, common A-V valve, primum ASD, inlet VSD
  - Intermediate: single annulus, A-V valve two orifices, primum ASD, inlet VSD
  - Partial: two annuli, cleft left A-V valve, primum ASD
- Associated defects: TOF, double-outlet RV, total PAPVD, pulmonary atresia

Common Atrioventricular (A-V) Valve

- There is a common A-V valve annulus, with two orifices. The leaflets covering the orifice are abnormal with two bridging leaflets (superior and inferior) in place of the anterior mitral valve and septal tricuspid valve leaflets.
- The "cleft" is the apposition line between septal attachments of superior and inferior bridging leaflets in the right A-V valve (tricuspid) and left A-V valve (or mitral).
- Leaflet chordae may directly attach the leaflet to the IVS. These chordae can be seen in the ME 5C and ME AV LAX view. Turbulent flow may be seen in the LVOT using color Doppler.

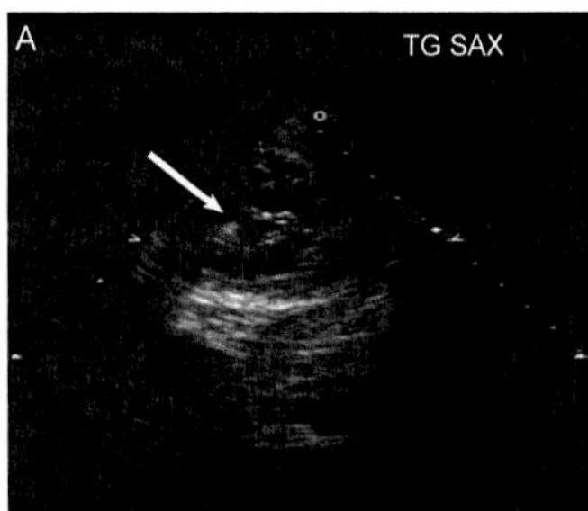

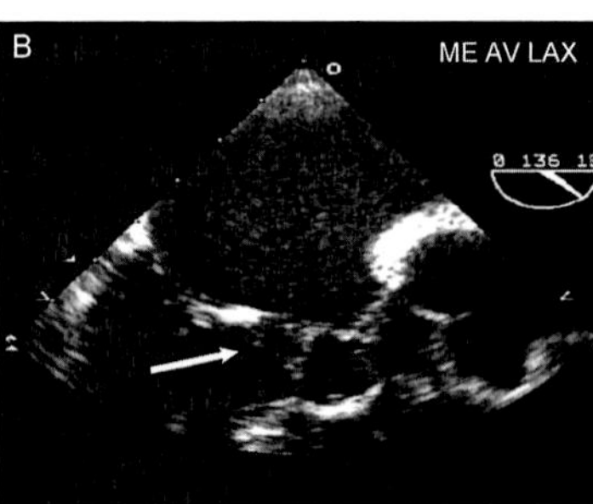

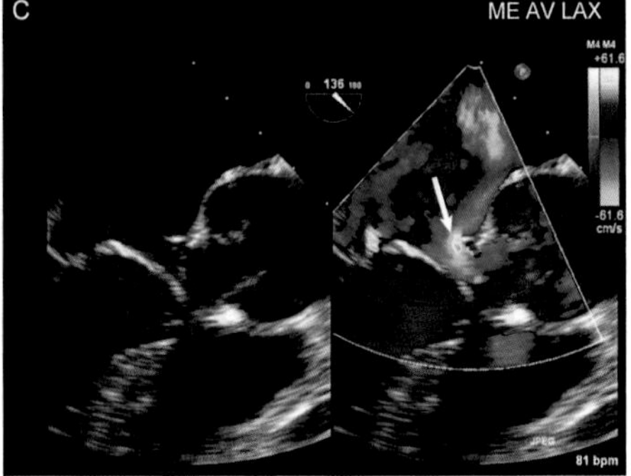

Partial AVSD examples. (**A**) Basal TG view shows the slit-like gap in the left A-V valve (arrow). (**B**) ME AV LAX view shows abnormal chordae attachment of leaflet tissue to the base of the IVS. (**C**) ME AV LAX view shows the abnormal chordal attachments to the IVS and cleft in the left A-V valve. Color Doppler shows an eccentric regurgitant jet (arrow) that originates at the cleft and another jet at the point of coaptation.

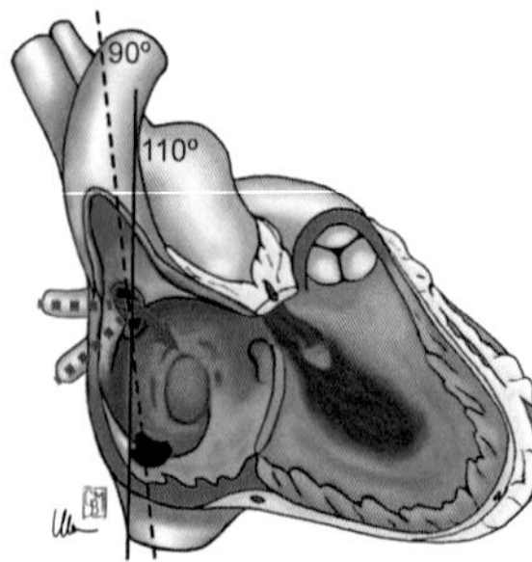

Sinus Venosus Defect

- This is not a true ASD (8%) as there is no defect in IAS tissue.
- This is a defect in the sinus venosus septum between the vena cava (SVC, IVC) and right pulmonary veins.
- This pathology has normal right pulmonary vein connections to the LA, but with abnormal drainage into the RA, which is termed partial anomalous pulmonary vein drainage (PAPVD).
    - SVC type defect: RUPV, RLPV
    - IVC type defect: RLPV

Modified bicaval view (109°) shows a discontinuity in the vena cava. (**A**) SVC type is seen between LA, SVC, and RA with the RPA in view. (**B**) Advancing the probe towards the liver images the IVC type. Measure the defect size (arrow). Color Doppler shows laminar blue flow from an unrestricted L→R shunt in both of these cases.

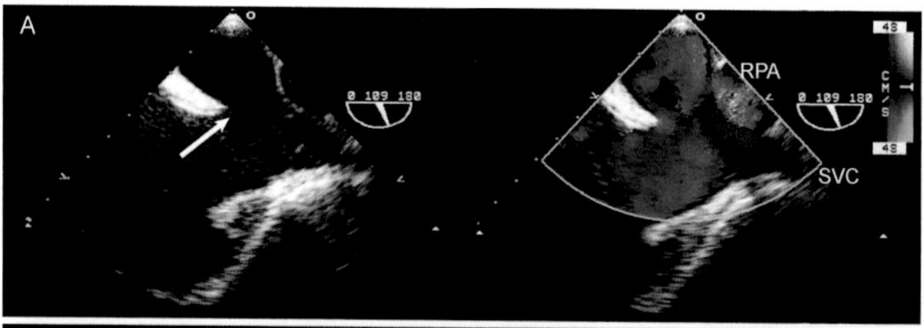

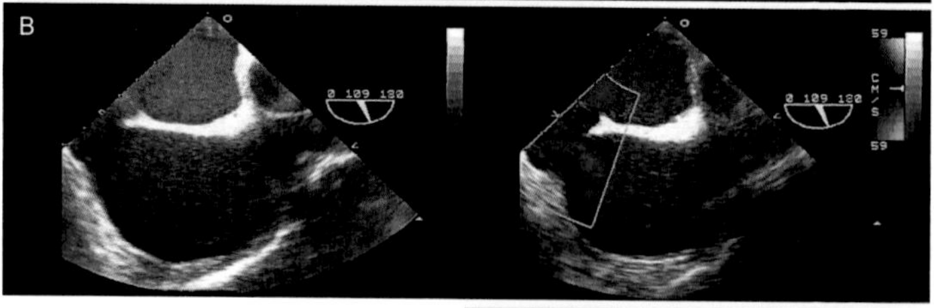

PAPVD of the RUPV may occur with the SVC type sinus venosus defect. (**C**) The teardrop sign in which the SVC assumes this shape is seen in the modified ME Ascending Aorta SAX view. Color Doppler shows flow from the RUPV into the SVC. (**D**) Color Doppler shows RUPV (red) flow enters the confluence of LA, SVC, and RA, with atrial flow going from the LA to RA (blue). (**E**) Post-repair, the RUPV (arrow) drains into the LA, while SVC flow enters the RA.

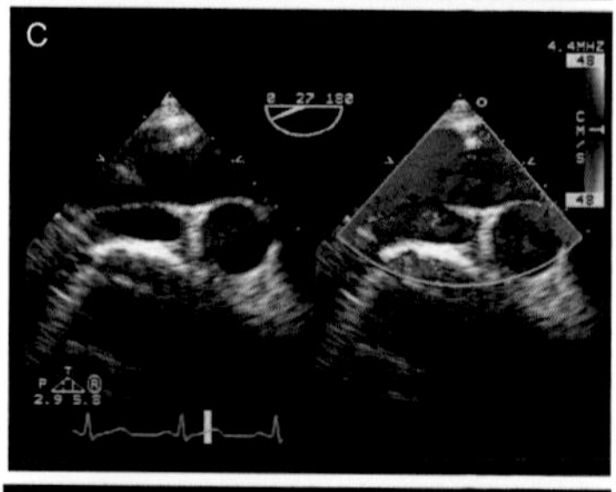

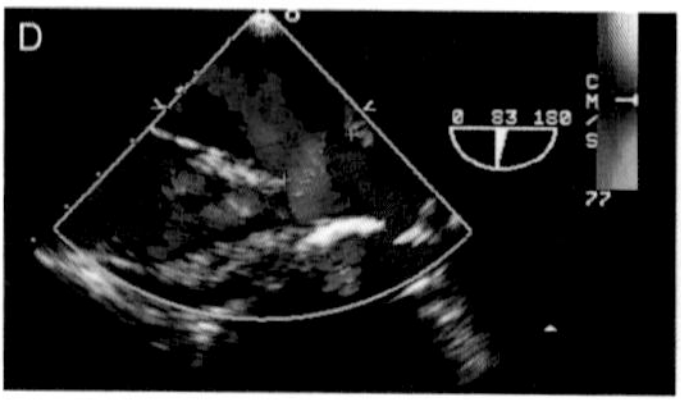

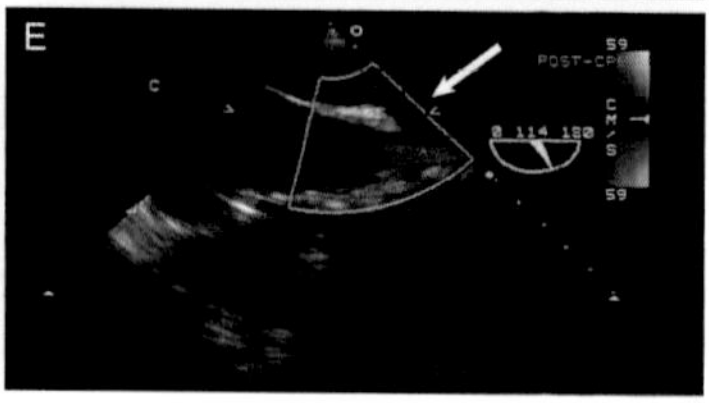

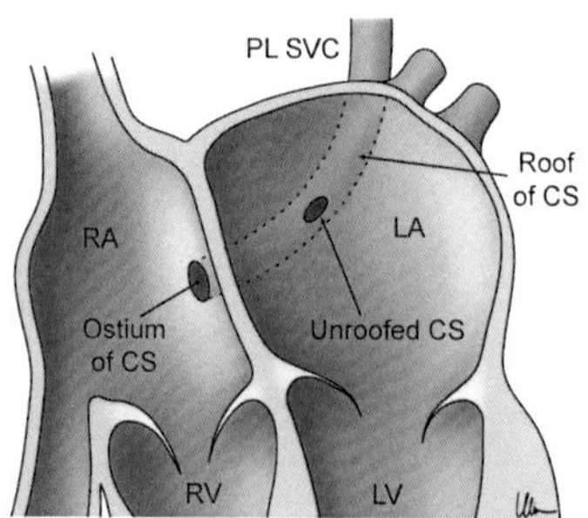

Coronary Sinus (CS) Defect

- This is not a true ASD as the IAS is often intact.
- This is a defect in the coronary sinus wall and the LA, termed unroofed CS.
- Four subtypes of unroofed CS
- There is flow directly from CS into LA.
- There may be flow from the LA into the RA via the CS (inter-atrial shunt).
- Rarest atrial shunt defect (2%)
- Associated lesions:
  - Persistent Left SVC (PLSVC)
  - Secundum ASD

A CS defect is a rare communication between the CS and the LA of which four subtypes have been described. The fossa ovalis may be intact, or there may be a secundum ASD. There is often an associated anomalous drainage of a left-sided superior vena cava into the CS (see p. 262), which dilates the CS.

Imaging a CS defect by TEE is challenging and often requires using modified views to see the defect. (**A**) Modified tricuspid valve (TV) view shows a CS defect (arrow) at the inferior posterior portion of the IAS. Color Doppler (Nyquist 19.3 cm/s) demonstrates flow from the CS into the LA and the RA. (**B**) Compare this image with a normal modified TV view to best appreciate these findings. (**C**, **D**) ME 2C view shows a large defect in the wall of the dilated CS (arrow), allowing deoxygenated blood to mix directly with oxygenated blood in the LA as demonstrated using color Doppler.

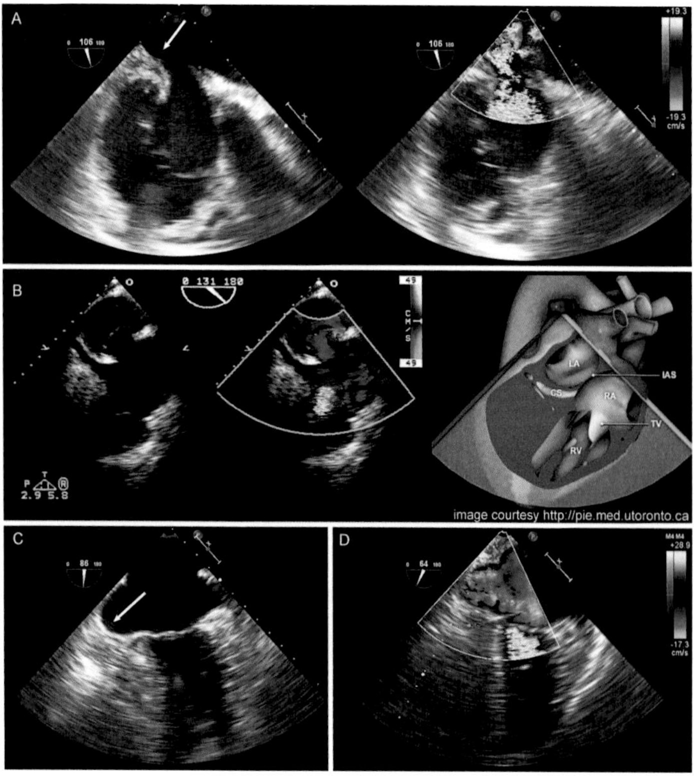

image courtesy http://pie.med.utoronto.ca

Types

A VSD forms from a deficiency in interventricular septal tissue. Different classifications and nomenclature have been used to describe VSDs, often with frequent overlap of the types. VSDs may be isolated or part of complex congenital heart disease.

- Perimembranous (70%, conoventricular, infracristal): occurs below the AV and lateral to the septal TV leaflet, often single and small
- Muscular (20%): occurs in any location in the muscular portion of IVS, surrounded by myocardium, multiple, variable in size
- Inlet (5%, A-V canal): occurs posterior to the membranous IVS, between TV/MV, associated primum ASD, A-V valve abnormality, or complete A-V canal defect
- Outlet (5%, supracristal, subarterial, infundibular, conal, subpulmonary, doubly committed): occurs in the RVOT above the crista terminalis anterior to the membranous IVS, below the aortic and pulmonic valves, single

2D Imaging

- 2D TEE views (see below), TTE is better than TEE to image the IVS
- Type, location, size
- Volume overload, dilates the left-sided structures (LA, LV) and PA:
  - LV size and function (see below)
  - PA dilatation and ± pulmonary hypertension
- RV is less dilated as most flow is into the RVOT (and PA) during systole
  - RVH if ↑ PAP or pressure overload in large VSDs
- IVS aneurysm may be present, appears as "windsock" (see p. 237)
- Associated lesions: PDA (6%), coarctation of aorta (5–10%)

Doppler

- Color Doppler helps identify the shunt location
- CW measure peak systolic pressure gradient between the ventricles to classify as restricted/unrestricted (see below), and shunt direction (L→R, R→L, bidirectional)
- Estimate RVSP from VSD velocity/pressure and systolic BP (SBP), or TR jet
  RVSP = SBP – VSD peak pressure gradient
  $RVSP = 4(TR\ vel)^2 + RAP$
- Shunt fraction Qp/Qs (see p. 61)

Indications for Surgery

- Symptomatic
- CHF failing medical treatment
- LV volume overload
- Reduced LV function
- Qp/Qs ≥2
- Endocarditis
- VSD with aortic insufficiency
- VSD with associated defects

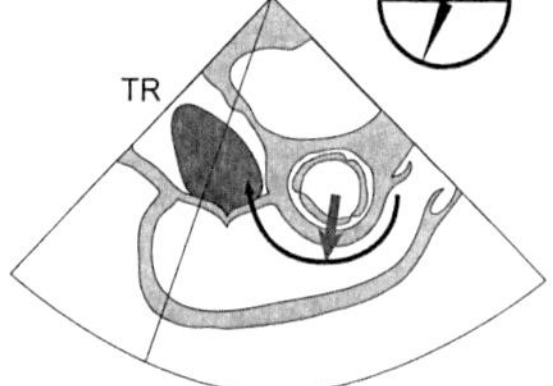

ME RV Inflow - Outflow

VSD	Peak pressure (mmHg)	LA or LV dilatation	Pulmonary artery pressures
Restrictive	>75	no	normal
Moderate restrictive	25–75	+	+
Non-restrictive	<25	++	++

VSD type	2D imaging/best in	Doppler
Muscular	Difficult to identify by 2D, use color ME 4C, ME LAX, TG SAX	Color Flow disturbance on RV side with L to R shunts
Inlet (post- to septal TV)	MV and TV in the same plane ME 4C	
Perimembranous (A + S TV leaflets (R + non AV cusps)	LVOT below AV Extend to inlet, outlet, muscular ME RVOT, 5C, AV LAX or SAX	Spectral CW shows high velocity L to R flow in systole
Outlet (below PV)	AV cusp herniation + AI ME RVOT, AV LAX	

What to Tell the Surgeon VSD	
PreCPB	**PostCPB**
• Location (type), size, number • Shunt direction • Shunt fraction (Qp:Qs) • Peak pressure gradient VSD • Associated findings – RVH, LA dilated, PASP • Ventricular function (RV, LV) • Associated pathology: – Complex congenital – AV cusp herniation/AI – Subaortic membrane	• Residual leak • Ventricular function (RV, LV) • Atrioventricular valve regurgitation • Aortic insufficiency • RVSP from TR jet

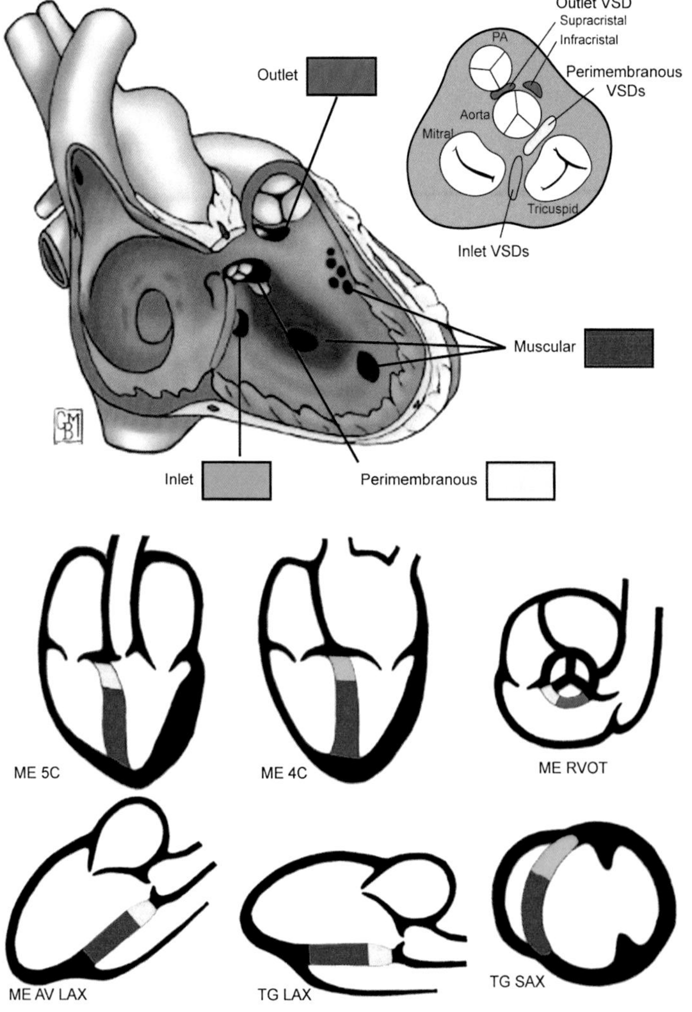

Perimembranous + Inlet VSD: (**A**) ME 4C view with MV and TV at the same level suggests an endocardial cushion defect. Color Doppler in the (**B**) ME RVOT and (**C**) ME AV LAX views shows mostly turbulent left (LV) to right (RV) flow through the VSD into the RVOT. (**D**) TG SAX view shows flow in the posterior part of the septum.

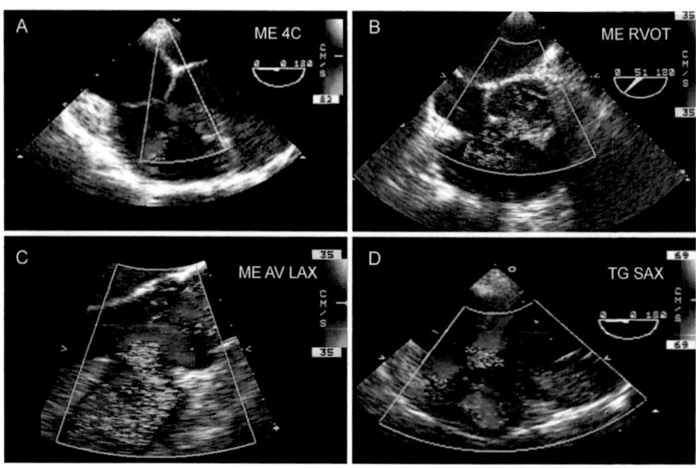

Perimembranous + Outlet VSD: (**A**) 2D ME 5C view (AV) shows a gap (arrow) in the IVS, and (**B**) Color Doppler shows mostly turbulent left to right flow through the VSD. (**C**) ME RVOT and (**D**) ME AV LAX views with color Doppler show flow is below the PV in the RVOT from LV to RV. (E,F) ME 4C views showing large muscular VSD.

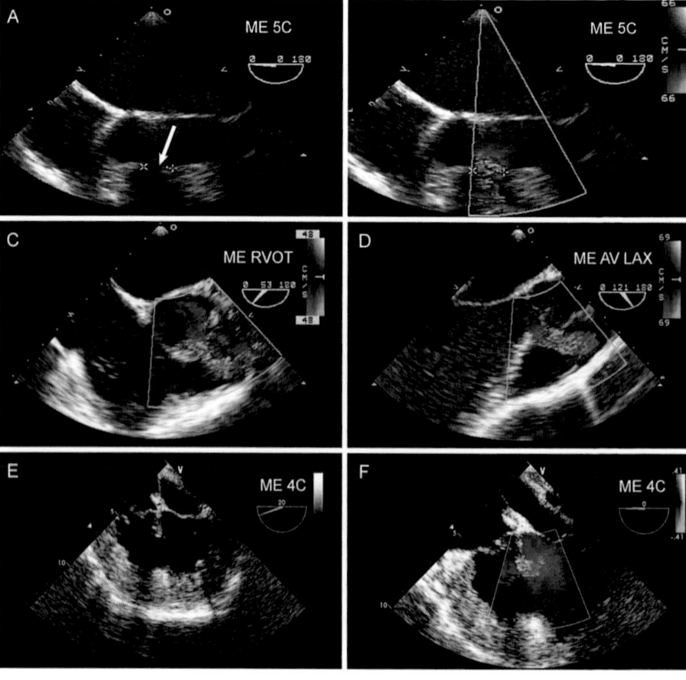

(**A**, **B**) Aneurysm of membranous IVS seen in ME 4C and AV LAX views. There may be an associated VSD, though none was present in this patient. (**C**) Aortic valve cusp prolapse through a subarterial VSD with and without color Doppler during diastole.

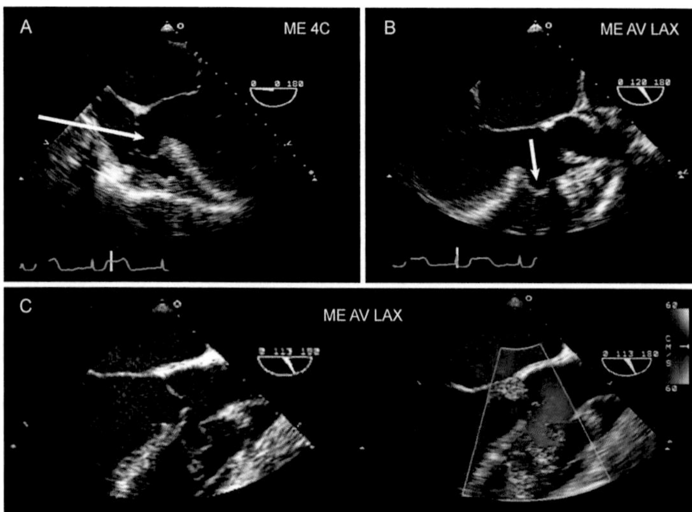

Doppler Flow Through VSD

Perimembranous VSD imaged in TG 2C view allows spectral CW Doppler alignment. Turbulent flow suggests a restrictive VSD which using CW Doppler shows high velocity systolic flow from LV to RV, with a peak pressure gradient of 64 mmHg. In the presence of a large unrestricted VSD, color flow would be laminar and spectral Doppler would show flow in both systole and diastole.

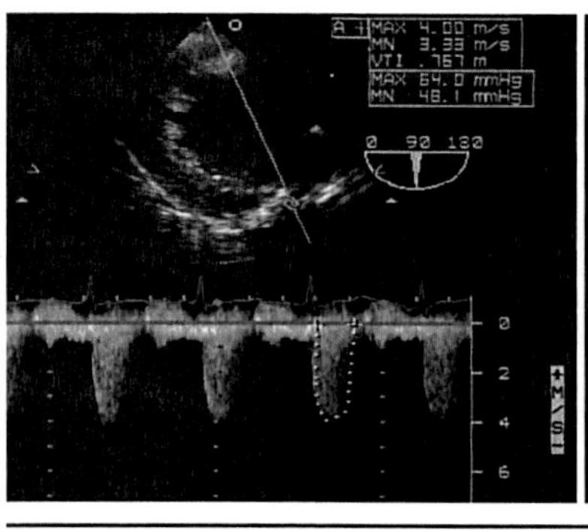

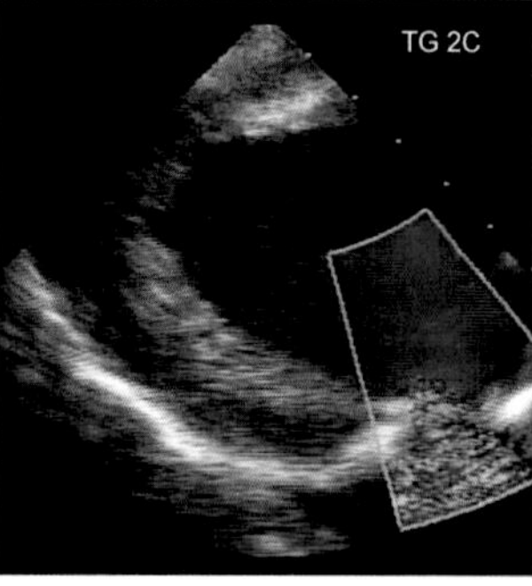

Gerbode Defect

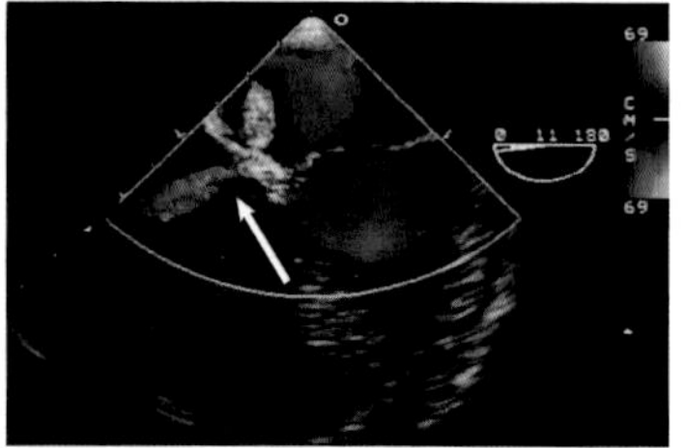

- Congenital: rare atrioventricular septal defect (AVSD) variant
- Acquired: post-MV surgery
- Shunt is directly between LV → RA
- Defect in superior portion of atrioventricular septum, between TV/MV
- Turbulent color flow (arrow) with high CW Doppler pressure gradient
- Distinguish from perimembranous VSD flow (LV → RV) and TR

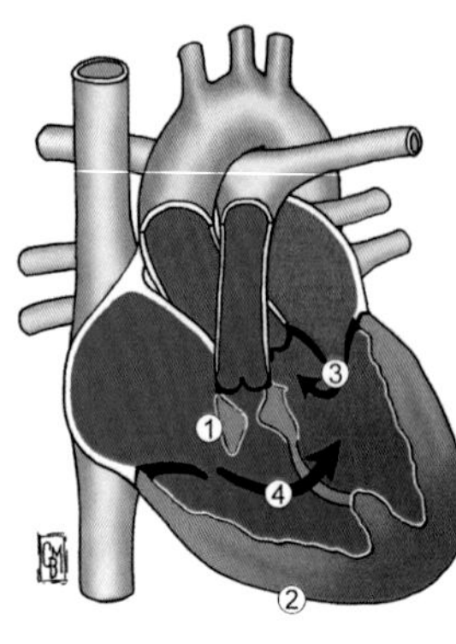

Tetralogy of Fallot Lesions

❶ RV outflow tract obstruction (infundibular)
❷ RV hypertrophy (RVH)
❸ Overriding aorta
❹ Ventricular septal defect (VSD), large

Associated Pathology

- ASD (= Pentalogy of Fallot) (25%)
- Right-sided aortic arch (25%)
- Pulmonic valve atresia (10%), see p. 240
- Second VSD (Down's syndrome)
- Coronary artery anomalies (10%)
- Systemic venous anomalies, Left SVC
- LVOT obstruction
- Aortic valve is large (75%) with AI

Surgery

Patients may have had a palliative shunt prior to a complete correction at a young age with a transannular patch or valved conduit.

- Palliative shunt: Blalock-Taussig, Watterson, Pott's
- Patch closure of VSD
- Repair RVOT/PV using a transannular patch, PV (valvotomy, replace)

Re-Operation

Patients may present again for surgery as an adult most often with pulmonary insufficiency (PI) causing RV dilatation and dysfunction, RVOT obstruction (from muscular hypertrophy), or a small VSD patch leak.

2D Imaging

- Aorta overrides the IVS and is doubly committed to both ventricles.
  - By definition, in TOF, the aorta is committed to the LV by at least 50%.
- VSD: large outlet/membranous, unrestricted mixing leads to RV volume overload
- RVH, RV function, muscular RVOT results in dynamic obstruction
- Pulmonic valve stenosis (bicuspid, doming), annulus size, if dilated, results in PI
- Check main PA size and branches, may be hypoplastic
- Large aortic valve and root with AI
- May have ASD, anomalous coronaries (LAD arises from RCA crosses RVOT)

Doppler

- RVOT obstruction:
  - ↑ Velocity + turbulence at level obstruction (valvular, subvalvular, supravalvular)
  - Color or PW Doppler to locate the level of obstruction
  - CW to estimate peak pressure (>80 mmHg)
- Pulmonic stenosis: peak + mean pressure gradients across pulmonic valve
- VSD pressure gradient (low as unrestricted), patch leak

What to Tell the Surgeon TOF	
PreCPB	**PostCPB**
• Uncorrected: VSD, RVOT level of obstruction, overriding aorta, RVH • Corrected: – Pulmonic valve (PS/PI severity) – VSD leak – RVOT obstruction • RV size and function – Aneurysmal RVOT if PI • TR severity (functional), may repair • Aortic valve (AI) • LV function • Origin coronary arteries • Size of pulmonary arteries – Branch stenosis	• Residual VSD patch leak • Pulmonic valve function (prosthetic) – Paravalvular leak – Pressure gradients • RV size and function • Residual RVOT obstruction • TR severity • RVSP estimate • Coronary blood flow • LV global regional function

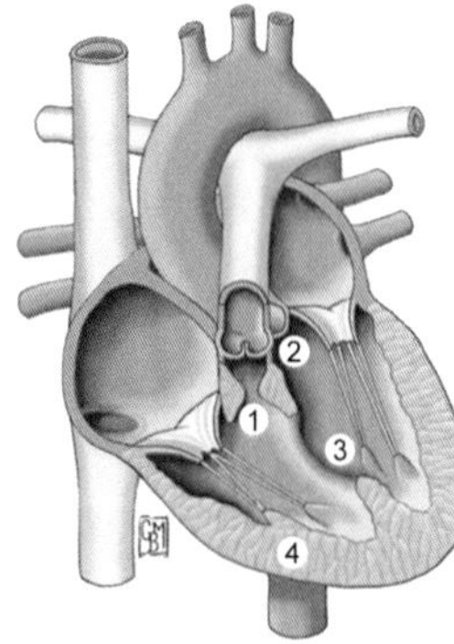

TEE imaging for TOF in adults depends on the previous surgical interventions. It is rare for an uncorrected TOF to present as an adult as the survival rate is only 3% at age 40. Features of TOF are readily identified using different TEE views:

❶ RV outflow tract obstruction (infundibular)
❷ Overriding aorta
❸ Ventricular septal defect (VSD), large
❹ RV hypertrophy (RVH)

Most patients are reoperated on for pulmonic insufficiency of the native or prosthetic valve, causing RV dilatation and dysfunction. Care is taken by the surgeon during PVR surgery to maintain coronary perfusion as TOF patients may have anomalous coronary arteries.

Uncorrected TOF

(**A**–**D**) These are TEE images in an adult with an uncorrected TOF. (**A**) ME 4C view shows RV hypertrophy from PS or RVOT obstruction. The free wall thickness is >5 mm with a small cavitary size. The overall RV systolic function is usually preserved. (**B**) The RVOT is narrowed in the ME RVOT view due to trabecular hypertrophy and antero-cephalad deviation of the outlet septum. Color Doppler shows turbulent RVOT flow. Surgery would include resection of the muscle bundles to improve flow through the RVOT. (**C**) The PV may be stenotic as shown here or insufficient. PV morphology is best seen in the ME RVOT or UE arch SAX view, which also allows good spectral Doppler alignment. (**D**) ME AV LAX view shows a large unrestricted VSD (arrow) and the aorta overriding the interventricular septum. Note the large AV. VSD patch closure is required.

Corrected TOF

(**E**) A patient with a previous corrected TOF including a VSD patch closure is shown. The VSD patch (arrow) appears bright and echogenic without shadowing artifact. Examine using color Doppler for a residual patch leak. Note the overriding aorta which is present.

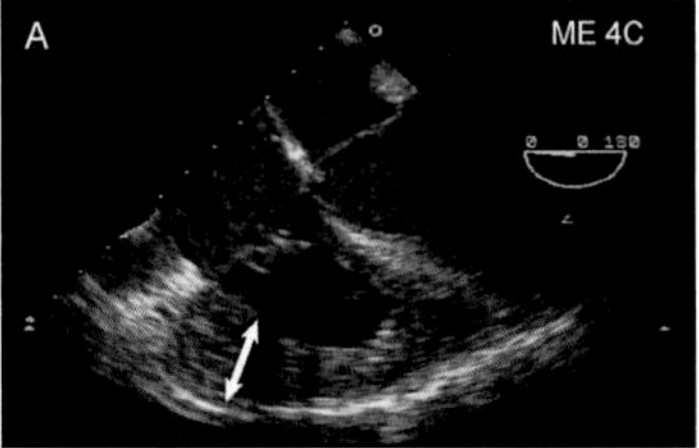

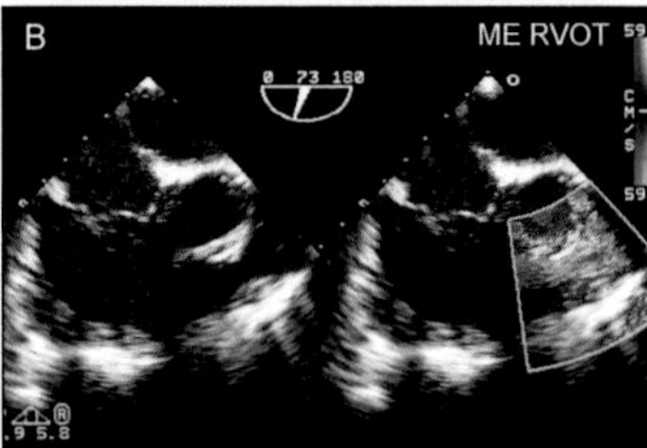

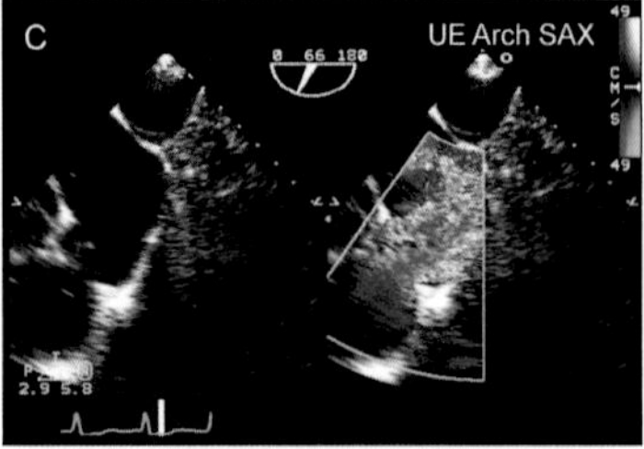

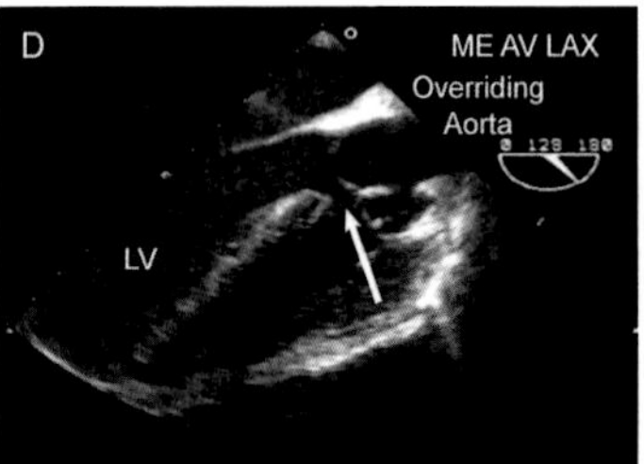

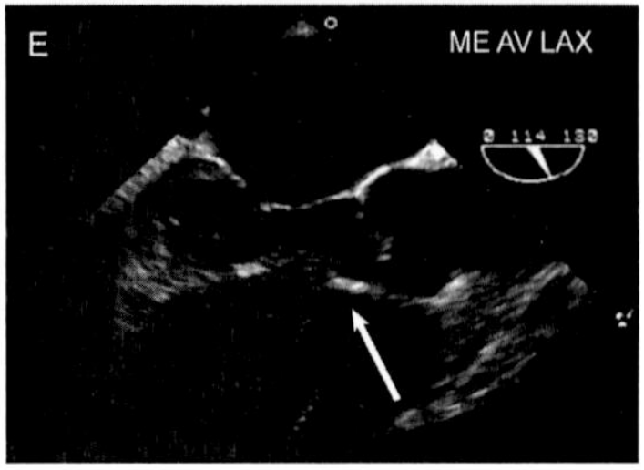

Pulmonary Atresia with VSD

These lesions represent the most severe form of TOF characterized by no continuity between the RV and PA. There are many variations in pulmonary artery blood supply, making surgical management challenging. The pulmonary arteries are considered 'confluent' when they maintain free communication with each other. If there is interruption of the continuity between the LPA and RPA, 'non-confluence' exists. The Rastelli procedure (see p. 241) is a surgical option if the RV and TV are developed.

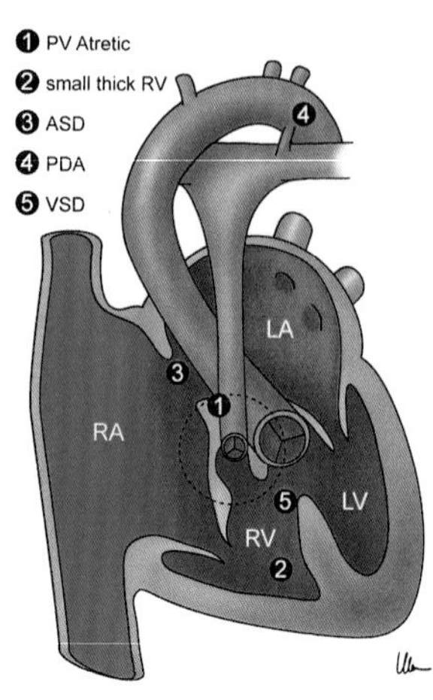

2D Imaging

- Overriding aorta, VSD
- RVH in ME AV LAX view
- VSD: large subaortic/membranous, unrestricted mixing
- No pulmonic valve (PV)
- Large AV and aortic root
- Check main PA size + branches, hypoplastic
- May have ASD, anomalous coronaries (LAD arises from RCA crosses RVOT)

Color/Spectral Doppler

- VSD pressure gradient (low as unrestricted), patch leak if previous repair
- AV for aortic insufficiency (AI)

(**A**) ME 4C view shows the large VSD. (**B**) No RVOT or pulmonic valve is seen in the ME AV SAX view. (**C**) ME AV LAX color compare view shows the overriding aorta and laminar color flow across the unrestricted VSD and out through the aorta.

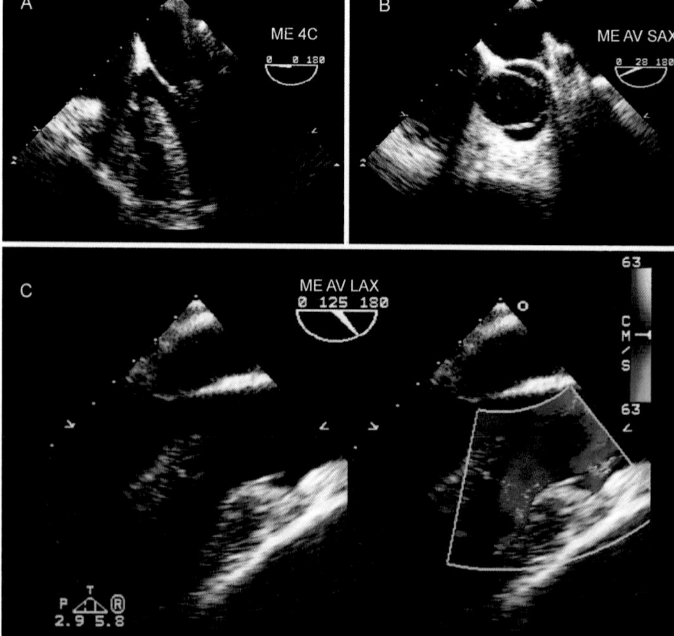

The Rastelli procedure connects the RV to the PA, using a valved conduit. It is indicated for patients with

- d-TGA (as shown here)
- Overriding aorta (TOF)
- DORV and VSD
- RVOT obstruction: pulmonic atresia, pulmonic stenosis, subpulmonary stenosis

Typically, flow is re-established from the RV to PA and LV to aorta with closure of any VSD or ASD, which may be present. Patients may return for surgery with failed conduits from valvular stenosis or regurgitation, requiring conduit replacement.

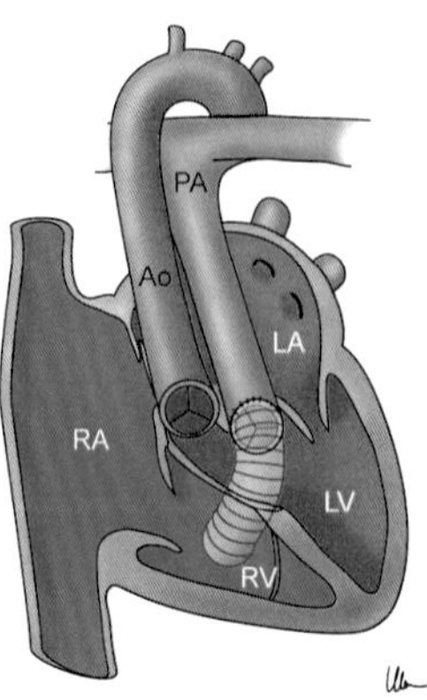

(**A**) The conduits are best imaged in the UE views as shown here, or (**B**) because they arise from the anterior wall of the RV in the TG views. Spectral Doppler alignment is good in either location.

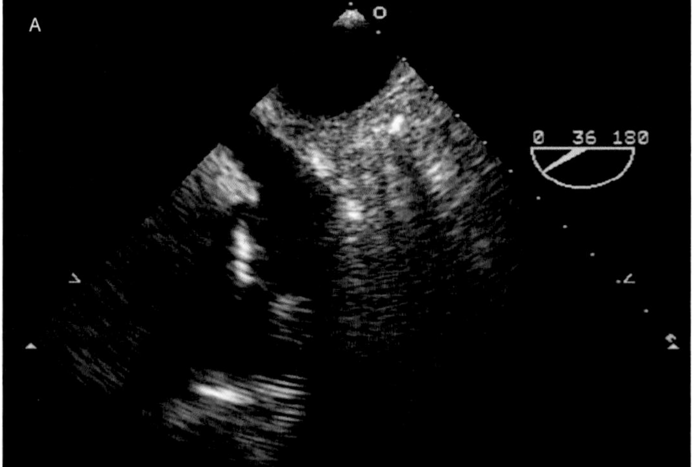

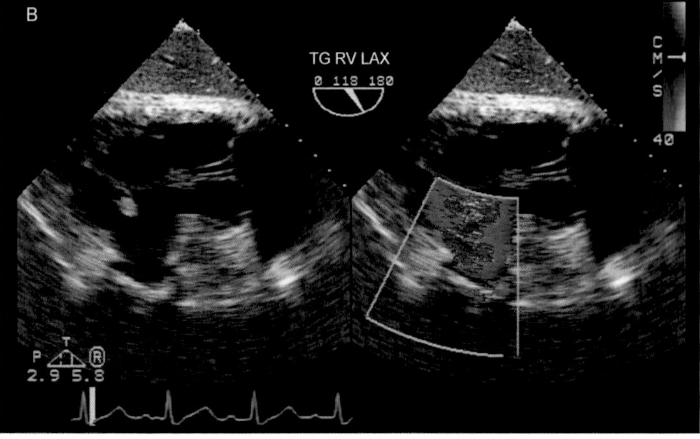

Transposition of the Great Arteries (D-TGA)

The pulmonary artery arises from the LV and the anterior aorta (with coronary arteries) from the RV. Systemic venous blood returns to the RA, from which it goes to the RV and then to the aorta. Pulmonary venous blood returns to the LA, from which it goes to the LV and then to the PA. Two separate circuits are formed–one that circulates oxygen-poor (blue) blood from the lungs back to the lungs, and another that recirculates oxygen-rich (red) blood from the body back to the body. This arrangement requires an ASD, VSD, or PDA for patient survival. The atria, atrioventricular valves, and ventricles are all positioned normally.

Normal	Transposition Great Arteries (d-TGA)
Perpendicular great vessels 1. Aorta from the morphologic LV, with the AV and coronary arteries 2. PA from the morphologic RV, muscular infundibulum	Parallel great vessels 1. Aorta from the morphologic RV via a muscular infundibulum, with the AV and coronary arteries 2. PA from the morphologic LV, PV is in fibrous continuity with the MV
RV (+ TV) is venous ventricle LV (+ MV) is systemic ventricle	RV (+ TV) is systemic ventricle LV (+ MV) is venous ventricle
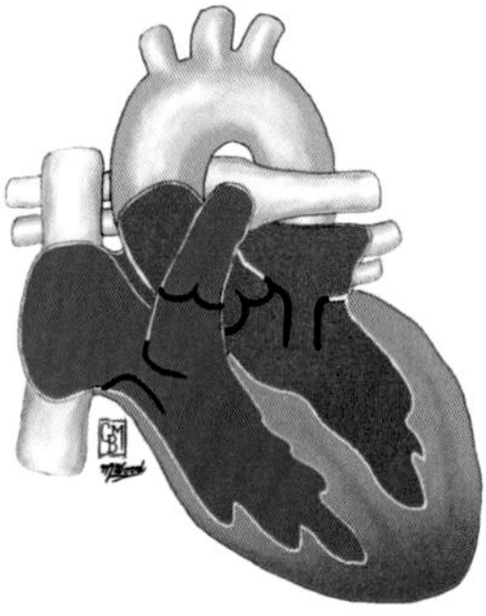	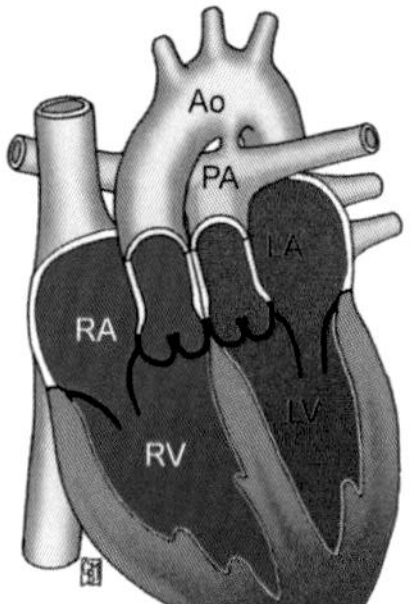 Ao PA LA RA RV LV

Associated Pathology
- ASD (size important for survival)
- VSD (40%), different types, may be multiple
- PDA
- LVOT or RVOT obstruction
- Obstructed pulmonary artery outflow
- Pulmonic or aortic valve stenosis
- Atrioventricular valve abnormalities
- Coronary artery anomalies
- Aortic arch anomalies (coarctation, interrupted)

2D Imaging
- Parallel great vessels, "double barreled"
- Systemic (morphologic RV) ventricle size + function:
  - dilated RV, RVH
- Venous (morphologic LV) ventricle size + function:
  - smaller, banana-shaped, IVS bulges into the LV
- Exclude:
  - LVOT obstruction from bowing of IVS into LVOT
  - Systolic anterior motion (SAM)
  - Premature closure of the pulmonic (systemic) valve

Color/Spectral Doppler
- Atrioventricular valve regurgitation (MR, TR)
- Assess PAP from venous atrioventricular valve (MR jet)
- Baffle leaks (see p. 245)
- Baffle obstruction

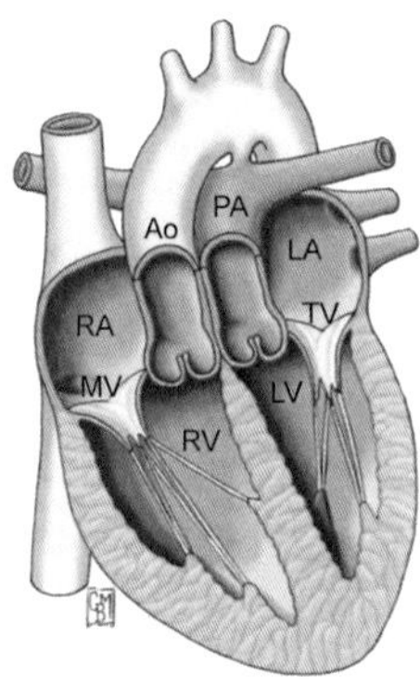

TEE imaging for D-TGA in adults depends on the previous surgical interventions.

- In the 1960s, patients will have had an atrial switch procedure either with native IAS tissue (Senning) or synthetic baffles (Mustard) see p. 244, and thus may return for revision of these procedures.
- Since the early 1990s, the arterial switch operation (Jatene procedure) has become the procedure of choice. In this procedure, the PA and aorta (with coronary arteries) are switched to attach to their corresponding ventricle.

The features of d-TGA can be appreciated by careful systematic examination of different TEE imaging planes.

(**A**) **ME 4C view,** Systemic ventricle (+ TV) is the morphologic RV (moderator band). Pulmonic ventricle (+ MV) is the morphologic LV. This is a patient with a Mustard procedure, the baffles prevent showing a classic ME 4C view.

(**B**) **ME RVOT view.** The pulmonic valve (PV) is central (shown here as a bicuspid valve) and AV is anterior which is opposite to the usual RVOT orientation. Note both valves are seen in SAX confirming the coplanar orientation.

(**C**) **ME AV LAX view.** Aortic arch arises from anterior ventricle (RV) + pulmonary artery, which is bifurcated from the posterior ventricle (LV). The ventricles are normally positioned, though the LV functions as the pulmonic ventricle with outflow to the centrally positioned PA.

(**D**) **UE Aortic Arch view.** The aorta and pulmonary artery (PA) are aligned in parallel, often termed "double barreled." In this view, the great arteries are both seen in LAX, instead of the usual orthogonal arrangement where the PA is seen in LAX and the aorta in SAX.

(**E**) **Modified TG view.** This view best shows the ventriculo-arterial connections, the LV connects to PA and RV to aorta. Note the parallel great arteries, and the normally positioned ventricles. Compare this view with the ME AV LAX view, from which it is rotated 90°.

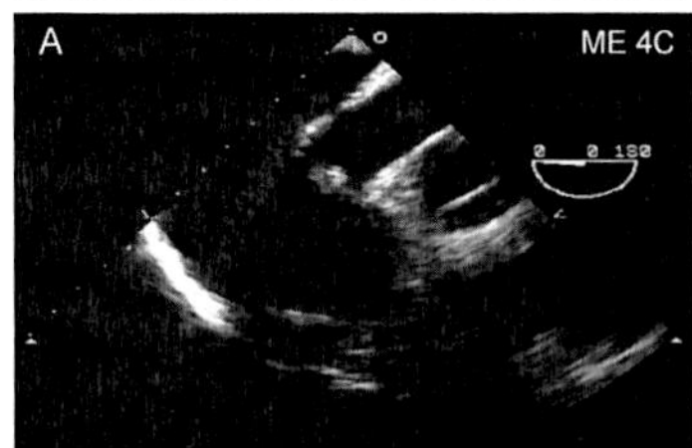

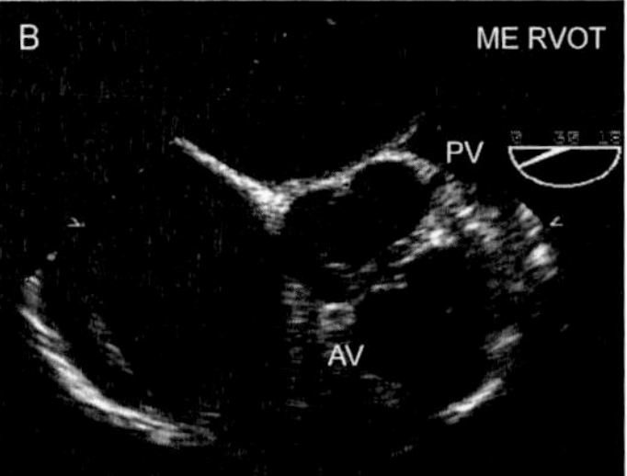

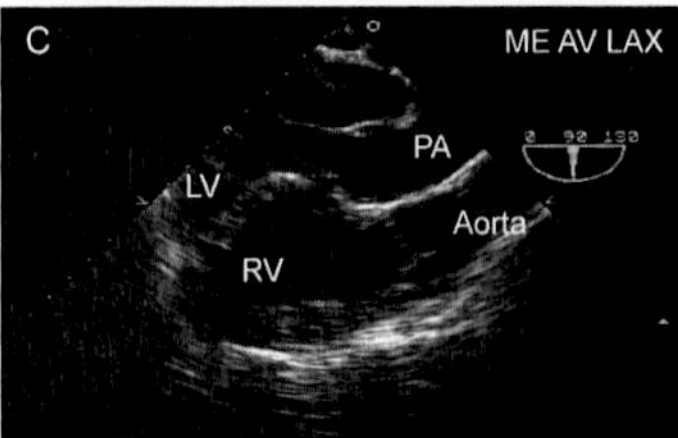

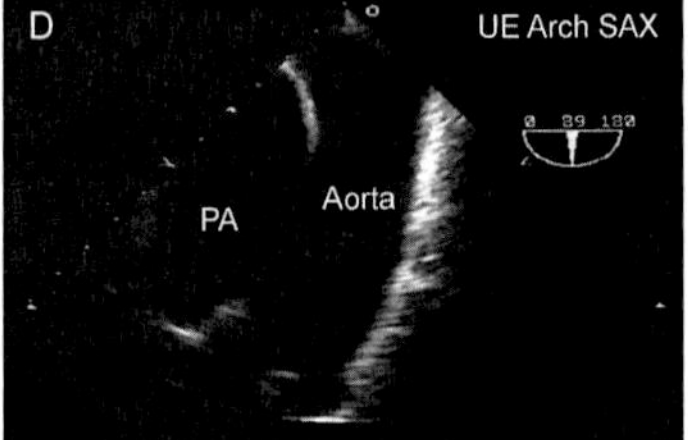

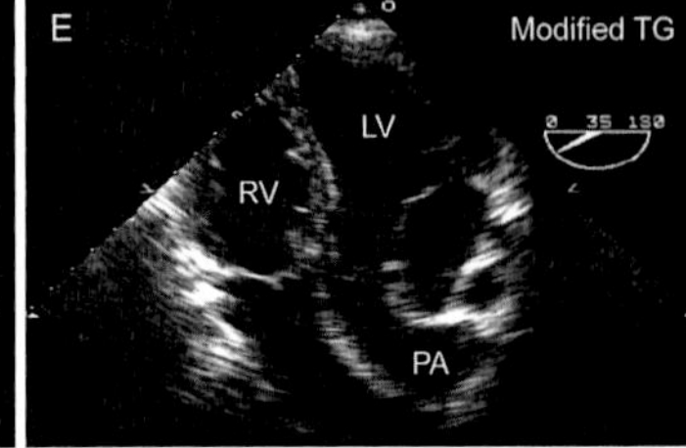

Mustard Procedure

Atrial switch (Mustard or Senning) procedure replaces the inter-atrial septum (IAS) with baffles that redirect blood flow to the ventricles. The IAS is excised; the coronary sinus drains into the LA. A pericardial patch is sutured to allow drainage of the pulmonary veins (oxygenated blood) into the pulmonary venous atrium and outflow through the tricuspid valve (TV) into the RV and aorta. The SVC, IVC, and CS drain into the systemic venous atrium with outflow through the mitral valve (MV) into the LV and PA.

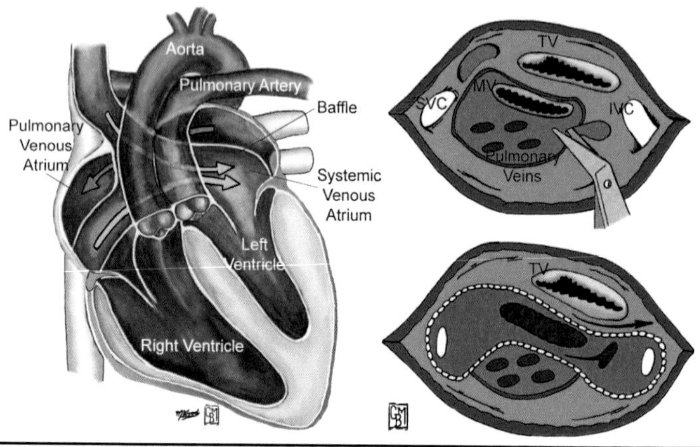

TEE Imaging Mustard Procedure

- Imaging begins with the ME 4C view to identify cardiac chambers and function.
- Flow into each of the chambers is traced by manipulating the TEE probe to show inflow into the ventricles.
- The systemic ventricle receives blood from the right and left pulmonary veins.
  - LUPV: usual location above the venous atrium (ME 4C)
  - RUPV: turn probe right to identify it draining into the systemic atrium
- The venous ventricle receives blood from the venous atrium (IVC and SVC).
  - IVC: advance probe from ME 4C to hepatic vein, IVC drains into venous atrium
  - SVC: seen in modified ME TV view (138°) as it drains into the venous atrium, a pacer wire (arrow) may be seen which passes through the MV.

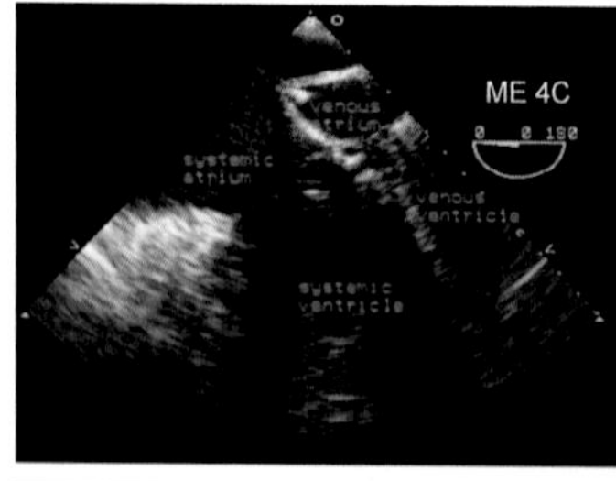

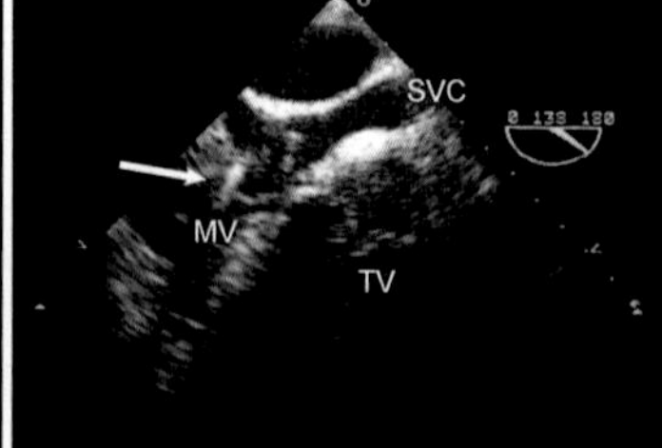

What to Tell the Surgeon D-TGA	
PreCPB	**PostCPB**
• Anatomy – Parallel great arteries – Coplanar valves – Apical displaced TV • ASD, VSD: location, size, flow • Ventricular size, function • A-V and aortic valve function • Coronary arteries	• Measure systemic (RV) size, function • Assess systemic A-V valve (TR) • Baffle obstruction by – Color Doppler – Spectral Doppler – Contrast • PASP from MR • Exclude LVOT obstruction

- Baffles are not imaged at the same level; advance and withdraw TEE probe.
- Baffle flows normally show:
  - Velocity (low)
  - Phasic flow
  - Respiratory variations
- Baffle obstruction has high velocity, non-phasic flow without respiratory variation.
- Baffle leaks are difficult to diagnose, but may see color across the baffle walls and can be confirmed with saline contrast.

Systemic Venous Baffle

This baffle returns systemic venous blood from the SVC and IVC to the sub-pulmonic ventricle (morphologic LV), which supplies blood via the PA to the lungs. The SVC forms the upper limb of the systemic venous baffle and is imaged in a ME 4C view. It appears in the middle of the display and may have pacer wires or catheters, making it easier to identify. The IVC forms the lower limb of the systemic venous baffle and is imaged at gastro-esophageal junction (lower ME) near the liver.

Obstruction usually occurs at the SVC and RA junction and results in SVC dilatation.

- Color Doppler shows continuous turbulent flow with loss of respiratory variation
- PW continuous (non-phasic) flow, suspicious if >1.2 m/s, more convincing >1.5 m/s
- Contrast injection in upper extremity is used to image the IVC
  - No obstruction: contrast fills the systemic venous atrium (SVA) from above and the IVC remains free of contrast
  - Partial obstruction: normal filling of SVC with gradual appearance of contrast material in the IVC from collaterals
  - Complete obstruction: SVC fills with contrast only from below by collaterals

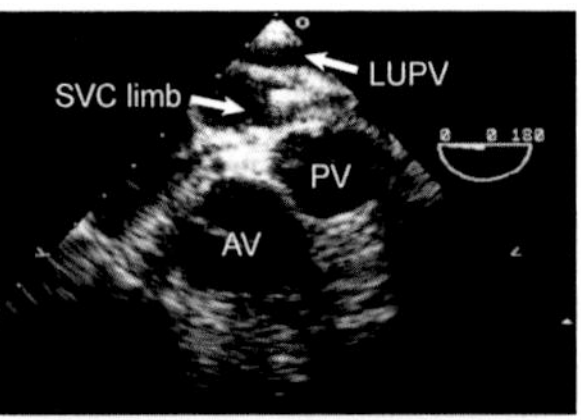

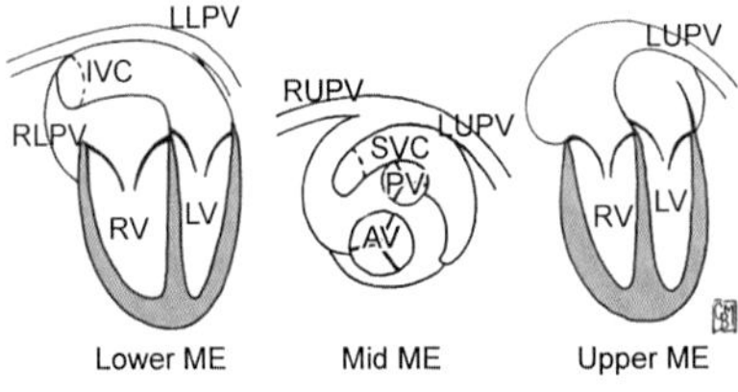

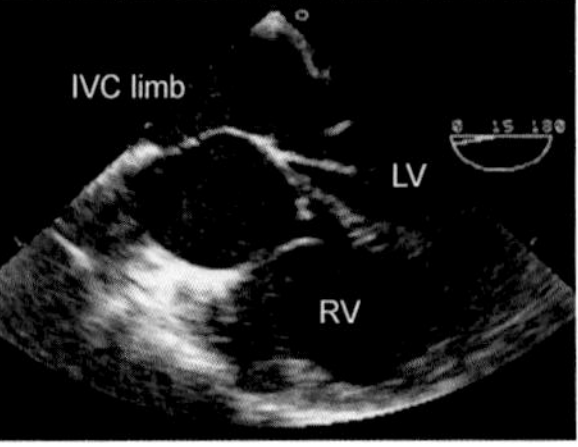

Pulmonary Venous Baffle

This baffle returns oxygenated blood from the pulmonary veins to the systemic ventricle (morphologic RV), which supplies the aorta. The LUPV is imaged in the usual position at 0–60°, above (posterior) the SVC baffle (upper ME). The right pulmonary veins (RUPV + RLPV) are imaged at 0–30° in their usual position.

Obstruction is usually mid-baffle or from isolated pulmonary vein stenosis

- Color Doppler lower velocity turbulent flow doesn't rule it out
- PW/CW: Diastolic velocity convincing if >1.5 m/s, loss of phasic flow

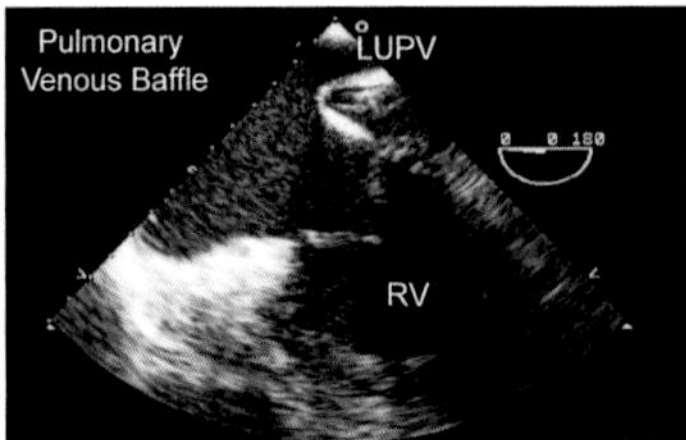

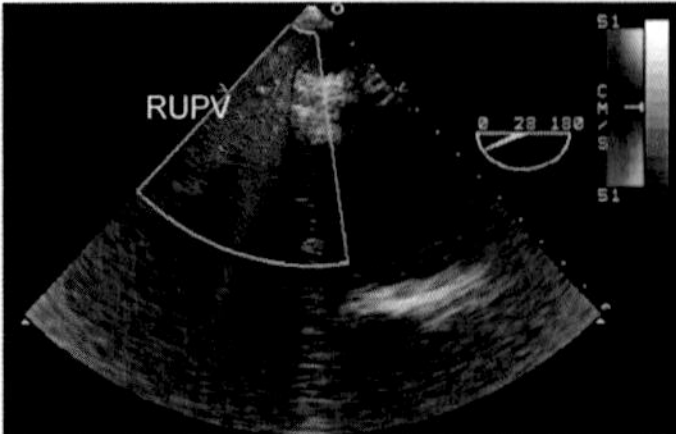

Double-Outlet Right Ventricle (DORV)

- This pathology has an abnormal ventriculo-arterial connection in which both great arteries are nearly or completely aligned with the RV. It is a spectrum of pathologies that are difficult to categorize.
- Classification can be based on the (1) VSD location or (2) relationship of the great vessels.
- A VSD is present and its relation to the great vessels determines the physiology and aids in describing the pathology.
  - Subaortic VSD (commonest type, 50%): similar to TOF but with no aortic-mitral continuity in DORV, mal-aligned IVS, repaired with VSD patch
  - Subpulmonic VSD (Taussig-Bing anomaly, 30%): similar to TGA with VSD (>50% of PA from LV) as blood from LV → PA and RV → aorta, mal-aligned IVS, repaired with arterial switch and VSD closure
  - Doubly committed (10%): infundibular septum is absent, so both AV and PV relate to the VSD, repaired with patch closure
  - Non-committed (10%): remote VSD is present, so blood mixes in RV, repair may involve Fontan procedure.
- Great Arteries: normal (crossed), TGA (parallel)
- Associated anomalies: A-V valve abnormalities, ASD, muscular VSDs, ventricular hypoplasia, coronary artery anomalies, right arch

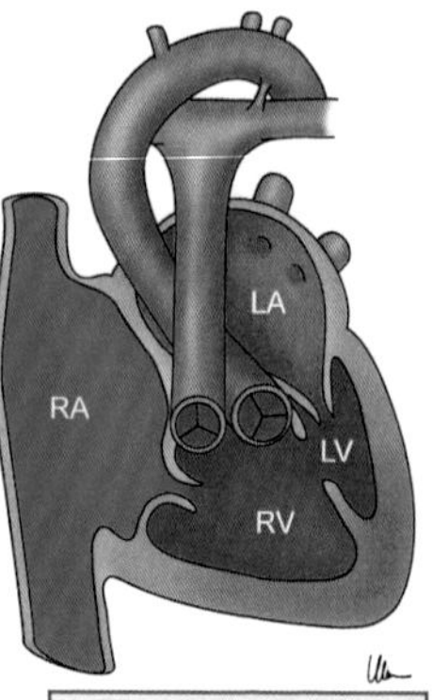

DORV Types
VSD Location
Subaortic
Subpulmonic
Double committed
Remote
Great Vessels
Normal (crossed)
TGA (parallel)

Deep TG view shows the subaortic VSD (arrow) and relationship to the both great vessels (crossed or parallel -TGA) exiting the RV. Compare with the diagram which is flipped vertically from the one shown above.

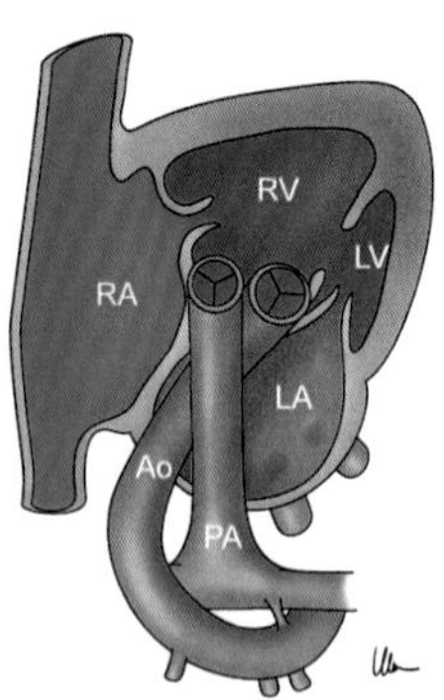

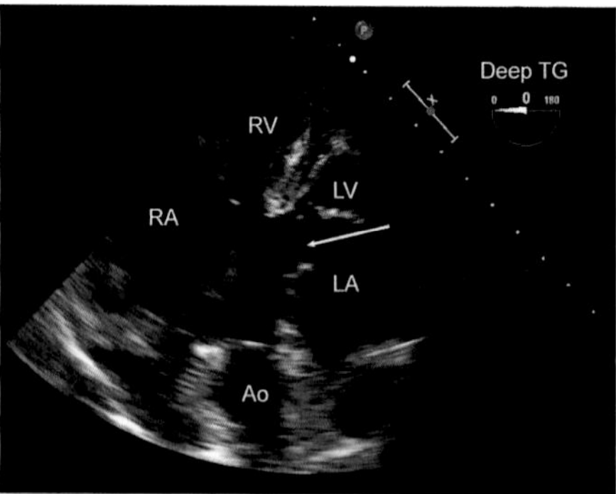

What to Tell the Surgeon DORV	
PreCPB	**PostCPB**
• VSD: location – Size relation to great vessel diameter – Shunt direction, Peak pressure • VSD relation to great arteries – Distance from IVS crest to AV • Great artery relation – normal (crossed), TGA (parallel) • Ventricular function • A-V valve straddling VSD – TV chordae insert into LV • Subpulmonic stenosis • Associated pathology	• Residual VSD leak • Ventricular function • Atrioventricular valve regurgitation • Aortic valve regurgitation • Conduits or baffles • Coronary blood flow

This is a heterogeneous group of pathologies related to the presence of a single functional ventricle, with atria and two great vessels. It is rare to have only one ventricle as, more often, the other ventricle is rudimentary. The ventricle often has a circular or spherical shape from volume overload. The ratio of PVR and SVR determines relative flows. Palliative shunts (ASD, Blalock-Taussig, Glenn) are used to augment pulmonary blood flow. The Fontan circulation is the final common circulation in these patients.

Univentricular Heart
Atretic valve (MV, TV)
Hypoplastic heart (HLHS)
Double-inlet A-V connection
Common A-V canal (unbalanced)
Single ventricle heterotaxy

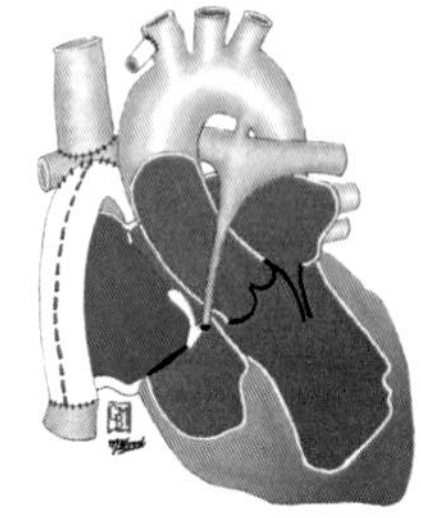

2D Imaging

- Single ventricle in ME views
  - Morphology: LV, RV, indeterminate
  - Ventricular size + function
  - Relationship to atrioventricular valve
  - Relationship to great arteries
- Atretic atrioventricular valve (MV, TV)
- Atria, ASD
- VSD
- PDA

Color/Spectral Doppler

- Valve regurgitation stenosis
- VSD: direction, gradient

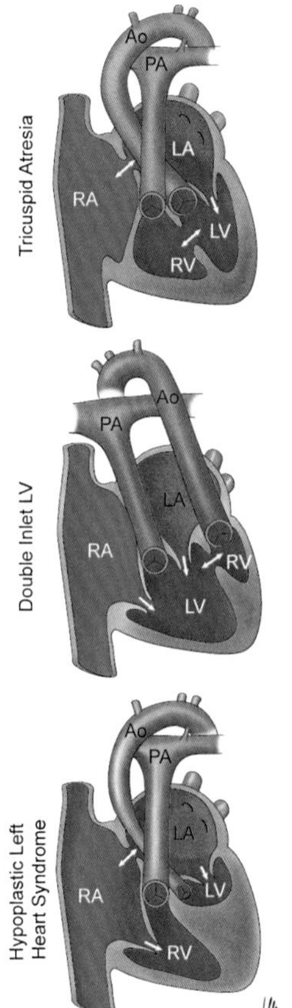

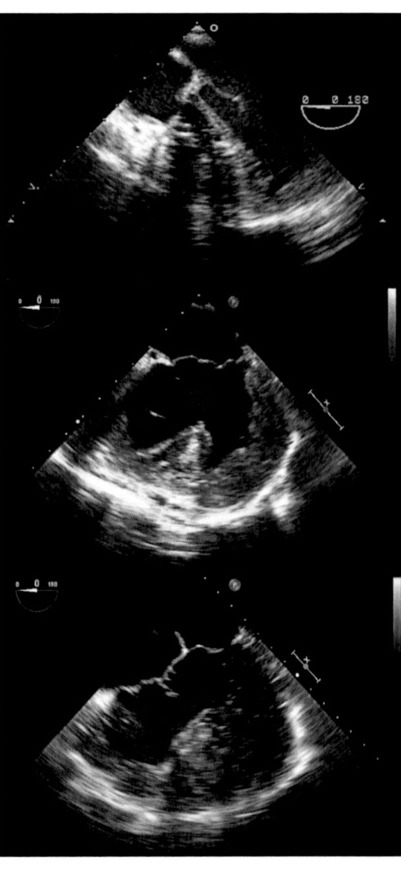

The Fontan procedure brings venous blood from the IVC to the PA. There is no pumping chamber in the Fontan circulation. It is a palliative procedure for an univentricular circulation. The first stage involves directing venous blood from the SVC into the pulmonary artery.

- Classic Glenn: SVC to right PA
- Bidirectional Glenn: SVC to PA bifurcation

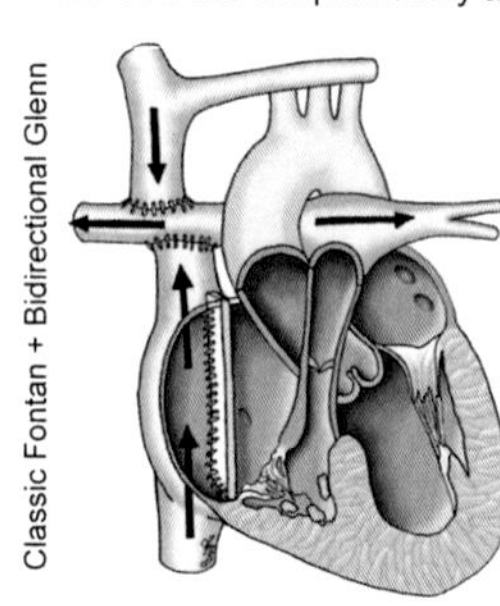

Many variations to the Fontan procedure.

- Early version incorporated the RA, which dilated, causing thrombus and arrhythmias.
- Later versions placed conduits inside or outside the heart.
- Many patients are upgraded to a total cavopulmonary circulation (TCPC) in which both cava are directly connected to the PA.

Classic Fontan

(**A**) RA to PA directly, side of main PA.
(**B**) RA to PA directly, end of main PA.

Modified Fontan

(**C**) RA to RV via pericardial patch.
(**D**) RA to RV via conduit (± valve).
(**E**) Total cavopulmonary anastomosis (IVC + SVC + RA) with intra-atrial (lateral tunnel).
(**F**) Total cavopulmonary anastomosis (IVC + SVC + RA) with extracardiac conduit.

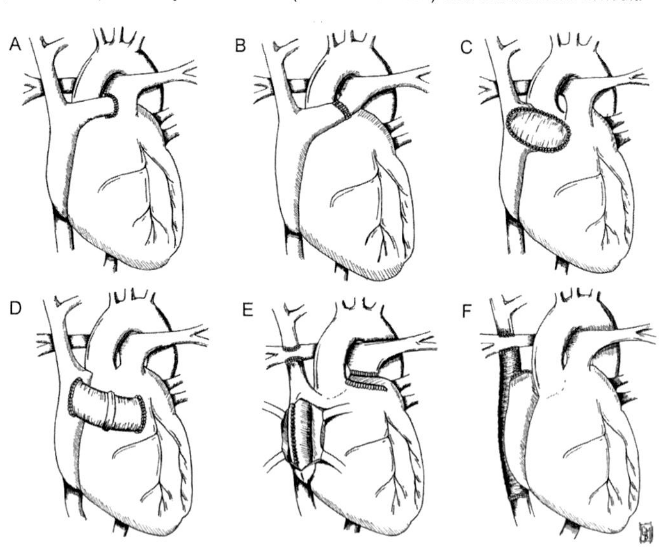

What to Tell the Surgeon Fontan	
PreCPB	**PostCPB**
• Assess ventricular size, function • Residual atrial leak • Systemic atrioventricular valve regurgitation • Pulmonary artery and vein Doppler • Fontan circulation: – Conduit location – Doppler velocity, respiratory variation – Mass/thrombus – Fenestration	• Conduit location • Doppler flow • Ventricular function • Atrioventricular valve function

(**A**) ME view of a classic atriopulmonary connection shows an enlarged right atrium (RA) with smoke. (**B**) Lateral tunnel connection in a ME view shows the conduit as it traverses the enlarged RA. Note the ASD (arrow). (**C**) An extracardiac conduit is seen in this ME 4C view outside the RA and a common atrium.

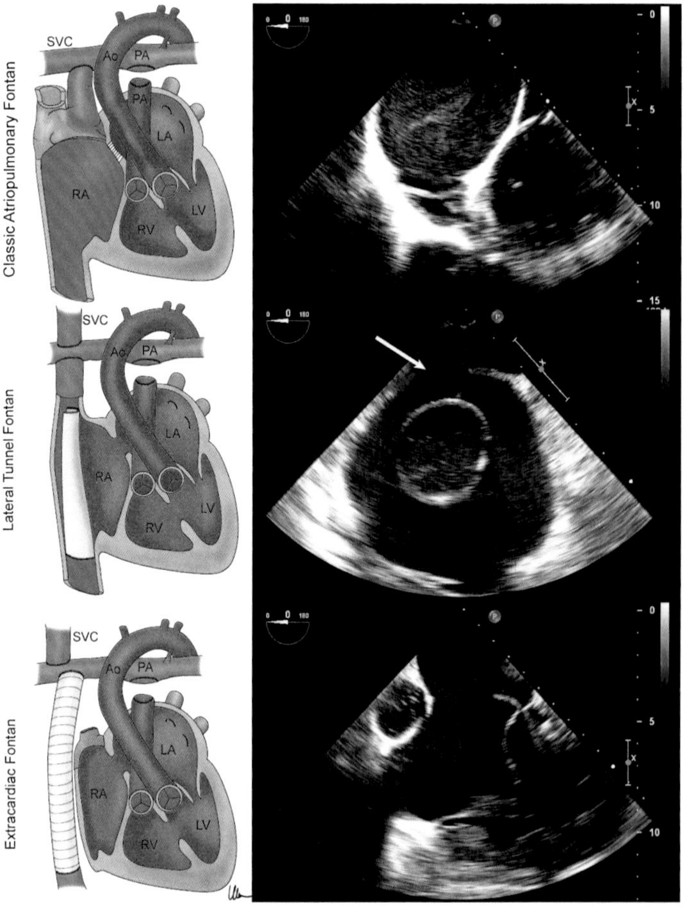

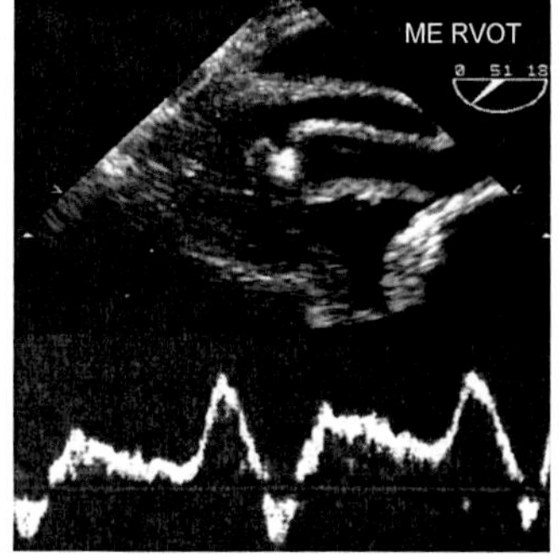

PW Doppler Trace (PA Conduit in RA)

- Low velocity ≤ 1 m/s
- Bi (or tri) phasic flow
  - Forward flow in atrial systole
  - Retrograde flow in early atrial relaxation
  - Lower velocity forward flow
- Respiratory variation, ↑ inspiration

Obstruction of Atriopulmonary Flow If:

- High velocity >1 m/s
- Turbulent
- Continuous flow
- Loss of respiratory variation

Ebstein's Anomaly

- Congenital malformation of TV and RV, from failure of TV to separate (delaminate) from RV wall.
- Progressive displacement of septal and posterior leaflets toward RV apex. Functional TV orifice is anterior and apical from true TV annulus.
- Dysplastic TV leaflets:
  - Large malformed anterior leaflet
  - Hypoplastic septal leaflet
  - Leaflets "tethered" to RV wall (>3 attachments)
- TR originates at the functional orifice below the true annulus in the RV cavity, variable severity
- Atrialization of RV (dilated), small functional RV
- RA enlarged

Associated Pathology

- ASD (50%), PFO
- L-TGA, Mitral valve prolapse

TEE Imaging (ME 4C View)

- Dilated RA
- Dilated true TV annulus
- Enlarged atrialized RV + small functional RV
- Large malformed anterior leaflet tethered to the RV wall, may be fenestrated
- Apically displaced hypoplastic septal leaflet with an increased distance from the MV annulus >20 mm or $\geq$8 mm/m^2

Doppler

- Color: Severe TR, origin below the TV annulus
- Spectral: RVSP

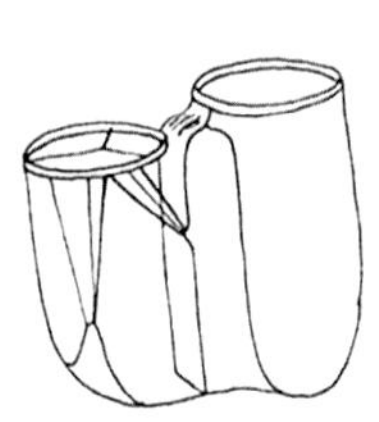
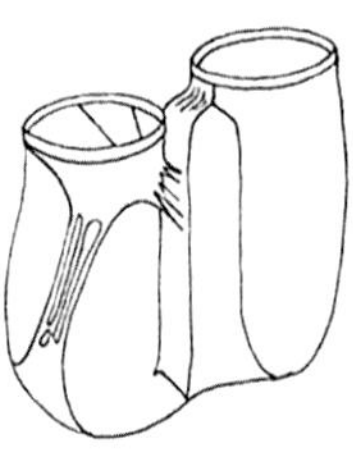
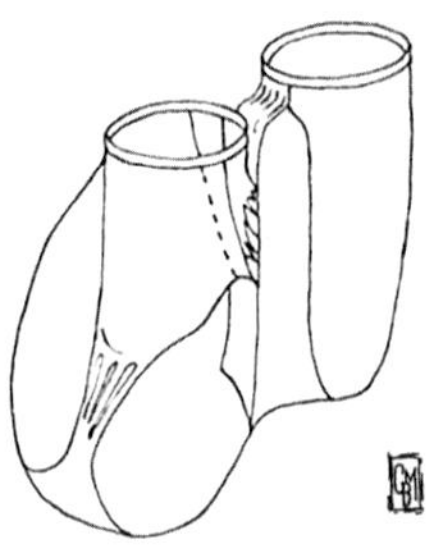

The mechanism of TV leaflet dysfunction involves progressive septal leaflet displacement and elongation of the anterior leaflet. The septal leaflet is tethered to the RV septal wall and the anterior leaflet becomes large and sail-like.

Surgical Repair

- Predicting the potential for TV repair is based on this scoring system.
- Challenging surgery which may involve:
  - Mobilize (untether) large anterior leaflet to coapt with small septal leaflet
  - Atrialized RV is plicated to reduce size
  - RA size is reduced
  - TV annuloplasty to reduce TR
- Cone Repair involves mobilizing the TV from the RV walls, retaining the chordal attachments, rotating the valve, and reattaching the leaflets to the true TV annulus, recreating the TV as a cone.

2-D echo features	
Tethered ant leaflet (severe)	3
Tethered ant leaflet (mild)	1
Restricted motion ant leaflet	2
Functional RV <35%	2
Absent septal leaflet	1
Displaced ant leaflet	1
Aneurysmal RVOT	1
RA diameter >60 mm/mm^2	1
Severe tricuspid prolapse	1

Index >5 predicts need for TV replacement as compared to repair
Source: Shiina A, et al. Circulation 1983; 68:534–44

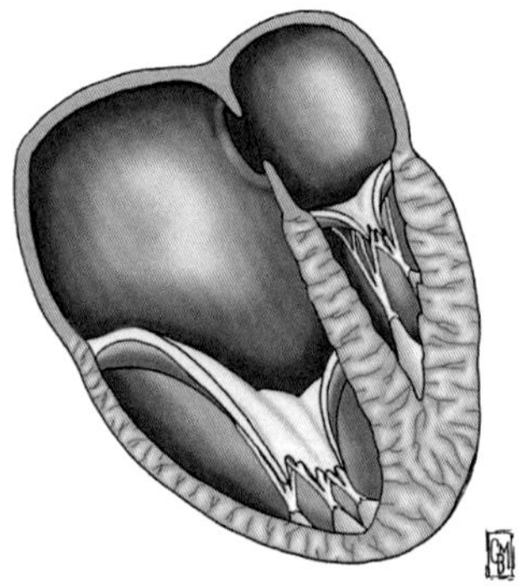

(**A**) The diagnosis of Ebstein's Anomaly is made from the ME 4C view which shows an apically displaced TV septal leaflet, as measured from the MV annulus in diastole. The insertion of the septal TV leaflet appears displaced from tethering to the IVS, though the anatomic TV annulus is not displaced. The functional RV is small; the remainder of the RV is atrialized. (**B**) The anatomic TV annulus measured during systole is severely dilated. The severe TR jet (arrow) starts well below the TV annulus at the functional orifice. (**C**) ME LAX view demonstrates a large atrialized RV in diastole. The IVS is displaced into the LVOT. This requires an image depth of 18 cm to show the entire RV. This may cause LVOT obstruction with SAM post-TV repair or replacement. (**D**) The ME RVOT view shows tethering of the posterior and septal TV leaflets to the RV walls. (**E**) Laminar retrograde (red) flow across the TV suggests severe TR with significant RV dysfunction.

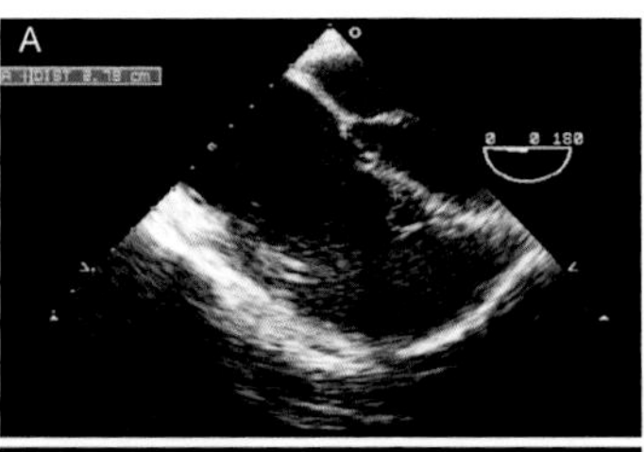

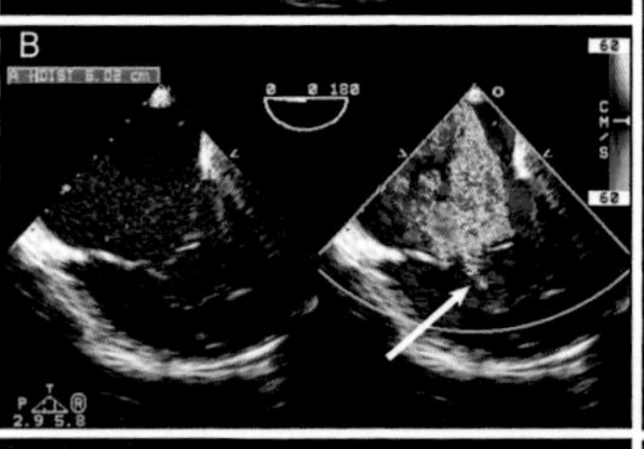

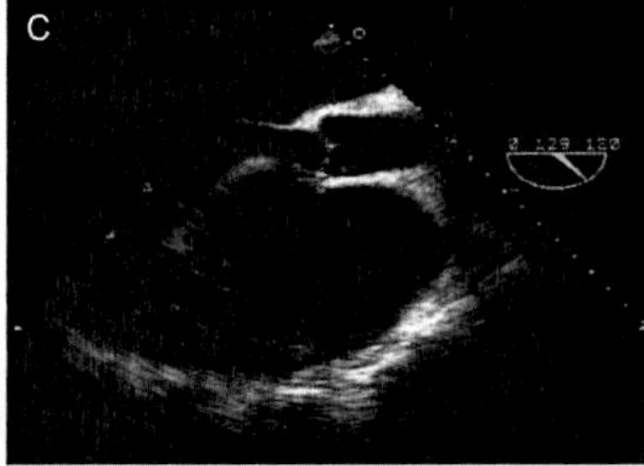

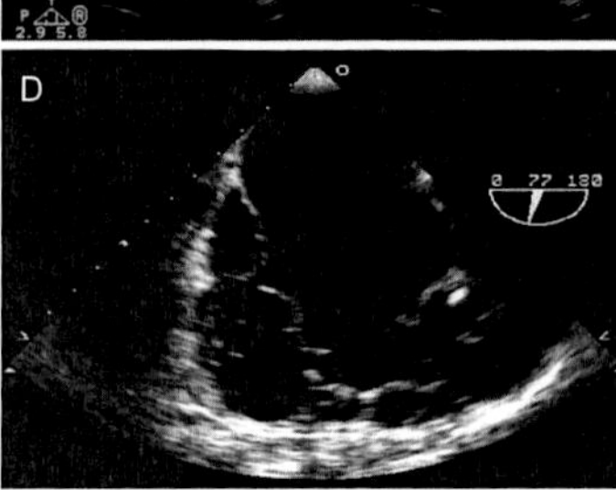

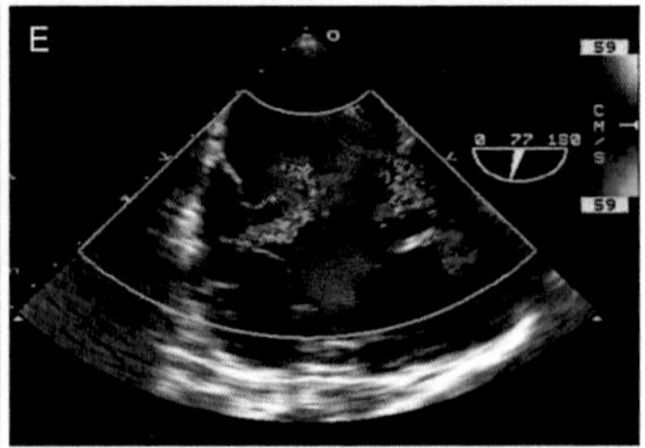

What to Tell the Surgeon Ebstein's Anomaly	
PreCPB	**PostCPB**
• Displaced septal leaflet >20 mm	• TV repair vs. replacement
• Anterior leaflet tethering	• Residual TR
• Absent septal leaflet	• RV function
• RV size and function	• RVSP
• RA size	• LVOT obstruction
• TV annulus diameter	• SAM
• TR severity	
• RVSP	
• Associated pathology	

In this pathology, the morphologic LV is the venous ventricle and gives rise to the PA, and the morphologic RV is the systemic ventricle and gives rise to the aorta. There is atrioventricular discordance + ventriculo-arterial discordance, so "2 wrongs make a right." The morphologic RV was not intended to support the systemic circulation. Patients are usually asymptomatic until they have systemic ventricular (RV) failure and atrioventricular valve (TV) regurgitation.

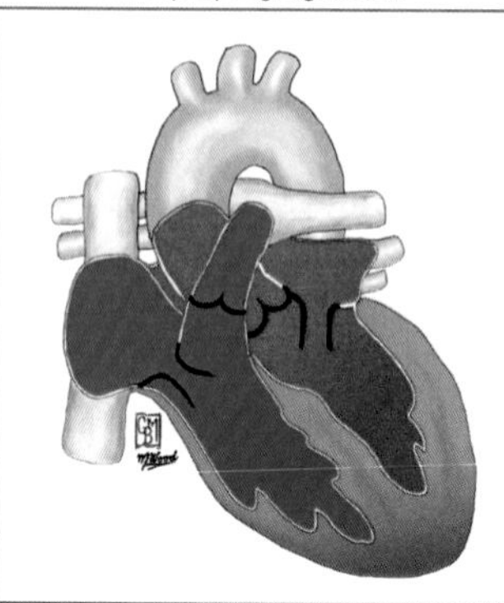	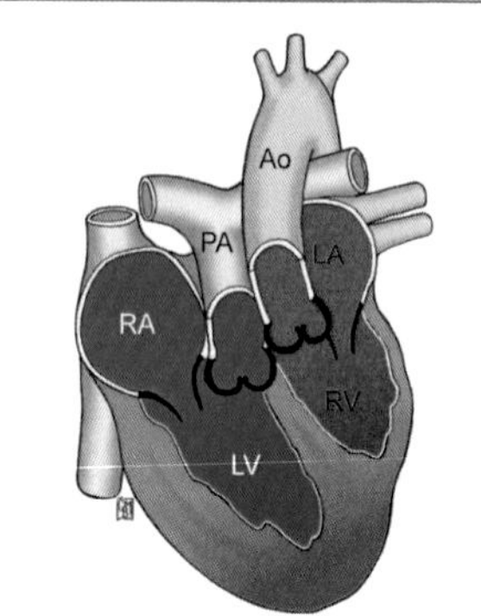
Normal	**L-Transposition of great arteries**
1. Perpendicular great vessels	1. Parallel great vessels
2. PA is anterior to aorta	2. Aorta is anterior to PA
3. RV (+ TV) is venous ventricle, PA from RV	3. LV (+ MV) is venous ventricle, PA from LV
4. LV (+ MV) is systemic ventricle, aorta from LV	4. RV (+ TV) is systemic ventricle, aorta from RV

The ME 4C view shows the morphologic RV on the right side of the display. The TV is apically displaced and is frequently regurgitant. The ME AV SAX view shows the aortic and pulmonic valves are coplanar, rather then being orthogonal.

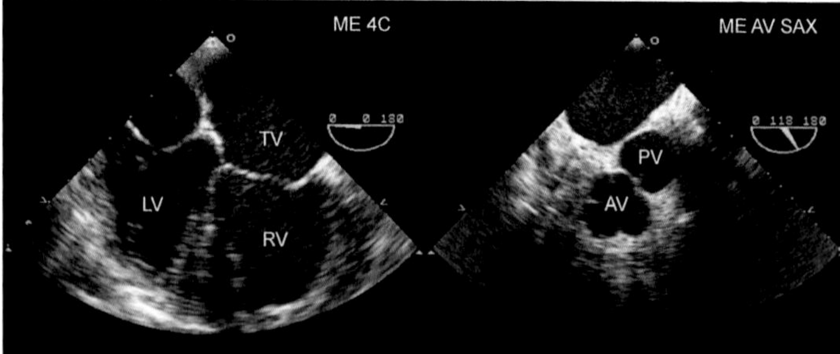

What to Tell the Surgeon L-TGA	
PreCPB	**PostCPB**
• Anatomy – Parallel great arteries – Coplanar valves – Apical displaced TV (identifies RV) • A-V valve function (MR, TR) • RVSP • Ventricular function: – Systemic (RV) – Pulmonic (LV)	• Residual A-V function • Ventricular function • RVSP • Intervention – PA band – Valve replacement

In this pathology, an intra-atrial membrane divides the LA into two parts:

1. Accessory pulmonary venous chamber into which the pulmonary veins drain
2. LA chamber contiguous with MV

The connection between the accessory chamber and true LA varies in size and may cause pulmonary vein obstruction.

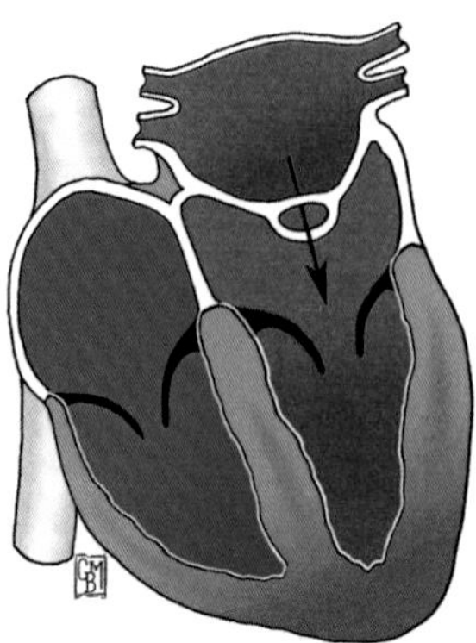

TEE Imaging

- Intra-atrial membrane seen in multiple views, inserts proximal to the LAA into the "coumadin ridge"
- Diastolic movement towards the MV
- May have RVH + RV dilatation
- May have associated PFO/ASD, persistent left SVC, AVSD, PAPVD, coarctation
- Color flow laminar or turbulent flow
- PW Doppler pressure gradient, significant if mean gradient >10–12 mmHg

Intra-atrial membrane seen in the LA in multiple views, ME 2C view above the LAA, ME 4C view attached to the IAS. The ME LAX and ME 2C views show a gap in the intra-atrial membrane with laminar color flow. The membrane, an incidental finding, was resected at the time of surgery.

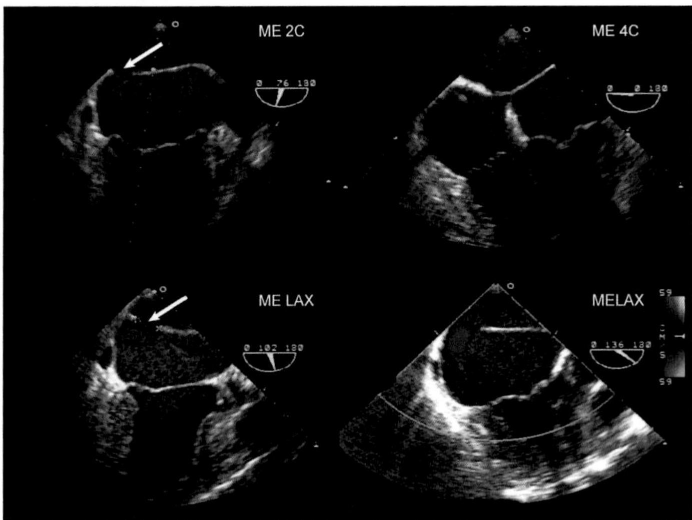

What to Tell the Surgeon Cor-Triatriatum	
PreCPB • Membrane in LA – Multiple ME TEE views • Flow across membrane – Color: Laminar, turbulent – PWD mean gradient >10–12 mmHg • Associated pathology – PFO/ASD, AVSD – Persistent left SVC – PAPVD – Coarctation	**PostCPB** • Absence of membrane

PDA is persistence beyond 10 days after birth of the normal fetal connection between the pulmonary artery (PA) and descending aorta. In utero, the ductus enables blood to bypass the lungs and perfuse the fetus. It usually closes spontaneously at birth. PDA is an uncommon isolated pathology, but may be present in complex congenital heart disease. If untreated, there is a L → R shunt with risk of endocarditis, increased pulmonary blood flow, pulmonary hypertension, LA, and LV volume overload. Treatment includes open surgical closure and percutaneous device closure.

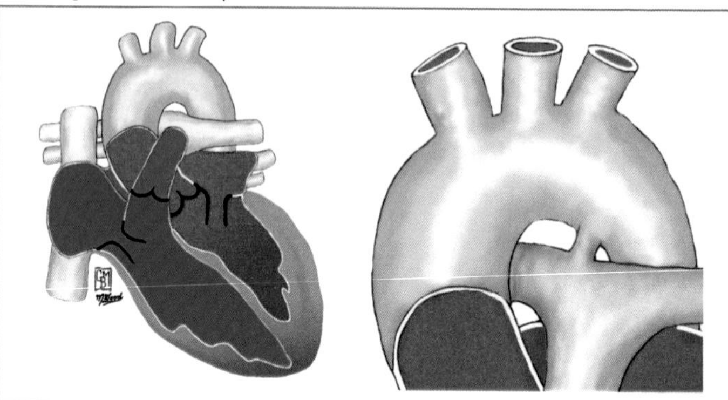

Findings PDA

1. Connection between PA and descending aorta at level of left subclavian artery. Variable in size, though usually restrictive with mosaic color.
2. LV and LA often dilated
3. PA may be dilated
4. RV affected if pulmonary hypertension
5. RVSP estimates pulmonary hypertension

UE Aortic Arch SAX color compare view (Nyquist 48 cm/s) shows turbulent flow from the aorta to the main pulmonary artery. The connection between both structures is seen in the 2D image. CW Doppler shows continuous high velocity (3 m/s) systolic and diastolic flow. Bidirectional flow suggests elevated PA pressures compatible with Eisenmenger's.

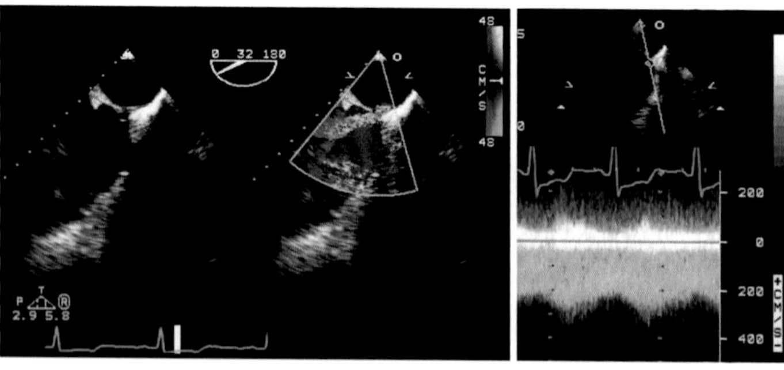

What to Tell the Surgeon PDA	
PreCPB	**PostCPB**
• Identify connection PA to aorta • Color Doppler turbulent flow • Spectral Doppler continuous flow • LV, RV size, and function • PA size • RVSP estimate	• Absence of flow • RV, LV size, and function • RVSP estimate

In this pathology, there is a single arterial trunk from which both the pulmonary artery (PA) and aorta (Ao) originate. Both ventricles have a single, common outlet and the truncal root overrides a VSD. Classification of this defect into four types (I, II, III, IV) is based on the origin of the PA(s) from the truncal root. The clinical manifestations of this lesion depend largely on the status of the pulmonary vascular resistance and the presence of any intrinsic stenosis in the PAs.

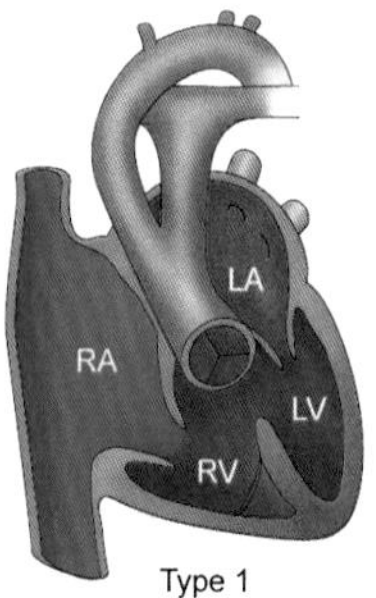

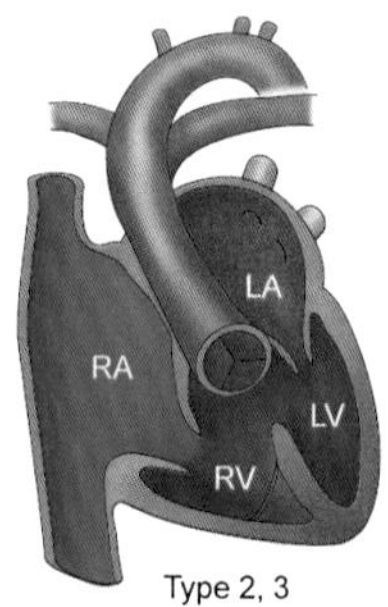

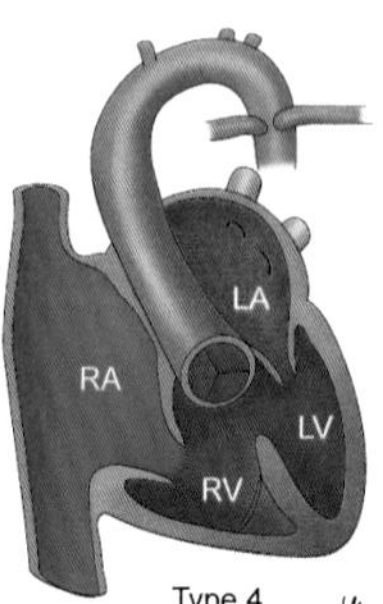

Associated Pathology
- Truncal valve anomalies
- Right aortic arch, interrupted arch
- Coronary ostial anomalies

2D Imaging
- Single trunk in ME AV LAX, TG views
- PA from single trunk
- Truncal valve (ME, TG views)
- VSD: large unrestricted
- Ventricle function

Color/Spectral Doppler
- Valve regurgitation stenosis
- VSD: direction, gradient

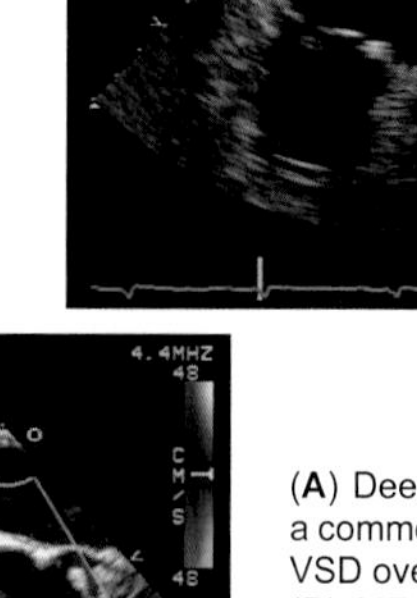

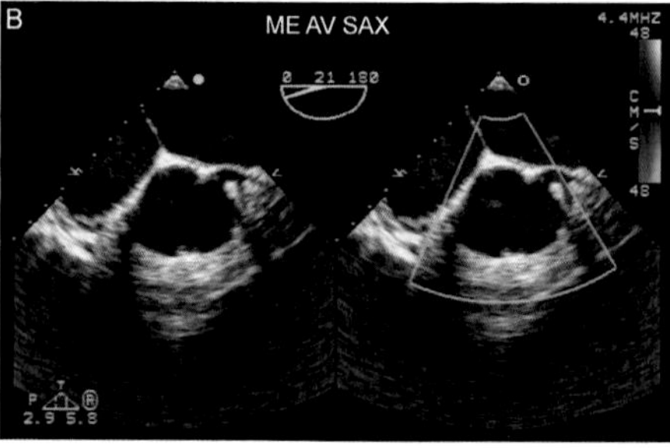

(**A**) Deep TG view showing a common truncal valve and VSD overriding the IVS.
(**B**) ME AV SAX view with color Doppler (Nyquist 48 cm/s) showing the single truncal valve with normal systolic flow into the left main coronary artery.

What to Tell the Surgeon Truncus Arteriosus	
PreCPB	**PostCPB**
• VSD: location, size, shunt direction, peak Pressure gradient • Single trunk, PA location • Truncal valve: regurgitation, stenosis • Ventricular function – Common: abnormal coronaries – Minor: LSVC, ASD, right arch – Major: AVSD, double aortic arch	• Residual VSD leak • Ventricular function – Global – Regional wall motion • Conduits or baffles

- A subaortic membrane is a fibrotic ridge of tissue that is present in the left ventricular outflow tract (LVOT) located just below the AV or lower down involving the anterior mitral valve leaflet. There may be a more acute ventriculo-aortic angle, greater separation of the AV and MV, and the AV overriding the IVS. The membrane is rigid and may result in a fixed LVOT obstruction and a pressure gradient. The AV may become damaged from turbulent flow after the membrane resulting in AI.
- Associated congenital heart defects are found in 25–50% of patients; VSD, PDA, coarctation, bicuspid AV, AVSD, Shone complex, interrupted aortic arch, and persistent left SVC.

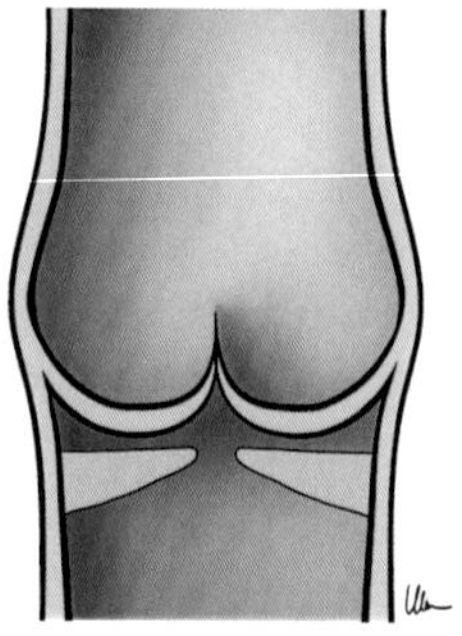

ME AV LAX views show turbulent flow starting below the AV in the LVOT during systole. (**A**) The 2D image shows tissue in the LVOT. (**B**) The narrowed LVOT is seen en-face in a 3D Live view of the LVOT and (**C**) the turbulent flow (and MR) is shown with 3D color full volume view.

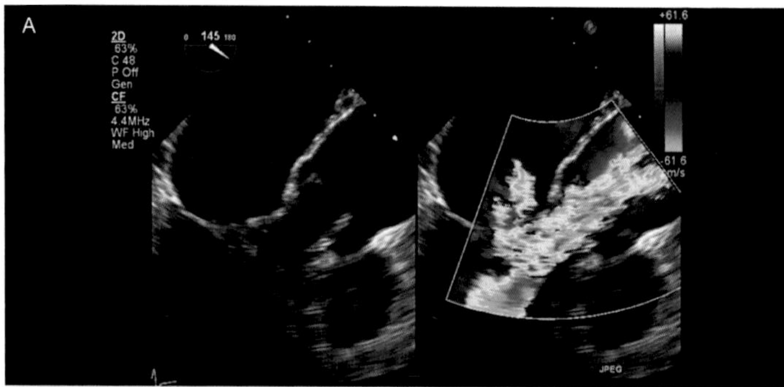

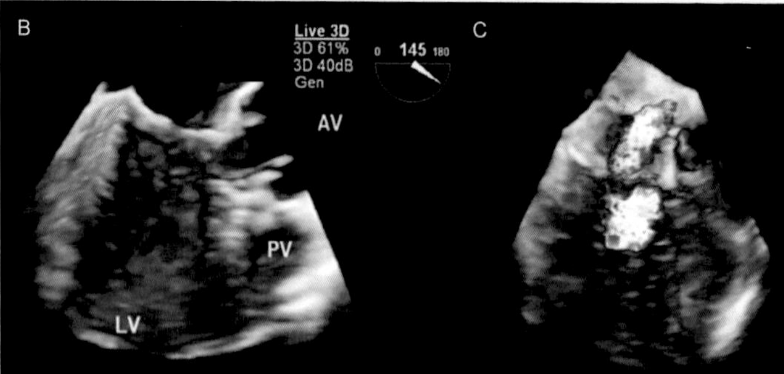

What to Tell the Surgeon Subaortic Membrane	
PreCPB	**PostCPB**
• Membrane in LVOT	• Residual tissue
• Turbulent color flow	• Laminar flow
• Pressure gradient	• Gradient in LVOT
• LV size and function	• LV function
• AV thickened, AI	• AV, AI
• MR	
• Associated pathology	

Subvalvular RVOT obstruction is common and usually dynamic from muscular hypertrophy. An isolated fibrous membrane in the RVOT is rare. Supravalvular pulmonary artery (PA) stenosis may be present from proximal narrowing of the main PA or, more commonly, from peripheral PA stenosis. Branch PA stenosis may result from congenital syndromes (Noonan's, Alagille's, or William's syndromes), systemic inflammatory disease (Behcet's), or thromboembolism. In certain patients, percutaneous PA stents may be inserted to relieve obstruction (see p. 265).

(**A**) ME RVOT view shows turbulent flow (color Doppler Nyquist 59 cm/s) in the RVOT that originates near the pulmonic valve. (**B**) TG RVOT view shows the turbulence is related to a supravalvular membrane in the main pulmonary artery. The main PA is dilated. (**C**) Spectral Doppler alignment accurately measures a peak pressure gradient of 35 mmHg in this TG view.

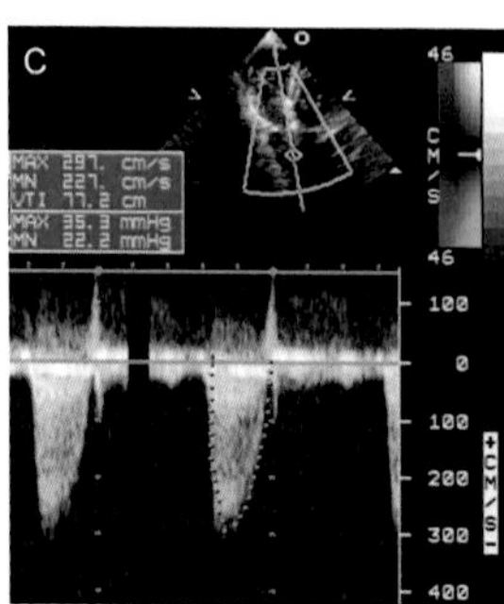

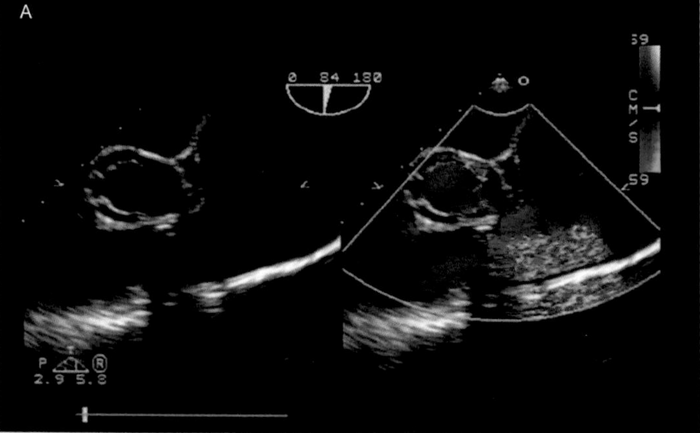

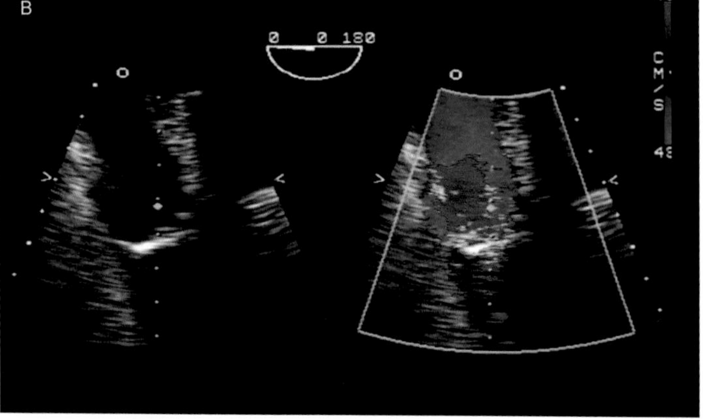

11
Variants, Foreign Material, Artifacts, Masses, Endocarditis

A. Vegas, *Perioperative Two-Dimensional Transesophageal Echocardiography*, https://doi.org/10.1007/978-3-319-60902-7_11

- Normal structures or their variants may mimic pathology resulting in errors in interpretation that may cause unnecessary clinical interventions. These imaging pitfalls are generally categorized as anatomic structures, echo-free spaces, or foreign material. Careful imaging using multiple imaging planes and knowledge of variants may help differentiate these from actual pathology.

Structures
• LA: Warfarin ridge, LAA (inverted, trabeculations, multi-lobed) • RA: Eustachian valve, Chiari network, Crista Terminalis, Thebesian valve, Pectinate muscles • RV: Crista superventricularis, Moderator band, Trabeculations • LV: False tendon, Trabeculations • AV: Nodule of Arantius, Lambl's excrescences • IAS: Lipomatous IAS, IAS aneurysm • Aorta: Innominate vein

Echo-Free Spaces	**Foreign Material**
• Persistent left SVC	• Catheters and Cannulae
• Transverse sinus	• Pacer wires
• Oblique sinus	• Sutures
• Effusions	• Stents

LAA, left atrial appendage; IAS, inter-atrial septum; SVC, superior vena cava

Left Atrium (LAA View 70°)

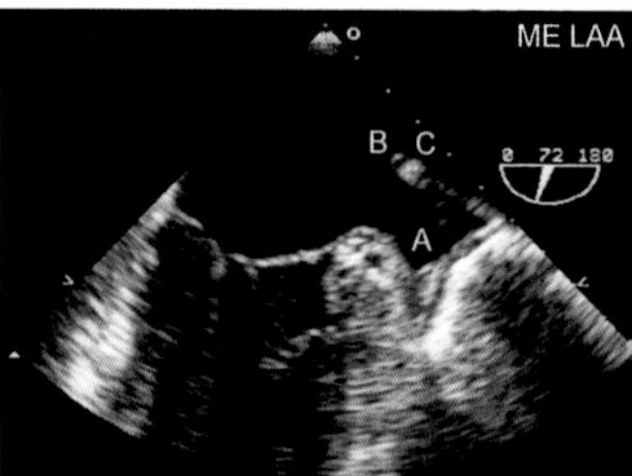

- LAA pectinate muscles (A) are trabeculations in the LAA which may be confused for thrombus.
- Coumadin ridge (B) is an echogenic "Q" tip-shaped tissue ridge that separates the (C) left upper pulmonary vein (LUPV) from the LA.
- Persistent left SVC (see p. 262) drains blood into a dilated coronary sinus

Right Atrium

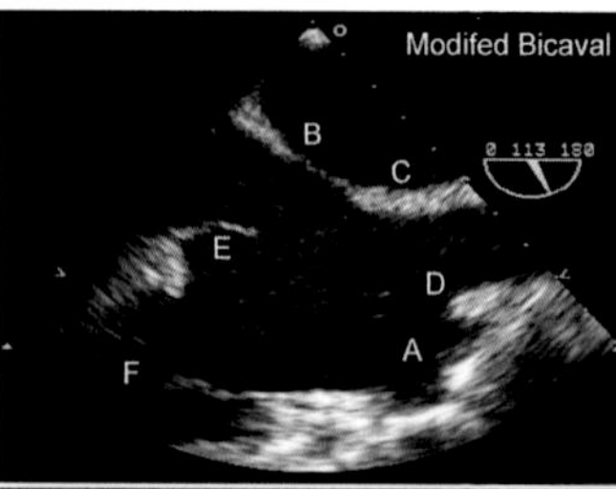

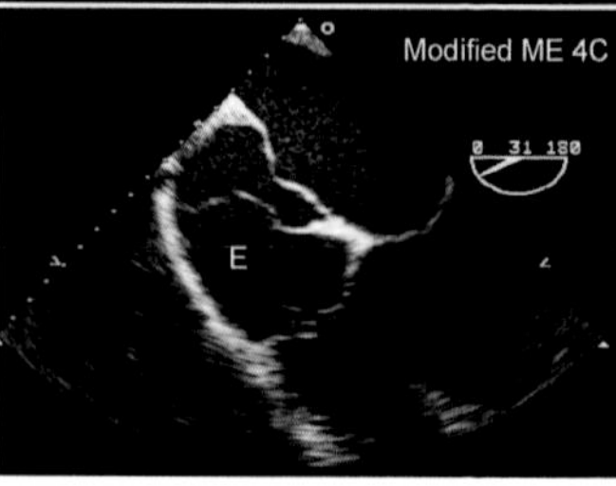

- Pectinate muscles (A) are thick muscle bundles that are not isolated to the RAA, but extend to the vestibule. These may be confused with RA thrombus.
- IAS foramen ovalis (B) is the thinned central portion of the IAS.
- Lipomatous hypertrophy of the IAS (C) is fatty infiltration of the IAS, not to be confused with tumor.
- Crista terminalis (D) is a muscle ridge that separates the SVC/RA.
- Eustachian valve (E) is a fine filamentous strand that attaches at the IVC/RA junction. In utero, it channels blood from the RA through the PFO. A prominent valve may complicate IVC cannulation.
- Chiari network (F) results from failure of resorption of right-sided sinus venosus valve which normally forms the valves of the IVC (Eustachian valve) and coronary sinus (Thebesian valve). It appears as a fenestrated network of tissue that may join the IVC, coronary sinus, and crista terminalis. May be associated PFO, IAS aneurysm, paradoxical emboli.
- Thebesian valve (not shown) is the valve to the coronary sinus, which prevents regurgitation of blood into the coronary sinus.

Right Ventricle

- RV trabeculations (A) are muscle bands in the RV that become more prominent with RV hypertrophy.
- Moderator band (B) is a prominent apical muscle band from the septum to the anterior papillary muscle. It is an important anatomic feature that distinguishes the RV from the LV.
- Epicardial fat (C) over the pericardium may make the RV free wall appear thickened or mimic a clot collection.

Left Ventricle

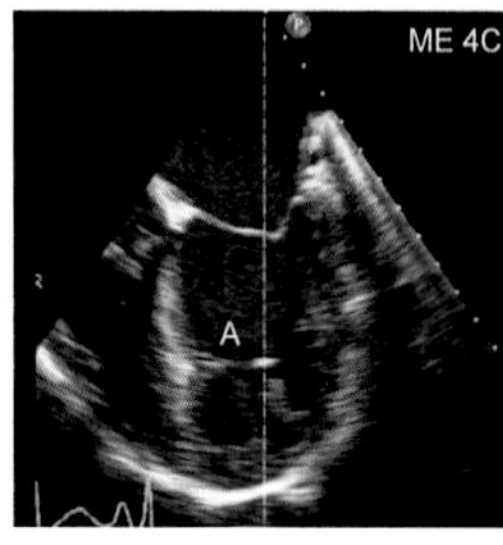

- False tendons (A) are fine filaments that traverse the LV cavity between the LV wall (free wall or IVS) and papillary muscle. These are located in the LV apex, do not attach to the MV, and are seen in more than one TEE view. These might mimic the moderator band seen in the RV.
- Papillary muscles normally there are two, but there may be more or even only one.
- Aberrant chordae may originate from the papillary muscles or even the ventricular walls and attach to the MV leaflets.

Aortic Valve

- Nodules of Arantius (A) are thickened points of coaptation at the edge of the AV cusps. The nodules may become calcified or be a source of excrescences.
- Lambl's excrescences (B) are degenerative fibrous strands (<1 mm thick, <1 cm long) originating from the nodules on either side of the valve cusps. These should not be confused with tumors or vegetations.

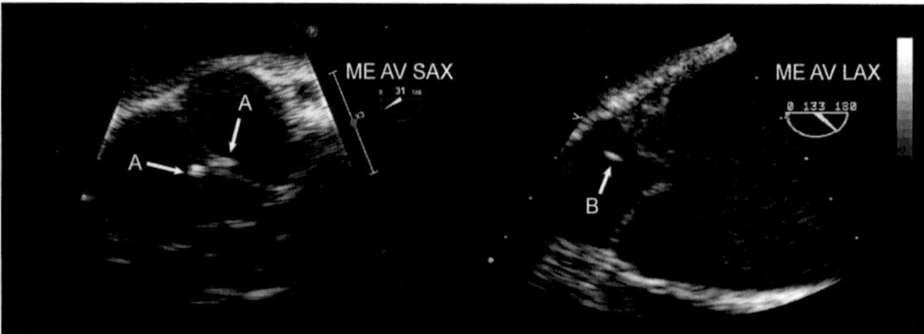

Pericardium

- Adipose tissue may appear as an epicardial fat pad around the RV (see above)
- Transverse sinus: space between posterior wall of ascending aorta and anterior LA (RVOT view). May appear as cystic mass differentiate from LAA, fibrin, or cyst.

Inter-Atrial Septum **(see p. 224)**

- Lipomatous hypertrophy IAS (A) makes the IAS echogenic "dumb bell shaped"
- IAS aneurysm (B) mobile septum >1.0 cm × 1.0 cm into atria, sigmoid shape

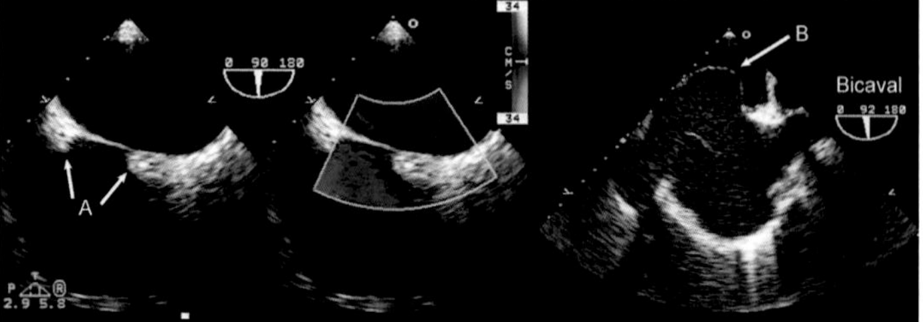

Persistent Left Superior Vena Cava (LSVC)

- A persistent LSVC results from failure of the left common cardinal vein to reabsorb.
- Incidence 0.5% general population, 10% in patients with congenital heart disease
- Subtypes of persistent LSVC exist.
  - 90% have both R and L SVC present
  - Rarely, there is absence of R SVC
  - Bridging innominate vein absent in 65%
- In 80–90% of patients, the persistent LSVC drains into the coronary sinus (CS) which enters the RA. It may, however, drain into the LA or pulmonary vein resulting in a L → R shunt.
- Associated with congenital heart disease: Coarctation of aorta, ASD (sinus venosus), VSD, cor-triatriatum.
- Persistent LSVC can complicate retrograde cardioplegia administration.

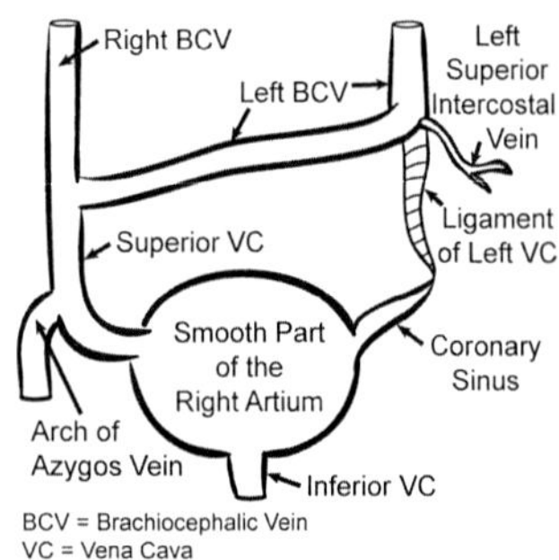

Source: Goyal SK, et al. Cardiovasc Ultrasound 2008; 6:50.

TEE Findings

- Dilated coronary sinus (>2 cm) is seen in multiple ME (4C, 2C) and lower esophageal views.
- Cystic structure appears between LUPV and LAA
- Color Doppler shows flow in the structure
- Agitated saline injection from the:
  - Left arm opacifies the CS than RA
  - Right arm opacifies the RA

Differential Dilated Coronary Sinus

- Persistent LSVC
- Elevated RAP
- Coronary arterio-venous fistula
- Partial anomalous pulmonary venous drainage
- Unroofed coronary sinus LA ↔ CS flow, shunt

(A) There is a cystic structure imaged between the LUPV and left atrial appendage (LAA) in the ME 4C view. Note in the LAA view, there appears to be 3 cystic structures: the LUPV, persistent LSVC, and LAA. (B, C) Color Doppler (Nyquist 48 cm/s) identifies flow in the structure. (D) The coronary sinus (CS) is dilated (> 2 cm) as seen in (D) LAX in the lower esophageal Coronary Sinus view or in (C) SAX in the ME 2C view. Agitated saline injected into the left arm enters from the left subclavian vein and rapidly appears in the CS. A PA catheter inserted in the left central veins may also appear in the CS.

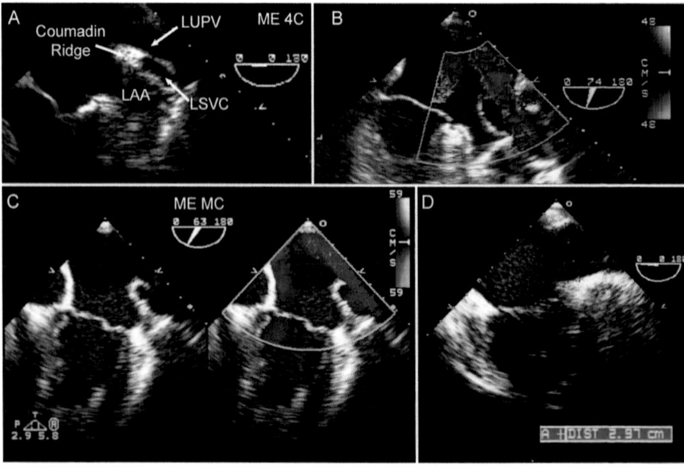

Pleural Effusions

- A collection of fluid may accumulate in the pleural space around either the right or left lung. The fluid may represent hydrothorax (serous/exudate fluid), hemothorax (blood), chylothorax (chyle), or pyothorax (pus).
- TEE can identify the presence, size, and nature of an effusion and guide drainage (thoracentesis). Ultrasound is more sensitive than CXR and CT in identifying fluid.
- The appearance of the fluid may help differentiate the type of effusion.

US Findings	Fluid Appearance	Fluid Type
Anechoic	Homogeneous	Transudate, exudate, acute hemothorax
Echoic	Particles	Exudate, hemothorax
Complex	Septated	Inflammatory

- Estimate volume by tracing the cross-sectional area (CSA): CSA: <20 cm^2 (<400 cc), 20–40 cm^2 (400–1200 cc), >40 cm^2 (>1200 cc)
- Formula: Axial length of effusion (probe proximal-distal limit) × CSA = volume

(A) Right pleural effusion is an echolucent space with the "tiger's claw" directed to the right above the liver. No aorta is present. This view is obtained by rotating the probe counter-clockwise from the ME descending aorta SAX view. (B) Left pleural effusion appears as an echolucent region immediately below the descending aorta in the ME Descending Aorta SAX view. The "tiger's claw" is directed left. Note left lung atelectasis (arrow). (C) A large complex right pleural effusion is shown with multiple septae and fibrous material. (D) A left hemothorax is seen in a patient in the immediate postoperative period. Note the echoic fluid surrounding the consolidated left lung. (E) Fluid in the stomach should not be confused with a left pleural effusion. Note there is no aorta seen. The fluid contains particulate matter. (F) Combined small pericardial effusion (arrow) medial to the left pleural effusion immediately below the aorta.

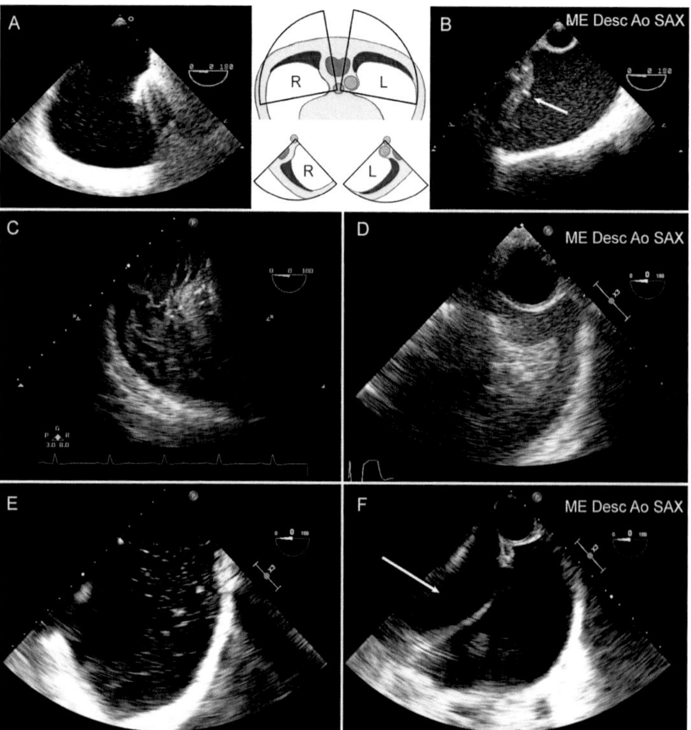

Cannulation

- During cardiac surgery, arterial and venous cannulae are placed by the cardiac surgeon to use cardiopulmonary bypass (CPB). Examination of cannulation sites pre- and postCPB is important to exclude complications.
- Other cannulae used in cardiac surgery include cardioplegia and vents.
- Cannulae are also used for extra-corporeal life support (see pp. 298–299).

(A) Standard cannulation includes placing an aortic cannula (arrow) in the distal ascending aorta as seen in the UE Arch LAX view. (B) A single double-stage venous cannula is placed in the RA and directed towards the IVC. Blood is drained from 2 regions, the distal end (IVC) and mid-portion (RA). (C) Bicaval cannulation places 2 single-stage cannulae separately in the SVC and IVC to drain all blood from the RA as seen in this ME Bicaval view. The IVC cannula should not be malpositioned in the hepatic vein as this will obstruct liver blood flow. (D) Coronary sinus cannula is used for retrograde cardioplegia and is positioned directly into the coronary sinus. In this ME Bicaval view, the balloon of this cannula is seen in the RA and should be redirected to the coronary sinus (arrow).

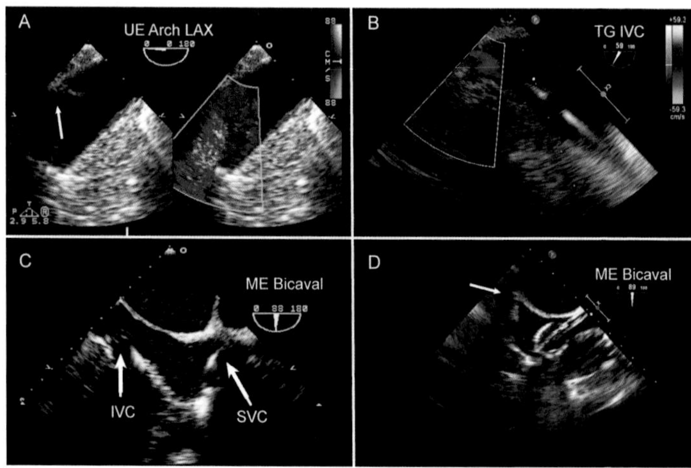

Catheters and Wires

- Various venous catheters can be seen in the right heart including, central lines, pulmonary artery catheters (PAC), and peripherally inserted central catheter (PICC) lines. These cannulae should be carefully examined for the presence of thrombus.
- TEE may help guide positioning of the PAC in the main PA by using different views (A) to show the catheter sequentially in the RA (ME Bicaval), RVOT (ME RV inflow-outflow), and PA (UE Arch SAX).
- Pacing wires may be seen entering the right heart (RA, RV) and coronary sinus. The wires may cause shadowing and have mobile masses consistent with thrombus or potential infection. (B) Pacer wire is positioned in the RAA in this ME-modified Bicaval view.

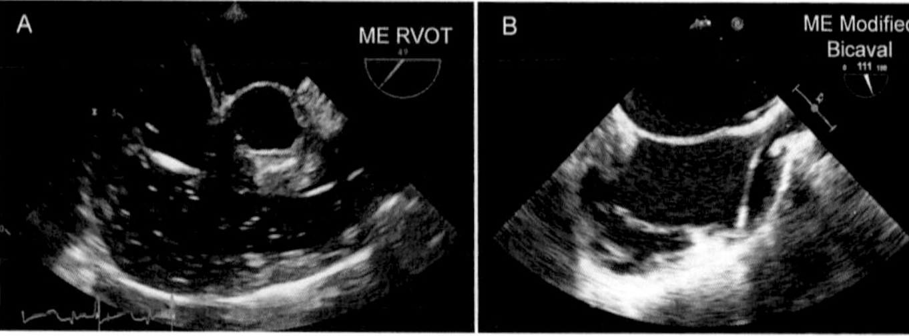

Intra-Aortic Balloon Pump Catheter

The IAB catheter tip is seen in the Descending Aortic SAX and LAX views. Optimal IAB catheter position is just below the left subclavian artery in the descending thoracic aorta imaged in both SAX and LAX.

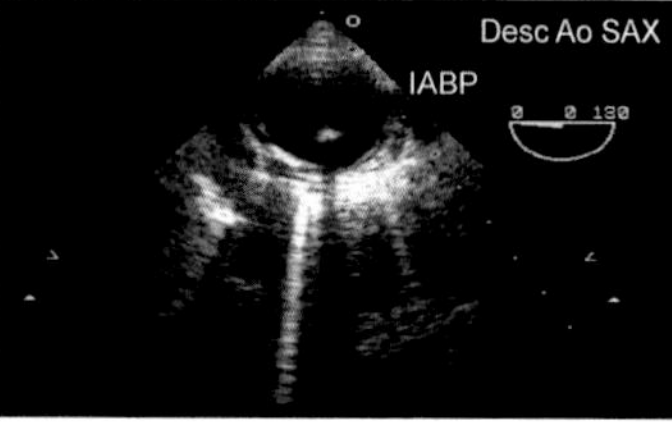

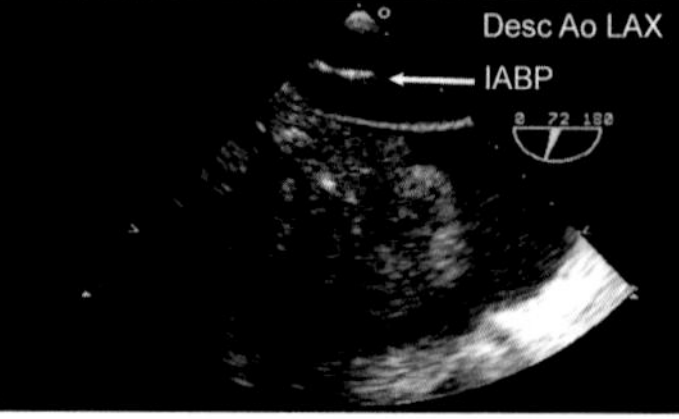

Elephant Trunk

The first stage of the procedure in a patient with mega-aorta syndrome involves replacement or sparing of the AV and Dacron graft for the ascending aorta and arch. The Dacron graft appears free floating in the dilated native aorta as imaged within the descending aorta in SAX and LAX views. The proximal end is attached to the distal aortic arch and the distal end is left unattached. The second stage uses an endovascular or open approach to secure the distal Dacron graft.

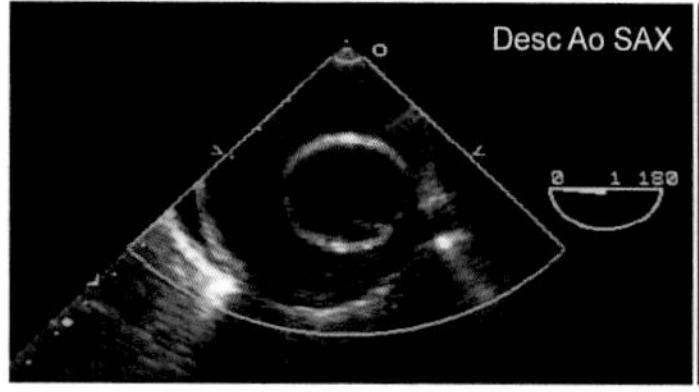

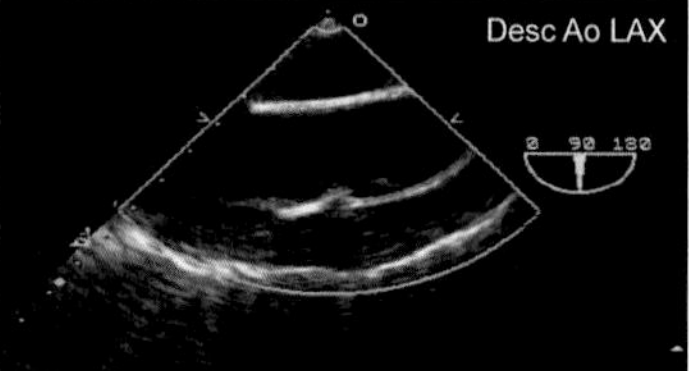

Coarctation Stent

This is located in the proximal descending aorta near the arch. It appears as a circular cluster of echogenic dots comprising the edges of the stent.

Pulmonary Artery (PA) Stent

A stent is positioned in the main PA using a percutaneous approach in a patient with congenital PA stenosis.

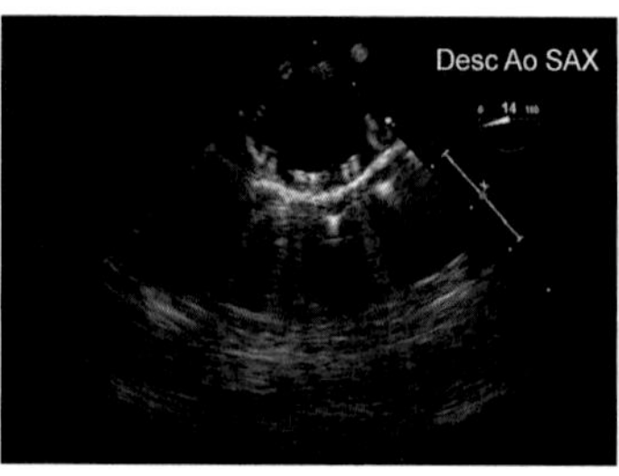

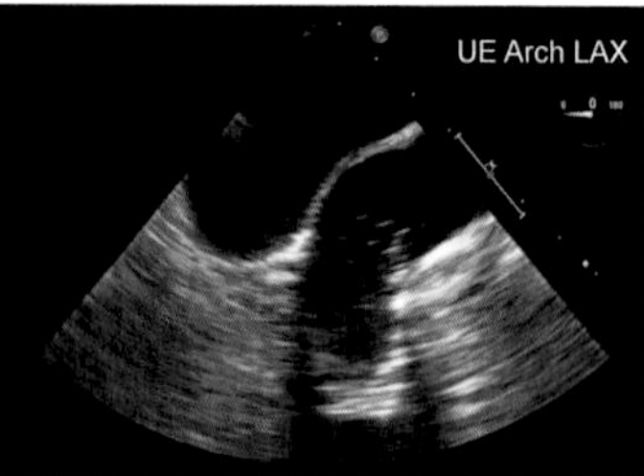

Pulmonary Artery Band

A band (arrow) is placed on the main PA to restrict flow in patient with L-TGA. Note there is distal turbulent flow after the band with color Doppler (Nyquist 60 cm/s).

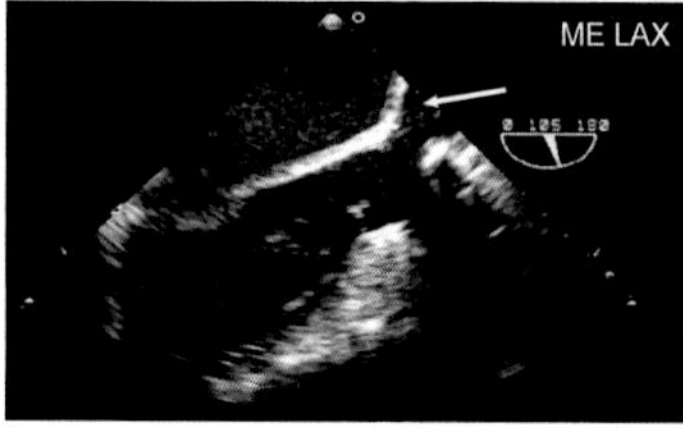

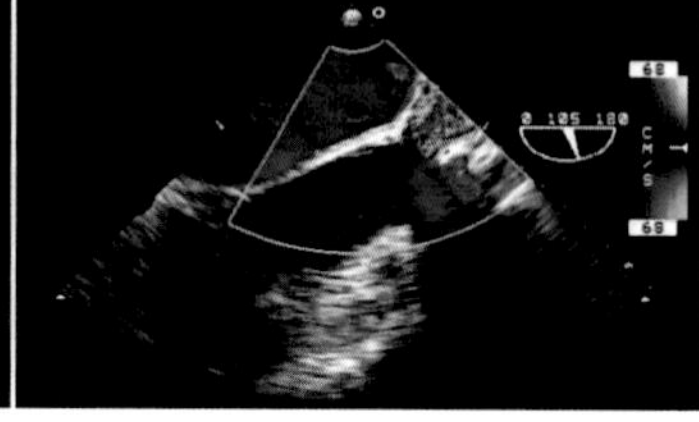

- Artifacts are defined as any structure in an image that does not correspond to an anatomic structure. This represents an error in imaging. The image can be tainted by structures:
  - that appear when they should not be there (false or extra echoes)
  - disappear when they should be there (missing or anechoic echoes)
  - are altered from reality: location (misplaced), size, shape, echogenicity
- It is crucial to distinguish this false information to avoid errors in diagnosis. Repositioning the probe or changing views will often eliminate artifacts from images.
- Artifacts result from violation of the basic assumptions of ultrasound, equipment malfunction, or operator error.
- Imaging artifacts can be categorized into groups based on the fundamental principles of US imaging. However, the terminology can often be confusing when various names are used to identify artifacts in the different imaging modes.

	Sound Assumptions
❶	Sound travels in a straight line.
❷	Sound travels directly to a reflector and back.
❸	Sound is constant 1540 m/s
❹	Imaging plane is extremely thin
❺	Reflections only from structures along the beam's main axis
❻	Reflected intensity is related to tissue characteristics.

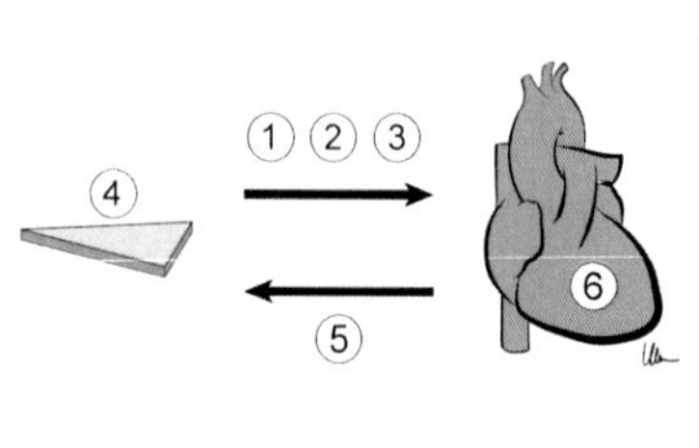

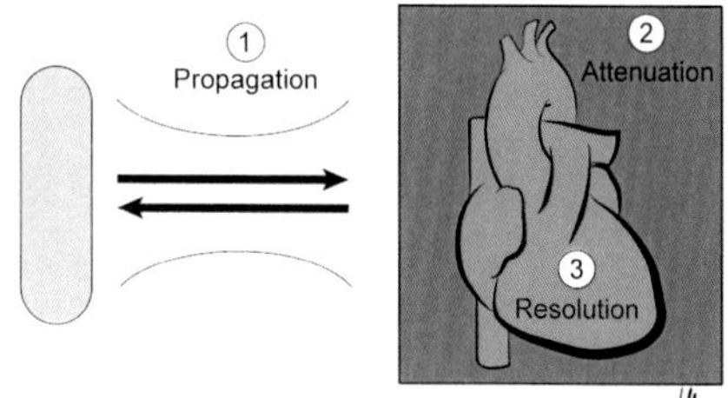

Artifacts by Sound Principles	
❶ Propagation Path	**❷ Attenuation**
Reverberation	Acoustic Shadowing
Mirror image	Enhancement
Comet tail	Focal Enhancement
Ringdown	**❸ Resolution**
Refraction	Axial Resolution
Ghosting	Lateral Resolution/Beam Width
Speed error	Slice/Beam Thickness
Edge shadowing	Dropout
Multipath	Speckle/Noise
Side lobe	Near-Field Clutter
Grating Lobe	
Range Ambiguity	

2D Imaging	Spectral Doppler	Color Doppler
Acoustic shadowing	Non-parallel intercept angle	Aliasing
Reverberations	Aliasing	Ghosting
Beam width	Range ambiguity	Shadowing
Lateral resolution	Crosstalk	Background noise
Refraction	Mirroring	Underestimate flow signal
Range ambiguity	Electronic interference	Intercept angle
Noise		Electronic interference

Propagation Path Artifacts

Reverberation Artifacts

- Bouncing of US beam (reflections) between 2 strong reflectors
- Appear as echoes of an echo
- Single or multiple artifacts
- Equally spaced lines of ↓ amplitude
- Parallel to the sound beam
- Deeper and along a straight line

Mirror Image

- Reverberation artifact
- Single reflection between a strong reflector and transducer along the same path
- 2nd copy of reflector at twice the distance
- Same structure in more than one place
- Color Doppler also appears
- UE Aortic arch LAX, Desc Aorta SAX/LAX
- Right PA within a large ascending aorta

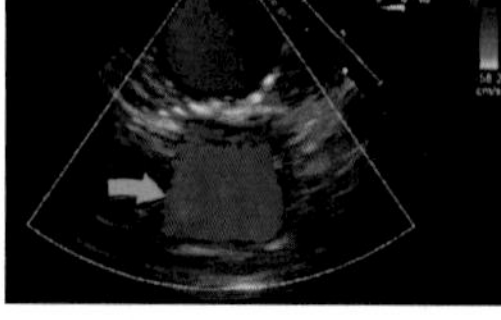

Comet Tail

- Reverberation artifact
- Small intense reflector (solid object) repeatedly reflected (resonates) in line with the US beam
- Aortic atheroma (is shown), mechanical valves
- Tail appears distal to the object
- Thin closely spaced discrete (clean shadow)
- Long hyperechoic line, parallel to sound beam

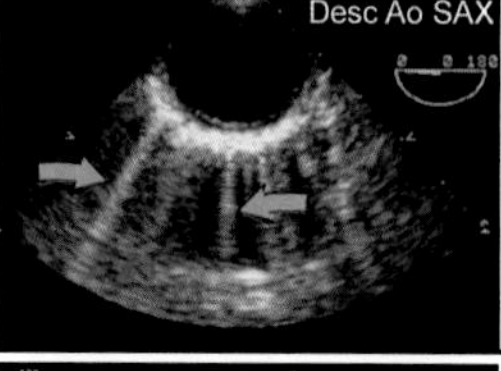

Ring Down

- Reverberation artifact
- Energy is trapped in tissue and slowly released
- Multiple reflections
- Small weaker reflector (**air**) has some transmission
- Adds streak to the end of the scan line
- Numerous, thin, closely spaced, but less discrete than comet tail (dirty shadow)

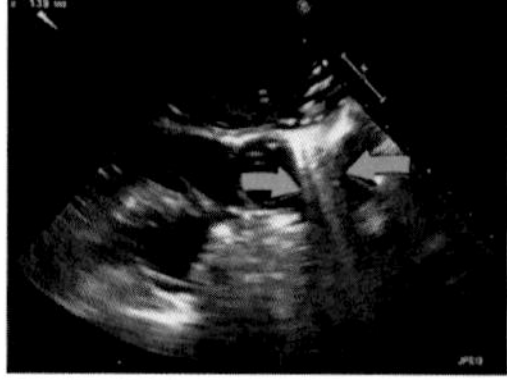

Refraction Artifacts

- Refraction is bending of transmitted and reflected waves.
- Sound changes direction when it strikes a boundary obliquely or when the media have different propagation speeds.
- US beam reflects off structures outside of beam planes.

Ghosting

- Refraction of sound striking boundary obliquely
- Second copy of true reflector appears side-by-side of the true anatomic structure.
- Objects appear in different position than they actually are.
- Extra echoes are present
- Degrades lateral resolution (edges appear blurred)

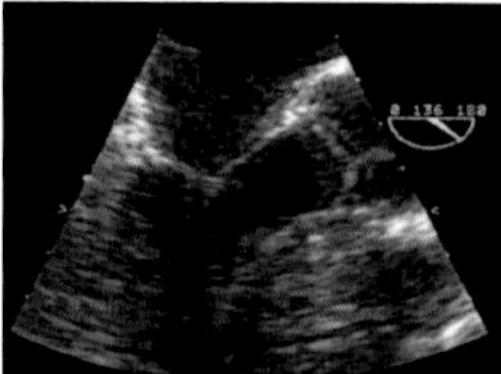

Propagation Speed Errors

- Refraction occurs from the difference in sound transmission through tissues (bone, liver)
- S(low) A(way) F(ast) T(owards)
  1540 m/s, reflector is shallower, narrower
  <1540 m/s, reflector is deeper, longer
- Displays a correct number of reflectors, but at incorrect depths.
- Structure edge appears "fractured" or cut

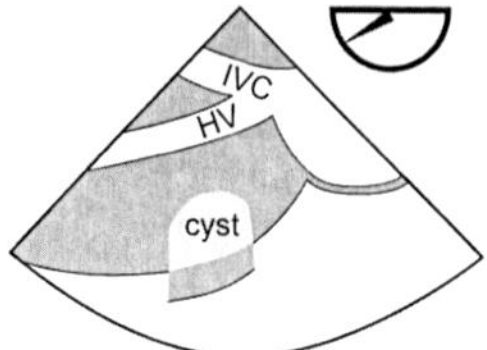

Refraction Artifacts

Edge Shadowing

- Refraction artifact
- Beam is bent at the edge of rounded structures, so there is no returning echo
- From high to low velocity gives a narrow shadow, opposite is true from low to high velocity
- Small dark areas appear beneath edges of circular structure (anechoic)
- ME Asc Aorta SAX view

ME Asc Ao SAX

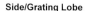

Side/Grating Lobe

- Side lobes are made by single element transducer
- Grating lobes are made by array transducers
- US is transmitted but not along the main beam
- Bounce off highly reflective structures (calcified aorta, mechanical valves, and catheters)
- Multiple structures are present on either side
- Appear as curved arc at same level of true object
- Hyperechoic, superimposed over structures

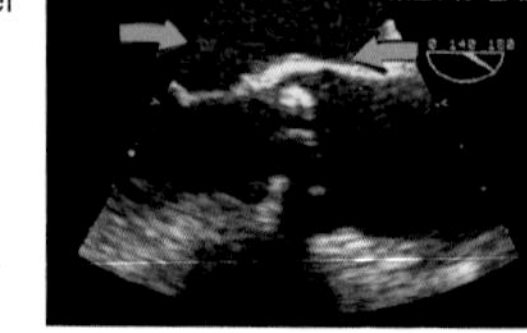

Range Ambiguity

- Pulsed sound returns late, after 2nd pulse sent
- Deeper structures appear closer to the transducer than their actual location.
- Late arriving reflection in display, even though reflector is beyond the scan area, results in an unexpected intra-cardiac echo.
- Changing the depth (PRF) may cause the artifact to disappear or change position.

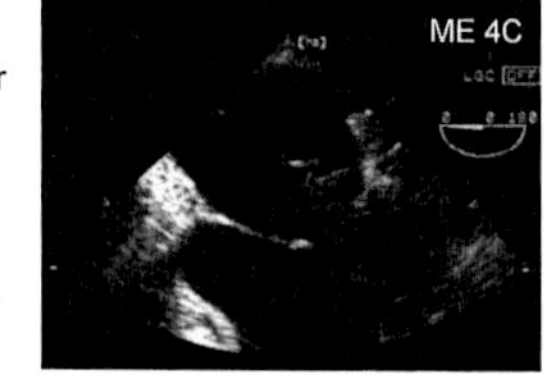

Attenuation Artifacts

Shadowing

- Loss of US beam transmission from high reflection or absorption
- High density structures (Ca^{2+}, prosthetic valves)
- Distal structures not seen (anechoic), or grey shadow
- Shape of shadow follows US path, a small structure close to the transducer casts a long shadow

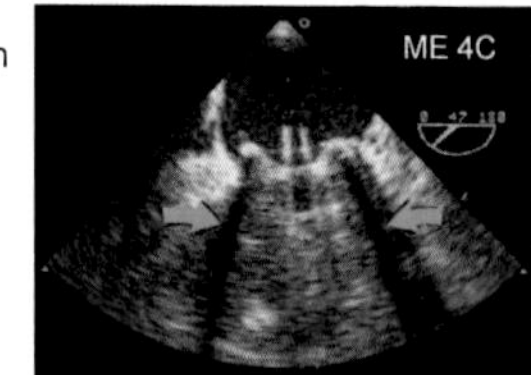

Enhancement

- Proximal structure has low sound absorption (< soft tissue), so distal structure has more energy reflected
- Hyperechoic region appears under tissue of low attenuation
- Distal structures appear brighter (hyperechoic)
- Transmitted object is darker (hypoechoic)
- This is the opposite of shadowing
- TG SAX view with anterior wall brighter

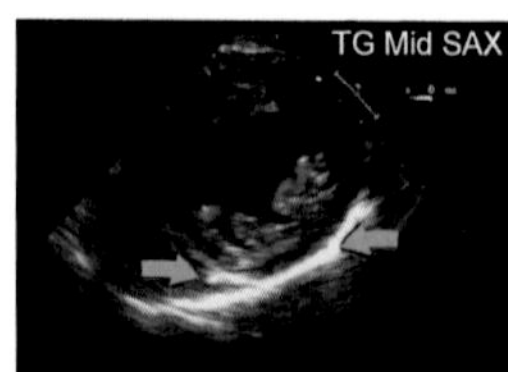

Focal Enhancement or Focal Banding

- Occurs around the focal zone
- Increased side by side intensity, extra echoes
- Too much band brightness compared to other depth
- Same appearance as incorrect TGC settings

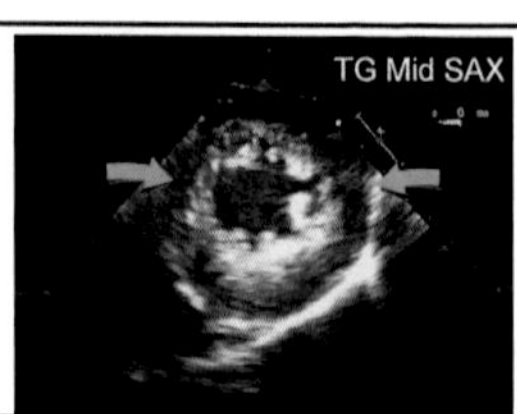

Resolution Artifacts

- This group of artifacts relates to image quality.
- Problems with:
  Dropout
  Speckle/noise
  Near-field clutter

Dropout

- Structures are not seen, anechoic
- Signal attenuation from
  Inadequate TGC/brightness or power
  Too high filters
  Use of high frequency transducer
- Imaging beam parallel to structure (anistrophy)
- TG SAX view poorly seen lateral + septal wall
- ME 4C view intra-atrial septum

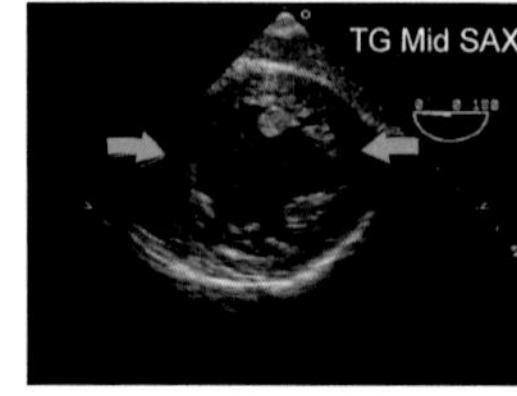

Noise

Acoustic (Acoustic Speckle)

- Created from interference of scattered sound waves, not reflection from tissues
- Extra small amplitude echoes, grainy image
- Improves with harmonic imaging (see below)

Electrical

- Repetitive geometric pattern

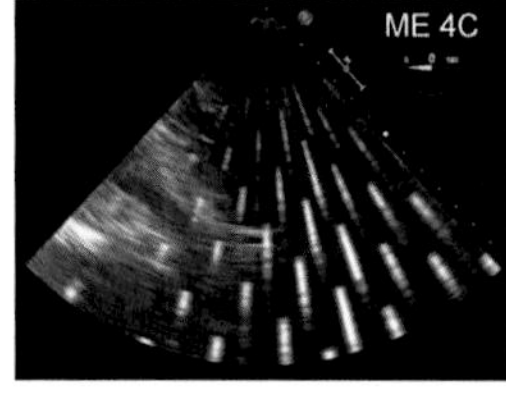

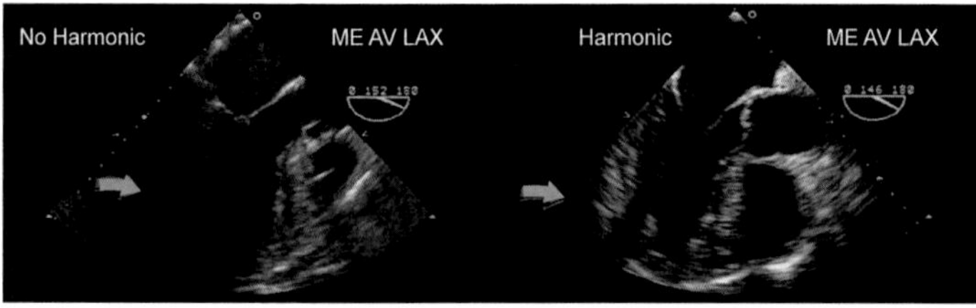

Near-Field Clutter

- High-amplitude oscillations of piezoelectric elements
- Extra echoes in the near field
- Difficulty differentiating near-field structures
- Common when imaging with an epiaortic probe
- Reduce by using stand-off such as a saline-filled glove

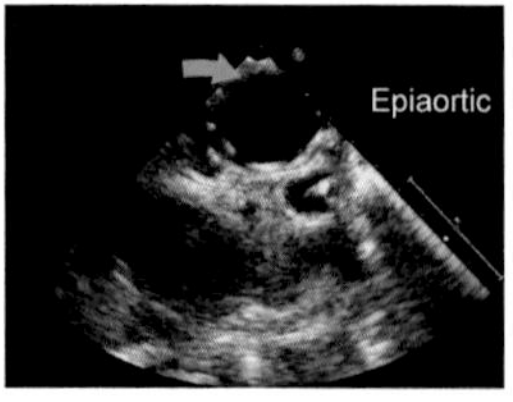

Beam Width

- US beam has finite width, smallest at focus
- Lateral resolution distinguishes 2 side by side structures. Two structures that are closer together than the lateral resolution will appear as a single reflector
- Can produce shape distortion like lateral stretching of small but strongly reflective echogenic objects (wires, gas bubbles)
- Strong reflector at the edge of the beam produces echo seen within the beam adjacent to the structure
- Can appear as unexpected intra-cardiac echo.

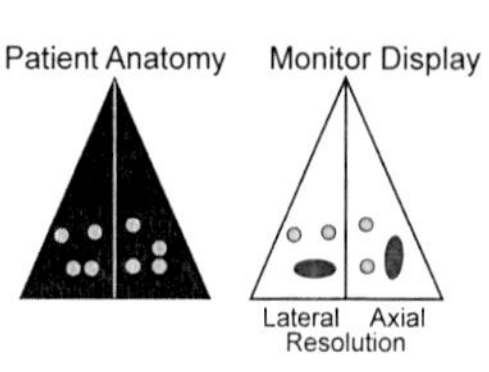

- Masses are abnormal structures within or adjacent to the heart.
- Pathologic masses should be distinguished from normal variants to avoid misdiagnosis (see pp. 260–261).
- Etiology of Masses (3 Types): Thrombus, Vegetations, Tumor

Thrombus	Vegetations	Tumor
Pacer wires Catheters LAA LV	Valves Myocardium Foreign material	Primary cardiac Benign Malignant Secondary metastatic
Spheroid or laminar Echogenic Laminar or mobile	Irregular shape and size Echogenic Independently mobile	Variable size Variable echogenicity Mobile or immobile

1° Benign Tumors (75%)	Incidence (%)	Location
Myxoma	30	LA > RA > RV = LV
Lipoma	10	LV, RA, IAS
Papillary fibroelastoma	9	AV > MV > TV
Fibroma	4	LV > RV, IVS
1° Malignant Tumors (25%)		
Angiosarcoma	9	RA, pericardium
Rhabdomyosarcoma	6	
Mesothelioma	2	
Fibrosarcoma	1	
2° Metastatic		
Direct extension	Lung, esophagus, breast	
Intravascular	SVC (bronchogenic, thyroid), IVC (renal, hepatoma)	
Hematogenous	Lymphoma, melanoma, leukemia	
Primary cardiac tumors are rare (0.03%), most are metastatic to the heart (1%). Over 75% of primary cardiac tumors are benign **Source: Tazelaar HD, et al. Mayo Clin Proceed 1992;67:957–65**		

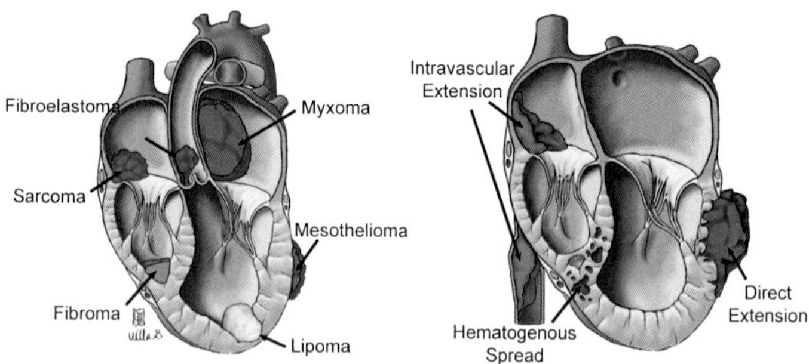

Diagnosis
- Appearance of the mass is not pathognomonic, need the clinical context
- Image mass by using echocardiography, CT, MRI
- Identify location (single or multiple, site of attachment, or direct extension)
- Measure size
- Assess mobility
- Effect: obstruction, LV/RV dysfunction, atrial fibrillation, emboli

Surgery Indications
- For diagnosis or excision
- Require complete excision and reconstruction if needed
- Avoid tumor manipulation to prevent embolization

Myxomas

- These are the commonest primary cardiac tumor.
- Myxomas have a gelatinous mucoid texture composed of mural endocardial cells in myxomatous stroma. Typically appear as irregular polypoid, pedunculated, or with a short broad-based attachment.
- Location
  - LA (75%) > RA (20%) > RV = LV (5%)
  - Majority solitary, multiple (3–5%)
  - Variable size
  - Pedunculated or sessile
  - Vacculations may appear as echolucent areas from tumor necrosis
  - Independently mobile, deforms during the cardiac cycle
- Result in
  - Valve obstruction: syncope or death
  - Valve regurgitation
  - Embolization from LA 30–40%, LV 50% to coronary, brain, periphery
- Syndrome myxoma = Carney's complex: familial
  - Cutaneous lesions: lentigines, blue nevi
  - Endocrine neoplasms: adenomas, Sertoli
  - Myxoma: cardiac involving multiple sites, but less often the LA

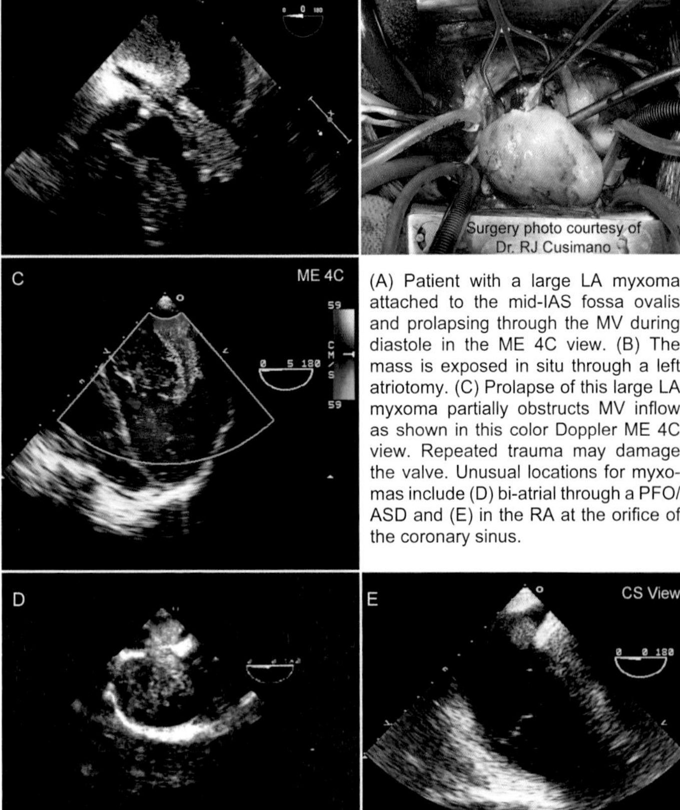

(A) Patient with a large LA myxoma attached to the mid-IAS fossa ovalis and prolapsing through the MV during diastole in the ME 4C view. (B) The mass is exposed in situ through a left atriotomy. (C) Prolapse of this large LA myxoma partially obstructs MV inflow as shown in this color Doppler ME 4C view. Repeated trauma may damage the valve. Unusual locations for myxomas include (D) bi-atrial through a PFO/ASD and (E) in the RA at the orifice of the coronary sinus.

Fibroelastomas

- This is the 2nd commonest cardiac tumor and the commonest valve tumor.
- Gross pathology resembles a sea anemone with frond-like projections.
- May involve any endothelial surface
  - Semilunar valves (ventricular side): AV (44%), PV (8%)
  - Atrioventricular valves (atrial side): MV (35%), TV (15%)
  - Mural endocardium
- Pedunculated: small size (1 cm), pom-pom appearance, narrow stalk, mobile
- Homogeneous speckled appearance
- Stippled edge from fronds, mobile undulating edges

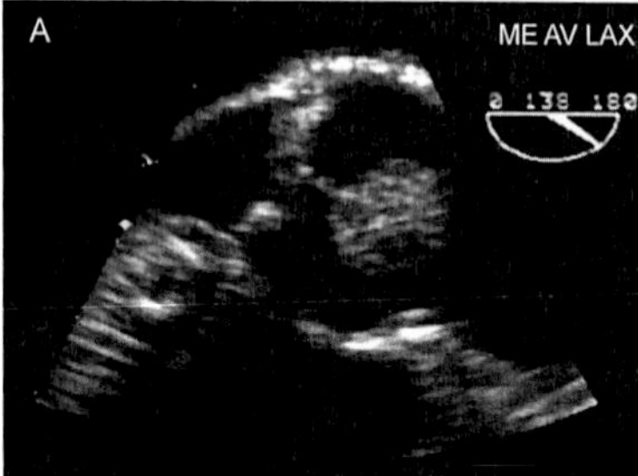

(A) Patient with typical "pom-pom" appearance of a pedunculated tumor on the aortic valve in this ME AV LAX view. (B) A small tumor (arrow) is present on the MV chordae in this patient as seen in the ME LAX view. (C) When exposed to saline, the tumor fronds become apparent and appear like a sea anemone.

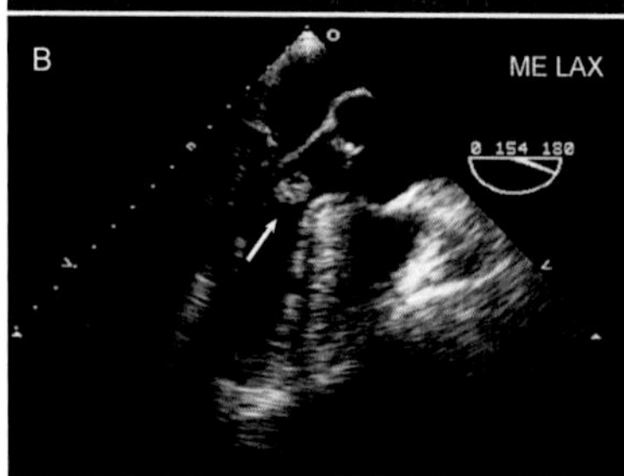

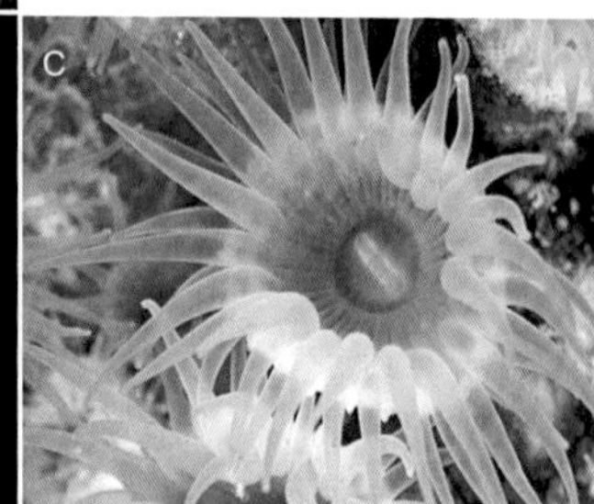

Lipoma

- This is a benign primary cardiac tumor.
- It occurs commonly in the body of the right atrium and left ventricle.
- Appear as sessile immobile masses, but occasionally may be pedunculated
- Well-demarcated homogenous and hyper-echogenic appearance

(A) Patient with a large hyperechoic LV mass shown in the (A) ME 4C and (B) ME AV LAX views. The mass was actually attached by a broad base to the IVS and not the LV apex. Pathology showed a lipoma.

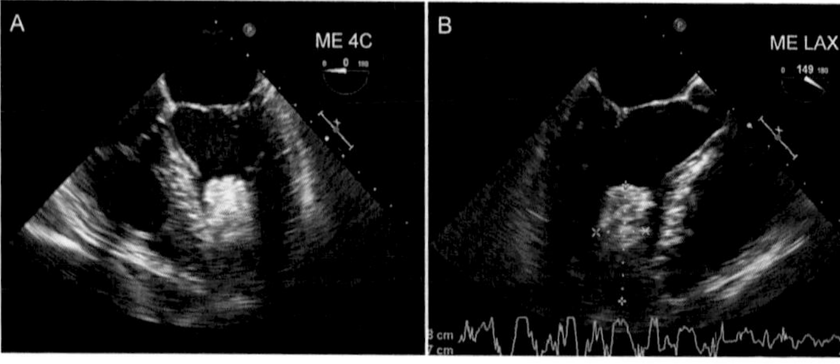

Fibroma

This patient presented with a RV tumor and underwent complete resection requiring RV reconstruction with a pericardial patch. Tumor extension into the RV as a hypoechoic mass is seen in (A) ME 4C view and (B) at the time of surgery. The anterior papillary muscle had to be resected and reimplanted. Pathology confirmed a fibroma.

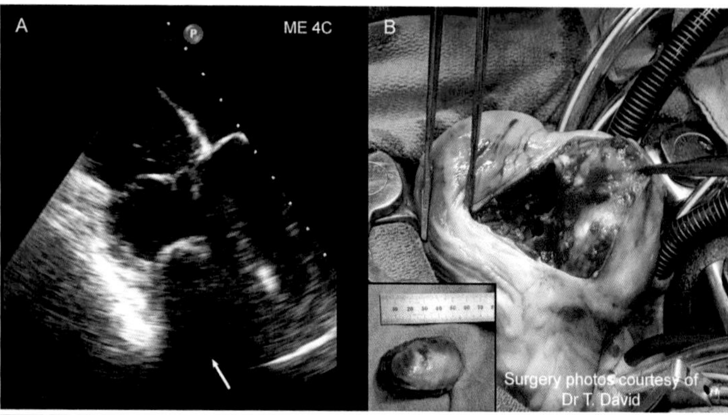

Sarcoma

- This is the commonest malignant primary cardiac tumor.
- More often in pediatric population
- Involves connective tissue
  - Angiosarcoma: blood vessels such as PA, aorta
  - Rhabdomyosarcoma: skeletal muscle
  - Fibrosarcoma: fibrous connective tissue
  - Liposarcoma: fat cells
  - Leiomyosarcoma: smooth muscle

Patient with a RA sarcoma at the junction of the inferior vena cava (IVC). The tumor location in the RA relative to the IVC is best shown in the (A) 2D ME bicaval and (B) Live 3D bicaval views. (C) The tumor is seen in situ at the time of surgery through a right atriotomy. Resection of the tumor and part of the IVC and RA was performed under circulatory arrest.

Surgical photo courtesy of Dr. RJ Cusimano.

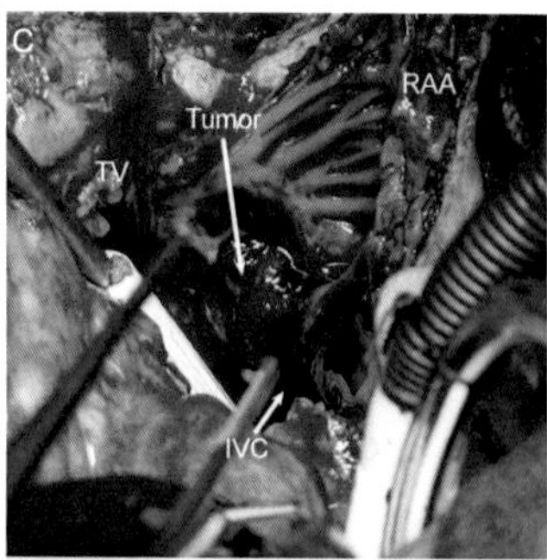

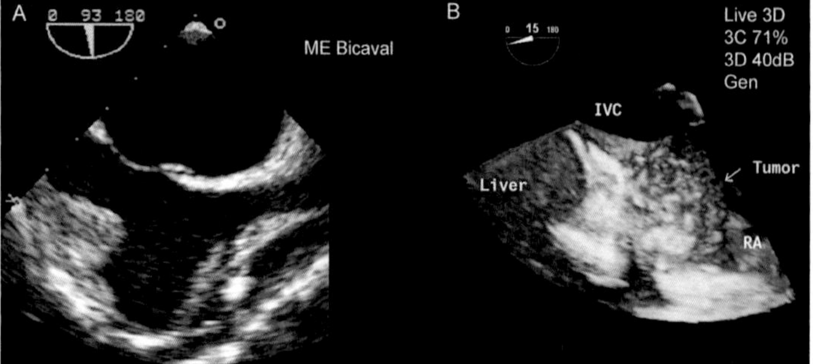

Metastatic Tumors

- These are the commonest of cardiac tumors.
- Mechanisms of tumor extension are by:
  - Intravascular extension
    SVC (bronchogenic, thyroid)
    IVC (renal, hepatoma)
  - Hematogenous spread
    lymphoma, melanoma, leukemia
  - Direct extension
    lung, esophagus, breast

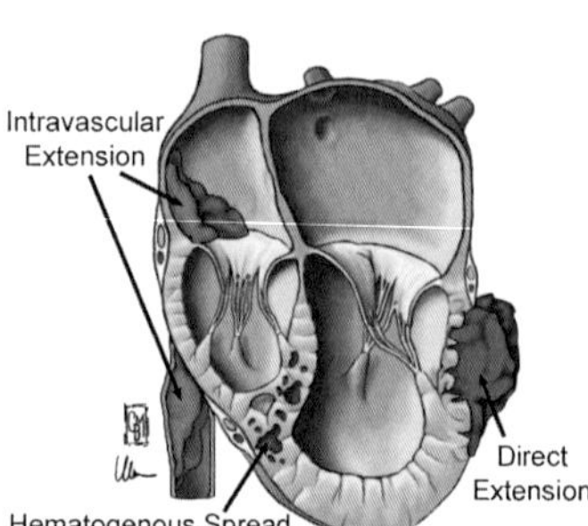

Intravascular Extension

(A) Patient with a renal cell tumor extending into the IVC just proximal (1.64 cm) to the hepatic vein. (B) Color Doppler demonstrates non-obstructive flow in the IVC and hepatic vein. (C) Another patient with renal cell carcinoma that extends via the IVC to the RA junction. Color Doppler does not show obstruction in the IVC at the RA junction. (D) The right kidney with tumor extension was removed without requiring CPB. (E) A large leiomyosarcoma of the IVC extends into the RA as shown in this color Doppler hepatic vein view. (F) Surgery required extensive resection of the mass and surrounding tissue with reconstruction of IVC.

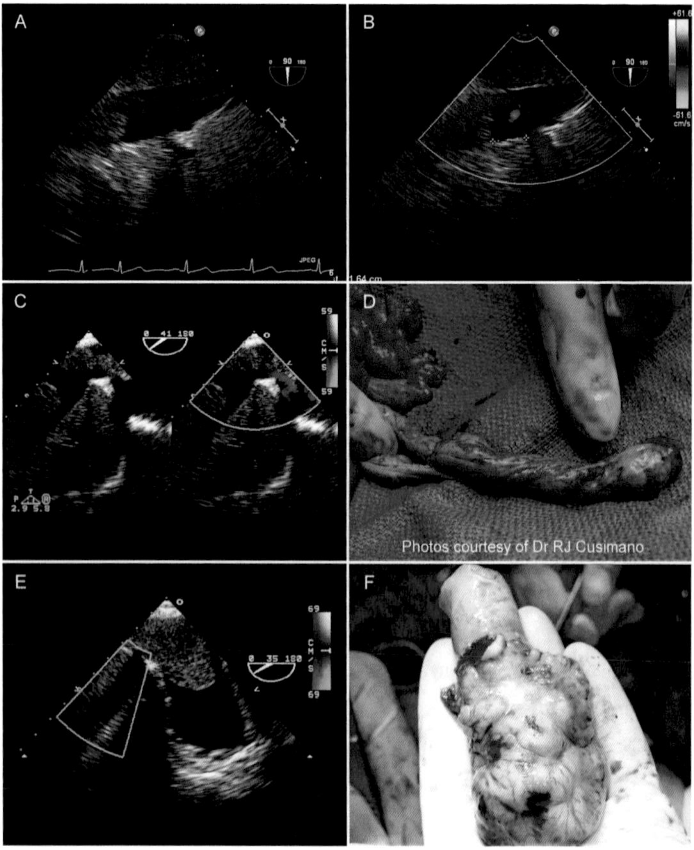

Photos courtesy of Dr RJ Cusimano

Hematogenous Spread

(A) Patient with metastatic melanoma of the LV apex. The ME 2C view shows a fullness in the LV apex with similar consistency to surrounding myocardium. (B) At the time of surgery, the tumor was remarkably well-encapsulated.

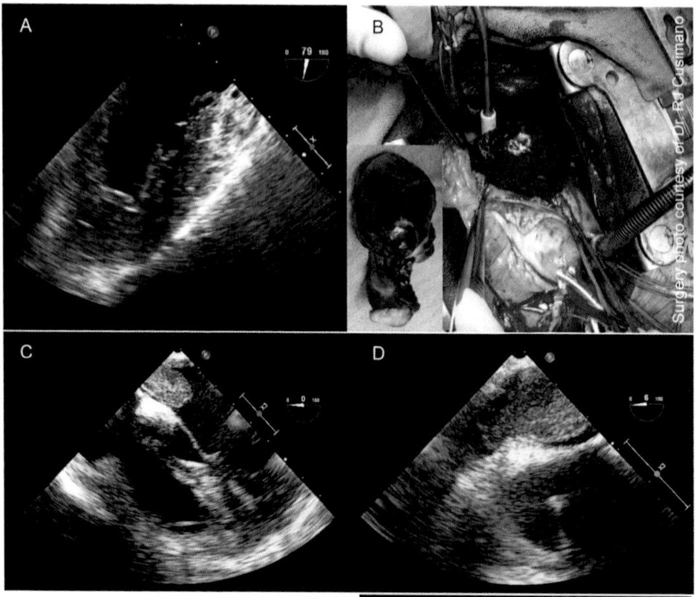

Surgery photo courtesy of Dr. RJ Cusimano

(C) Patient with metastatic uterine carcinoma seen in the left atrium in the ME 4C view. (D) The tumor originated from the right upper pulmonary vein (RUPV) as seen in this modified 4C view rotated to the right. (E) Despite the large size of the mass, flow into the LA from the RUPV was unobstructed by color Doppler (Nyquist 59 cm/s).

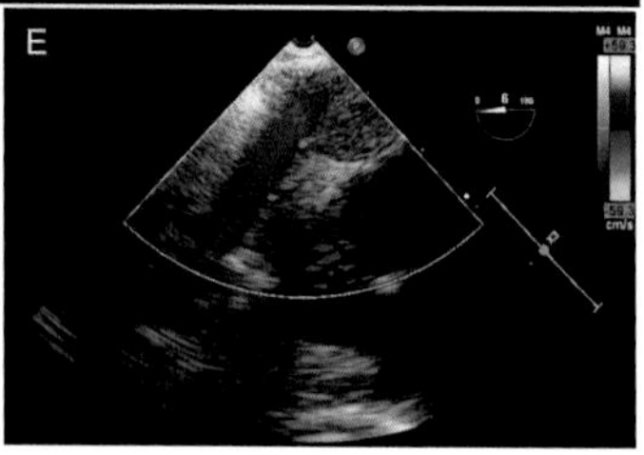

Direct Extension

Patient with sarcoma of the upper lobe of the left lung. MRI suggested extension into the LUPV. (A) Imaging of the LUPV in the ME 2C view did not show any tumor in the proximal LUPV. (B) Epicardial exam directly on the more distal portion of the LUPV demonstrates the tumor (arrow).

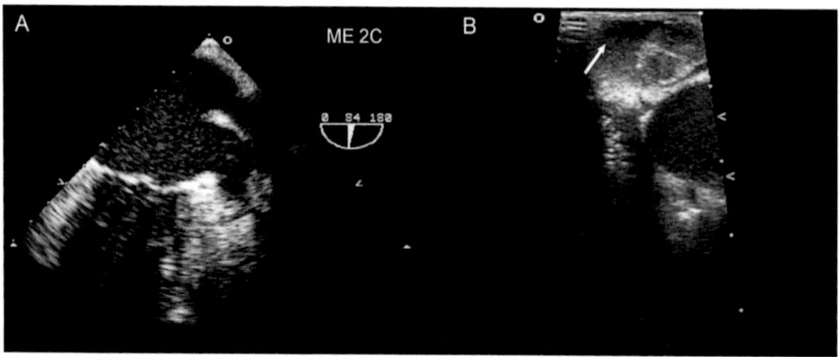

- Cardiac thrombi can result from either primary cardiac, hematologic, or rheumatologic (Behcet's syndrome) etiologies.
- Thrombi can be present:
  - in areas of stasis: LA (MS, atrial fibrillation), LV (abnormal wall motion)
  - on a catheter or device related (RA, RV, coronary sinus)
  - as thrombus in transit (RA, RV, PA)
- TEE has variable sensitivity for diagnosing thrombus.

LAA Thrombus

- LA enlarged + spontaneous echo contrast
  - Highest incidence in mitral stenosis (MS) and atrial fibrillation
  - Lower incidence with MR as the regurgitant jet disrupts blood stasis
- Blood flow in LAA
  - NSR or atrial flutter: velocity > 40 cm/s
  - Atrial fibrillation: low velocity flow (see below)
  - Thrombus risk increases with decreasing LAA velocities: <20 cm/s (29%), 20–40 cm/s (10%), and >40 cm/s (1%)
- TEE has high sensitivity + negative predictive value for LA thrombus
  - Appear as echogenic mass (arrow in image below)
  - May be laminated or spheroid
  - Immobile
  - Seen at multiple transducer angles, distinguish from pectinate muscles

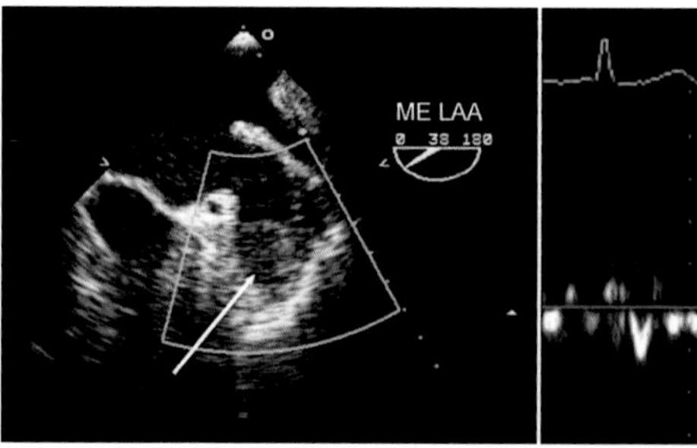

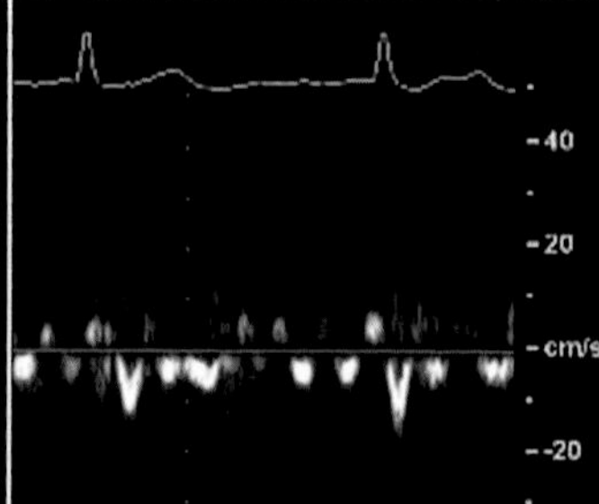

LV Thrombus (see p. 113)

- Increased risk with stasis: dilated LV (EDD > 60 mm), underlying wall motion abnormality, aneurysm, ECLS
- Homogenous laminated or layered
- LV apex looks thicker (arrow) than the other LV walls
- Avascular masses, no color Doppler flow within
- TTE is the diagnostic test of choice as the probe is closer to the LV apex

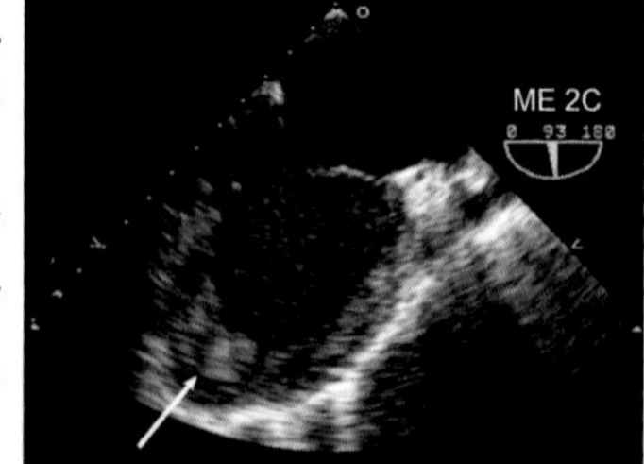

RV Thrombus

- Increased risk with stasis: dilated RV, poor RV function, mechanical assist, ECLS, catheters, and pacing wires
- Homogenous laminated appearance
- Avascular masses so no flow with color Doppler

Despite systemic anticoagulation, this patient developed a massive thrombus filling the entire RV cavity while on venous-venous (VV) ECMO.

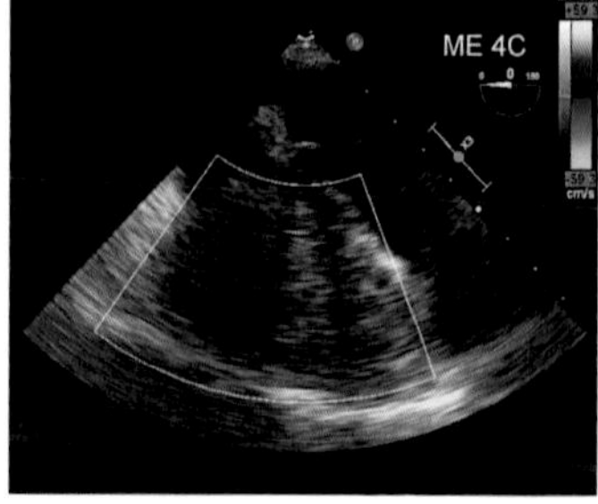

Pacer/Catheter Thrombus

- Difficult to differentiate thrombus from infection, so need clinical correlation.
- May require extraction if the thrombus is large or a PFO is present.
- Mass may be allowed to embolize to PA if there is no PFO.

(A) Large thrombus encasing a ventricular pacer lead is shown in the ME 4C view and during surgery. (B) Patient with a small thrombus attached to a permanent pacing wire as well as thrombus formation on the PA catheter (arrow).

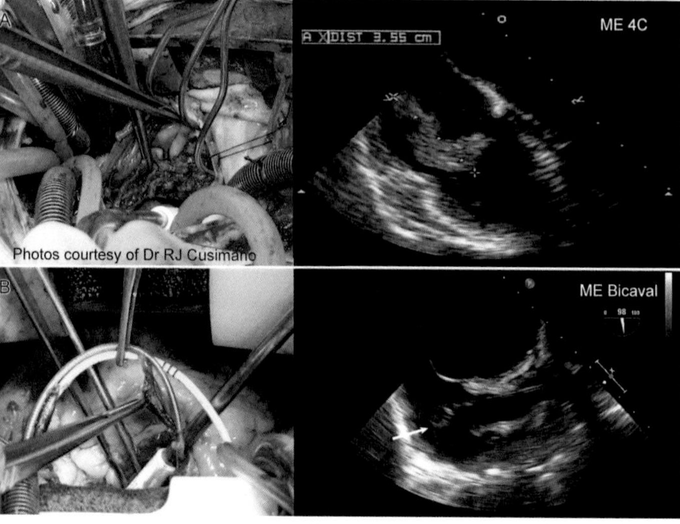

Thrombus in Transit

- Worm-like appearance on echocardiography
- Freely mobile in RA, RV, and PA, but may become entrapped in a PFO

(A) The ME 4C view shows a worm-like floating right heart thrombus in transit which was removed without requiring CPB. (B) A thrombus trapped in a PFO is seen in a ME view and at the time of surgery.

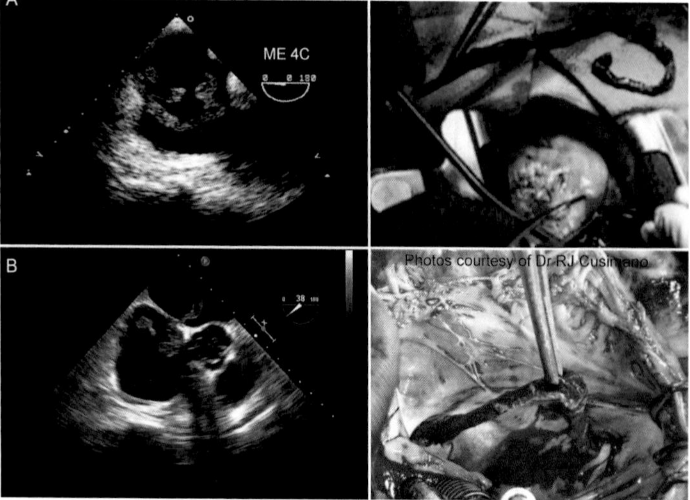

Pulmonary Emboli

- Risk: blood stasis + hypercoagulable + intimal damage
- Diagnostic tests are chosen based on convenience and cost
- Echocardiographic suspicion of PE is raised by finding indirect signs that mainly involve the right heart and not by direct visualization of clot. Overall, TEE is better than TTE to visualize clot, but is insensitive compared with other imaging.

Diagnostic Test	Sensitivity (%)	Specificity (%)
CT Pulmonary Angiography	96–100	97–98
MRI	77	98
TTE	68	89
TEE	70	81
Ventilation/Perfusion (V/Q) scan	98	10

- Findings differ depending on whether the embolism is acute or chronic. In both, PAP (and PVR) increase so the RV must compensate.

Indirect Findings	Acute	Chronic
RV size	Dilated	Dilated, hypertrophy
RV systolic function	Dysfunction Reduced strain McConnell's sign	Dysfunction Reduced strain
RV diastolic	↑ IVRT, ↑ IVCT, ↑ RVMPI	↑ IVRT, ↑ IVCT, ↑ RVMPI
LV Function	Normal LVMPI	↑ IVRT, ↑ IVCT, ↑ LVMPI
TR	Mod-severe	Variable
PAP (RVSP)	Normal, low	Elevated
60/60 sign	PA mid-systolic notch	
IVS	Flattened diastole	Flattened systole
McConnell's sign: hypokinetic mid/basal-free wall with normal/hyperkinetic apex 60/60 sign in acute PE: TR PG ≤ 60 mm Hg, PA acceleration time ≤ 60 ms MPI, myocardial performance index; IVCT, isovolumic contraction time; IVRT, relaxation time		

(A) ME Ascending Aorta view of the main pulmonary artery (PA) shows a large pulmonary embolus (arrow). (B) Pulmonary artery acceleration time (normal ≥130 ms) measurement from a PA spectral Doppler trace. (C) Descending thoracic aorta view shows thrombus (arrow) in the left pulmonary artery (LPA) and a left pleural effusion with lung consolidation. The LAX view confirms that this is the LPA as the Ascending Aorta LAX view would show the RPA above the ascending aorta.

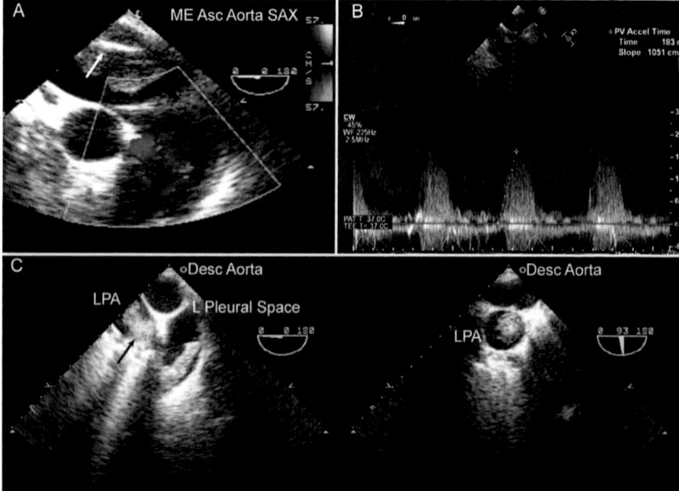

Pulmonary Thromboendarterectomy (PTE)

Chronic thromboembolic pulmonary hypertension (CTEPH) is a form of pulmonary vascular disease that is caused by chronic pulmonary thrombus. Surgery is the only definitive therapy for CTEPH, with pulmonary thromboendarterectomy (PTE) being the surgical procedure of choice. PTE is performed on CPB with deep hypothermic circulatory arrest.

- RV: size and function (ME 4C, TG SAX)
  - Dilated
  - Hypertrophied, flattened IVS (TG view)
  - RV FAC, strain, TAPSE
- Dilated PA
- Thrombus in main PA, RPA, LPA
- Quantification of tricuspid regurgitation
- Estimate RVSP from TR (PASP)
- Detection PFO (25–35% of patients)
- Complete remainder of full TEE exam

TEE for PTE Procedure

Pre
- RV: size and function
- TR severity
- Estimate RVSP
- Detection PFO
- Identify thrombus

Post
- Air
- RV function

(A) ME 4C view shows a dilated and hypertrophied RV consistent with RV pressure overload. (B) TG SAX view shows D-shaped interventricular septum flattened during systole. (C) ME Ascending aorta SAX view shows a dilated main and right pulmonary artery (RPA). (D) ME view of the distal RPA shows a portion of the thrombus (arrow). (E) Surgical photos show the emboli at surgery (arrow). The total amount of emboli removed from the pulmonary arteries are shown.

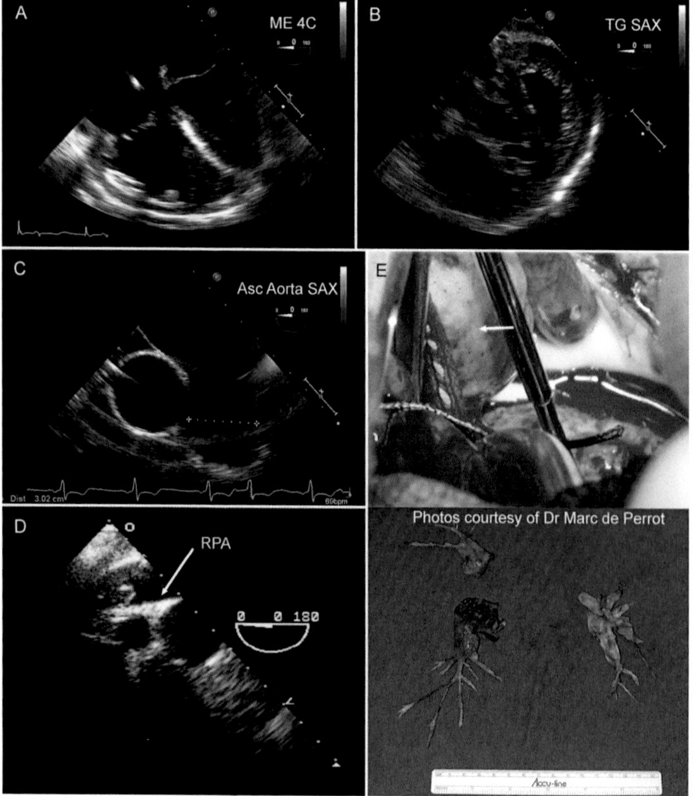

- Infective endocarditis (IE) is a microbial infection of the endocardial heart surface.
- The 3–20% incidence depends on the population (native vs. prosthetic valves).
- Echocardiography has a prominent role in the diagnosis, but also need blood and clinical information (Duke Criteria). Prompt diagnosis improves outcome.
- TTE is an inappropriate screening test unless there is a clinical suspicion of IE.
- TEE is preferred for patients at moderate to high risk of IE.
- A negative TEE does not rule out IE, as the vegetation may be small (<2 mm) or have already embolized. If there is a high clinical suspicion of IE, repeat the TEE in 7–10 days.
- When the TTE and TEE are both negative, the negative predictive value for IE is 95%.

TEE Indications for IE
- Difficult to image patients
- Small vegetations <10 mm
- Prosthetic valve endocarditis
- Clinical suspicion of IE
- High risk for IE complications

Duke Criteria	
Pathologic criteria: micro-organisms in vegetations Clinical criteria: 2 major or 1 major +3 minor or 5 minor	
Major	**Minor**
1) Blood cultures positive 2) Echo findings • Vegetations: thickened leaflets, mobile masses move through the valve during a cardiac cycle • New partial valve dehiscence • New valvular regurgitation	1) Predisposition (see below) 2) Fever >38 °C 3) Vascular 4) Immunologic 5) Microbiologic 6) Echo findings • Valve perforations • Nodular thickening • Non-mobile mass
Source: Durack DT, et al. Am J Med 1994;96:200–9	

Predisposition for Endocarditis		
High Risk (Use Antibiotics)	**Moderate Risk[a]**	**Low Risk[a]**
• Prosthetic valve or repair • Previous endocarditis • Heart transplant with cardiac valvulopathy • Congenital heart – Uncorrected cyanotic – Repair prosthetic material within 6 months – Repair with residua at site of prosthetic material	• Acquired valve – Rheumatic disease – Degenerative disease – MVP with/out MR • Congenital heart – Post-repair ASD, VSD – PDA after 6 months – Complex heart defects • HOCM	• ASD (isolated) • Atheroma • CABG • Pacemakers
[a]Antibiotics are no longer recommended **Source: Circulation 2007; 116:1736–54**		

Complications of Endocarditis
- Heart failure: LV/RV function greatest predictor of mortality
- Embolization: mitral > aortic vegetations
- Abscess: echoic area in adjacent tissue without communication with cardiac chamber or vessel, non-pulsatile, no color Doppler flow
- Fistula: abnormal communication between chambers, seen with color Doppler flow
- Pseudoaneurysm of intervalvular fibrosa: echo-free area between aortic annulus and base of AMVL, pulsatile with systolic flow from LVOT

What to Tell the Surgeon Endocarditis
- Vegetations (location, size, number)
- Valve pathology (preexisting)
- Valve function (obstruction, regurgitation)
- Complications (abscess, pseudoaneurysm, fistula)
- LV/RV function
- Infected devices (pacemaker leads, catheters)

Vegetations

- Soft tissue density echo
- Composed of platelets, fibrin, and microbes
- Irregular shape, size
- Mobile, independent of underlying cardiac structure
- Valves: AV > MV > TV > PV, check all valves
- Low pressure side of regurgitant jet
  AI jet → LV side AV, chordae MV
  MR jet → LA side MV, LA wall
  TR jet → RA side TV
  VSD orifice → orifice facing RV, 2° on PV and TV
- Implanted material
- Obstruction of normal valve function
- Incompetent valve function
- Embolization risk (20–50%)
  - Valve: Mitral (25%) > Aortic (10%)
    - Size >10–14 mm, AMVL attachment
  - Micro-organisms: *S. aureus*, *Candida*, HACEK
  - Within first 2–4 weeks of antibiotic therapy

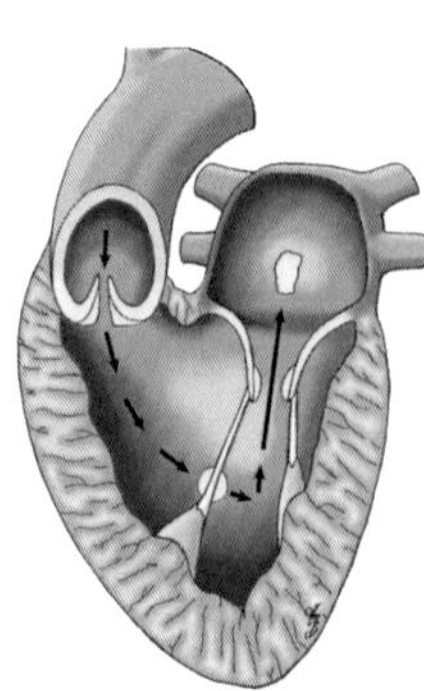

Source: Baddour L, et al. Circulation 2005;111:e394–e434.

(A) Tricuspid valve vegetations (arrows) are shown in the ME RVOT view and at the time of surgery through a right atriotomy. (B) Aortic valve vegetations (arrow) cause flail AV cusps with severe aortic insufficiency that fills the entire LVOT as seen with color Doppler (Nyquist 59 cm/s) in the ME AV LAX view. (C) Patient with an aortic valve vegetation (arrow) prolapsing through an outlet VSD into the RVOT in this color compare ME RVOT view (Nyquist 48 cm/s).

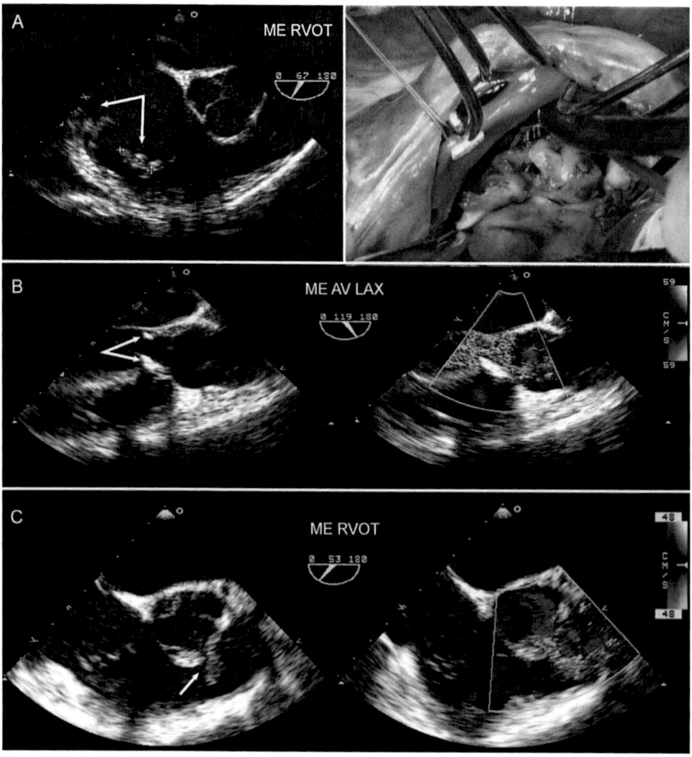

Complications of IE that involve the prosthetic valve bed include:

- Abscess: hypo/hyperechoic area in adjacent tissue without color flow
- Fistula: abnormal communication with flow between 2 sites
- Dehiscence: abnormal rocking motion of valve independent of surrounding tissue
- Pseudoaneurysm: echo-free space between aortic annulus and base of AMVL

Abscess

This is a pus-filled cavity that may involve the annulus, myocardium, or intervalvular fibrosa. It is seen as an echo-dense or echolucent area typically without any color flow.

(A) Shown here is a intraoperative photo of a paravalvular abscess surrounding the annulus of a prosthetic St Jude AVR and in the ME AV SAX view (B) without and (C) with color Doppler. (D, E) Abscess of the anterior MV leaflet (arrow) has echolucent cavities with a perforation and central MR with color Doppler.

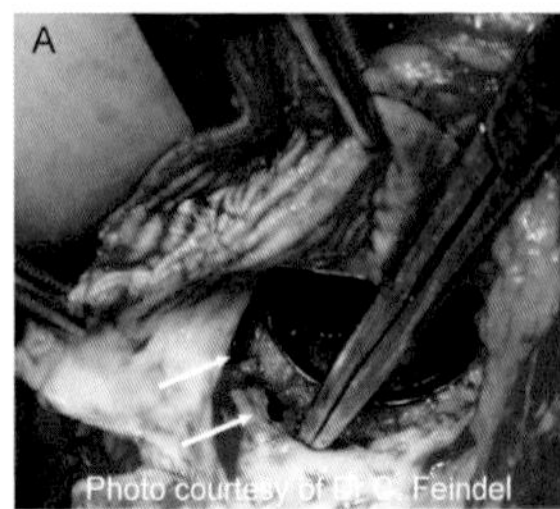

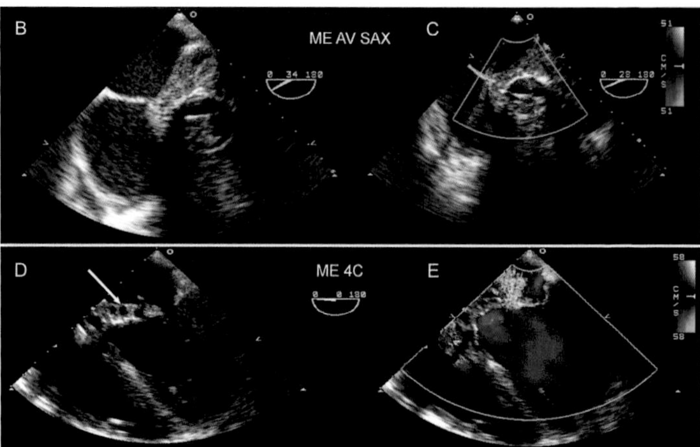

Fistula

This is an abnormal connection between 2 cavities as a result of an abscess or pseudoaneurysm rupture. Flow occurs through the connection.

(A) Photo at the time of surgery shows a fistula at the base of the anterior mitral valve leaflet. (B) ME AV LAX view shows a "wind sock" deformity (arrow) connecting the aortic root to the LA. (C) Color Doppler (Nyquist 58 cm/s) shows flow through the fistula from the aorta into the LA during systole in the ME AV LAX view.

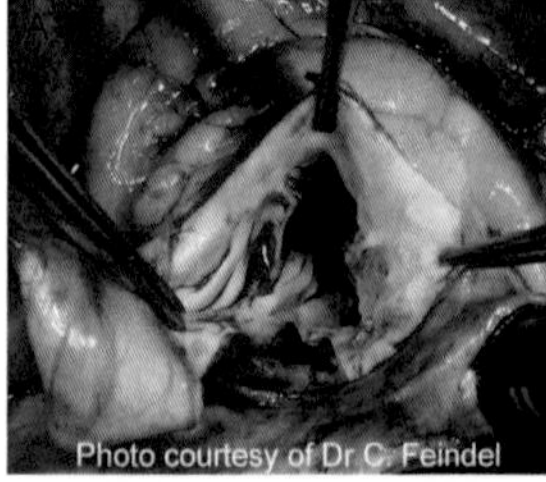

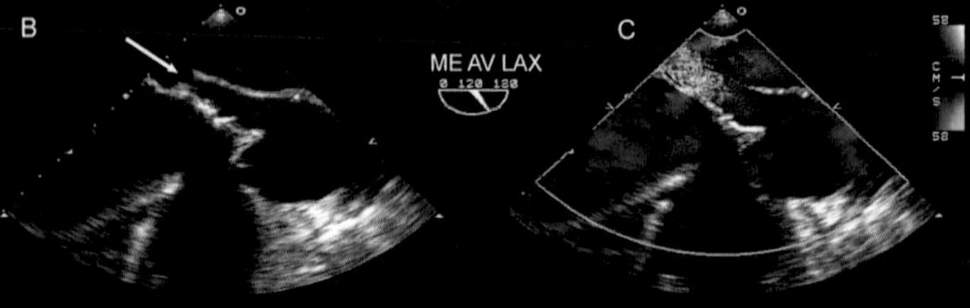

"Jet Lesion"

This is a mycotic aneurysm of the anterior mitral valve leaflet (AMVL), with a perforation resulting in MR. This forms as a result of the impact on the AMVL of the aortic insufficiency jet related to AV endocarditis.

(A) Surgical photo of a hole in the AMVL. (B) ME AV LAX view shows a "wind sock" deformity (arrow). Color Doppler (Nyquist 63 cm/s) shows flow through the AMVL in this region, resulting in severe MR with flow acceleration. This will require surgical correction, as a MV repair or replacement.

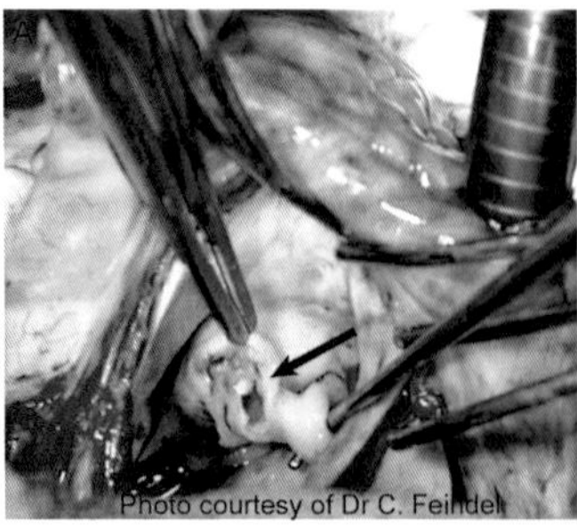

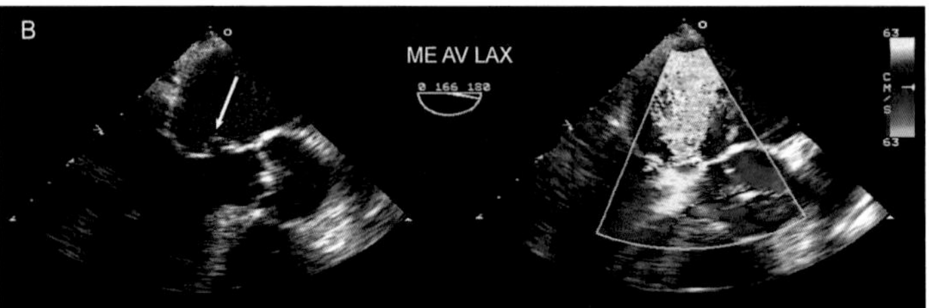

Dehiscence

There is a gap along the suture line used to attach the prosthetic valve or ring to the underlying tissue. The sutures are separated from underlying tissue resulting in a paravalvular leak. If a large enough gap is created, the prosthetic valve becomes unstable. This presents on echocardiography as an abnormal rocking motion of the prosthetic valve independent of surrounding structures.

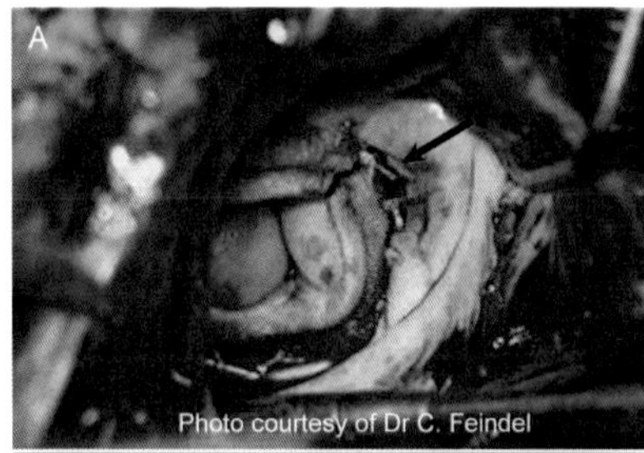

(A) A gap between the tissue and sewing ring of a prosthetic tissue valve as seen at surgery. (B) ME MC view shows destruction of a tissue MV. Color Doppler (Nyquist 59 cm/s) shows both severe valvular MR and a paravalvular leak. (C) This patient had a MV ring annuloplasty which has become dehisced with significant paravalvular regurgitation, causing severe MR.

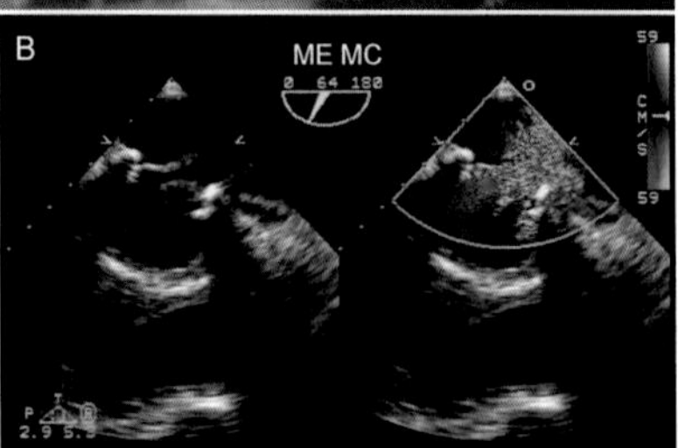

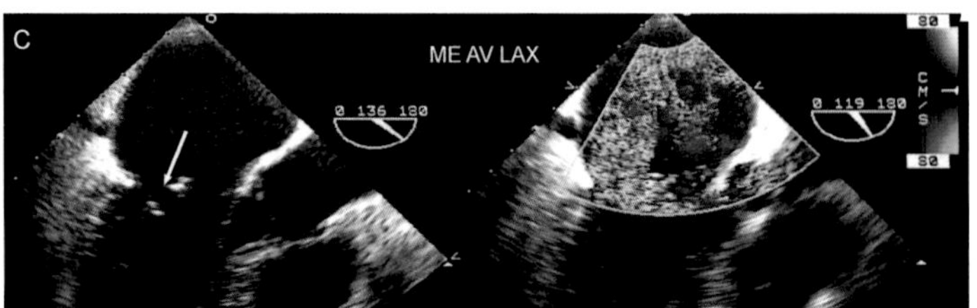

Pseudoaneurysm

- Intervalvular fibrosa pseudoaneurysm (arrow) is an echo-free area between aortic annulus and anterior mitral valve leaflet (AMVL) base.

(A) The space is dynamic expanding during systole and is (B) smaller during diastole. Color flow shows early systolic flow and early diastolic emptying.

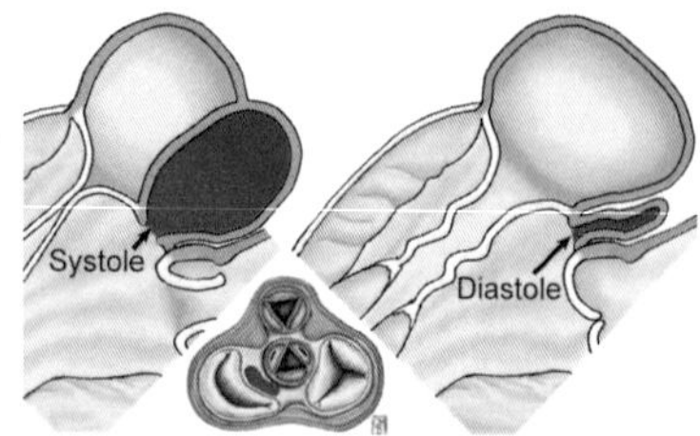

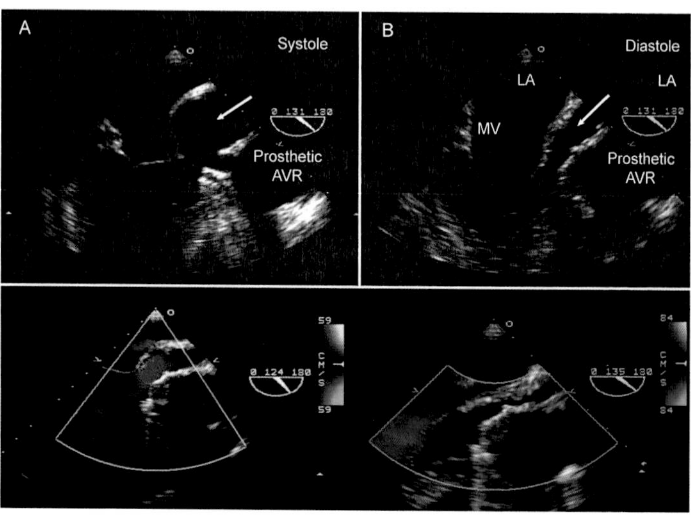

Abscess of the intervalvular fibrosa is an echo-free area between aortic annulus and LA in a patient with a mechanical AVR. Compare (A) 2D ME AV SAX and LAX (B) color Doppler AV LAX, (C) 3D ME AV SAX views, and the (D) intraoperative findings.

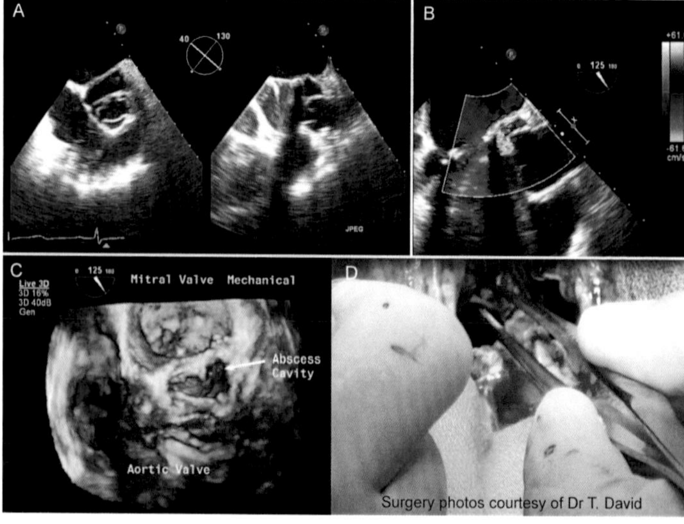

Pseudoaneurysm Fistula

- The aortic root shares an intimate relationship with surrounding structures including the right atrium (RA) and left atrium (LA).
- An aortic root abscess or pseudoaneurysm may rupture into surrounding chambers creating a fistula.
- Color Doppler (Nyquist 40–50 cm/s) shows flow between chambers.
- Surgery is required to repair the tract.

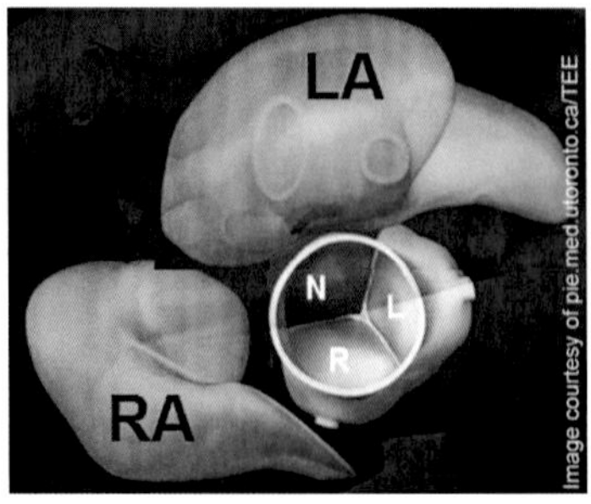

Patient after a Bentall procedure developed a pulsatile suprasternal mass. (A) CT reconstruction shows an anterior pseudoaneurysm (double arrows) comprised mostly of blood. (B) ME AV SAX view also shows a posterior pseudoaneurysm (arrow) that has ruptured into the LA creating a fistula. (C) Both pseudoaneurysms anterior (double arrow) and posterior (arrow) are seen in the ME AV LAX view. (D) There is a communication from the pseudoaneurysm into the LA. During systole color Doppler in the ME AV LAX view shows flow through the LVOT that enters the pseudoaneurysm (arrow) and from there into the LA, creating a LVOT to LA fistula. (E) Another patient with a homograft has a pseudoaneurysm which connects with the RA as shown in this ME AV SAX view and (F) zoomed view.

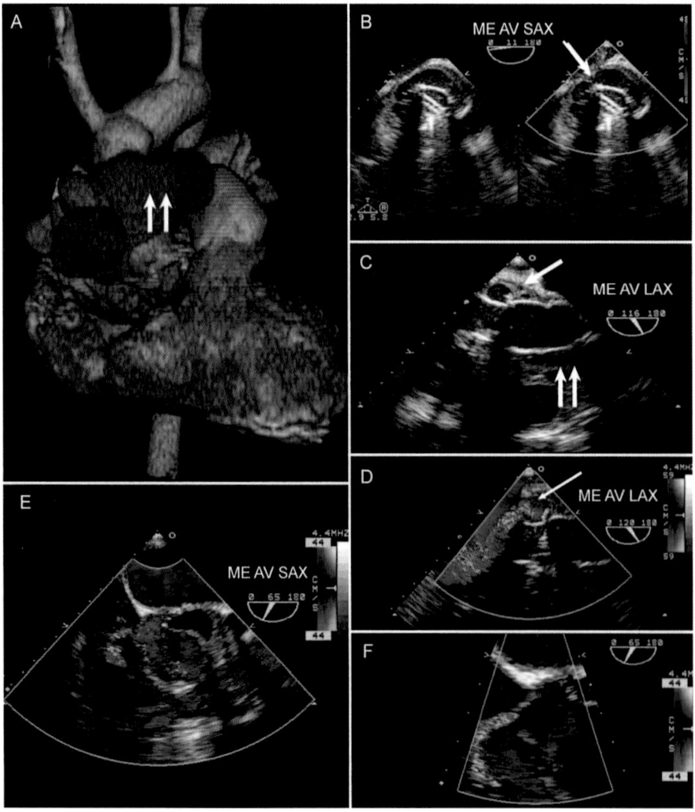

12
Mechanical Support, Heart Transplant

A. Vegas, *Perioperative Two-Dimensional Transesophageal Echocardiography*, https://doi.org/10.1007/978-3-319-60902-7_12

- There is a range of cardio-respiratory support from simple intra-aortic balloon catheters, ventricular assist devices (VADs), total artificial heart (TAH), and ventilation membranes, to advanced extracorporeal life support (ECLS) circuits.
- The choice of device depends on the patient's cardiac status and whether the patient has adequate ventilation (CO_2 elimination) and oxygenation.
- Mechanical circulatory support for patients with advanced heart failure has evolved considerably and is standard therapy at many medical centers.
- Echocardiography can help assess the need, implementation, detect complications, and weaning of mechanical support.

Circulation	Ventilation	Circulation and Ventilation
Intra-Aortic Balloon Pump (IABP) Ventricular Assist Device (VAD) Percutaneous VAD (pVAD) Total Artificial Heart (TAH)	VV ECMO Avalon Elite® Novolung®	VA ECMO BiVAD + oxygenator
ECMO; extracorporeal membrane oxygenation; VV venous-venous, VA; venous-arterial		

Ventricular Assist Devices

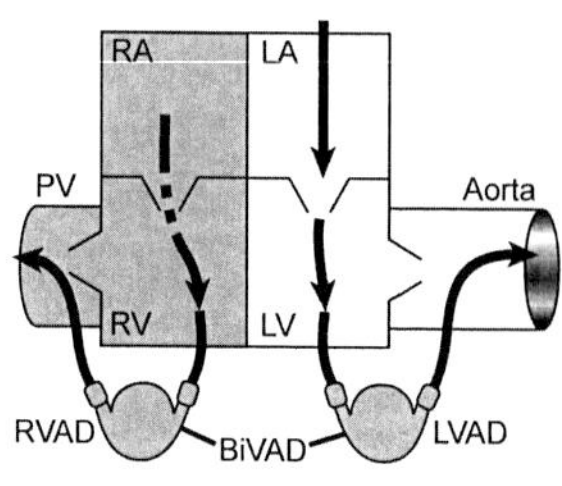

- Mechanical ventricular assist devices can support the LV (LVAD), RV (RVAD), or both ventricles (BiVAD).
- The devices rely on an inflow cannula into the device (outflow from patient) typically placed in the supported ventricle (RVAD or LVAD) or atrium (RA for RVAD). The outflow cannula from the device (inflow into the patient) is placed in the aorta (LVAD) or PA (RVAD). The devices can be positioned within the body (intracorporeal), beside the body (paracorporeal), or outside and away from the body (extracorporeal).
- Smaller more durable continuous flow devices have replaced the original bulkier pulsatile devices.
- Patients may receive VAD devices as a bridge to transplantation (BTT), bridge to recovery (BTR), bridge to candidacy (BTC), or as destination therapy (DT). The devices provide temporary (days) and long-term support (months, years).
- Continuous flow percutaneous VAD devices (pVAD) can be inserted at the bedside (Impella® and TandemHeart®).

Pulsatile Flow VAD	Continuous Flow VAD	
	Axial	Centrifugal
Intermediate to Long-Term Support (Months to Years)		
Berlin EXCOR® Thoratec® PVAD	HeartMate II® LVAD CentriMag® Jarvik 2000® Berlin INCOR®	HeartWare® HVAD HeartMate 3™ LVAD
Short-Term Support (Days to Weeks)		
	Impella®	TandemHeart®

Pulsatile VADs

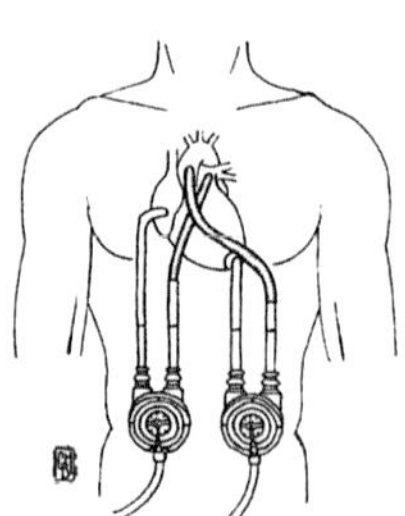

- These first-generation devices (HeartMate® XVE, Thoratec VAD) are now mostly of historical significance as they have been replaced by smaller more efficient devices.
- Current pulsatile devices are the Thoratec® PVAD and Berlin EXCOR®, both used in pediatric patients. The device is implanted paracorporeal with cannula connecting to provide LVAD and/or RVAD support.
- The pump has valves to provide asynchronous (to the native heart) positive displacement of blood into the patient's systemic circulation.

Continuous Flow VADs

- Continuous flow devices are small, durable, and totally implantable. They have a simple valveless design with either axial or centrifugal blood flow.
- Axial flow devices have a propeller screw-type design rotating at rapid rates to push blood continuously forward.

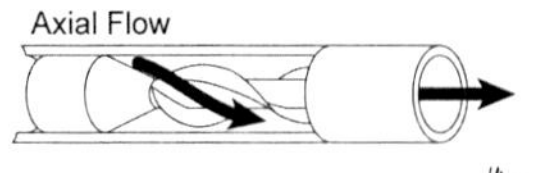

- Centrifugal pumps have an impeller suspended by magnetic and hydrodynamic forces, which has contact-free impeller rotation at rapid rates.

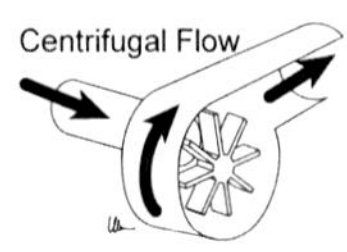

- Speed in rotation per minute (rpm) determines device flow (2–6 L), higher rotational speed has more flow.
- Devices are attached directly to the LV apex for inflow into the device and an outflow cannula is attached to the ascending aorta or descending aorta (Jarvik 2000®).

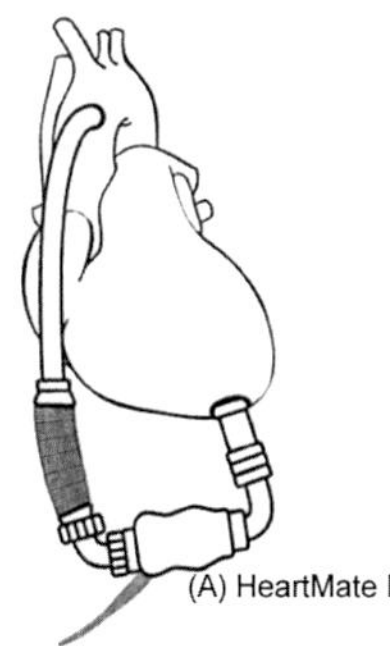
(A) HeartMate II

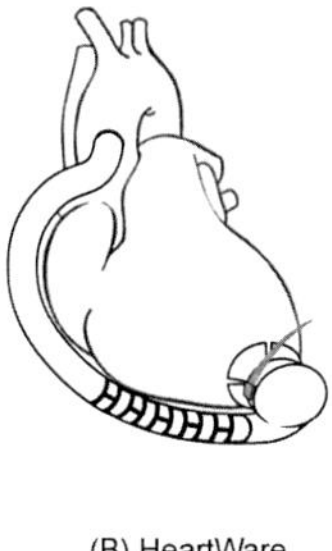
(B) HeartWare

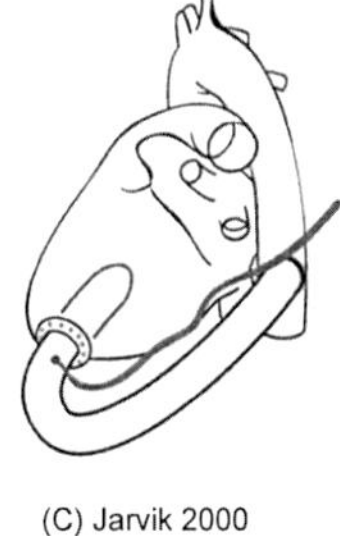
(C) Jarvik 2000

Images by permission of Frances Yeung modified by Willa Bradshaw

---

Total Artificial Heart (TAH)

- SynCardia CardioWest Total Artificial Heart (SynCardia, Inc., Tucson, AZ) is an implantable orthotopic pneumatic biventricular, pulsatile device.
- TAH consists of 2 artificial ventricles made of semi-rigid polyurethane. Each ventricle has mechanical inflow and outflow valves (Medtronic-Hall tilting disc) to provide unidirectional blood flow.
- Blood fills the artificial ventricles and is pneumatically pumped into the pulmonary and systemic circulations. Stroke volume is 70 cc, flow is up to 9.5 L per minute.
- The patient's native ventricles and all valves are removed, connectors are sewn to the native MV and TV annulus, PA, and aorta. The TAH attaches to the connectors.
- The TAH is indicated as a bridge to transplant in patients who may not be candidates for VAD support (intra-cardiac thrombus, small LV cavity, Fontan circulation).
- TEE findings are summarized below.

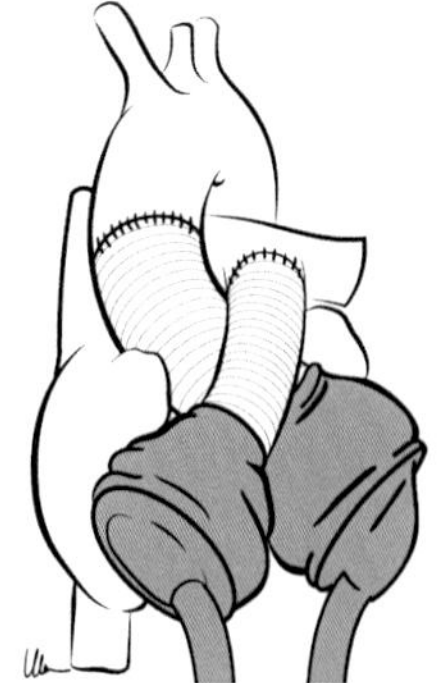

TEE preCPB TAH	TEE postCPB TAH
Central venous line (not in RA) PFO, ASD Atrial thrombus IVC size Pulmonary veins location, flow	Problems: no ECG, shadowing Deairing Mechanical valve function Decrease device filling Kink IVC Kink pulmonary veins >1.1 m/s

Source: Mizuguchi KA, et al. Anesth Analg 2013;117:780–4

- TEE is useful during insertion of Ventricular Assist Devices (LVAD, RVAD, BiVAD).
- Continuous flow LVAD devices are implanted with the device positioned at the LV apex and outflow cannula in the ascending aorta.
- Adequate device function relies on unimpeded LV filling, drainage into the device, and outflow back into the aorta. Device flow is preload- and afterload-sensitive.
- PreCPB TEE screens for the presence of any diseases that may contraindicate or alter the implantation technique. TEE exam focuses on conditions which will compromise device function:
  - ❶ LV apex to exclude aneurysm or thrombus.
  - ❷ PFO post-device hypoxemia.
  - ❸ Aortic insufficiency post-device recirculation loop
- PostCPB TEE determines adequate device function, residual cardiac function, and excludes complications. Shadowing and electrical interference from the device complicate TEE assessment.

TEE preCPB VAD	TEE postCPB VAD
LV size, function	Deairing
RV size, function	Repeat PFO assessment
Shunt: PFO, ASD, VSD	Cannula position
Aortic Insufficiency	Device function/flows
Intra-cavitary thrombus (LV, LAA)	LV decompression
TR, MS	Aortic valve opening
Aorta atheroma	Aortic Insufficiency
Aortic dissection	RV size and function
Prosthetic valve	TR
Sources: Stainback R, et al. J Am Soc Echocardiogr 2015;28:853–909. Chumnanvej S, et al. Anesth Analg 2007;106:583–401	

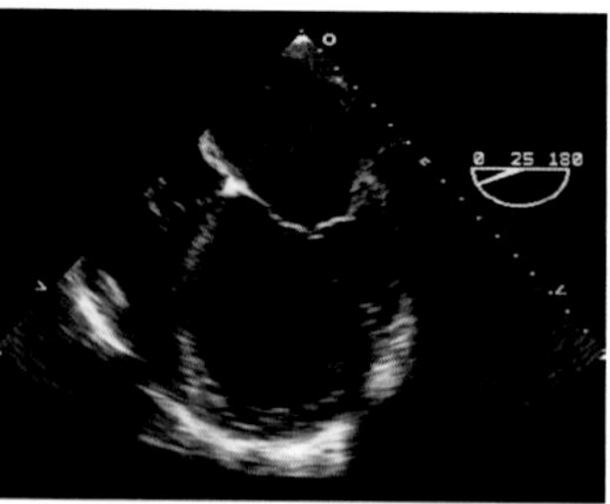

LV Size and Function

- LV size is dilated with poor function
- IVS position, it is often shifted right
- Examine the LV apex for thrombus or thinned aneurysm
- Baseline measure of LV internal diameter (LVID) in diastole for post-VAD comparison
- Small, highly trabeculated cavity may make implantation more challenging

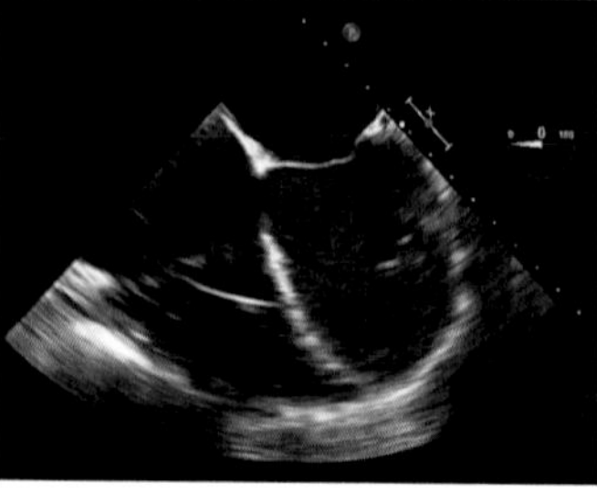

RV Size and Function

- RV function determines LVAD filling
- RV size and function is an important determinant of overall patient morbidity and mortality post-VAD
- The presence of existing RV dysfunction may require BiVAD support
- Quantification of RV function includes
  - RV FAC
  - TAPSE
  - TDI TV S′
- TR may alter RV function
- RVSP estimate from TR

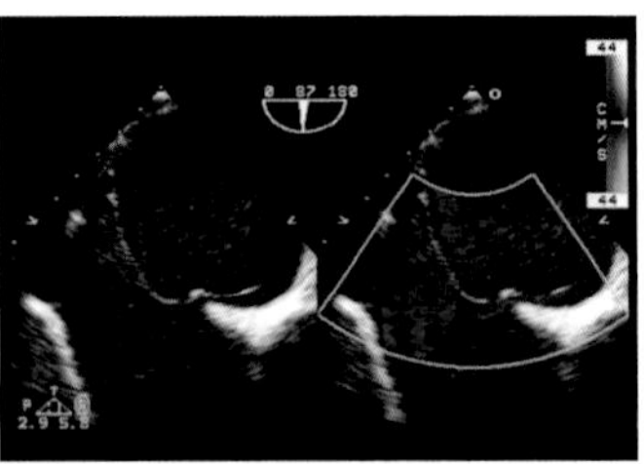

Patent Foramen Ovale (PFO)

- Post-LVAD hypoxemia R → L shunt
- Paradoxical emboli
- May be difficult to detect as
  - LAP > RAP
  - Septum bowed to right and immobile
- Valsalva will increase RAP
  - Color Doppler ± Valsalva
  - Bubble study ± Valsalva
- If PFO is present, it needs to be closed
- Recheck for PFO post-CPB

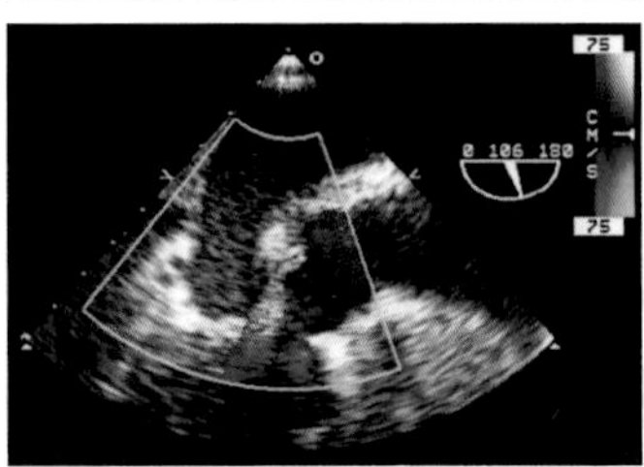

Aortic Insufficiency (AI)

- LVAD loop → poor systemic perfusion
- Underestimate AI severity preCPB as have reduced transaortic valve gradient from low aortic pressure - high LVEDP
- Can check AI on CPB (as shown here) as the aortic pressure is high like with LVAD flow
- LV vent drain >1.5 L/min is significant
- Repair or replace the AV if there is moderate to severe AI.

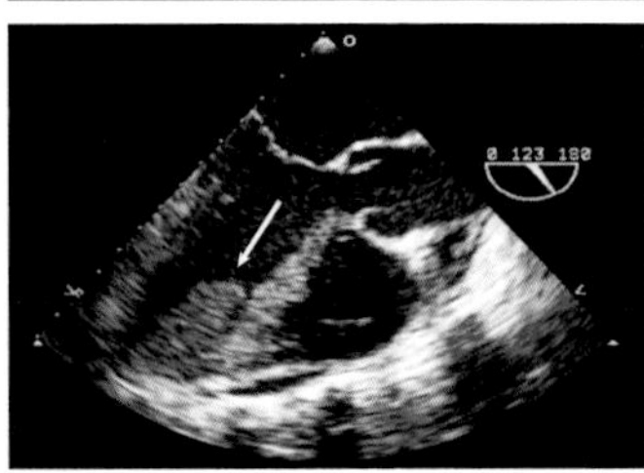

Intra-Cavitary Thrombus

- Smoke indicates low flow in the: ventricles, atria, aorta
- LAA clot: tie off LAA
- LV clot (arrow): carefully remove as
  - May occlude cannula
  - May embolize with heart manipulation
- Significant amount of clot may preclude device insertion

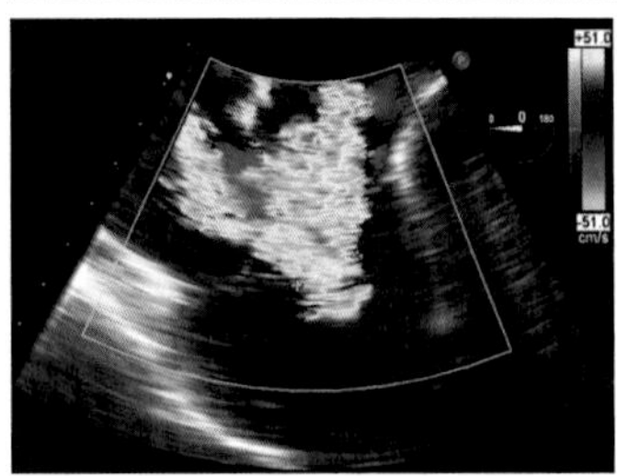

Tricuspid Regurgitation (TR)

- Impairs RV function post-VAD
- Determine if functional or primary cause
- Quantify TR severity
- May improve or worsen with LVAD flow
- Severe TR requires surgical repair

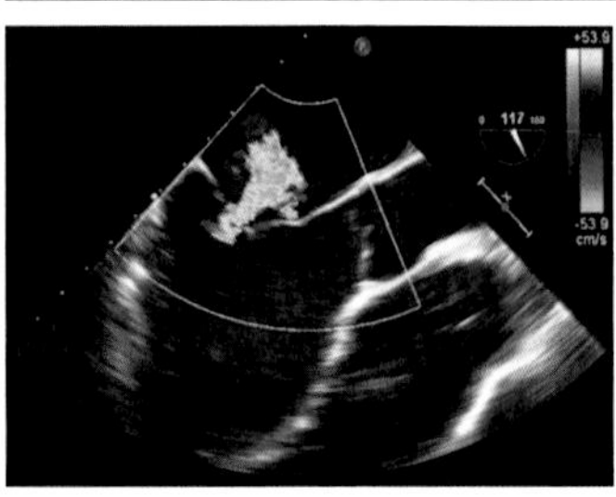

Mitral Valve (MV) Disease

- LVAD filling depends on MV function
- Mitral stenosis (MS) needs to be fixed by MV replacement as it impedes LVAD filling
- Mitral regurgitation (MR) is not a problem as the LV volume fills the LVAD
- Rarely, MR may worsen after an LVAD if the inflow cannula interferes with chordae

- TEE assessment post-VAD implantation begins prior to weaning from CPB with deairing of the device.
- Adequate device function requires proper positioning of cannula. Cannula patency is assessed using Doppler (color and spectral).
- LV should decompress. Device speed is adjusted to optimize LV size with IVS in a neutral position.
- RV function is important for LVAD filling and may worsen after a LVAD.
- Changed hemodynamics may unmask a PFO, AI, or worsening TR.

TEE Post-CPB LVAD
Dearing
RV size and function
LV decompression
Aortic valve opening
AI
TR
Reassess for PFO
Cannula position
Device function/flows

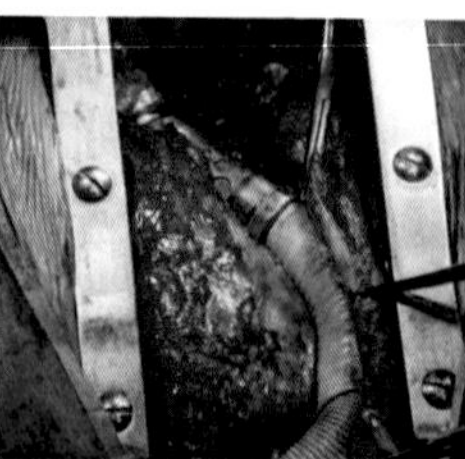

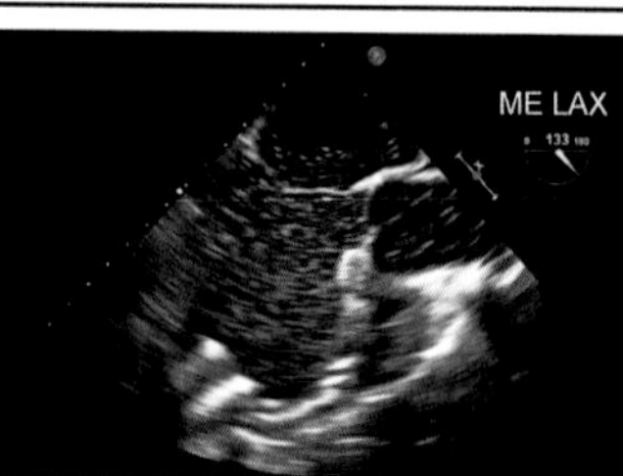

Device Deairing

- The device is started on CPB.
- Air appears in the LV, ascending aorta, proximal to the aortic conduit.
- Air may traverse the right coronary artery to further impair RV function.
- If continuous air is present, consider air entrainment through an open suture line or cannula displacement.

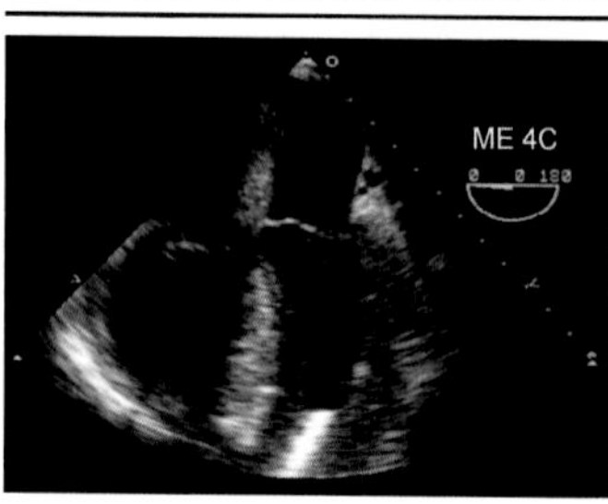

LV Decompression

- Reduced LV cavity size
- Pulsatile devices nearly empty the LV
- Continuous flow devices partly empty LV
- Monitor interventricular septum position
- Suction event:
  - Negative pressure in pump
  - With cavity obliteration, LV myocardium partially occludes the LV cannula
  - Treat by giving volume and reducing the pump speed

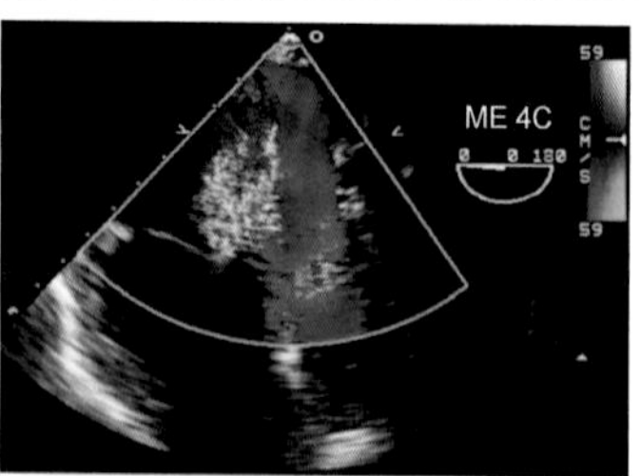

RV Function

- Septal position important to RV function
  - Left bowed: LV too decompressed
  - Right bowed: LV not decompressed
  - Neutral: best position optimizes RV
- RV function may
  - Worsen with ↑ preload
  - Improve ↓ afterload
- Tricuspid regurgitation is variable
- RVSP estimate

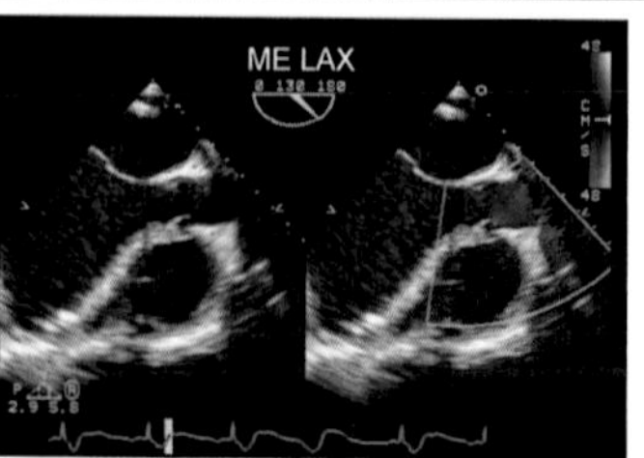

Aortic Valve (AV) Function

- AV intermittently opens every 3rd beat
  - Adjust device speed to open
  - Unopened AV has risk of sclerosis
- Assess for the presence of AI
  - Intermittent or continuous AI flow
  - Can use color m-mode for duration
- Grade AI severity
  - Use vena contracta (VC) width
  - Do not use: PHT, aortic flow reversal

LV Apical Cannula

- Device inflow, patient outflow
- Positioned away from IVS + LV walls, towards MV, seen in 2 orthogonal views
- Color: laminar unidirectional flow
- Spectral Doppler (PW or CW):
  - Pulsatile: discrete, <2.3 m/s
  - Continuous: not to baseline (arrow) 1.0–2.0 m/s
  - HeartWare® device has electrical interference which prevents the adequate assessment by color Doppler and the spectral Doppler trace is unreadable.

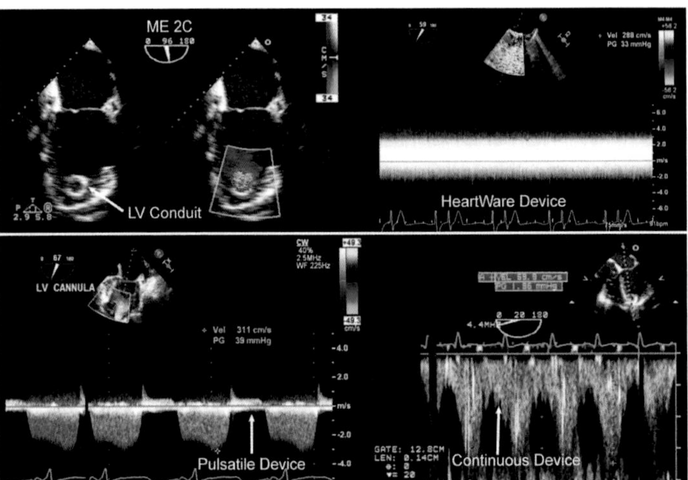

Aortic Cannula

- Device outflow, patient inflow
- Position in antero-lateral ascending aorta, angulated, withdraw TEE probe to see
- Color: turbulent unidirectional flow
  - Assess for the presence of aortic insufficiency (AI)

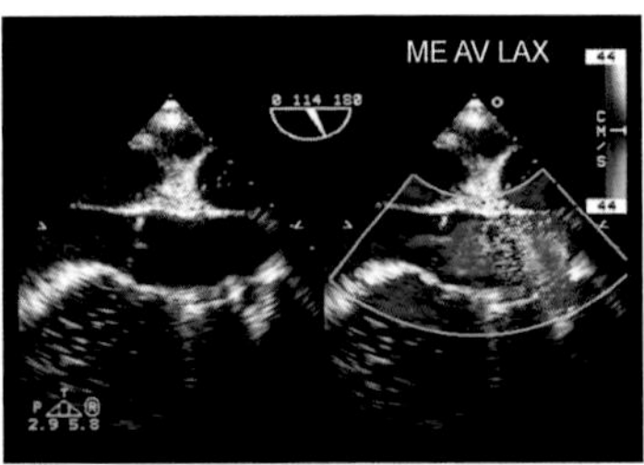

Spectral Doppler (PW or CW):

- Pulsatile:
  - Discrete, 2.1 m/s
  - Asynchronous to ECG
- Continuous:
  - Not to baseline (arrow) 1.0–2.0 m/s
  - Pulsatile pattern is from LV contraction synchronous with ECG

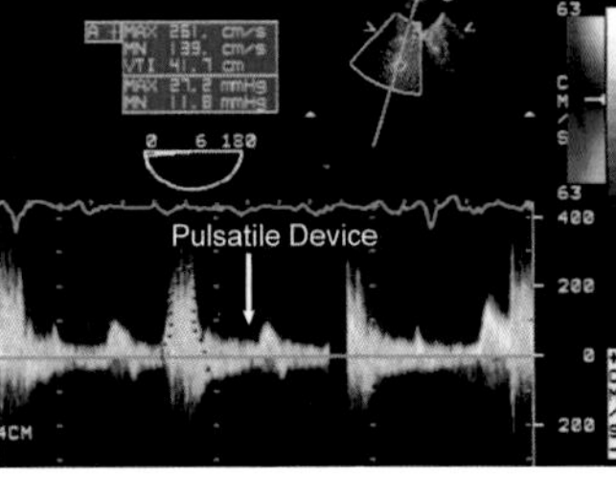

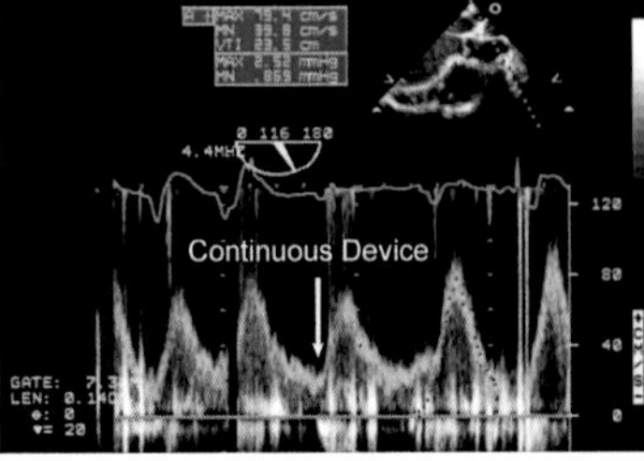

VAD Complications

- Device low output
  - ❶ Hypovolemia (empty RV, LV)
  - ❷ RV failure (dilated, hypofunction, TR)
  - ❸ Cardiac tamponade
  - ❹ Inflow cannula obstruction
  - ❺ Device failure
  - ❻ Outflow cannula obstruction
- Device high output
  - Sepsis
  - Aortic insufficiency
- Thrombus
- Hypoxemia

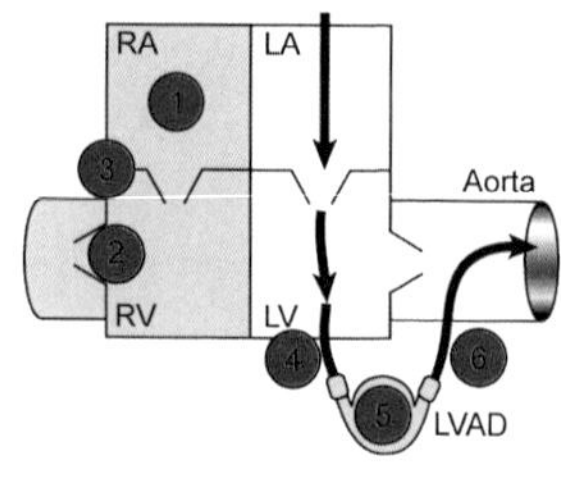

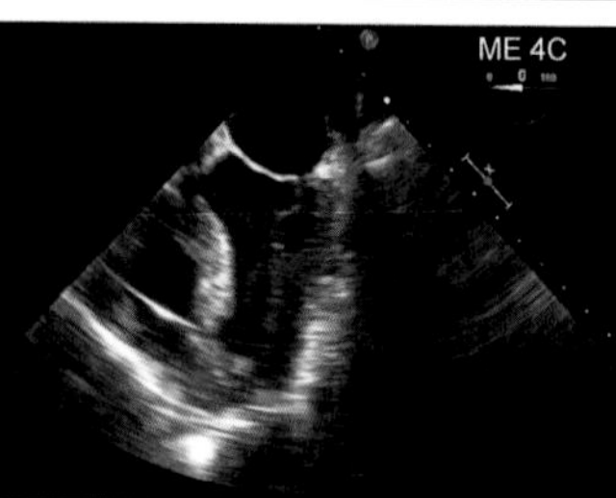

Suction Event
- Myocardium "sucked" into cannula
  - Hypotension, arrhythmias
  - Low VAD flows
  - Chattering lines
- Caused by
  - Hypovolemia
  - RV failure
  - Cardiac tamponade
- LV cavity obliteration, IVS to left
- Treat: ↓ VAD flows, underlying cause

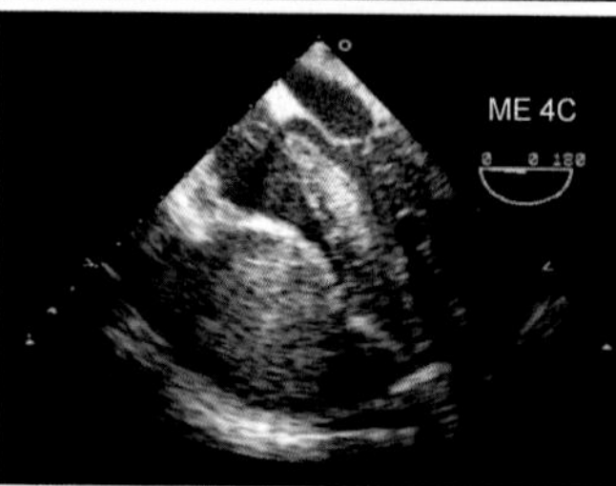

Cardiac Tamponade
- Local or circumferential pericardial effusion
- Chamber compression: RA, RV (shown)
- Compromise LVAD filling, low flow
- Common early or late problem as patients require anticoagulation postoperatively and are prone to bleeding
- Require drainage of fluid or surgical evacuation of hematoma

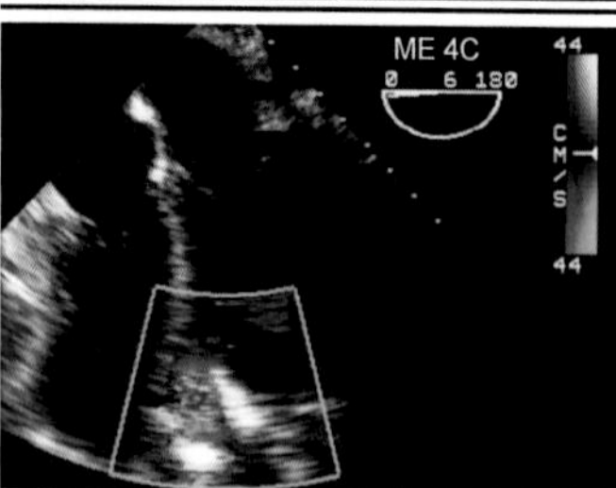

Inflow Cannula Obstruction
- Etiology of obstructed orifice:
  - Malposition towards LV wall (shown)
  - Hypovolemia results in chamber collapse around cannula
  - Thrombus occluding cannula
- Doppler
  - Color: turbulent flow
  - Spectral: velocity >2.3 m/s
- Cause of device low flow

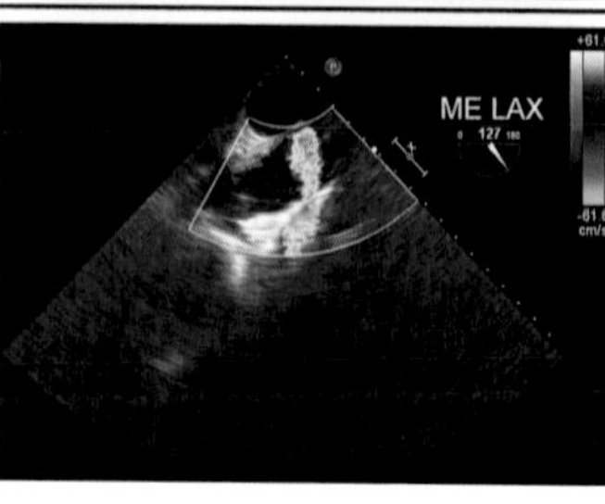

Outflow Cannula Obstruction
- Etiology of obstructed orifice:
  - Malposition
  - Kinking graft
  - Thrombus occluding cannula
- Doppler
  - Color: turbulent flow
  - Spectral: velocity >2.3 m/s
- Cause of device low flow

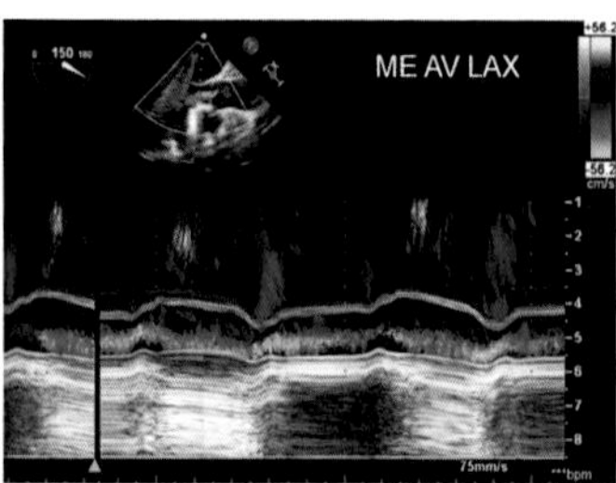

Aortic Insufficiency (AI)

- Continuous high pressure in aorta
- Continuous or intermittent AI
  - Assess duration with color M-mode
- High device output as create a circuit of LVAD filling and emptying
- Difficult to quantify severity
  - Use vena contracta (VC) width
  - Do not use: PHT, aortic flow reversal
- Difficult to manage, reduce afterload, consider AV replacement

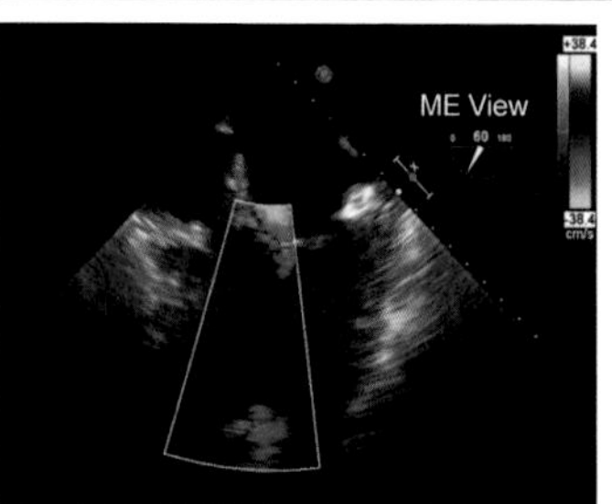

Device Thrombus

- 1–4% of patients
- Risk factors: atrial fibrillation, LV thrombus, subtherapeutic anticoagulation, low pump flows
- Suspect if hemolysis, heart failure
- Device: ↑ Power
- Echo low Doppler inflow, shown here as laminar color Doppler inflow despite low Nyquist
- RAMP study to assess device function
- May require device exchange

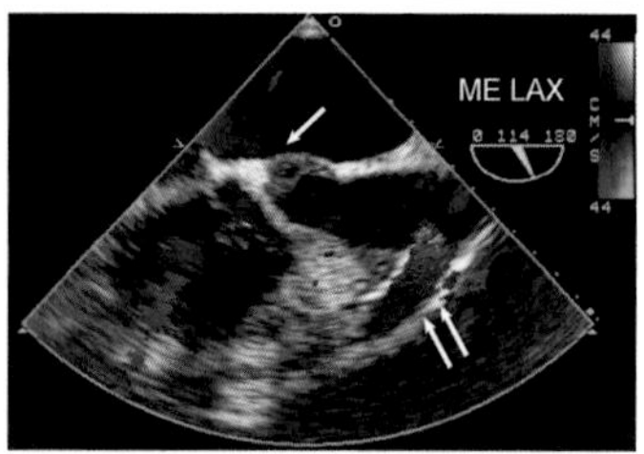

Valve Thrombus

- Thrombi may form in stagnant areas
- If the AV always remains closed, there is a risk of thrombus formation (arrow) and valve dysfunction
- Flow from VAD outflow cannula (double arrow) in ascending aorta should prevent this, as well as intermittent AV opening and closing
- Risk of systemic embolization

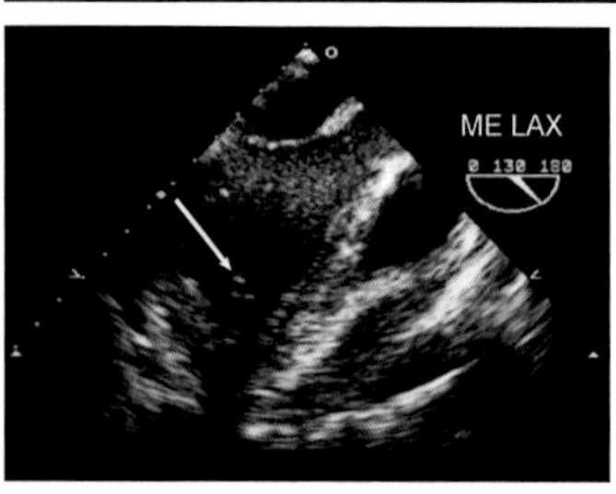

Cannula Thrombus

- Thrombus may form on the cannula tip or in the cannula
- May obstruct cannula inflow
- Cause of device low flow
- Shown is a small thrombus on the tip of LV cannula (arrow)
- Anticoagulation is often required to prevent thrombus formation

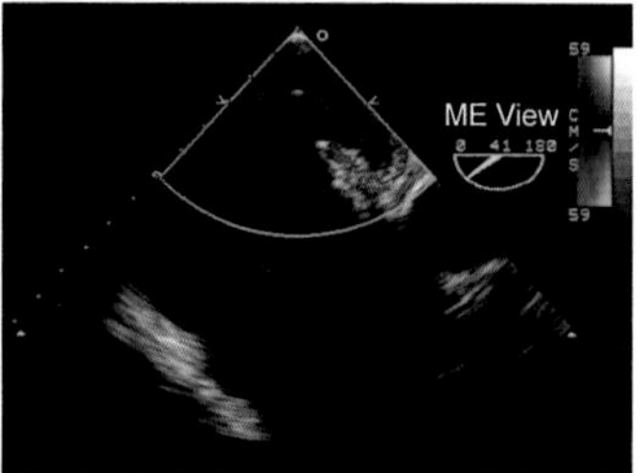

Hypoxemia

- From persistent cardiac shunt: PFO, ASD, or VSD
- Unmasked with changes in intra-cardiac pressures
- Echo diagnosis with saline contrast
- Change in pump speed may temporarily improve condition
- May require percutaneous device closure. Shown here is residual shunt flow after device closure which resolves after device endothelialization.

RVAD or BiVAD

- Patients can receive biventricular VAD (BiVAD) support when both ventricles fail:
  - Continuous flow systems: CentriMag®
  - Pulsatile systems: Berlin Heart EXCOR®, Thoratec® PVAD™
- These devices are positioned outside the body:
  - Extracorporeal: CentriMag
  - Paracorporeal: Berlin Heart, Thoratec® PVAD™
- BiVAD support uses 2 devices and cannulation to support inflow and outflow for each of:
  - Right heart: Inflow (RA, RV) → Outflow (PA)
  - Left heart: Inflow (LA, LV) → Outflow (aorta)
- Device inflow cannula: RA or RV
- Device outflow cannula: PA
  - Velocity 1.0–2.0 m/s
  - Discrete or continuous flow
- Devices can provide flows up to 9.9 L/min

CentriMag™ Pump

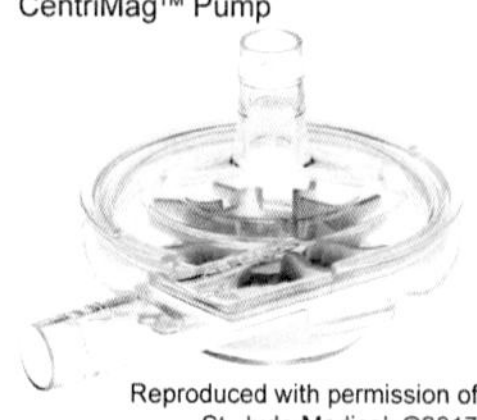

ME 4C RA Cannula

ME RVOT PA Cannula

ME MC LV Cannula

ME LAX Aorta Cannula

RA Inflow Cannula Pulsatile Device

PA Outflow Cannula Pulsatile Device

LV Inflow CentriMag

Aorta Outflow CentriMag

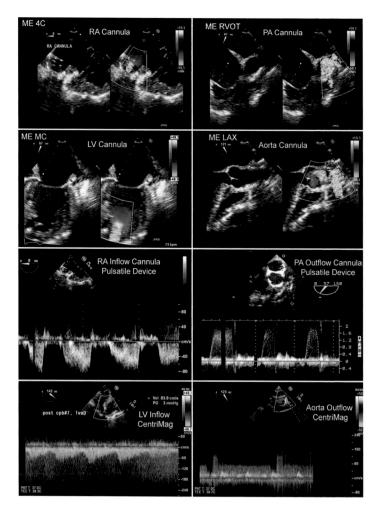

Percutaneous Ventricular Assist Device (pVAD)

- Percutaneous VADs provide temporary (5–14 days) partial or total circulatory support.
- Devices are inserted into the femoral artery and continuously recirculate oxygenated blood from the left heart into the systemic circulation.
- Indications are for cardiogenic shock, unload LV, support of circulation.

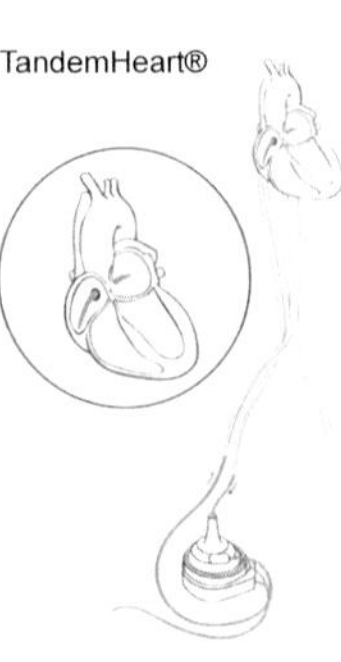

TandemHeart® pVAD (CardiacAssist, Pittsburgh, PA)

- This is a continuous flow extracorporeal pVAD system consisting of 3 parts which unloads the LV.
- Oxygenated blood is aspirated from the LA and returned via a femoral artery (flow 3-5 L/min).
- A 21F femoral venous cannula is inserted into the RA and directed trans-septal into the LA under fluoroscopy or TEE guidance. This cannula is attached as inflow to an extracorporeal centrifugal pump.
- Outflow from the pump is a 15–17F catheter inserted in the right femoral artery to the aortic bifurcation.

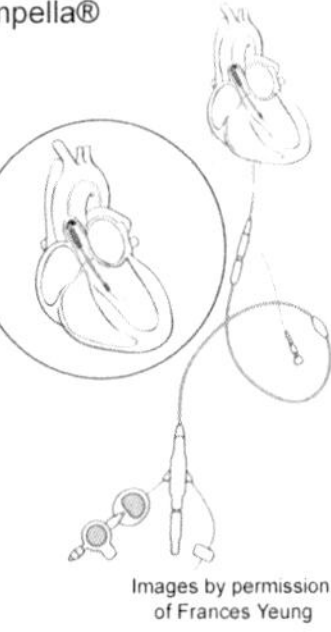

Images by permission of Frances Yeung

Impella® (Abiomed, Danvers MA)

- Range of LV unloading catheters that contain a microaxial flow pump. Oxygenated blood is drawn from the LVOT into the distal inlet portion of the catheter, passes through the pump, and is expelled into the ascending aorta.
- 2.5–5.0 L/min LV support depending on catheter selected
- Catheter is inserted retrograde via a femoral artery and is positioned across the AV.
- Correct positioning of the catheter is with the:
  - Inflow port in the LVOT 3–4 cm from the AV
  - Outflow port 1.5–2.0 cm distal to sinus of Valsalva
- Poor catheter position can be identified by TEE.
- Impella RP® supports the RV (4.0 L flow) by placing a catheter in the IVC, aspirating blood, and expelling it into the PA.

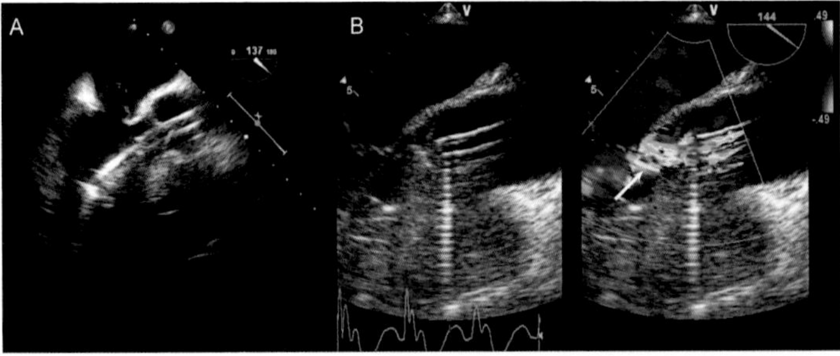

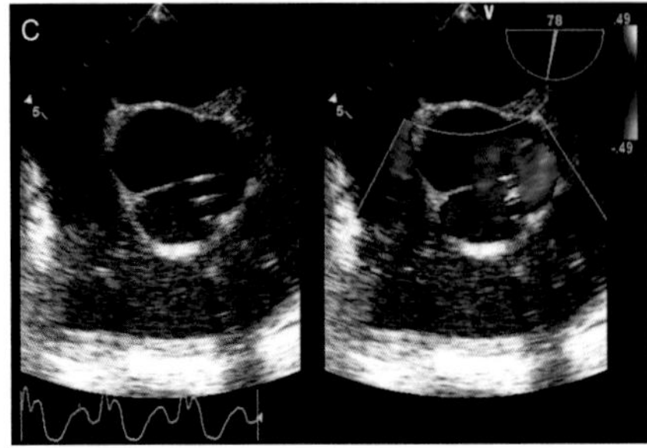

(A) ME LAX view shows an Impella® catheter positioned through the AV, but too far into the LV. (B) ME AV LAX view with color Doppler shows continuous flow drawn through the distal portion of the catheter (arrow) and expelled into the ascending aorta. (C) ME AV SAX view with color Doppler shows an Impella® catheter positioned in the center of the AV.

Extracorporeal Life Support (ECLS)

- This is a growing medical field that assists the failing lungs, heart, or both by providing ventilatory and circulatory support.
- ECLS often involves the positioning of percutaneous cannula in the central or peripheral circulation. Different configurations are used.
- Echocardiography can help assess the need, implementation, detect complications and weaning of ECLS.

Venous-Venous (VV) ECMO

- This configuration provides ventilatory support and relies on the native heart to pump oxygenated blood.
- Cannulation is often percutaneous or by cut-down of peripheral vessels with long cannulae positioned more centrally.
- Adequate venous drainage requires optimal drainage cannula position in the RA just beyond the caval-atrial junction. Cannula malposition may damage structures:
  - Too far: damage to TV, IAS
  - Not far enough: damage to IVC
- Need adequate distance between the return and drainage cannula to avoid recirculation.

Venous-Arterial (VA) ECMO

- This configuration provides cardio-respiratory support and does not rely on the native heart or lung function.
- VA ECMO involves placement of a venous cannula for drainage and arterial cannula for return of oxygenated blood.
- Peripheral venous cannula is in the femoral vein to the IVC/RA junction, return cannula is in the femoral artery to iliac artery.
- Central cannulation retains the cannula position of CPB, venous cannula in the RA, and arterial cannula in the ascending aorta.

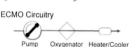

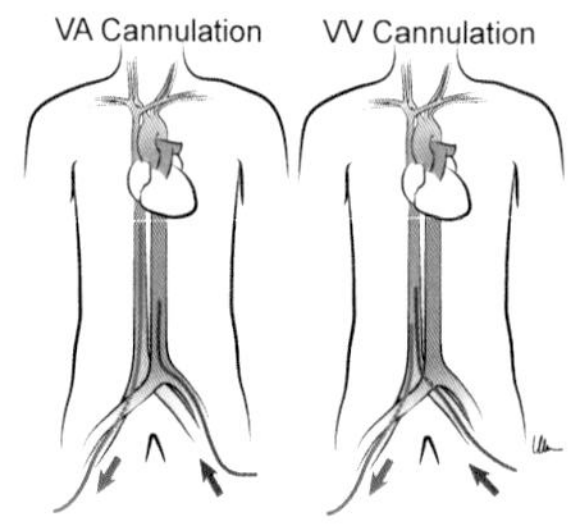

ECMO Circuitry

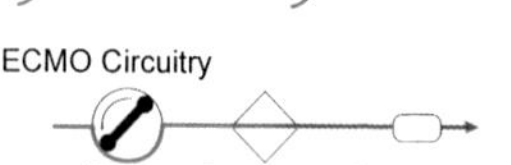

Venous-Venous (VV) ECMO			Venous-Arterial (VA) ECMO	
Respiratory failure			Cardio-respiratory failure	
Cannulae 2 veins or 1 vein			Cannulae vein and artery	
	Drainage	**Return**	**Drainage**	**Return**
Femoroatrial	Fem (IVC/RA)	IJ (SVC/RA)	Femoral vein	Femoral artery
Femoral-Femoral	Fem (mid IVC)	Fem (RA)	RA	Aorta
Internal Jugular (IJ)	IJ (SVC, IVC)	IJ (RA)		

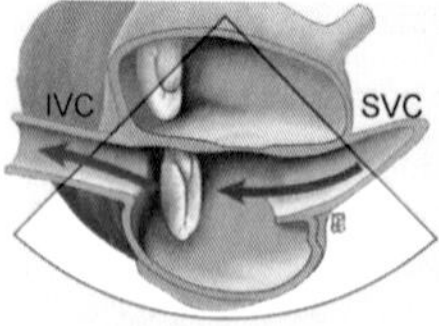

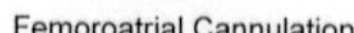
Femoroatrial Cannulation

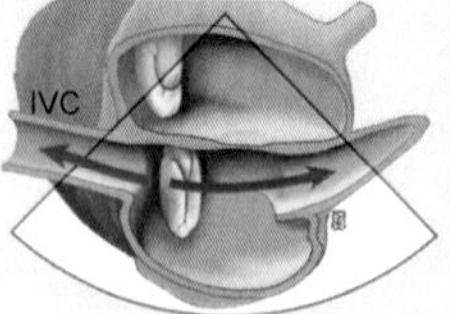

Femoral-Femoral Cannulation

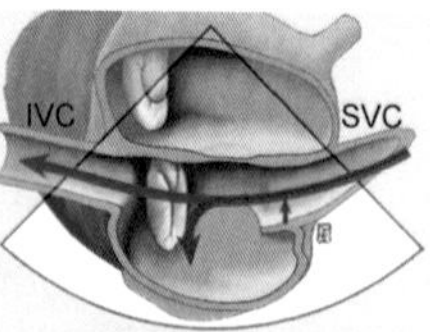

Internal Jugular Cannulation

TEE ECLS		
Pre-insertion	**Post-insertion**	**Weaning**
LV size, function	Cannula position	LV size, function
RV size, function	Pericardial effusion	LVEF >20%
Valvular TR	Aortic dissection	S′ > 6 cm/s
PFO, ASD	Chamber size	Aortic VTI > 10 cm
IVC, SVC size	LV distension	RV size, function
Atheroma	Thrombus	AV function
Chiari network	AV opening	TR, RVSP
Source: Doufle G, et al. Critical Care 2015;19:326		

Venous Cannulation

Percutaneous venous cannulae for ECLS are inserted into the femoral veins or internal jugular veins. Cannulae are positioned to allow unobstructed flow.

(A) ME Bicaval view shows an internal jugular venous return cannula in the SVC and advanced to the RA for VV ECMO. (B, C) ME bicaval views without and with color Doppler show the femoral venous drainage cannula positioned at the junction of the IVC and RA.

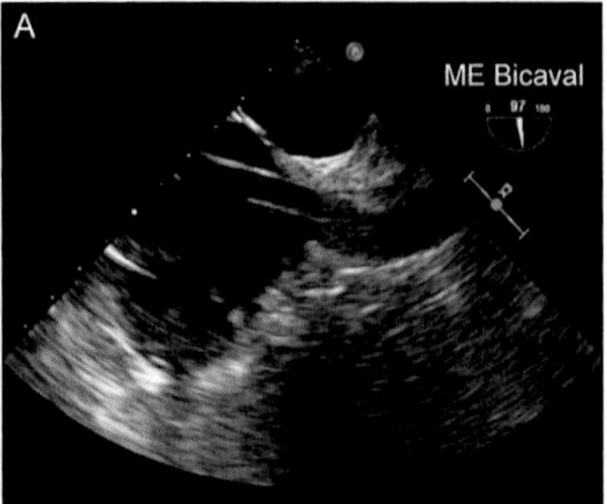

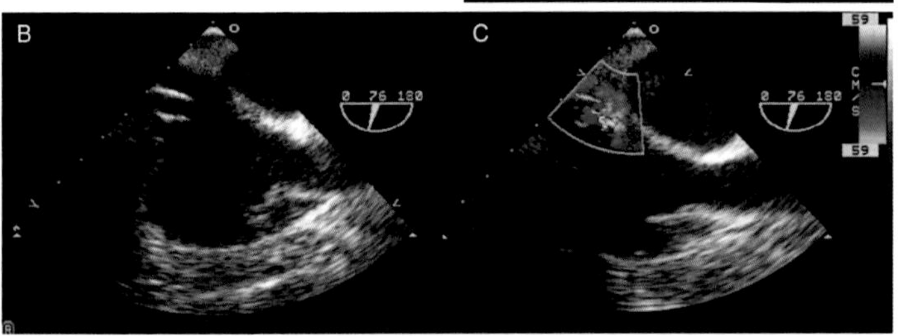

Avalon Elite® Catheter (Maquet, Rastatt, Germany)

- This is a double lumen cannula that drains blood from both cava (IVC, SVC) and returns oxygenated blood into the RA.
- Percutaneous insertion of this catheter is via the RIJ vein into RA.
- Position the tip at RA/IVC junction.
- Orientate the catheter so outflow (red arrow) is towards the TV, and not the IAS (ME Bicaval view).
- Provides single cannulation for VV ECMO to minimize recirculation, maximize blood flow.

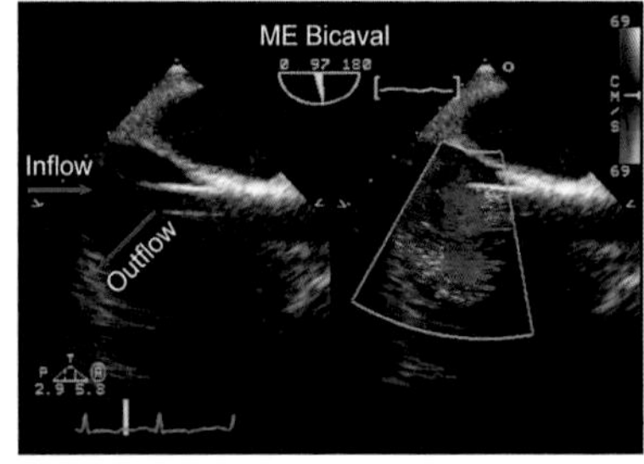

Novalung® iLA Membrane Ventilator (XENIOUS AG, Germany)

- This external ventilation support device is primarily designed to eliminate CO_2.
- Blood is drained from the body into an oxygenating membrane and returned.
- Peripheral cannulation is via the femoral artery and vein.
- Central cannulation (PA to LA) can be a bridge to lung transplantation in patients with primary PA hypertension, provides pressure decompression + gas exchange.

(A) ME RV Inflow-Outflow view with color Doppler shows cannula positioned in the main pulmonary artery (arrow). (B) ME-modified Bicaval view with color Doppler shows the inflow cannula in the right upper pulmonary vein entering the left atrium.

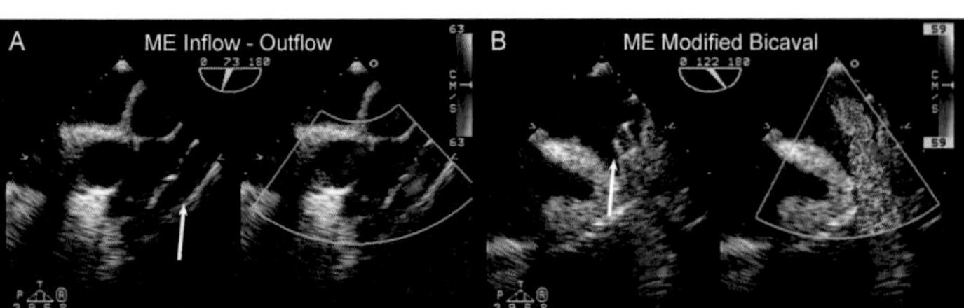

Orthotopic Heart Transplantation

- This is the gold standard surgical procedure to manage refractory heart failure.
- The procedure involves the explant of the native heart and implant of the donor heart, using 1 of 2 techniques (see p. 301).
- TEE is of limited use preCPB
  - Estimate pulmonary vascular resistance (PVR)
    PVR = TRmax × VTI RVOT × 10 + 0.16
- TEE is most useful to assess early graft function, diagnose potential complications, and help guide the institution of mechanical support if required.
- Biventricular dysfunction may represent primary graft failure or early rejection.

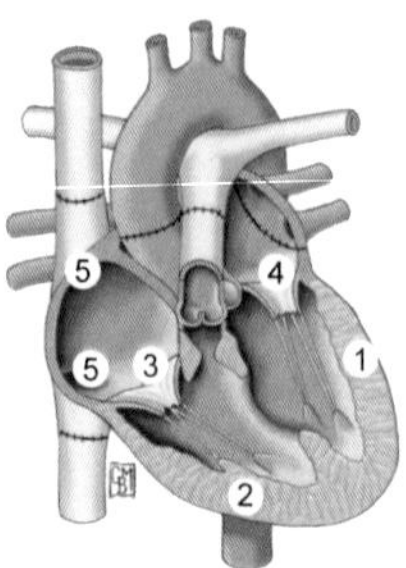

TEE PreCPB Heart Transplant	TEE PostCPB Heart Transplant
Dilated Ventricles	Deairing
Thinned myocardium (<6 mm)	❶ ❷ Ventricular function (R,L)
Smoke, thrombus	Global
Caval size	Regional
Persistent left SVC	❸ TR (estimate PASP), MR
Tricuspid Regurgitation (TR)	Anastomotic sites
Estimate PASP, PVR	❹ LA, pulmonary vein
VAD explant (LVAD, BiVAD)	❺ SVC
Pleural effusion	❻ IVC
Pacer wires	PFO

Anastomosis

- Bicaval anastomosis requires careful examination of the SVC, IVC to measure size and by color Doppler to ensure laminar flow. It is difficult to obtain adequate spectral Doppler alignment to assess velocity in these structures. The surgeon should be informed if turbulent flow is present. SVC obstruction requires clinical correlation and may necessitate surgical revision. IVC stenosis may benefit from postoperative stent deployment.
- LA anastomosis for adequate filling of the LV, through the MV and pulmonary veins.
- Aorta, PA anastomosis rarely has problems.

(A) ME 4C view shows LA anastomotic stenosis (arrow) with turbulent flow above the MV restricting LV filling. (B) ME bicaval views showing turbulent flow in the IVC (arrow) that required a postoperative stent and in the SVC (double arrow).

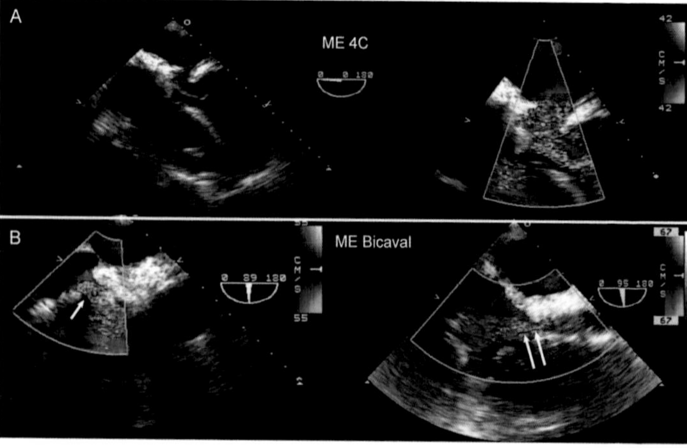

Heart Transplant Technique

Bi-atrial (Lower-Shumway)

Part of recipient RA, LA, pulmonary veins (blue) are preserved and sutured to donor RA and LA (red).

Bicaval (Wythenshawe)

Recipient native RA is removed and anastomosis is between donor (red) and native (blue) SVC, IVC and LA.

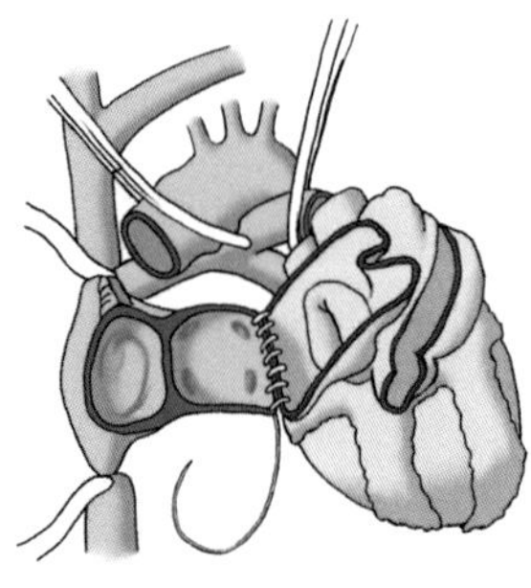

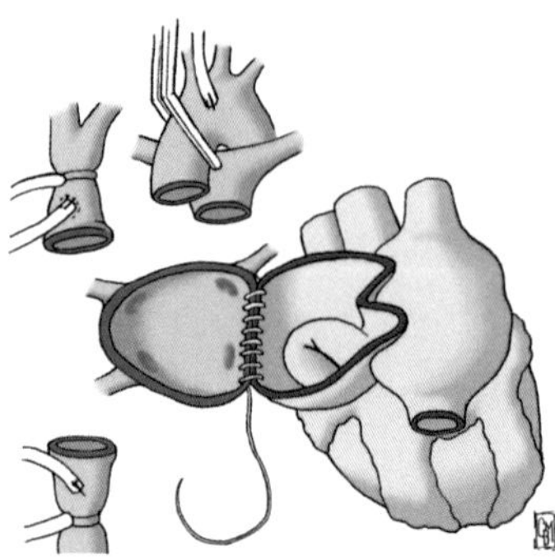

RV Function

- Donor RV function is often decreased after heart transplantation from multiple reasons: donor myocardial dysfunction, hypervolemia, prolonged ischemic time, preexisting elevated PAP, and possible rejection.
- Findings suggestive of RV dysfunction are listed.
- Reduced RV function has prognostic implications.
- Avoid excessive volume which worsens RV function.

RV Failure
Dilated
Wall motion abnormal
IVS septal bowing
Reduced TAPSE
TR severe (also RVSP)
RV-free wall strain

(A) ME 4C view shows a dilated RV with the IVS bowed into the LV. (B) ME Inflow-Outflow view with color Doppler (Nyquist 59 cm/s) shows significant laminar TR that indicates severe RV dysfunction.

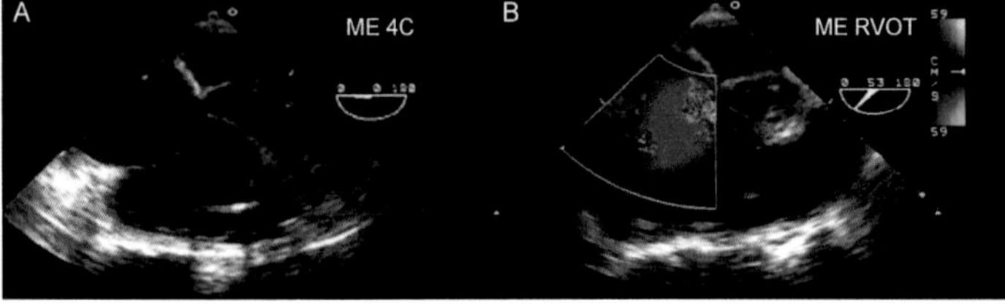

Pericardial Effusion, Tamponade

- Bleeding is common after heart transplantation from preexisting coagulopathy and the presence of multiple new suture lines.
- A blood collection may be loculated and compress cardiac chambers or nearby structures.
- Atrioventricular valve flow is assessed for respiratory variation to diagnose tamponade.

ME 4C view shows compression of the left upper pulmonary vein (arrow) as it drains into the LA. This is from a collection of blood in the oblique sinus compressing the LA.

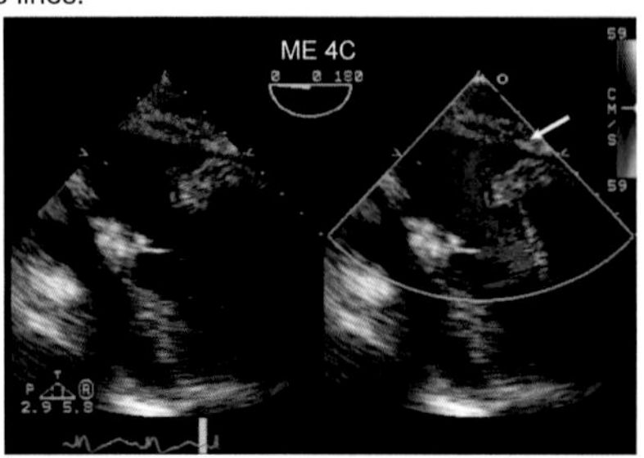

13
Cardiomyopathies

Page

A. Vegas, *Perioperative Two-Dimensional Transesophageal Echocardiography*, https://doi.org/10.1007/978-3-319-60902-7_13

- Cardiomyopathies are diseases of the myocardium that result from structurally and functionally abnormal heart muscle causing cardiac dysfunction, in the absence of coronary artery disease (CAD), hypertension, valvular, and congenital heart disease. These can be familial (genetic mutations) or non-familial.
- There is no universally agreed upon classification of cardiomyopathies as each tries to integrate anatomy, physiology, and genetics. The one shown here is the simplified European version.
- Each type may have multiple causes.
- Echocardiography can easily identify different cardiomyopathies by assessing ventricular function (systolic and diastolic), wall thickness, and chamber size.
- Alternative diagnostic approaches are endomyocardial biopsy and heart catheterization.

Cardiomyopathy Types
Dilated (DCM)
Restrictive (RCM)
Hypertrophic (HCM)
Arrhythmogenic RV dysplasia
Unclassified:
  Takotsubo
  LV non-compaction
Source:
Eur Heart J 2008;29: 270–6.

Dilated Cardiomyopathy (DCM)

- DCM is defined by the presence of LV dilatation and systolic dysfunction in the absence of abnormal loading conditions (hypertension, valve disease) or CAD.
- DCM is the commonest cardiomyopathy (60%, 5–8/100,00) originating from multiple causes with an unfortunate high mortality 50% (2 year), 75% (5 year).
- DCM has a dilated ventricle (either or both) with systolic and diastolic dysfunction. Reduced contractility from thinned myocardium causes a decreased cardiac output, increased EDP, and EDV. Valvular dysfunction (MR/TR) results from annular dilatation. Elevated LAP leads to pulmonary hypertension. LVEDD >4 cm/m^2 and RV function importantly predict prognosis.
- Echo is likely to make the diagnosis of DCM, but is unlikely to distinguish the specific etiology. Serial echoes help follow progression and determine management.

Etiology DCM
Idiopathic
Familial
Myocarditis:
  Infective/toxic/immune
Kawasaki disease
Eosinophilic
Viral persistence
Drugs
Pregnancy
Endocrine
Nutritional (thiamine)
Alcohol

TEE Dilated Cardiomyopathy
2D
Chamber dimensions
EDD, spherical shape
Thin myocardium
Reduced EF (<45%)
↑ Ventricular mass (eccentric hypertrophy)
Apical LV thrombus, SEC
Doppler
Valvular regurgitation (MR, TR)
PAP (RVSP from TR jet)
LV diastolic filling (MV + pulmonary vein)
Early abnormal relaxation
Pseudonormalization
Reduced aortic ejection velocity

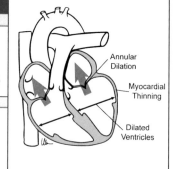

Annular Dilation
Myocardial Thinning
Dilated Ventricles

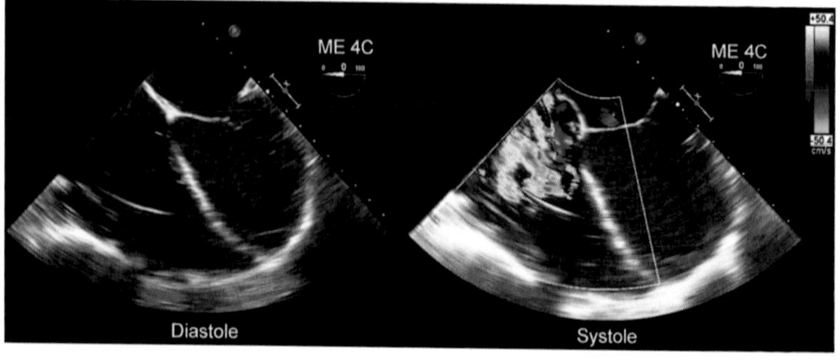

Restrictive Cardiomyopathy (RCM)

- RCM is the least common cardiomyopathy. It is defined by restrictive ventricular physiology from a stiff ventricle with normal systolic, but impaired diastolic function. RCM is characterized by normal or reduced diastolic and systolic volumes (of one or both ventricles) and normal ventricular wall thickness. Pseudohypertrophy from infiltrates, not myocardial hypertrophy, may make the ventricle walls appear thick.
- Isolated LV involvement results in pulmonary congestion from impaired diastolic filling (↑ LVEDP) and RV involvement causes right heart failure (edema, ascites).
- RCM may be idiopathic, familial, or result from various systemic disorders and endocardial pathology (fibrosis, fibroelastosis, thrombosis). Fibrous endocardial lesions of the RV and/or LV inflow tract cause atrioventricular valve incompetence. There are specific echocardiographic findings related to each etiology.

Etiology RCM
Familial
Amyloid
Scleroderma
Carcinoid heart disease
Metastatic cancers
Radiation
Drugs (anthracyclines)
Endomyocardial fibrosis
Hypereosinophilic
Idiopathic
Chromosomal
Drugs: serotonin
Methysergide
Ergotamine

Amyloidosis Commonest RCM Amyloid deposits	• Echogenic infiltrates (speckled appearance) • Thick heart (walls + valves) • Infiltrates in atrial walls (+ IAS) and RV, thrombi in atria
Sarcoidosis Granulomatous infiltrates	• Localized thinning + LV dilatation, usually near base • IVS involvement of conduction system leads to HB, papillary muscles results in MR
Hemochromatosis Iron deposits	• Early thickened ventricle (spares valves) • Later have non-specific findings, similar to DCM
Carcinoid syndrome Serotonin deposits	• Right heart and rarely left heart • Valves + RA/RV wall infiltrate • Thick retracted TV + PV leaflets severe regurgitation
Hypereosinophilic syndrome	• LV thrombus despite good LV function • Late stage have MV + TV subvalvular regurgitation or stenosis

TEE Restrictive Cardiomyopathy	
• Nondilated thickened LV and RV	**Restrictive pattern DD**
• Normal systolic function	MV Inflow
• Diastolic dysfunction (DD): restrictive pattern	E/A > 2
Constrictive pericarditis: (TDI) E' > 8 cm/s	Short DT < 150 ms
Restrictive cardiomyopathy: (TDI) E' < 8 cm/s	Short A-wave duration
• Bi-atrial enlarge (LA > 60 mm independent risk)	Pulmonary Vein Flow
• ↑ PAP (TR, paradoxical septal motion)	PV D < 30 cm/s
• Doppler: TR (↑ PAP)	PV S/D < < 1
Pulmonary vein flow	PV Ar > 35 ms
MV Inflow	PV Ar/MVI Ar > 0.6

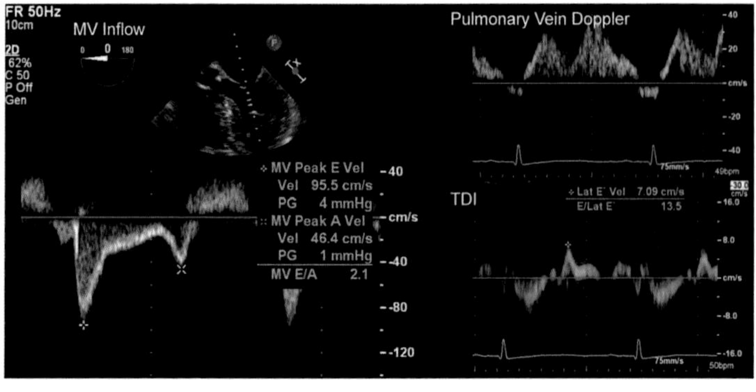

Arrhythmogenic Right Ventricular Cardiomyopathy (ARVC) or Dysplasia (ARVD)

- ARVD is a histological diagnosis from progressive replacement of RV myocardium with adipose and fibrous tissue. It is often confined to a triangle of dysplasia involving the anterior infundibulum (outflow), apex, and inferior (inflow) parts of the RV. It is related to an autosomal-dominant gene mutation and, though uncommon, it is a cause of sudden cardiac death. There may be LV involvement.
- Echocardiography is sensitive but not specific for diagnosing ARVD, as it does not assess adipose in the myocardium. Echocardiographic features consistent with ARVD are as listed. Diagnosis of ARVD requires an integrated assessment using ECG, echocardiography, cardiac MRI/CT, and angiography.
- Original 1994 ARVD diagnostic criteria have been updated in 2010.

ARVD TEE
RV + RA dilatation
Isolated RVOT dilatation (> 30 mm)
Hypokinetic/dyskinetic inferobasal
Segmental RV wall aneurysms
Highly reflective moderator band

Diagnostic Criteria Arrhythmogenic RV Dysplasia (ARVD)	
Major Criteria	**Minor Criteria**
RV Dysfunction	
• Severe RV dilatation + ↓ RV EF with little or no LV impairment • Localized RV aneurysm • Severe segmental RV dilatation	• Mild global RV dilatation ± ↓ EF with normal LV • Mild segmental RV dilatation • Regional RV hypokinesis
Source: McKenna WJ, et al. Br Heart J. 1994; 71:215–218	
• Regional RV akinesia, dyskinesia, aneurysm • One of following (end-diastole): PLAX RVOT ≥32 mm, PLAX/BSA ≥19 mm/m² PSAX RVOT ≥36 mm, PLAX/BSA ≥21 mm/m² Fractional area change ≤33%	• Regional RV akinesia, dyskinesia • One of following (end-diastole): PLAX RVOT 29–31 mm, /BSA 16–18 mm/m² PSAX RVOT 32–35 mm, /BSA 18–20 mm/m² Fractional area change 34–40%
Source: Marcus FI, et al. Circulation 2010; 121:1533–41	
Fibrofatty replacement of myocardium by endomyocardial biopsy	
ECG	
• Epsilon waves V1–V3 • Localized prolonged QRS (> 110 ms) V1–V3	• Inverted T-waves in V2 + V3 no RBBB • Late potentials signal averaged ECG • Ventricular tachycardia with a LBBB • Frequent PVCs (>1000 PVCs/24 h)
• Familial disease confirmed on autopsy or surgery	• Family history (FMH) of ARVD • FMH sudden cardiac death < age 35

RVOT
30mm
Moderator
Band
Focal
Aneurysm
Epsilon
Wave

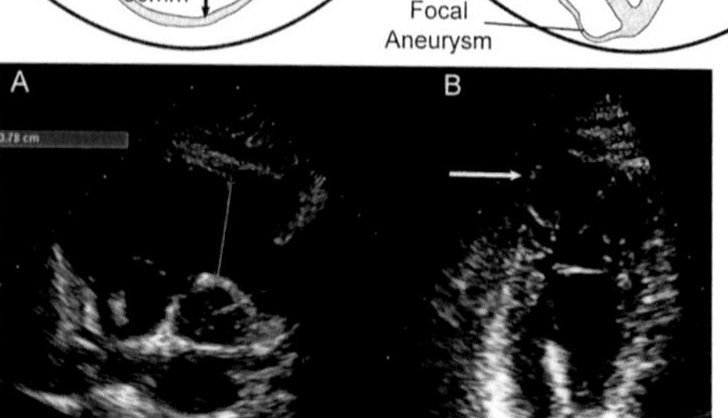

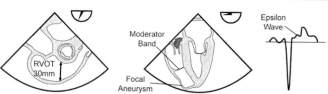

(A) This TTE RV inflow-outflow view shows RVOT dilatation of >30 mm. (B) This TTE apical 4C view isolated on the RV shows the presence of an apical aneurysm (arrow) and prominent moderator band. Both these findings are consistent with ARVD.

Left Ventricular Non-Compaction (LVNC)

- LVNC is characterized by prominent LV trabeculae and deep intertrabecular recesses (spaces) that involve the LV apex. The epicardial layer is thin with thickened myocardial and endocardial layers.
- LVNC is often familial and considered a congenital cardiomyopathy. It occurs in isolation and in association with congenital cardiac disorders (Ebstein's anomaly or complex cyanotic heart disease) and some neuromuscular diseases.
- Diagnosis can be made with echocardiography, cardiac MRI, or LV angiography. Two echocardiographic criteria (Chin and Jenni) are used for diagnosing LVNC by quantifying the depth of penetration of the intertrabecular recesses. The Jenni criteria describe the LV wall as being made up of 2 layers, an outer compacted layer, contiguous with the epicardium, and an inner non-compacted layer.
- Other TEE findings consistent with LVNC include:
  - Numerous, excessively prominent trabeculations + deep intertrabecular recesses
  - Mid LV (especially inferior + lateral) and apical segments
  - Intertrabecular recesses perfused by intraventricular blood (color Doppler)
  - Preserved LV systolic function, or global or regional LV and RV dysfunction

LVNC TEE
Trabeculae + recesses
Mid + apical segments
Color Doppler
LV function

Chin Criteria
X-to-Y ratio ≤ 0.5 in LVNC X = epicardial surface to trabecular recess trough Y = epicardial surface to trabecular peak

Jenni criteria
End-systolic thickness of non-compacted (NC) and compacted (C) layer is taken at the area of maximal LV wall thickness in the LV SAX view. A ratio of NC/C > 2 is LVNC

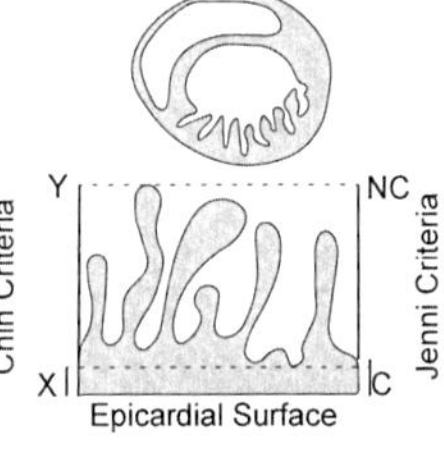

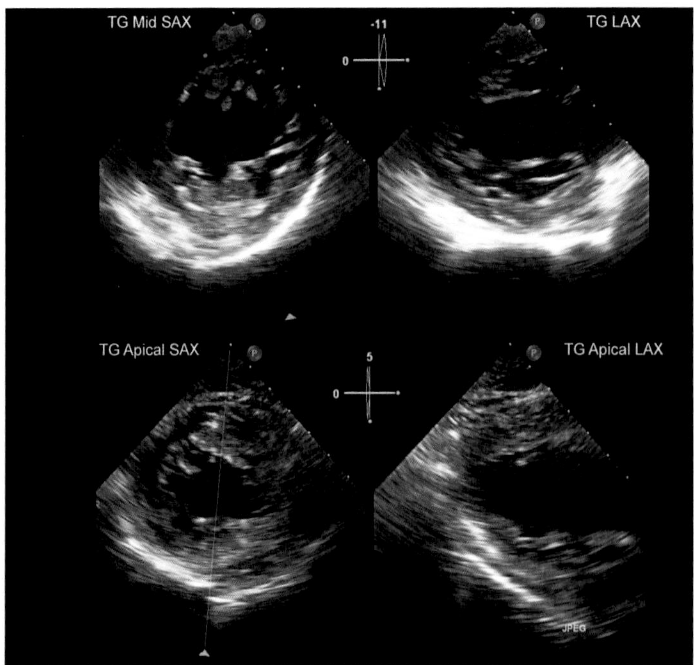

Takotsubo Cardiomyopathy

- Transient LV apical ballooning, broken heart syndrome, or stress cardiomyopathy is characterized by transient (reversible) regional systolic dysfunction involving the LV apex and/or mid-ventricle in the absence of obstructive CAD on angiography.
- Patients present with
  - An abrupt onset of angina-like chest pain
  - Diffuse ECG changes (T-wave inversion, ST elevation)
  - Mild cardiac enzyme elevation
- Stress is a precipitant and it may occur with acute cerebral vascular accidents.
- LV function usually normalizes over a period of days to weeks and recurrence is rare. Treatment is supportive.
- Formal diagnostic criteria have been proposed but lack general acceptance:
  - LV wall motion abnormalities are beyond a single major coronary artery
  - Nonobstructive CAD (<50% stenosis) by angiography within 24 h of symptoms
  - New ECG changes such as transient ST-segment elevation and/or diffuse T-wave inversions or troponin elevation.

> **TEE in Takotsubo Cardiomyopathy (TC)**
> - LV wall motion abnormalities of apical and/or mid-ventricular dyskinesis.
> - In systole, the inferobasal wall contracts normally but the apex balloons out, giving the appearance of an octopus trap (takotsubo in Japanese).
> - Variants include:
>   - Inverted Takotsubo Cardiomyopathy: basal ballooning with apical hyperkinesis
>   - RV involvement has more severe LV dysfunction and pleural effusions

(A, B) TTE apical 4 chamber views of patients with Takotsubo cardiomyopathy are shown in diastole and systole, (A) without and (B) with contrast. Note the normal basal contraction and apical ballooning seen during systole.

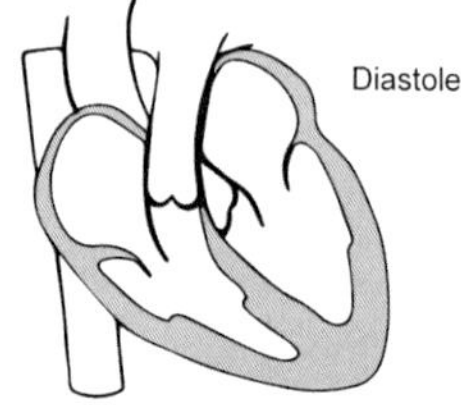

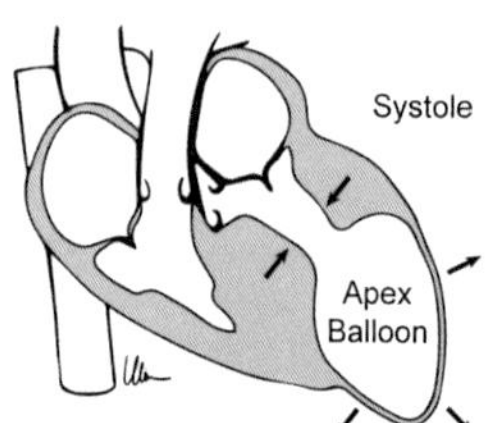

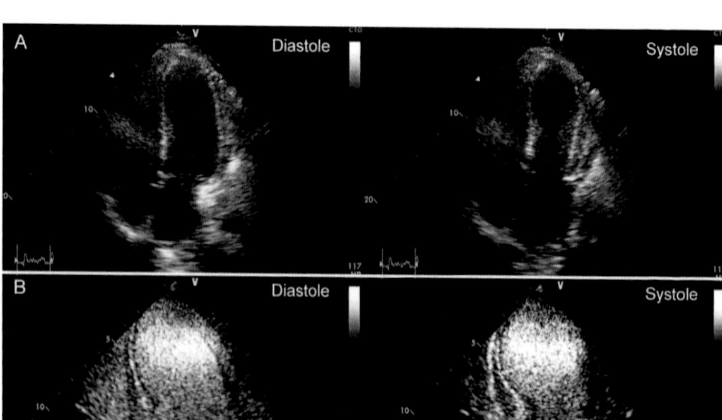

Myocarditis

- Myocarditis is an inflammation of the myocardium. It is most often due to viral infection, but can result from bacterial infections, medications, toxins, and autoimmune disorders.
- The gold standard for the diagnosis is biopsy. MRI is also useful. Echocardiography has non-specific findings, but is important for prognosis.
- Myocarditis has been described in relation to the onset after systemic illness as fulminant (1–2 day), acute (days to weeks), and chronic (weeks to months). Most often, patients present with heart failure and systolic dysfunction, sometimes systolic function is preserved.
- Fulminant myocarditis is an inflammatory process of the myocardium that is characterized by the sudden onset of severe heart failure soon after a viral prodrome. This is distinct from a nonfulminant process which is less severe, but more often results in dilated cardiomyopathy.
- There is thickening of the LV wall from myocardial edema related to lymphocyte infiltration and myocardial necrosis.
- In fulminant myocarditis, the LV internal cavity is normal or small and the LV wall thickened from "pseudo-concentric hypertrophy." In the nonfulminant form, the LV internal diameter is often enlarged with thin myocardium.
- Serial echocardiographic exams can track progression or regression of LV wall thickness and cavity size.

Sigmoid Septum

- This is a defect of aorta and IVS alignment that is common in the elderly.
- It should not to be confused with basal septal hypertrophy (HCM, see pg 310).
- It is formed by an abnormal aortic angle with the IVS, which makes the septum appear sigmoid in shape and project into the LVOT, creating a unique profile.
- It rarely causes dynamic LVOT obstruction.
- It is more pronounced in hypertensive patients. Following an infero-posterior MI, there could be further collapse of the IVS into the LVOT.
- This is a benign condition, so no treatment is needed.
- The aortoseptal angle is the angle between a line along the septum and a line through the long axis of the aortic root. Reduced angle values represent increasing angulation as seen with a sigmoid septum.
  - Normal angle >125°
  - Reduced angle 100–110°

(A) Normal relation of aorta and IVS with an obtuse aortoseptal angle is shown in this ME LAX view. (B) Patient with asymmetric septal hypertrophy and a septal measure of 2.0 cm. The aortoseptal angle is normal and the same as the patient in (A). (C) Patient with a sigmoid septum bulging into the LVOT with a reduced aortoseptal angle. Though reduced in diameter, there is no obstruction in the LVOT.

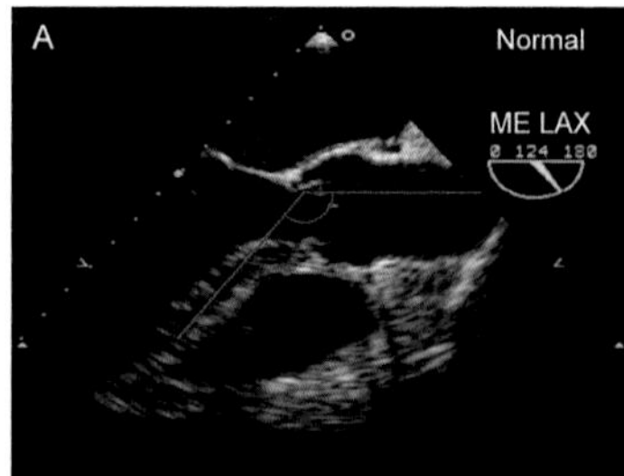

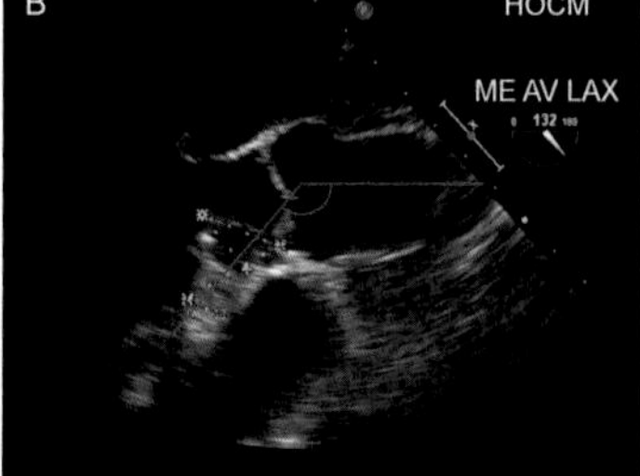

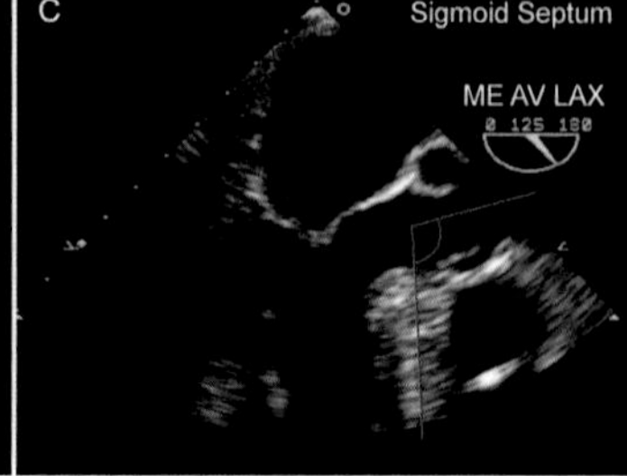

Pathophysiology

- This is a genetic disorder resulting in abnormal myocytes that cause left ventricle hypertrophy (LVH). It is familial autosomal dominant with variable penetrance, related to abnormalities of the B myosin heavy chain resulting in mis-shapen myocytes. Incidence of 1:500.
- There is symmetric or asymmetric LVH with obstruction to LV flow (LVOT or mid-cavitary), abnormal diastolic function, and mitral regurgitation (MR). There is often normal or supranormal systolic function that becomes impaired late in the disease.

> **HCM Pathology**
> LV thick wall
> LV obstruction
> Diastolic dysfunction
> SAM, MR

Hypertrophy

- Different patterns of hypertrophy have been described:

A. Reverse curvature septum HCM shows a predominant mid-septal convexity toward the LV cavity, making it appear as a crescent-shaped cavity. SAM can occur.
B. Sigmoid septum HCM shows the septum concave to the LV cavity and a prominent basal septal bulge creating an ovoid-shaped cavity. SAM can occur.
C. Neutral septum HCM shows a straight septum that is neither predominantly convex nor concave toward the LV cavity. SAM can occur.
D. Mid-ventricular HCM shows predominant hypertrophy at the mid-ventricular level. There is mid-cavity obstruction without SAM.
E. Apical HCM shows a predominant apical distribution of hypertrophy.

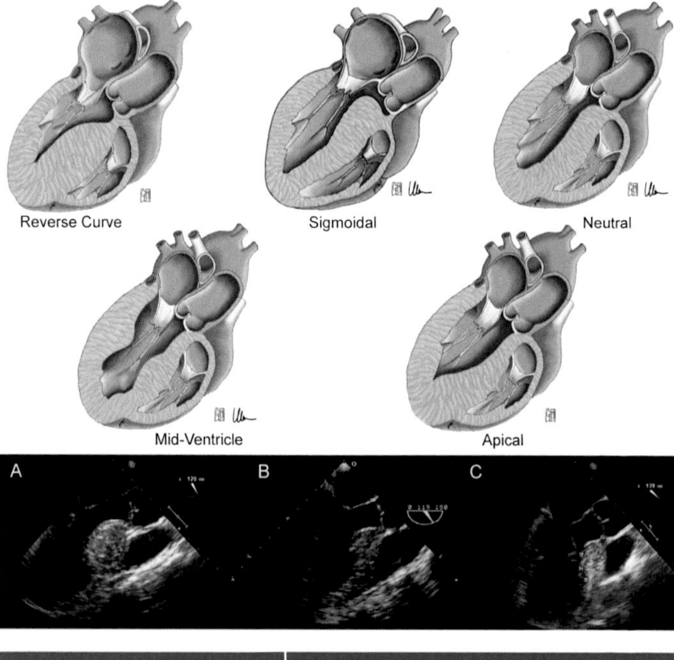

Asymmetric Hypertrophy	Symmetric Hypertrophy
Familial	Hypertension
Sigmoid shaped in elderly	Aortic stenosis
Eisenmenger's	Infiltration (amyloid, glycogen, sarcoid)
Septal sarcomas	Metabolic (Cushing, diabetes)
LVH with lateral wall infarct	Renal disease
Pulmonary hypertension + RVH	Athletic heart, obesity
Hypertension	Congenital (Fabray, Noonan, Friedrich's Ataxia)
Hemodialysis	

Differential SAM
HOCM
LVH post-AVR
Post-MV repair
RV dysfunction

Obstruction

- Despite LVH, flow through the LV may be nonobstructive, labile (or provoked), or obstructive at rest.
- Obstruction to flow may occur at different levels: LVOT, mid-ventricular or apical, and at rest or with provocation. Assess the LVOT gradient clinically at rest or after provocation.
- In the normal heart, the LVOT is formed by the IVS and anterior mitral valve leaflet (AMVL). Most often in HCM, the thick septum protrudes into the LVOT below the AV, causing narrowing which results in turbulent flow and a dynamic late peaking (dagger) high velocity systolic gradient.

Increase LV Obstruction	Decrease LV Obstruction
↓ Preload: Valsalva, amyl nitrate	↑ Preload: fluids
↑ Contractility: Post-PVC, inotrope	↓ Contractility: B blockers
↓ Afterload: amyl nitrate	↑ Afterload: phenylephrine

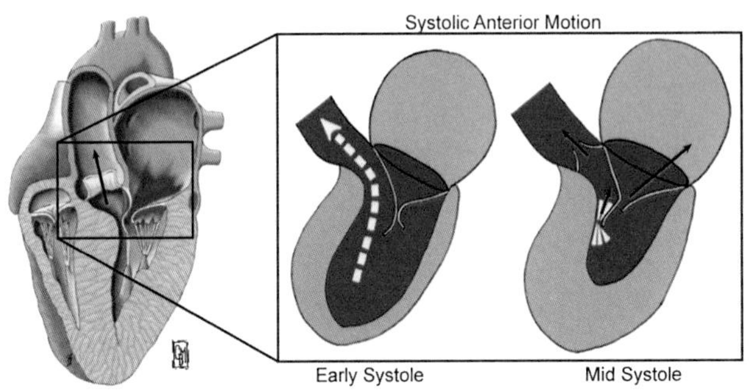

Mitral Regurgitation (MR)

- In patients with septal hypertrophy, the LVOT is narrowed, the papillary muscles are anteriorly displaced, and the MV leaflets elongated. During early systole, the body of the AMVL coapts with the tip of the posterior mitral valve (PMVL). The AMVL tip is dragged into the LVOT by the Venturi effect of mid-systolic flow; this is termed systolic anterior motion (SAM).
- The displaced AMVL results in poor MV leaflet coaptation and eccentric posterior-directed MR in mid to late systole.
- MR severity relates to the degree of LVOT obstruction.

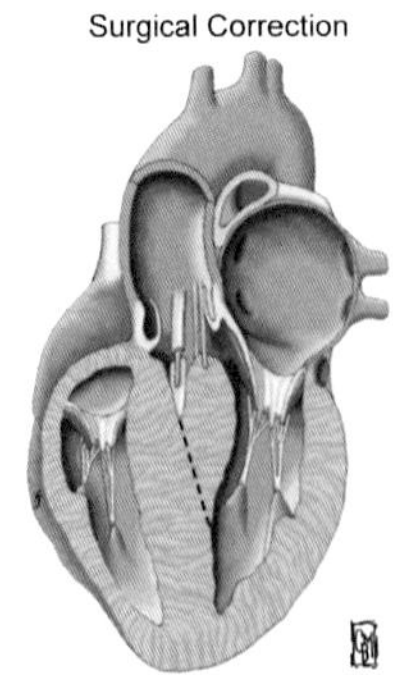

Diastolic Dysfunction (DD)

- The LV wall is thickened resulting in different grades of DD from impaired relaxation to restricted filling patterns.
- The presence of restrictive filling worsens prognosis.
- No single Doppler modality is superior in assessing DD in the setting of HOCM.

Clinical

- Patients are usually asymptomatic, though presenting symptoms include LVOT obstruction (syncope, sudden death), myocardial ischemia (angina), and diastolic dysfunction (pulmonary congestion and shortness of breath).
- Surgery involves a transaortic septal myectomy with a parallel excision of the IVS below the right coronary cusp to the papillary muscles.

Surgical Indications HOCM	Complications	%
• Obstructive disease from SAM	Atrial arrhythmia	26
• Peak PG >50 mm Hg at rest or provoked	Ventricular arrhythmia	7
• Symptoms (angina, heart failure, syncope) refractory to medical therapy	Heart block	10
	Left ventricular rupture	1
	Ventricular septal defect	0.6

Pre-Myectomy TEE
- Septal measures
- AV flutter
- MV morphology
- SAM
- MR
- Peak gradient LVOT
- LA size
- LV function (S,D)

TEE Findings PreCPB

2-D Imaging
- Identify LV wall thickness
  - Symmetric or asymmetrical, septal, and lateral walls
  - Septal:free wall ratio > 1.3:1
  - >15 mm thickness is abnormal
- Assess mitral valve (MV):
  - No intrinsic MV disease
  - SAM of anterior MV leaflet (AMVL)
- Aortic valve cusps fluttering, with mid-systolic closure
- Anomalous papillary muscle insertion directly into the leaflet, 10% of patients
- ↑ LA size >40 mm or >20 cm^2 in ME 4C
- LV and RV systolic function is normal or hyperdynamic
- Measurements of septal size are made at end-diastole (both AV and MV closed) from ME AV LAX view. Goal is to provide surgeon with measures of the myectomy.
  - Align perpendicular to the IVS, the AV should appear symmetric
  - Echogenic region on the IVS is the septal contact point (fibrotic IVS)
- Measure LVOT diameter in systole
- Measure AMVL length
  - use ME AV LAX view (see next page)
  - if >35 mm consider plication
- Septo-aortic angle between IVS and aorta
  - HOCM: obtuse angle >125°
  - Sigmoid septum: acute angle 100–110°

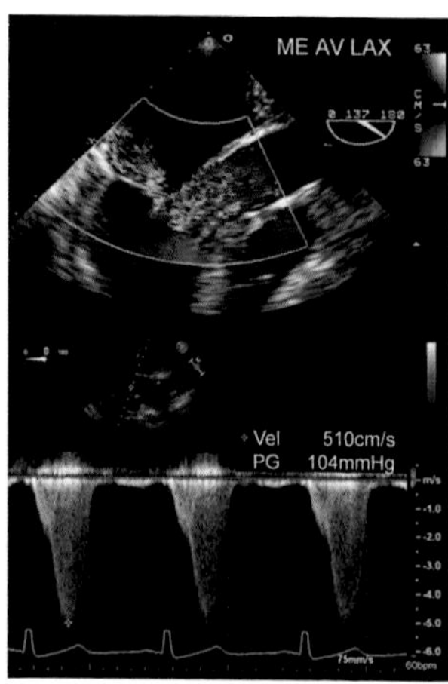

Color Doppler
- Turbulent LVOT flow (Nyquist 50–60 cm/s)
- Turbulent mid-cavitary flow
- Mitral regurgitation
  - Eccentric posterior directed jet
  - Central jet implies other MV pathology
  - Difficult to quantify due to jet eccentricity

Spectral Doppler
- PW for peak gradient (mid-cavitary, LVOT)
- CW peak and mean LVOT gradient
  - Late peaking systolic (dagger shape)
  - Significant if peak >30 mmHg at rest
  - Gradient ↑ post-PVC or amyl nitrate
- LV has diastolic dysfunction with different patterns from impaired relaxation to restrictive filling as assessed by:
  - MV Inflow: E > A
  - Pulmonary vein: S < D
  - Tissue Doppler: E' < 8 cm/s, E/e'

HOCM Measurements (End-Diastole)
(A) Distance RCC to maximum thickness
(B) Maximal septal thickness
(C) Distance RCC to distal narrowing
(D) Distal narrowing
(E) RCC to septal contact point

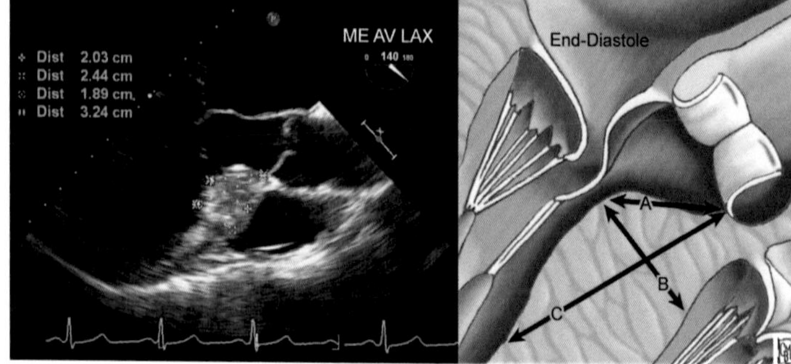

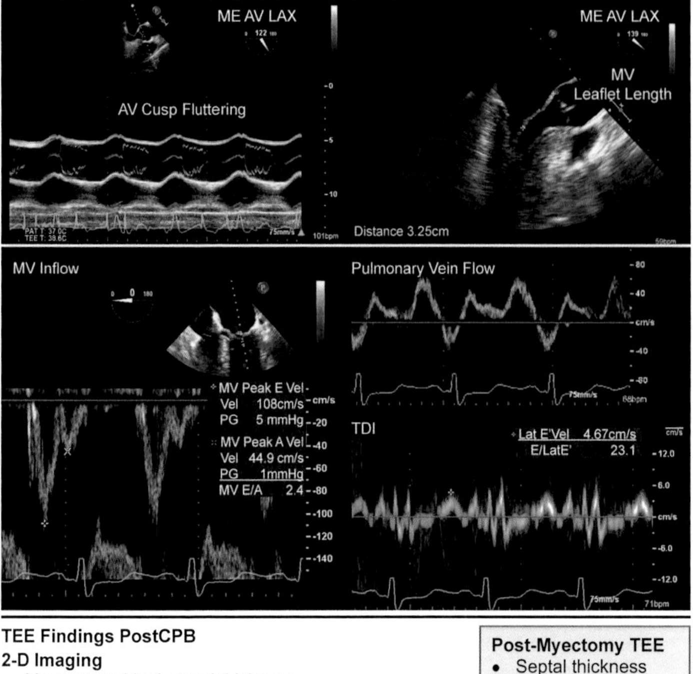

TEE Findings PostCPB

2-D Imaging
- Measure residual septal thickness
- SAM and residual MR (adequate ventricular filling + BP)
- LV/RV systolic function (LAD muscle bridge)

Color Doppler
- Laminar systolic LVOT flow
- MR minimal or from intrinsic valve disease
- Septal perforator flow into LV during diastole
- VSD (<3 mm IVS) absent, high velocity L to R flow in systole

Spectral Doppler
- CW peak LVOT gradients (rest, post-PVC)
- Mid-ventricular cavitary obstruction
- Diastolic function

Post-Myectomy TEE
- Septal thickness
- LVOT diameter
- Residual SAM
- Residual MR
- Peak gradient LVOT
- VSD absent
- Aortic valve (AI)

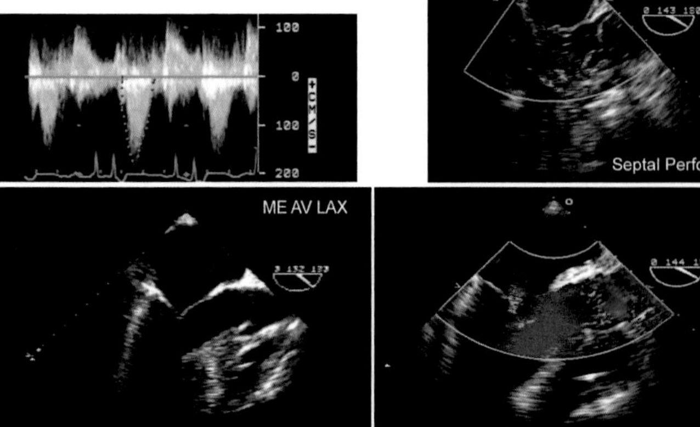

14 Pericardium

Page

A. Vegas, *Perioperative Two-Dimensional Transesophageal Echocardiography*, https://doi.org/10.1007/978-3-319-60902-7_14

Pericardial Anatomy

- Normal pericardium is an avascular sac composed of inner serous and outer fibrous pericardium. The serous pericardium comprises the (a) outer parietal layer adherent to the fibrous pericardium and the (b) inner visceral layer that reflects back onto the heart surface.
- The potential space between the visceral and serous parietal pericardium is the pericardial cavity. Normally, 15–50 cc of clear pericardial fluid is in the pericardial sac to reduce friction between pericardial surfaces.

Pericardial Sinuses

- The parietal and visceral pericardium are continuous where the major vessels enter and leave the heart. There are 2 blind sacs: the smaller transverse and larger oblique sinuses.
- The oblique sinus lies behind the left atrium (LA) so that the posterior LA wall is actually separated from the pericardial space. A posterior pericardial effusion behind the LA and LV is easily seen in a supine patient.
- The transverse sinus is the connection between two tubes of pericardium that envelop the great vessels. The aorta and pulmonary artery (PA) are enclosed in one antero-superior tube, and the vena cava and pulmonary veins are enclosed in a more posterior tube.
- Pericardial fluid located in the superior recess should not be mistaken for an intimal flap of an aortic dissection.

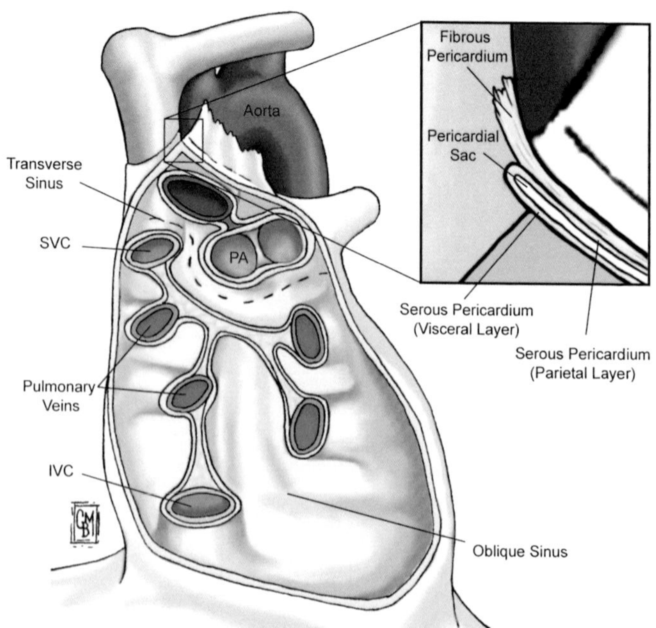

Physiology

- Pericardium has a number of different functions
  - Fixes the heart in the chest
  - Protects the heart from surrounding structures
  - Limits chamber overfilling
  - Couples ventricular function in diastole
  - Pericardial fluid provides lubrication

Pericardium Functions
Restrain in chest
Constrain filling
Ventricular interdependence
Protection
Fluid lubrication

- Direct transmission of intra-thoracic pressures to intra-pericardial pressure alters cardiac filling during both spontaneous respiration and mechanical ventilation.
  - During spontaneous inspiration, intra-thoracic pressure is low which better fills the right heart, shifting the IVS, and reducing LV stroke volume (SV).
  - In spontaneous expiration, intra-thoracic pressures are higher, reducing right heart volumes, shifting the IVS back, improving LV filling and SV.
- These changes are reflected in the spectral Doppler patterns of valve inflow.
  - Different inflow patterns are seen during spontaneous or positive pressure ventilation and are exacerbated with disease processes.
  - In a normal heart, there is <10% change in Doppler signals with ventilation

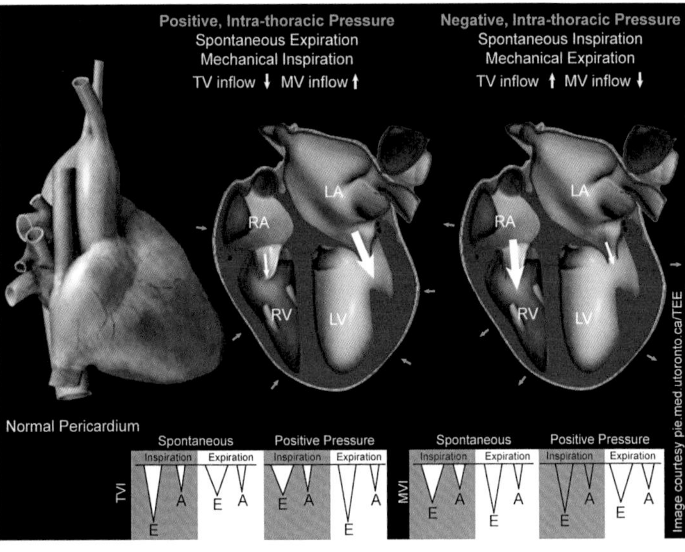

Pericardial Pathology

- Pathology of the pericardium includes common findings such as effusions and thickening.
- Tumors of the pericardium are rare, benign occur more often than malignant (mesothelioma).
- Congenital absence of the pericardium is rare.
  - 30% have an associated congenital abnormality
  - Absence can be complete or partial
    - 80% involve the left heart
    - Total absence is asymptomatic
    - Partial absence of the left heart is dangerous
  - Excessive heart motion has echo findings of:
    - Heart shifts to the left, so the RV appears dilated
    - Paradoxical IVS motion occurs during systole with exaggerated posterior wall motion causing anterior displacement of the IVS.
- Pericardial cysts usually appear as a localized, spherical echolucent space of variable size at the RA border.

Pericardium Pathology
Pericarditis
Effusion
Thickening
Constriction
Cyst
Tumor
Congenital absence

TEE of the Pericardium

- Normal pericardium surrounds the heart surface and is indistinguishable from the epicardium by echocardiography.
- As the pericardium surrounds the heart, it is visible in multiple TEE views from the ME (4C, 2C, and LAX) and TG (SAX and LAX) views.
- Echocardiography is the initial diagnostic test of choice to assess pericardial pathology. CT and MRI are also useful additional or alternative imaging modalities.
- Normally, a small amount of pericardial fluid (50 cc) is seen in the transverse sinus only in systole. Separation of the pericardial layers that is present throughout the cardiac cycle represents an effusion of >50 cc.
- TEE can accurately measure pericardial thickening.
- TEE can be used to guide and assess the success of various cardiac procedures.

TEE Indications
Pericardial window
Pericardiectomy
Pericardiocentesis

ME 4C view shows a small circumferential pericardial effusion which appears as a black echolucent stripe surrounding the heart during systole. Fluid is also present behind the LA.

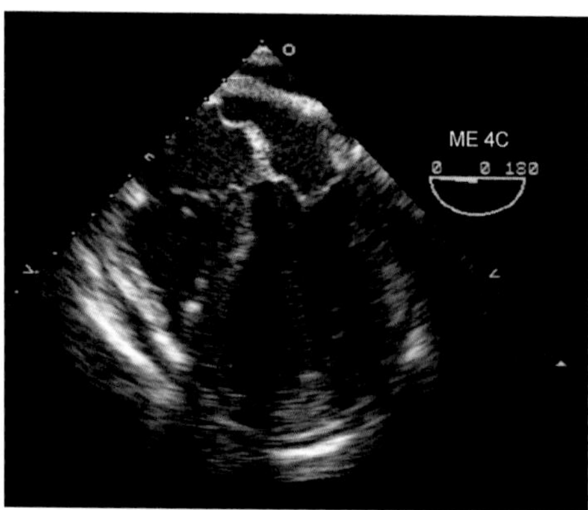

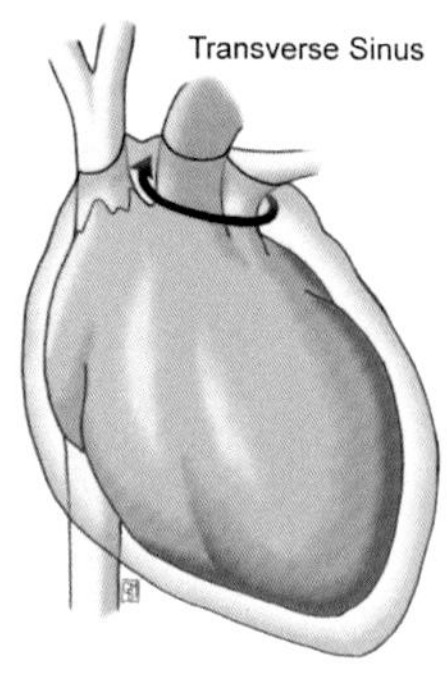

Epicardial Fat Pad

- The epicardial fat pad has a similar consistency to blood when imaged with echocardiography. It is typically located along the atrioventricular groove, interventricular groove, and over the anterior RV (RVOT, free wall). Epicardial fat contains the coronary arteries, lymphatics, and nerve tissue.
- Epicardial fat is brighter than underlying myocardium and moves with the heart
- Epicardial fat may be difficult to differentiate from a small hemopericardial effusion, particularly in the post-cardiac surgery setting.
- Measurement of RV wall thickness is best made in the TG views, not the ME views, to avoid including epicardial fat in the measurement.

(A) ME 4C view shows RV epicardial fat pad (arrow) compared with (B) a small pericardial hemopericardium with blood and clot (arrow) around the RV.

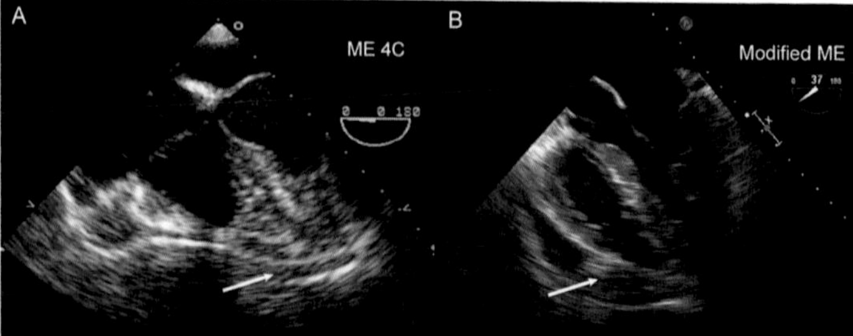

Pericardial Thickening

- Pericardial thickening is a pericardial thickness >5 mm.
- The pericardium appears bright echogenic and may be calcified in different views.
- Thick pericardium may be associated with constrictive pericarditis.

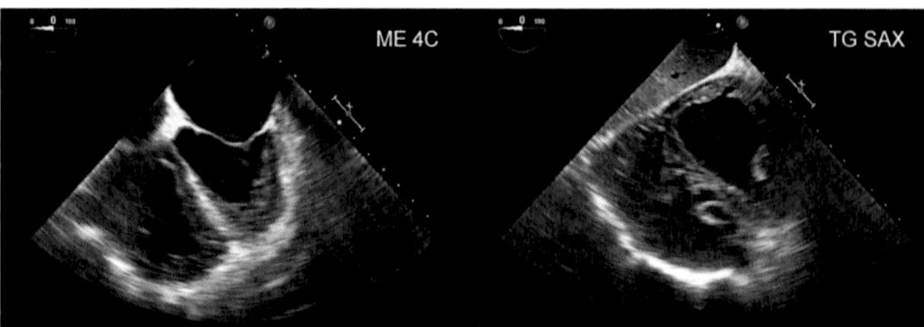

Pericardial Sinuses

Transverse Pericardial Sinus

- Transverse pericardial sinus is the space between the great vessels of the heart and can easily be seen in the ME AV SAX, ME RVOT, and ME AV LAX views.
- ME RVOT view shows the left atrial appendage (LAA) and a small amount of pericardial fluid (arrow) in the transverse sinus. This is the space between the pulmonary artery and LA.
- (B, C) Transverse sinus is shown at the level of the ascending aorta and right pulmonary artery (RPA) in ME AV LAX and Ascending Aortic LAX views. The space may appear filled with thrombus (arrow in B) or fluid (arrow in C).

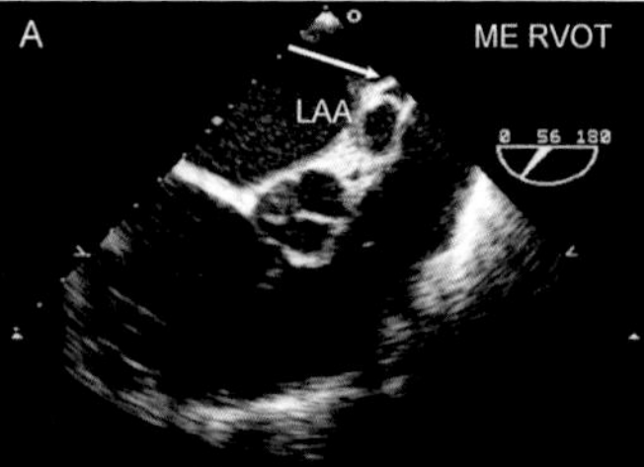

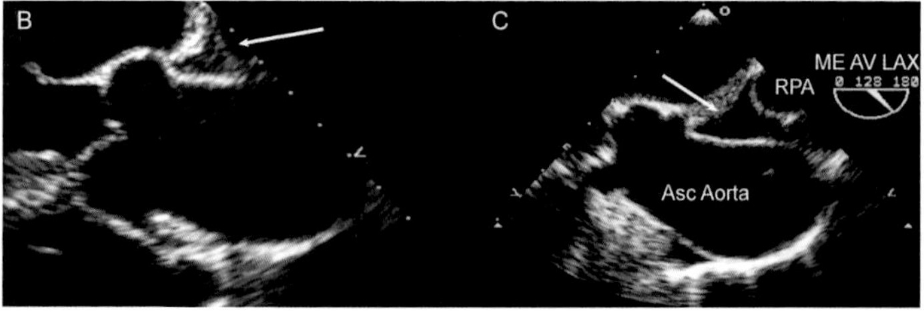

Oblique Pericardial Sinus

- This pericardial space is located behind the LA.
- The oblique pericardial sinus is best seen in the ME AV LAX view behind the LA.
- It often fills with fluid just before weaning from CPB.

(A) Modified ME view showing a collection of blood (arrow) in the oblique sinus. (B) ME LAX view showing pericardial fluid (arrow) behind the LA in the oblique sinus.

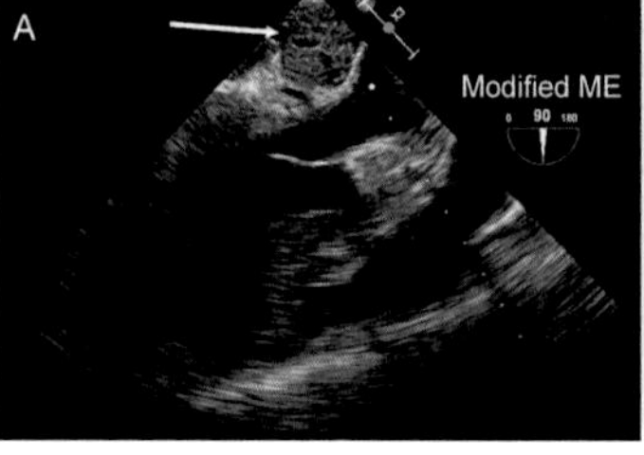

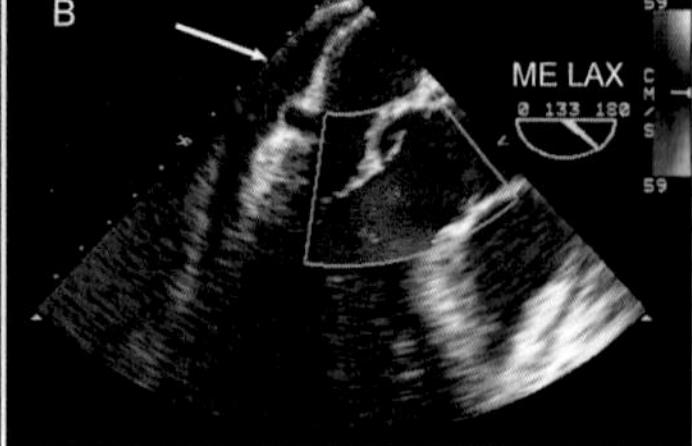

Pericardial Effusion

- Increased fluid produced by the serous pericardium or blood separates the visceral and parietal layers resulting in a pericardial effusion.
- Fluid types: transudate (serous), exudate (cells), pyopericardium (pus), or hemopericardium (blood)
- Etiology from various causes is listed.
- Location (circumferential, loculated)
  - Circumferential effusion surrounds the heart
  - Loculated effusion is adjacent to a cardiac chamber and may occur after cardiac surgery, inflammatory, or metastatic disease

Etiology
Inflammatory
Infectious
Neoplastic
Post-MI
Trauma
Post-surgery

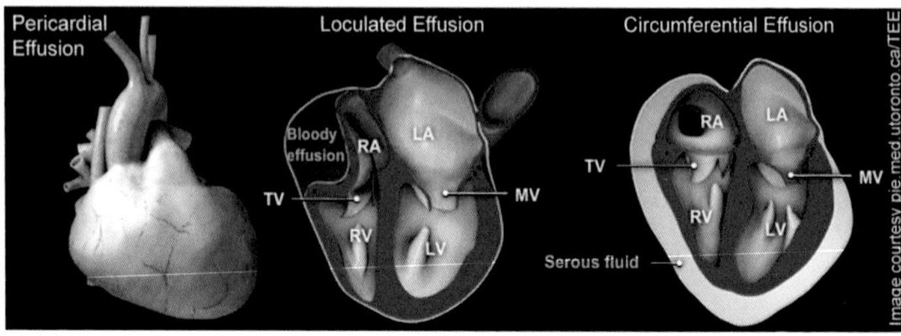

TEE Pericardial Effusions

- Echo-free (echolucent) stripe between visceral and parietal pericardium
  - Small amount of fluid is often seen during systole
  - Anterior effusion is imaged in ME views, posterior effusion in TG view
  - ↓ Echo gain setting to identify pericardial interface (brightest reflector)
  - Isolated anterior echo-free space may be an epicardial fat pad
  - Fibrin strands in long-standing effusions or from metastases
  - Hematoma frequently has a similar echo-consistency as myocardium
- Linear measurement of effusion size semi-quantitatively estimates volume.
- A left pleural effusion (PE) is easily seen in the ME desc aortic SAX view as an echo-lucent space anterior to the descending aorta. A left PE extends posterolateral, whereas a pericardial effusion track anterior to the descending aorta.

Severity	Width (mm)	Volume (cc)	Localization
Small	< 5	< 200	Behind posterior wall
Medium	5–20	200–500	Lateral and apical extension
Large	> 20	> 500	Circumferential

Clinical

- Physiological effects depend on the rate and volume of accumulation
  - Slowly expanding effusion can be quite large with little ↑ in pericardial pressure.
  - Rapid accumulation of a small fluid volume can markedly ↑ pericardial pressure.
- Heart translation in the pericardial sac results in electrical alternans in the ECG.
- Echo guidance can facilitate pericardial effusion drainage (pericardiocentesis).

(A) It may be difficult to identify the needle tip (arrow) in the effusion. (B) Injecting agitated saline (echo contrast, double arrow) will help confirm its location.

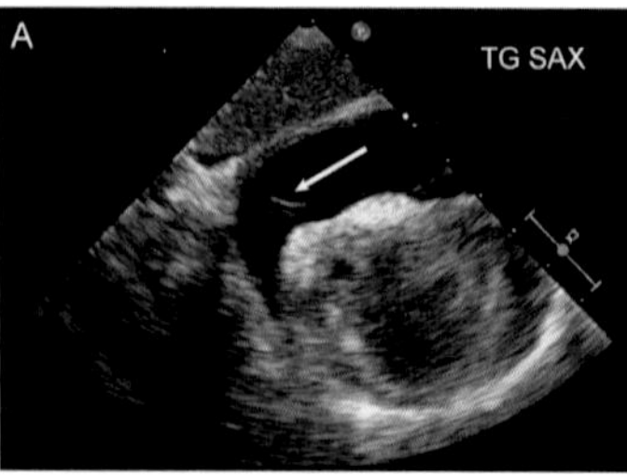

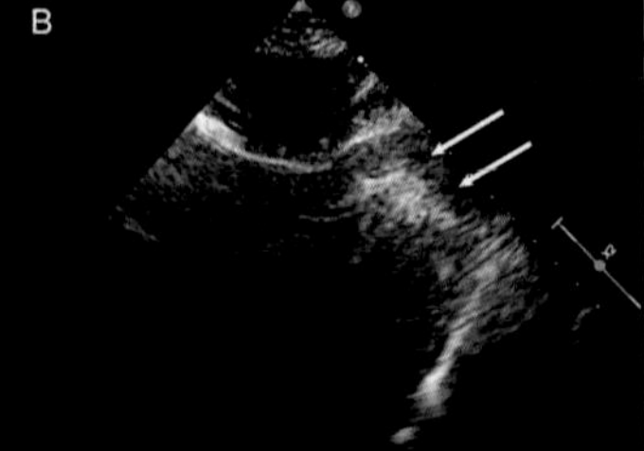

(A, B) A large pericardial effusion is seen (A) posteriorly in the TG mid SAX view and (B) laterally in the ME 4C view in a patient at 1 week after a mechanical MVR. This patient underwent surgical drainage of the effusion. (C) Another patient with a medium-sized circumferential pericardial effusion with fibrous strands mostly around the LV. (D) A patient soon after cardiac surgery develops a loculated pericardial effusion (hematoma) that compresses the right atrium (RA), restricting filling of the RV. This patient required surgical exploration for evacuation of the hematoma.

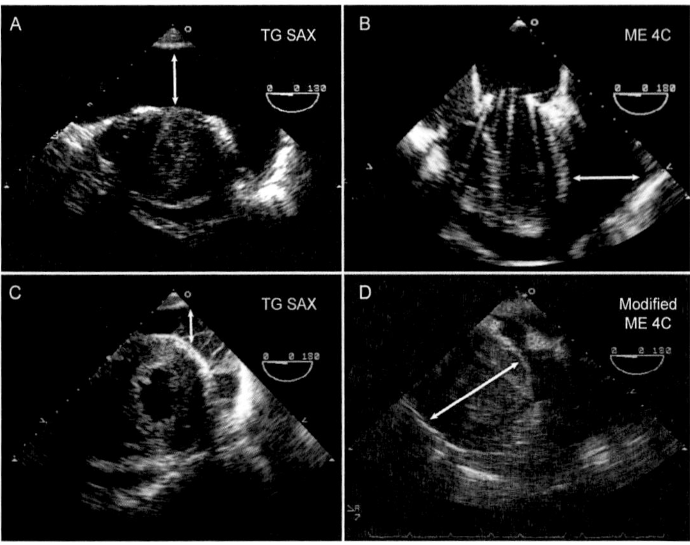

It is important to distinguish a pericardial effusion from other fluid collections such as a pleural effusion and ascites. (A) Patient with a left pleural effusion and pericardial effusion is seen in the Descending Aorta SAX view. The pleural effusion is immediately anterior to the aorta, the pericardial effusion is adjacent to the heart. (B, C) Two patients with ascites are shown in TG mid-SAX views. (B) The arrow points to a small amount of ascites around the liver and there is a tiny amount of pericardial fluid around the heart. (C) This patient with constrictive pericarditis has ascitic fluid (arrow) around the liver, a bright pericardium but no pericardial effusion.

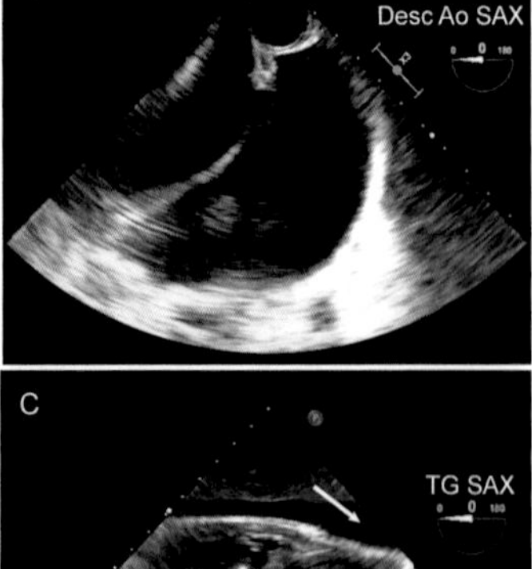

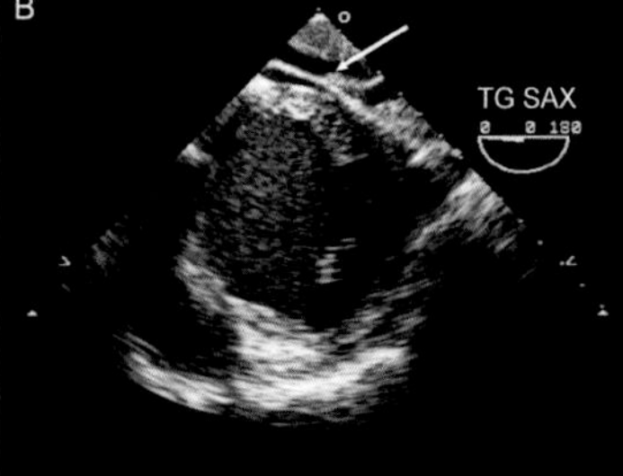

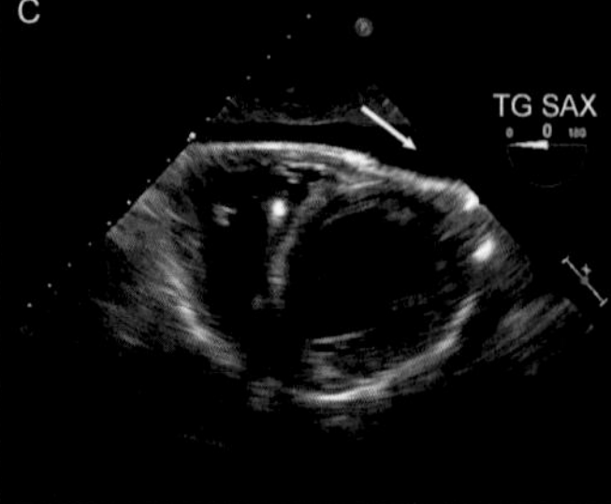

- Cardiac tamponade is a clinical diagnosis, TEE can help exclude the diagnosis.
- Clinical findings that support the diagnosis of tamponade are listed.
- Tamponade physiology occurs when pericardial pressure exceeds intracardiac chamber pressures impairing cardiac filling. Filling pressures become elevated and diastolic pressures equalize in all cardiac chambers.
- Chamber compression happens when the chamber pressure is the least, atrium (systole) and ventricle (diastole).
- Pulsus paradoxus is >10 mmHg variation in arterial pressures between inspiration and expiration.
  - Results from ↑ in venous return during inspiration → ↑ RV filling with left shift of IVS and ↓ LV stroke volume
  - Differential includes: tamponade, pulmonary embolism, cardiogenic shock, tension pneumothorax, SVC obstruction

Tamponade Clinical
Hypotension
Tachycardia
Low cardiac output
  Acidosis
  Low urine output
High CVP (=PAD)
Pulsus paradoxus

TEE Diagnosis

- Pericardial effusion
  - May be of variable size moderate-large, loculated
  - "Dry" tamponade can occur without a pericardial effusion if the pericardium is closed after cardiac surgery and is too tight, compressing the heart.
- Chamber collapse
  - RA systolic free wall collapse is an early sensitive sign, and more sensitive (>94%) /specific (100%) if the duration is >1/3 of systole.
  - RV diastolic free wall collapse is less sensitive (60%), but more specific (85–100%) than RA collapse.
  - Rarely, LA or LV collapse can occur unless there is a loculated collection.
- Respiratory variation in diastolic filling
  - Flow varies with spontaneous and is reversed in mechanical ventilation
  - Ventricular (MVI, TVI) and atrial filling (PVF, HVF) spectral Doppler profiles are exaggerated in tamponade. Absence of HVF indicates imminent cardiac arrest.

TEE Tamponade
Pericardial effusion
RA systolic collapse
RV diastolic collapse
Respiratory TV/MV
IVC plethora

Tamponade Doppler Flows

		Ventricular Filling		Atrial Filling	
		MVI	TVI	PVF	HVF
SP	I	↓ < 25%	↑ > 40%	↓ S,D	↑ S,D
	E	↑	↓	↑ S,D	↓ S,D
PPV	I	↑ > 40%	↓ < 25%	↑ S,D	↓ S,D
	E	↓	↑	↓ S,D	↑ S,D

PPV, positive pressure ventilation; SP, spontaneous ventilation; I, inspire; E, expire; MVI, mitral valve inflow; TVI, tricuspid valve inflow; PVF, pulmonary vein flow; HVF, hepatic vein flow; S, systole; D, diastole

Tamponade Spontaneous
Expiration Inspiration
Tricuspid E A E A
Mitral E A E A

- IVC plethora (dilated >2.0 cm)
  - <50% inspiratory collapse with spontaneous ventilation is a sensitive (97%) but nonspecific (40%) indicator of tamponade physiology
- Diastolic Dysfunction
  - Restrictive filling pattern due to elevated LVEDP
  - Prolonged IVRT, DT duration <160 ms, ↑ Emax velocity, E/A ratio >2, ↑ pulmonary venous A wave (>30 ms)
  - Mitral annular E′ wave is normal since myocardial function is not impaired.

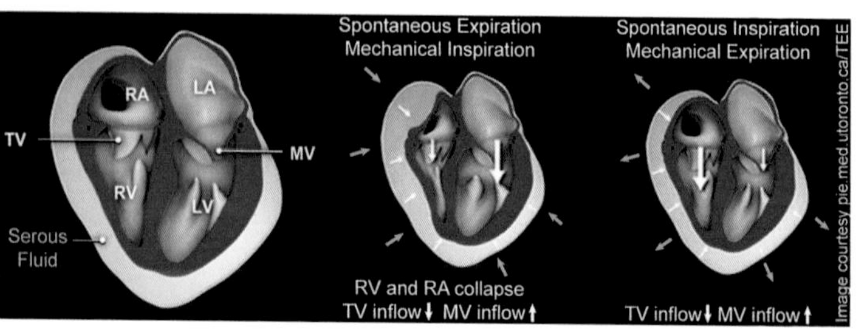

(A) ME 4C shows large extra-cardiac hematoma compressing the RA and TV. The hematoma is echodense, a common appearance after cardiac surgery. (B) ME 4C view shows a large circumferential pericardial effusion. (C) Pericardial effusion (PE) surrounding the right atrium (RA), which collapses during systole, is best shown with (D) M-mode (arrow). (E) TG SAX view of a patient anticoagulated after cardiac surgery with a large circumferential pericardial effusion. Both the RV and LV are small in size. (F) The IVC is dilated without significant respiratory variation in a ventilated patient. Additional findings include (G) 40% respiratory variation in MV inflow (MVI) and (H) respiratory variation in hepatic vein flow with prominent A wave.

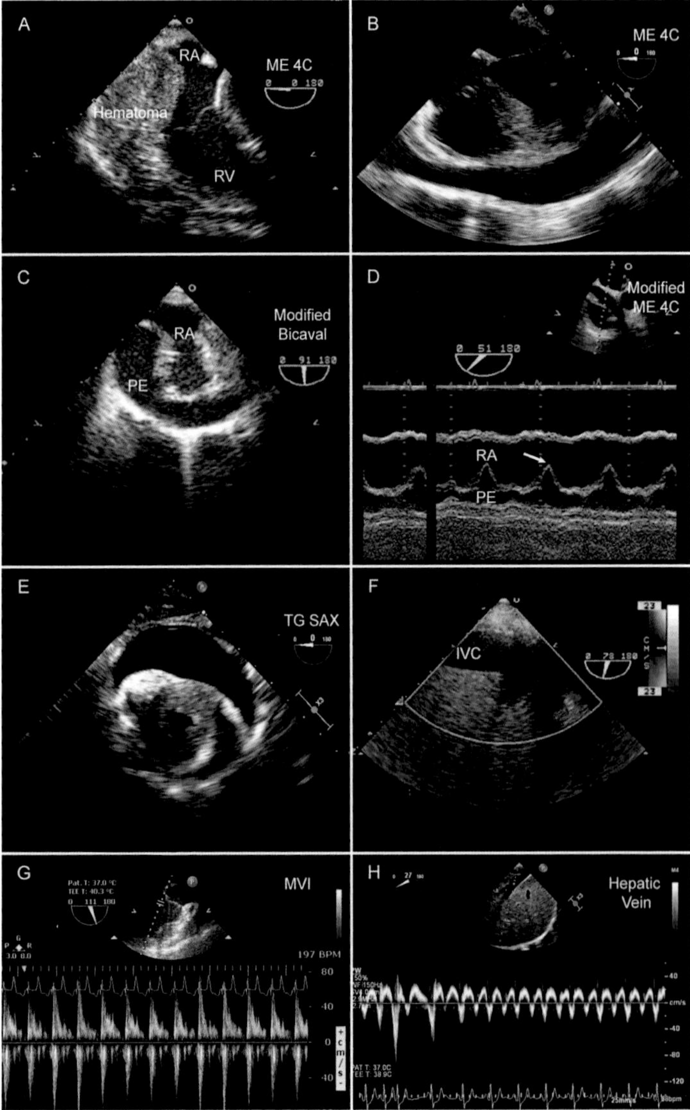

Constrictive Pericarditis

- Fusion of thickened visceral and parietal layers results in impaired diastolic ventricular filling. Early diastolic filling is rapid and abruptly stops as diastolic pressure rises when the ventricle is "full."
- Etiology: idiopathic, radiation, trauma, post-cardiac surgery, tuberculosis, renal failure
- Pericardial thickening >4 mm, visceral and parietal layers fused, no effusion
- Surgery involves a sternotomy without CPB. Cross-hatching of visceral pericardium is performed on the LV before RV to minimize hemodynamic instability.

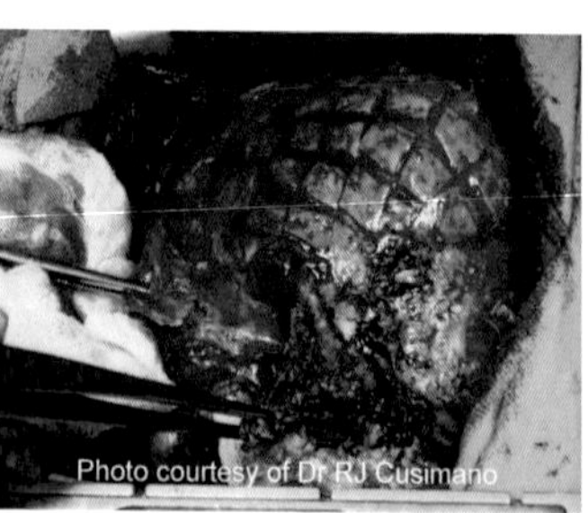

Echo Findings in Constrictive Pericarditis	
2D Imaging	
• Normal LV size and function – LA, RA can be normal or enlarged – Normal or increased MV annulus TDI velocity – Difficult TG views due to pericardial calcification • Pericardial thickening (> 4 mm) • Abrupt IVS motion (septal bounce) towards the RV, early diastole in inspiration • Flat pattern of diastolic posterior wall motion • Dilated IVC, hepatic veins, ascites	
Spectral Doppler: Respiratory Variation in Spontaneous Ventilation	
MV inflow (MVI)	Inspiration: Decrease E > 25%, ↑ early diastolic filling (E> > A)
Pulmonary Vein	Expiration: Blunted systolic "s" wave (S < D), prominent "a" wave
TV inflow (TVI)	Inspiration: Increase E > 40–50%
Hepatic vein (HV)	Expiration: Prominent "a" wave, blunted or reversed D wave
Source: Klein AL, et al. J Am Soc Echocardiogr 2013;26:965–1012	

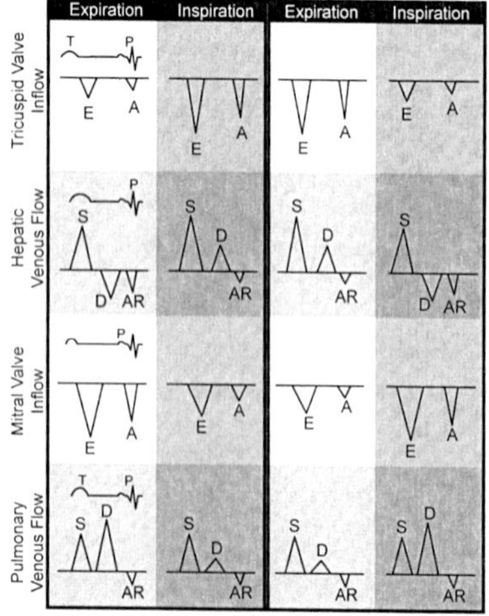

(A) ME 4C and (B) TG SAX views show bright echogenic pericardium predominantly surrounding the RA and RV in a patient with constrictive pericarditis. The LV is of normal size and function, while the LA and RA are dilated. No pericardial effusion is present. (C) The IVC is dilated at 2.26 cm in this TG hepatic vein (HV) view. (D) The patient presented with heart failure and a large left pleural effusion. Doppler inflows of the (E) tricuspid valve inflow (TVI) and (F) mitral valve inflow (MVI) show respiratory variation. (G) Spectral Doppler tracings confirm the presence of restricted filling pattern and preserved LV function (S′ TDI MV annulus). The MVI shows an E wave much larger than the A wave (E> >A). The pulmonary vein Doppler flow shows a prominent "A" wave, and S > D during expiration in this mechanical ventilated patient.

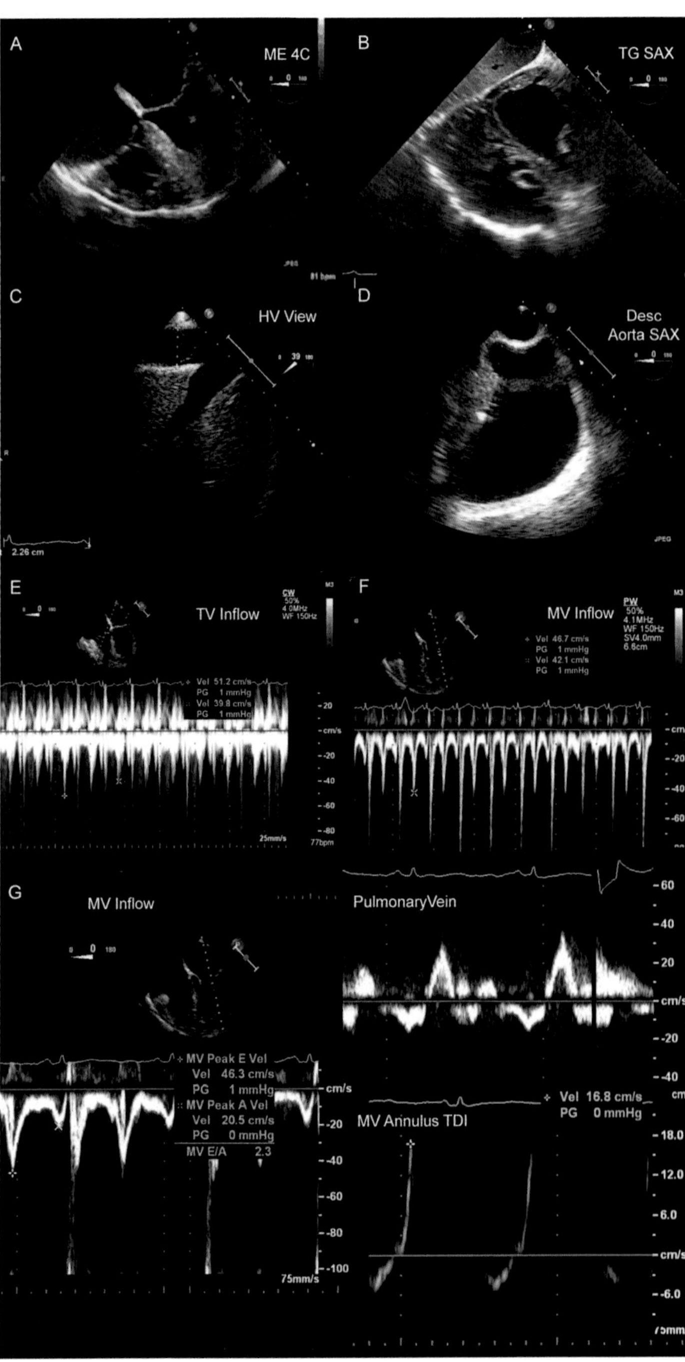
A
ME 4C
B
TG SAX
C
HV View
D
Desc
Aorta SAX
2.26 cm
E
TV Inflow
Vel 51.2 cm/s
PG 1 mmHg
Vel 39.8 cm/s
PG 1 mmHg
25mm/s
77bpm
F
MV Inflow
Vel 46.7 cm/s
PG 1 mmHg
Vel 42.1 cm/s
PG 1 mmHg
G
MV Inflow
MV Peak E Vel
Vel 46.3 cm/s
PG 1 mmHg
MV Peak A Vel
Vel 20.5 cm/s
PG 0 mmHg
MV E/A 2.3
75mm/s
PulmonaryVein
MV Annulus TDI
Vel 16.8 cm/s
PG 0 mmHg

Key Features	Tamponade	Constrictive	Restrictive
2D	Effusion Chamber collapse	Thick pericardium	Thick ventricle Dilated atria
Respiratory variation	+	+	–
Diastolic dysfunction	No/impair	Restrictive	Impair/restrict
IVC plethora	+	±	–

- Echocardiography and other imaging modalities are used to assess constrictive pericarditis (CP), restrictive cardiomyopathy (RCMP) and cardiac tamponade.
- Clinical and specific echo findings can distinguish CP, a pericardial disease, from RCMP a myocardial abnormality. All these diseases have impaired LV filling with an elevated LVEDP from different mechanisms.
- The most reliable method for differentiation is tissue Doppler imaging (TDI) which is reduced in RCMP and normal in CP.
- Another key finding present with pericardial diseases is the respiratory variation in Doppler flows.
  - Respiratory variations are opposite depending on spontaneous or positive pressure ventilation.
  - Respiratory changes occur only in normovolemia and may be absent in hypovolemia or hypervolemia.
  - 20% of patients with CP lack respiratory changes in the presence of mixed constrictive-restrictive disease and/or markedly increased LAP.

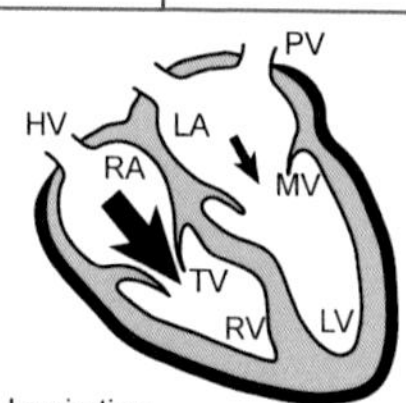

Inspiration

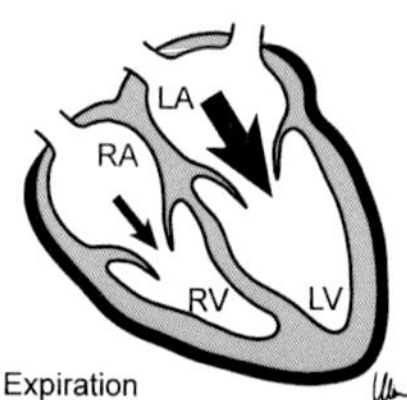

Expiration

Pericardial Tamponade	Constrictive Pericarditis	Restrictive cardiomyopathy
	Etiology	
Idiopathic, Infectious, Uremia, Neoplastic, Inflammatory, Radiation, Trauma, MI, Surgery	Idiopathic, Surgery Chronic pericarditis, Radiation, Infection	Amyloid, Sarcoid, Glycogen storage, Hemochromatosis, Endomyocardial fibrosis
	Clinical	
↓ CO, ↓ BP, ↑ JVP Pulsus paradoxus	↑ JVP Distant heart sounds Ascites, edema Pericardial knock	Fatigue Dyspnea Angina
	Diagnosis	
Echocardiography Pericardiocentesis ECG: Electrical alternans	CT or MRI Fluoroscopy R + L heart Cath	Endomyocardial biopsy
	Pressures	
↑ RAP ↑, RV = LV Normal PAP	↑ RAP ↑, RV = LV ↑ PAP (35–40 mmHg) >1/3 peak RV Pressure	↑ RAP ↑, RV > LV ↑↑ PAP (> 60 mmHg) <1/3 peak RV pressure
	Echocardiography	
Moderate to large PE RA systolic collapse RV diastolic collapse RV > LV volumes IVC plethora, no collapse	Pericardial thick (no PE) Normal LV size / function ↑ LA, RA size Flat diastolic PW motion Septal bounce Dilated IVC + HV PV premature opening	LVH (concentric), RVH Normal systolic function Impaired diastolic filling Pericardial effusion ↑ LA, RA size ± MR/ TR

HV, hepatic vein; LVH, left ventricular hypertrophy; MI, myocardial infarction; MR, mitral regurgitation; PE, pericardial effusion; PV, pulmonic valve; PW, posterior wall; RVH, right ventricular hypertrophy; TR, tricuspid regurgitation

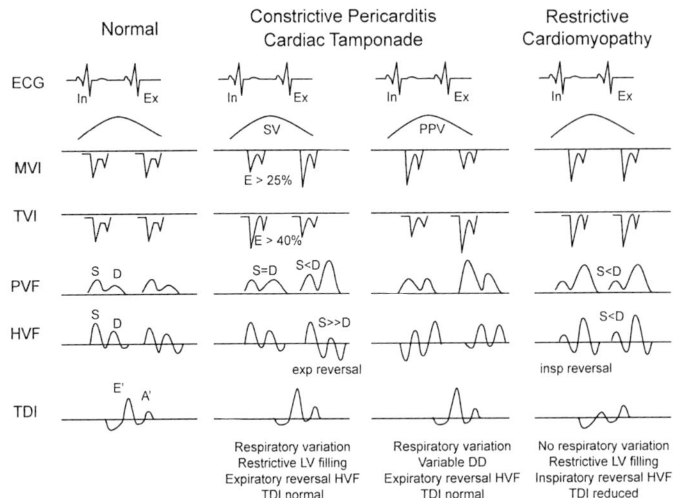

Examples of ME 4C views demonstrate many of the 2D findings associated with different pathologies compared to (A) normal. Basic assessment is made for chamber size, myocardial thickness, and the presence of a pericardial effusion. (B) Constrictive pericarditis shows a bright echogenic pericardium surrounding small-sized ventricles, enlarged atria, and no pericardial effusion. (C) Transthoracic apical 4C view shows the bright thickened myocardium associated with amyloidosis. The ventricles are of normal size, atria are enlarged, and a small pericardial effusion is present around the right atrium. (D) A large pericardial effusion is seen with normal-sized atria and ventricles. Doppler interrogation was consistent with cardiac tamponade.

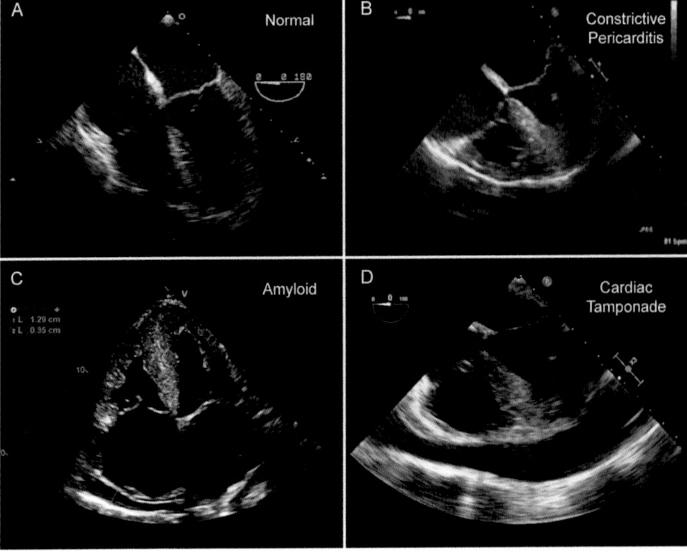

Suggested Readings

1. **TEE Views**
   - Hahn R, et al. Guidelines for Performing a Comprehensive Transesophageal Echocardiographic Examination: Recommendations from the ASE and the SCA. J Am Soc Echocardiogr 2013; 26:921–64.
   - Flachskampf FA, et al. Guideline from the Working Group: Recommendations for Performing Transesophageal Echocardiography. Eur J Echocardiograph 2001; 2:8–21.
   - Shanewise JS, et al. ASE/SCA Guidelines for performing a comprehensive intraoperative multiplane transesophageal echocardiography examination. Anesth Analg 1999;89:870–84.
2. **Doppler and Hemodynamics**
   - Quinones MA, et al. Recommendations for quantification of Doppler echocardiography: a report from the Doppler Quantification Task Force of the Nomenclature and Standards Committee of the American Society of Echocardiography. J Am Soc Echocardiogr 2002;15:167–84.
   - Skubas N. Intraoperative Doppler tissue imaging is a valuable addition to cardiac anesthesiologists' armamentarium: a core review. Anesth Analg 2009;108:48–66.
3. **Left Ventricle**
   - Cerqueira M, et al. Standardized myocardial segmentation and nomenclature for tomographic imaging of the heart: a statement for healthcare professionals from the Cardiac Imaging Committee of the Council on Clinical Cardiology of the American Heart Association. Circulation 2002;105:539–42.
   - Hu K, et al. Methods for Assessment of Left Ventricular Systolic Function in Technically Difficult Patients with Poor Imaging Quality. J Am Soc Echocardiogr 2013;26:105–13.
   - Lang RM, et al. Recommendations for Cardiac Chamber Quantification by Echocardiography in Adults: An Update from the American Society of Echocardiography and the European Association of Cardiovascular Imaging. J Am Soc Echocardiogr 2015;28:1–39.
   - Lang RM, et al. Recommendations for chamber quantification: a report from the American Society of Echocardiography's Guidelines and Standards Committee and the Chamber Quantification Writing Group, developed in conjunction with the European Association of Echocardiography, a branch of the European Society of Cardiology. J Am Soc Echocardiogr. 2005;18:1440–63.
   - Mor-Avi V, et al. Current and Evolving Echocardiographic Techniques for the Quantitative Evaluation of Cardiac Mechanics: ASE/EAE Consensus Statement on Methodology and Indications Endorsed by the Japanese Society of Echocardiography. J Am Soc Echocardiogr 2011;23:277–313.
   - Schiller NB, et al. Recommendations for quantitation of the left ventricle by two-dimensional echocardiography. American Society of Echocardiography Committee on Standards, Subcommittee on Quantitation of Two-Dimensional Echocardiograms. J Am Soc Echocardiogr 1989;2:358–87.
4. **Right Ventricle**
   - Haddad F, et al. The right ventricle in cardiac surgery, a perioperative perspective: I. Anatomy, physiology, and assessment. Anesth Analg 2009;108:407–21.
   - Horton KD, et al. Assessment of the Right Ventricle by Echocardiography: A Primer for Cardiac Sonographers. J Am Soc Echocardiogr 2009;22:776–792.
   - Rudski LG, et al. Guidelines for the echocardiographic assessment of the right heart in adults: a report from the American Society of Echocardiography endorsed by the European Association of Echocardiography, a registered branch of the European Society of Cardiology, and the Canadian Society of Echocardiography. J Am Soc Echocardiogr 2010;7:685–713.
   - Silverton N, et al. Speckle Tracking Strain of the Right Ventricle: An Emerging Tool for Intraoperative Echocardiography. Anesth Analg 2017;125:1475–8.
5. **Coronary Artery Disease**
   - Agricola E, et al. Ischemic mitral regurgitation: mechanisms and echocardiographic classification. Eur J Echocardiogr 2008;9:207–21.
   - Ender L, et al. Visualization of the Circumflex Artery in the Perioperative Setting with Transesophageal Echocardiography. Anesth Analg 2012;115:23–26.
   - Hauser M. Congenital Anomalies of The Coronary Arteries. Heart 2005;91:1240–1245.
   - Rallidis LS, et al. Right Ventricular Involvement in Coronary Artery Disease: Role of Echocardiography for Diagnosis and Prognosis. J Am Soc Echocardiogr 2014;27:223–9.

6. **Diastology**
   - Denault A, et al. Left and right ventricular diastolic dysfunction as predictors of difficult separation from cardiopulmonary bypass. Can J Anesth 2006;53: 1020–9.
   - Matyal R, et al. Perioperative assessment of diastolic dysfunction. Anesth Analg 2011;113:449–72.
   - Nagueh SF, et al. Recommendations for the Evaluation of Left Ventricular Diastolic Function by Echocardiography: An Update from the American Society of Echocardiography and the European Association of Cardiovascular Imaging 2016. J Am Soc Echocardiogr 2016;29:277–314.
   - Nagueh SF, et al. Recommendations for the evaluation of left ventricular diastolic function by echocardiography. J Am Soc Echocardiogr 2009;2:107–33.
   - Rudski LG, et al. Guidelines for the echocardiographic assessment of the right heart in adults: a report from the American Society of Echocardiography endorsed by the European Association of Echocardiography, a registered branch of the European Society of Cardiology, and the Canadian Society of Echocardiography. J Am Soc Echocardiogr 2010;7:685–713.
7. **Native Valves**
   - Anyanwu A and Adams D. Etiologic classification of degenerative mitral valve disease: Barlow's disease and fibroelastic deficiency. Semin Thorac Cardiovasc Surg 2007;19:90–96.
   - Baumgartner H, et al. Echocardiographic assessment of valve stenosis: EAE/ASE recommendations for clinical practice. J Am Soc Echocardiogr 2009;22:1–23.
   - Baumgartner H, et al. Recommendations on the Echocardiographic Assessment of Aortic Valve Stenosis: A Focused Update from the European Association of Cardiovascular Imaging and the American Society of Echocardiography. J Am Soc Echocardiogr 2017;30:372–92.
   - Cohen GI, et al. Reference values for normal adult transesophageal echocardiographic measurements. J Am Soc Echocardiogr 1995;8:221–30.
   - Eriksson MJ, et al. Mitral annular disjunction in advanced myxomatous mitral valve disease: echocardiographic detection and surgical correction. J Am Soc Echocardiogr 2005;18:1014–22.
   - Ho SY. Structure and anatomy of the aortic root. Eur J Echocard 2009;10:i3–10.
   - Lancellotti P, et al. Recommendations for the echocardiographic assessment of native valvular regurgitation: an executive summary from the European Association of Cardiovascular Imaging. Eur Heart J Cardiovasc Imag 2013; 14:611–644.
   - Nishimura RA, et al. 2014 AHA/ACC Guideline for the Management of Patients With Valvular Heart Disease: executive summary: a report of the American College of Cardiology/American Heart Association Task Force on Practice Guidelines. JACC 2104;63(22):e57–188.
   - Omran AS, et al. Intraoperative transesophageal echocardiography accurately predicts mitral valve anatomy and suitability for repair. J Am Soc Echocardiogr 2002; 15:950–7.
   - Wilkins G. Percutaneous balloon dilatation of the mitral valve: an analysis of echocardiographic variables related to outcome and the mechanism of dilatation. Br Heart J 1988; 60:299–308.
   - Zoghbi W, et al. Recommendations for evaluation of the severity of native valvular regurgitation with two-dimensional and Doppler echocardiography. J Am Soc Echocardiogr 2003;16:777–802.
   - Zoghbi W, et al. Recommendations for noninvasive evaluation native valvular regurgitation. J Am Soc Echocardiogr 2017;30:303–371.
8. **Prosthetic Valves, Transcatheter Valves, Valve Repairs**
   - Cohen GI, et al. Color Doppler and two-dimensional echocardiographic determination of the mechanism of aortic regurgitation with surgical correlation. J Am Soc Echocardiogr 1996;9:508–15.
   - El Khoury G, et al. Functional classification of aortic root/valve abnormalities and their correlation with etiologies and surgical procedures. Curr Opinion Cardiol 2005; 20:115–21.
   - Foster GP, et al. Accurate localization of mitral regurgitant defects using multiplane transesophageal echocardiography. Ann Thoracic Surg 1998; 65:1025–31.
   - Hahn R, et al. Recommendations for Comprehensive Intraprocedural Echocardiographic Imaging During TAVR. J Am Coll Cardiol Img 2015;8:261–87.

- Klein AA, et al. Controversies and Complications in the Perioperative Management of Transcatheter Aortic Valve Replacement. Anesth Analg 2014;119:784–98.
- Mahmood F and Maytal R. A Quantitative Approach to the Intraoperative Echocardiographic Assessment of the Mitral Valve for Repair. Anesth Analg 2015;121:34–58.
- Maslow A. Mitral Valve Repair: An Echocardiographic Review: Part 1. J Cardiothorac Vasc Anesth 2015;29:156–77.
- Van Dyck MJ, et al. Transesophageal echocardiographic evaluation during aortic valve repair surgery. Anesth Analg 2010;111(1):59–70.
- Zoghbi W, et al. Recommendations for evaluation of prosthetic valves with echocardiography and Doppler ultrasound: a report From the ASE Guidelines and Standards Committee and the Task Force on Prosthetic Valves, developed in conjunction with the ACC Cardiovascular Imaging Committee, Cardiac Imaging Committee of the AHA, the European Association of Echocardiography, a registered branch of the ESC, the Japanese Society of Echocardiography and the Canadian Society of Echocardiography, endorsed by the ACC Foundation, AHA, European Association of Echocardiography, a registered branch of the ESC, the Japanese Society of Echocardiography, and Canadian Society of Echocardiography. J Am Soc Echocardiogr 2009; 22:975–1014.

9. **Aorta**
   - Evangelista A, et al. Echocardiography in aortic diseases: EAE recommendations for clinical practice. Eur J Echocardiogr 2010;11(8):645–58.
   - Glas K, et al. Guidelines for the performance of a comprehensive intraoperative epiaortic ultrasonographic examination: recommendations of the American Society of Echocardiography and the Society of Cardiovascular Anesthesiologists; endorsed by the Society of Thoracic Surgeons. J Am Soc Echocardiogr 2007;11:1227–35.
   - Goldstein S, et al. Multimodality Imaging of Diseases of the Thoracic Aorta in Adults: From the American Society of Echocardiography and the European Association of Cardiovascular Imaging Endorsed by the Society of Cardiovascular Computed Tomography. J Am Soc Echocardiogr 2015;28:119–82.
   - Katz ES, et al. Protruding aortic atheromas predict stroke in elderly patients undergoing cardiopulmonary bypass: experience with intraoperative transesophageal echocardiography. J Am Coll Cardiol 1992;20(1):70–7.
   - Orihashi K, et al. Aortic arch branches are no longer a blind zone for transesophageal echocardiography: a new eye for aortic surgeons. J Thor Card Surg 2000;120:460–72.
10. **Congenital Heart Disease**
   - Ayres NA, et al. Indications and guidelines for performance of transesophageal echocardiography in the patient with pediatric acquired or congenital heart disease: report from the task force of the Pediatric Council of the American Society of Echocardiography. J Am Soc Echocardiogr 2005; 18:91–8. 25.
   - Cohen MS, et al. Multimodality Imaging Guidelines of Patients with Transposition of the Great Arteries: A Report from the American Society of Echocardiography Developed in Collaboration with the Society for Cardiovascular Magnetic Resonance and the Society of Cardiovascular Computed Tomography. J Am Soc Echocardiogr 2016;29:571–621.
   - Russell IA, et al. Congenital heart disease in the adult: a review with internet-accessible transesophageal echocardiographic images. Anesth Analg 2006;102:694–723.
   - Shiina A, et al. Two-dimensional echocardiographic-surgical correlation in Ebstein's anomaly: preoperative determination of patients requiring tricuspid valve plication vs replacement. Circulation 1983; 68:534–44.
   - Silvestry FE, et al. Guidelines for the Echocardiographic Assessment of Atrial Septal Defect and Patent Foramen Ovale: From the ASE and Society for Cardiac Angiography and Interventions. J Am Soc Echocardiogr 2015;28:910–58.
   - Vegas A and Miller-Hance WC. (2015) Chapter 12: Transesophageal Echocardiography in Congenital Heart Disease, in Anesthesia for Congenital Heart Disease (eds) D. B. Andropoulos, S. Stayer, E. B. Mossad and W. C. Miller-Hance, John Wiley & Sons.
11. **Variants, Foreign Material, Masses, Endocarditis**
   - Baddour L, et al. Infective endocarditis: diagnosis, antimicrobial therapy, and management of complications: a statement for healthcare professionals from the Committee on Rheumatic Fever, Endocarditis, and Kawasaki Disease, Council

on Cardiovascular Disease in the Young, and the Councils on Clinical Cardiology, Stroke, and Cardiovascular Surgery and Anesthesia, American Heart Association: endorsed by the Infectious Diseases Society of America. Circulation 2005;111:e394-e434.

- Durack DT, et al. New criteria for diagnosis of infective endocarditis: utilization of specific echocardiographic findings. Duke Endocarditis Service. Am J Med 1994;96:200–9.
- Goyal SK, et al. Persistent left superior vena cava: a case report and review of literature. Cardiovasc Ultrasound 2008; 6:50.
- Habib G, et al. Recommendations for the practice of echocardiography in infective endocarditis. Eur Heart J 2010;11:202–219.
- Konstantinides S, et al. 2014 ESC Guidelines on the diagnosis and management of acute pulmonary embolism. Eur Heart J 2014;35:3033–69.
- Le HT, et al. Imaging Artifacts in Echocardiography. Anesth Analg 2016;122:633–46.
- Tazelaar HD, et al. Pathology of surgically excised primary cardiac tumors. Mayo Clin Proceed 1992;67:957–65.
- Wilson W, et al. Prevention of infective endocarditis: guidelines from the American Heart Association: a guideline from the American Heart Association Rheumatic Fever, Endocarditis, and Kawasaki Disease Committee, Council on Cardiovascular Disease in the Young, and the Council on Clinical Cardiology, Council on Cardiovascular Surgery and Anesthesia, and the Quality of Care and Outcomes Research Interdisciplinary Working Group. Circulation 2007; 116:1736–54.

12. **Mechanical Support and Heart Transplantation**
    - Chumnanvej S, et al. Perioperative echocardiographic examination for ventricular assist device implantation. Anesth Analg 2007;106:583–401.
    - Douflé G, et al. Echocardiography for adult patients supported with extracorporeal membrane oxygenation. Critical Care 2015;19:326.
    - Mizuguchi KA, et al. Transesophageal Echocardiography Imaging of the Total Artificial Heart. Anesth Analg 2013;117:780–784.
    - Platts DG, et al. The Role of Echocardiography in the Management of Patients Supported by Extracorporeal Membrane Oxygenation. J Am Soc Echocardiogr 2012;25:131–41.
    - Stainback RF, et al. Echocardiography in the Management of Patients with Left Ventricular Assist Devices: Recommendations from the American Society of Echocardiography. J Am Soc Echocardiogr 2015;28:853–909.
13. **Cardiomyopathies**
    - Elliot P, et al. Classification of the cardiomyopathies: a position statement from the European society of cardiology working group on myocardial and pericardial diseases. Eur Heart J 2008; 29:270–276.
    - Jenni R, et al. Echocardiographic and pathoanatomical characteristics of isolated left ventricular non-compaction: a step towards classification as a distinct cardiomyopathy. Heart 2001;86:666–71.
    - Marcus FI, et al. Diagnosis of Arrhythmogenic Right Ventricular Cardiomyopathy/Dysplasia: Proposed Modification of the Task Force Criteria. Circulation. 2010;121:1533–1541.
    - McKenna WJ, et al., on behalf of the Task Force of the working group myocardial and pericardial disease of the European Society of Cardiology and of the Scientific Council on Cardiomyopathies of the International Society and Federation of Cardiology. Diagnosis of arrhythmogenic right ventricular dysplasia cardiomyopathy. Br Heart J. 1994;71:215–218.
    - Nageuh S, et al. American Society of Echocardiography Clinical Recommendations for Multimodality Cardiovascular Imaging of Patients with Hypertrophic Cardiomyopathy. J Am Soc Echocardiogr 2011;24:473–98.
    - Hensley N, et al. Hypertrophic Cardiomyopathy: A Review. Anesth Analg 2015;120:554–69.
    - Sherrid MV and Arabadjian M. Echocardiography to Individualize Treatment for Hypertrophic Cardiomyopathy. Prog Cardiovasc Dis 2012;54:461–476.
    - Wood MJ and Picard MH. Utility of Echocardiography in The Evaluation Of Individuals With Cardiomyopathy. Heart 2004;90:707–712.
14. **Pericardium**
    - Adler Y, et al. 2015 ESC Guidelines for the diagnosis and management of pericardial diseases: The Task Force for the Diagnosis and Management of

Pericardial Diseases of the European Society of Cardiology (ESC). Endorsed by: The European Association for Cardio-Thoracic Surgery (EACTS). Eur Heart J 2015;2921–2964.

- Dal-Bianco JP, et al. Role of Echocardiography in the Diagnosis of Constrictive Pericarditis. J Am Soc Echocardiogr 2009;22:24–33.
- Klein A, et al. American Society of Echocardiography Clinical Recommendations for Multimodality Cardiovascular Imaging of Patients with Pericardial Disease. Endorsed by the Society of Cardiovascular Magnetic Resonance and Society of Cardiovascular Computed Tomography. J Am Soc Echocardiogr 2013;26:965–1012.
- Maisch B, et al. ESC Guidelines: Guidelines on the Diagnosis and Management of Pericardial Diseases Full Text. Eur Heart J 2004;25:587–610.
- Yared K, et al. Multimodality Imaging of Pericardial Diseases. J Am Coll Cardiol Img 2010;3:650–60.

Index

A. Vegas, *Perioperative Two-Dimensional Transesophageal Echocardiography*, https://doi.org/10.1007/978-3-319-60902-7